HANDBOOK
FAMILY MEDICINE

VOLUME 1

CORE FOUNDATIONS OF PRIMARY CARE PRACTICE

Prof. (Dr.) Sujata K. Das

ALLIED
HEALTH
PRESS

Handbook Family Medicine
Volume 1: Core Foundations of Primary Care Practice

Author: **Prof. (Dr.) Sujata K. Das**

Allied Health Press
4164 Lakeshore Road
Burlington ON L7L 1A4
Canada
www.alliedhealthpress.com
Email: orders@arclereducation.com

ISBN: 978-1-77956-852-6

ABOUT THE AUTHOR

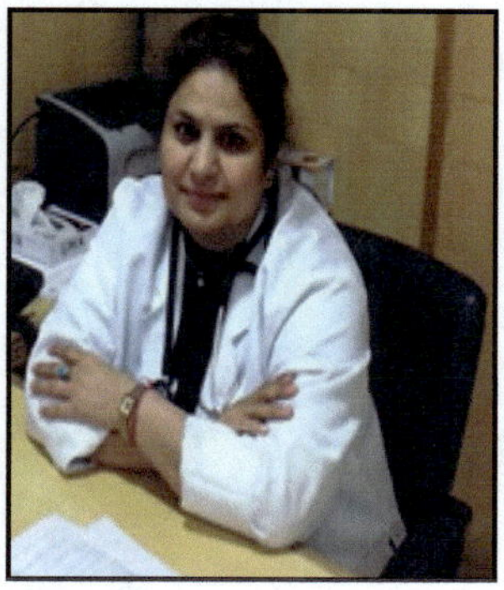

Prof (Dr) Sujata K. Dass, M.B.B.S, D.N.B, Ph.D. (Medicine) is a distinguished neuro-physician and academician, currently serving as an Attending Consultant in the Department of Neurology, B.L. Kapur Hospital, a renowned super-specialty medical institution in the New Delhi. Her illustrious career in medicine and research spans over three decades, characterized by her profound contributions to neurology and her unwavering commitment to medical education. Dr. Dass began her educational journey at Flushing High School in New York, USA, and completed her High School Diploma thereafter she joined Queens College of the City University of New York as an undergrad student. With a passion for medicine, she pursued her MBBS degree at King George Medical College, Lucknow, U.P., India. Her academic prowess and dedication to medicine were evident early on, setting the stage for a remarkable career. Dr Dass worked under the supervision of Dr M.S. Bains, M.D. as a Visiting Fellow in cardio-thoracic surgery at Memorial Sloan Kettering Cancer Research Center, New York, USA. Dr. Dass furthered her medical training by obtaining a D.N.B. (Family Medicine) and conducted significant research on hematological changes in malaria. Her quest for knowledge and excellence led her back to New York, where she completed her Ph.D. (Medicine) at the Department of Obstetrics & Gynecology, The New York Hospital-Cornell University Medical Center under the mentorship of Prof. Brij B. Saxena. Her groundbreaking work on Sn-Proto and Sn-Mesoporphyrin and the chemoprevention of neonatal jaundice culminated in the award of her D.Sc. (Medicine). Dr. Sujata Dass joined as the BR Ambedkar Chair Professor in July 2002 in the Institute of Biomedical Sciences, Faculty of Medicine, Bundelkhand University, Jhansi. Her tenure was marked by her dedication to advancing medical research and education. She also served as UGC National Research Award (Professor) at V.P. Chest Institute, University of Delhi. Throughout her career, Dr. Dass has received numerous awards and accolades on a global level. Notable among these are the UGC Research Award, the Fast Track Young Scientist Award from the Department of Science and Technology (DST), and the Women's Award of Highest Honour from Soka University, Japan. She has also received numerous research grants from DST, DBT and ICMR, UGC etc. These awards and grants underscore her exceptional contributions to medical science and research. Dr. Dass is a respected member of various scientific and administrative bodies like Planning Board (IGNOU), Executive Council - Bhagat Phool Singh Mahila Vishwavidhlaya, Haryana (2008-2011) where she continues to influence the medical community with her insights and expertise. Her commitment to guiding and mentoring students in their master's and doctoral thesis highlights her dedication to nurturing the next generation of medical professionals. Dr. Dass remains a beacon of excellence and a role model for aspiring medical professionals worldwide.

Brief Table of Contents

Getting Started with This Book

Chapter Openers

A list of Chapter Outline is presented providing a brief Introduction to what will be covered in the chapter.

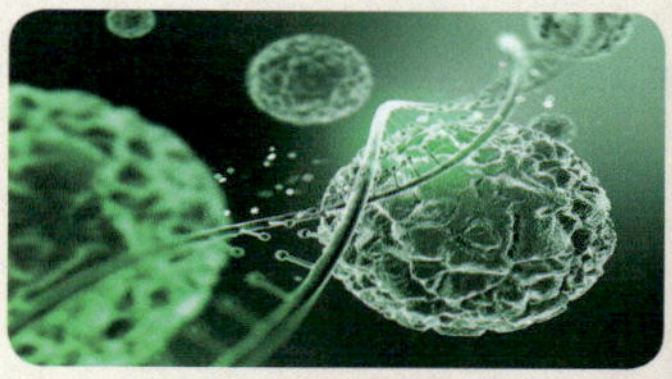

Introduction

Often referred to as the science of life, biology is a broad field of study aimed at comprehending the several kinds of life on Earth, from tiny creatures to sophisticated multicellular entities. Comprising several subfields, including molecular biology, ecology, and evolutionary biology, each of which advances our knowledge of living systems, this field clarifies the mechanisms controlling life events, including development, reproduction, and interaction with the surroundings, which is the central goal of biology. Moreover, biology fills in the void between the natural sciences and medicine by offering a necessary understanding of health, illness, and the interactions between organisms and their environments. Dealing with urgent global issues such as climate change, biodiversity loss, and new diseases depends on an awareness of these complex biological interactions, therefore highlighting the critical part biology plays in modern civilization. Fundamentally, biology explores and tests ideas about the living world using the scientific method. Through methodical observation and experimentation,

LEARNING OBJECTIVES

After studying this chapter, you will be able to:

1. Discuss the scientific method in biology;
2. Explain the cell theory;
3. Discuss the genetics and heredity;
4. Evolution and natural selection;
5. Focus on ecology and ecosystems;
6. Learn about human biology;
7. Evaluate the plant biology;
8. Explain the microbiology;
9. Focus on current trends in biology.

1.1. The Scientific Method in Biology

Learning Outcome

1. Describe the steps of the scientific method;
2. Focus on hypothesis formation;
3. Learn about experimental design.

Learning Outcomes

The beginning of each section of every chapter contains a set of Learning Outcomes that inform students of concepts they should understand. These outcomes help students understand what they should be able to do if they have mastered the material in that section.

Test Your Knowledge

Throughout each chapter, Test Your Knowledge cues you to note which topics have been covered and to self-test your understanding of the material presented.

Test Your Knowledge

1. Explain why correlation does not imply causation in scientific experiments.
2. How does the scientific method help reduce the influence of personal opinions in research?

Chapter Summary

The Summary Section appear at the end of each chapter and summarize main concepts covered throughout the chapter. These points provide key concepts in an engaging and meaningful way.

Summary

The investigation of biological principles highlights the importance of a comprehensive view of life by reflecting the intricate interactions that occur within living systems. The complexity of biology goes beyond individual species or systems, as this essay highlights; it also includes the interactions that mold ecosystems and affect biodiversity. Researchers can conduct in-depth analyses of metabolomic data using sophisticated technologies like MetaboAnalyst, which offer insights into the molecular mechanisms underlying these interactions. As demonstrated by the developments in MetaboAnalyst, for example, the integration of diverse omics data promotes a thorough understanding of metabolic pathways and helps identify important biological markers necessary for research on development and disease (Chong et al., 2018). Additionally, the phenomenon of ecological invasions is a key component of biological research and a vital field of study. The introduction of non-native species into unfamiliar habitats has significant ramifications and calls for multidisciplinary management strategies. Examining the origins and effects of these biological incursions, invasion science has become a crucial field that highlights the need to comprehend ecological dynamics and community interactions. As interest in biological invasions increases, new findings are emerging that put conventional ecological theories and practices to the test. The importance of incorporating various scientific viewpoints is shown by this developing discipline, which also highlights how invasive species shape ecosystems and advances our knowledge of ecological resilience (David et al., 2013). When taken as a whole, these discoveries from invasion science and metabolomics highlight the value of multidisciplinary biology research. Fostering cross-disciplinary collaboration and utilizing technological breakthroughs to improve our comprehension of intricate biological interactions are crucial as we look to the future of biological research. In addition to deepening our understanding of the complexities of life, this method lays the groundwork for tackling urgent environmental issues. Future studies can ensure the continued relevance of biology in a world that is constantly changing by acknowledging the interconnection of biological systems and opening the door to creative solutions that support sustainability and biodiversity conservation. We might imagine a thorough comprehension of life that serves both academia and society at large through ongoing investigation and integration of scientific knowledge.

Knowledge Assessment

The chapter includes material designed to review and reinforce each content. It includes Critical Thinking Questions to help test of your understanding of information presented in the chapter and Short answer Questions to review your understanding of the key concepts presented in the chapter.

Critical Thinking Questions

1. **Who is known as the "Father of Modern Biology"?**
   a. Aristotle
   b. Charles Darwin
   c. Gregor Mendel
   d. Louis Pasteur
2. **What is the basic unit of life?**
   a. Atom
   b. Molecule
   c. Cell
   d. Organism
3. **Which branch of biology studies the interaction of organisms with their environment?**
   a. Genetics
   b. Ecology
   c. Physiology
   d. Botany
4. **Which macromolecule is the main source of energy for living organisms?**
   a. Proteins
   b. Lipids
   c. Carbohydrates
   d. Nucleic acids
5. **DNA is primarily responsible for which function in living organisms?**
   a. Energy production
   b. Protein synthesis
   c. Storing genetic information
   d. Regulating body temperature

Short Answer Questions

1. What is biology, and why is it important to study biology?
2. What are the three main domains of life, and how are they different from one another?
3. Define homeostasis and give an example of how it works in living organisms.
4. What is the cell theory, and why is it fundamental to biology?
5. How do autotrophs and heterotrophs differ in the way they obtain energy?
6. What is the scientific method, and how is it applied in biological research?
7. Discuss how biology helps address global challenges such as climate change, disease, and food security.
8. Explain the levels of biological organization from the smallest unit to the largest. Provide examples at each level.
9. Describe the relationship between structure and function in biology, giving specific examples from cells or organs.
10. How has the discovery of genetics shaped our understanding of inheritance and variation among organisms?

Supplementary Materials

Key Terms: A list of key terms is given for quick reference

KEY TERMS FROM THIS CHAPTER

Annotation enrichment analysis	Biological structure	Cell
Cell theory	Cellular structure	Ecology
Ecosystems	Genetics	Human biology
Microbiology	Natural selection	Organism
Plant biology		

Further Resources: Recommendations for additional readings, websites, and multimedia resources.

References

1. Argelaguet, R., Velten, B., Arnol, D., Dietrich, S., Zenz, T., Marioni, J. C., Buettner, F., et al. (2018). Multi-omics factor analysis—A framework for unsupervised integration of multi-omics data sets. *Molecular Systems Biology, 14*. https://doi.org/10.15252/msb.20178124.
2. Bacher, S., Blackburn, T. M., Essl, F., & Genovesi, P. (2017). *Socio-Economic Impact Classification of Alien Taxa (SEICAT)*. https://core.ac.uk/download/286567949.pdf (accessed on 8th March 2025).
3. Barnett, R., Brace, S., Cucchi, T., & Dobney, K. (2013). *Divergent Evolutionary Processes Associated with Colonization of Offshore Islands*. https://core.ac.uk/download/20664364.pdf (accessed on 8th March 2025).

Detailed Table of Contents

LIST OF FIGURES

PREFACE

Family medicine is an essential part of the health system, typically the initial point of contact for individuals at all stages of life. It is predicated on continuity, comprehensiveness, and coordination of care and thus is an essential part of any functioning health system. Unlike other specialties that are predicated on a specific organ system or age, family medicine addresses the whole person, integrating medical science with the psychological, social, and cultural dimensions of illness. Its scope ranges from the management of chronic illness through the surveillance of chronic disease, preventive treatment, and palliative treatment—bridging gaps between specialties and reconciling healthcare provision with the day-to-day experience of patients and families.

Over the last decades, an enormous increase has been observed in the demand for accessible, patient-focused primary care, again highlighting the important role of family physicians. These specialists are generally assigned to diagnose a variety of ailments, develop long-term care plans, and oversee referrals for patients who will need complex treatment. Family practice requires a balance between clinical breadth and compassionate communication, as well as the ability to cope with uncertainty and complexity in decision-making. In diverse and dynamic communities, the family physician must remain both clinically competent and culturally sensitive, providing care that is individualized yet also addresses broader public health demands.

Handbook of Family Medicine—Volume 1: Core Foundations of Primary Care Practice is organized as a reference core to acquaint the reader with the basic concepts, functions, and domains of clinical practice essential to family practice. It acquaints readers with the standards that define the specialty and offers comprehensive reviews of common medical conditions encountered in routine clinical practice. This book synthesizes evidence-based knowledge and clinical experience to aid learners and practitioners in the development of their diagnostic proficiency and treatment planning skills. This is both an educational text and an actual working resource for clinicians committed to delivering effective, patient-driven care across the lifespan.

Chapter 1 presents the specialty of family medicine through an integrated review of its history, principles, and characteristics that distinguish it from other medical specialties. The chapter emphasizes the necessity for continuing care, preventive care, and the long-term physician-patient relationship.

Chapter 2 accentuates the wide variety of roles and responsibilities of a family physician, including patient advocacy, coordination, management of diverse medical conditions, and provision of input into the healthcare activity in the community. It also establishes the ethical and professional standards necessary in clinical practice.

Chapter 3 discusses respiratory disorders commonly encountered in family medicine practice, such as asthma, COPD, bronchitis, and pneumonia. The chapter provides diagnostic clues, treatment advice, and referral to specialty care.

Chapter 4 discusses cardiovascular disorders with a focus on hypertension, ischemic heart disease, arrhythmias, and heart failure. It takes the clinician step-by-step through risk stratification, lifestyle modifications, pharmacotherapy, and follow-up.

Chapter 5 covers ,endocrine diseases such as diabetes mellitus, thyroid illness, and adrenal illness. It integrates diagnostic strategies with patient instruction and chronic disease self-management programs.

Chapter 6 covers gastrointestinal diseases such as dyspepsia, gastroesophageal reflux disease, peptic ulcer disease, irritable bowel syndrome, and liver illness. It focuses on symptom evaluation, diagnostic testing, and institution of treatment.

Chapter 7 covers musculoskeletal disorders that are most frequently encountered in primary care, ranging from acute trauma to chronic back and joint disease. Particular attention is devoted to physical examination techniques, functional rehabilitation, pain control, and referral.

Chapter 8 covers dermatologic disorders that family physicians, including infections, rashes, eczema, acne, and skin cancers most often treat. It covers visual diagnosis, dermatologic procedures, and patient counseling.

Chapter 9 discusses pediatric care, including immunization schedules, growth and developmental milestones, frequent infections, and parent counseling. The chapter encourages early intervention and continuity of care during childhood.

Chapter 10 discusses adolescent medicine, including topics such as puberty, mental health, drug abuse, sexual health, and risk-taking behavior. It encourages the importance of confidentiality and rapport in the treatment of adolescent patients.

Chapter 11 covers women's health problems, such as menstrual disorders, conception, menopause, osteoporosis, and screening for cancer and infection. Both problem-focused and prevention approaches are explained.

Chapter 12 discusses obstetrics in family practice, including antenatal care, labor care, postpartum assessment, and counseling for the mother. The chapter emphasizes continuity of care from conception to childbirth and thereafter.

This guidebook is beneficial to a wide variety of students such as medical students, postgraduate trainees, general practitioners, nurse practitioners, and allied health professionals who need an orderly overview of family medicine. Policy-makers and public health practitioners who are interested in enhancing primary care systems will also find it useful. Used in schools or in daily practice, this guidebook provides a solid basis for building the clinical judgment, empathetic communication, and holistic care approaches required in the practice of family medicine.

INTRODUCTION TO FAMILY MEDICINE

1

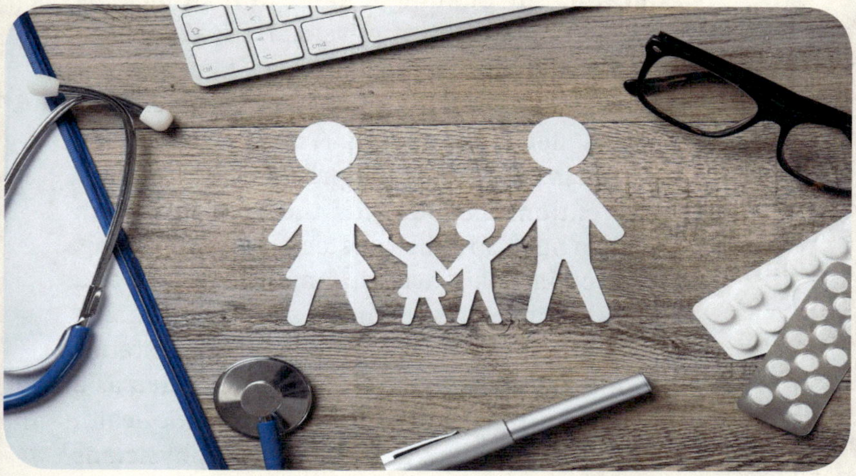

Introduction

Family medicine is a medical specialty that deals with the overall, individualized care of individuals at all stages and ages of life. Family physicians or family medicine practitioners provide comprehensive care for the whole family, addressing preventive care and chronic disease management. Family medicine, as opposed to specialties that focus on treating specific diseases or organ systems, integrates a number of aspects of care that involve physical, emotional, and social health. This model lies at the center of developing wellness and health, and of treating acute disease and caring for chronic conditions, within the context of family and community structures. Family physicians are often the first point of contact in the healthcare system, and hence their contribution is valuable for early diagnosis and timely treatment (Srivastava et al., 2020). The family medicine domain also extends beyond the individual patient to include familial and community health perspectives. The specialty is based on a biopsychosocial model that considers the interactions among biological, psychological, and social

LEARNING OBJECTIVES

After studying this chapter, you will be able to:

1. Understand the role of family physicians
2. Describe the family medicine training and education
3. Understand the concept of patient-centered care
4. Address common health issues
5. Discuss family medicine in different settings
6. Describe the challenges in family medicine

factors that influence health outcomes. By building long-term relationships with patients, family doctors become deeply aware of their patients' histories, values, and particular needs, which enables individually tailored health interventions. Family medicine also places the highest value on preventive care and health education, which are key pillars to reducing healthcare spending and improving people's and families' health. The emphasis on continuity of care facilitates the establishment of trust between physicians and patients, leading to improved patient satisfaction and adherence to treatment plans (Feldker et al., 2020). With ongoing advancements in healthcare, the role of family medicine is increasingly recognized as essential to addressing public health problems. Family physicians are not only clinicians but also patient advocates, engaging with community health and policymaking to enhance healthcare systems. This may include work to expand access to care, advocate for health equity, and address the social determinants of health that create health disparities. Further, as the medical field evolves, family medicine adapts to incorporate new methods and technologies, such as telehealth, which enhances access to care while maintaining patient-centeredness. Finally, family medicine is a system of care that is intended to be accessible, comprehensive, and responsive to the multifaceted populations (Srivastava et al., 2020) (Figure 1.1).

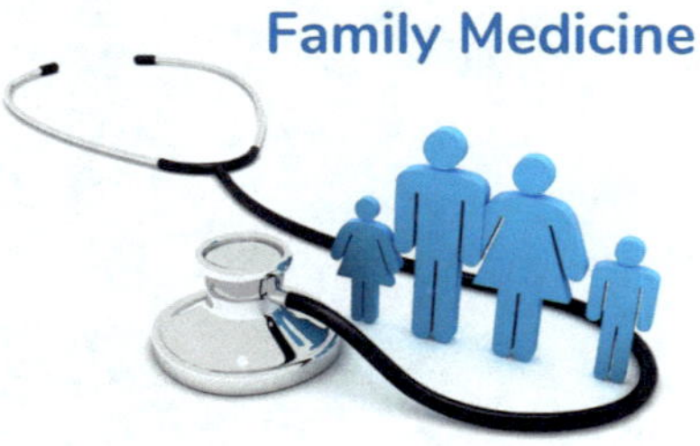

Figure 1.1. Family medicine.

Source: https://medicaldialogues.in/h-upload/2022/04/22/174803-family-medicine-2.jpg.

Overview of Family Medicine as a Specialty

Family medicine is a specialized field in medicine, characterized by its integrated approach to patient care. This specialty focuses on managing the health of individuals and families across all ages, genders, and disease states. Family physicians treat a broad spectrum of ailments, from acute complaints to chronic diseases, with a focus on disease prevention and health education. By building long-term relationships with patients, family physicians learn about their patients' medical history, family lives, and social situations, which is conducive to clinical decision-making. This continuity of care is essential, enabling practitioners to tailor interventions not just for the specific health problem but also to help foster general wellbeing, as a growing evidence base in primary care and family medicine research has shown (Singhal et al., 2023). The art of family medicine extends beyond mere treatment; it is now regarded as a key to preventing and controlling endemic health conditions in communities. Family physicians typically serve as the initial point of entry in the health system, providing a basis for a patient-centered approach. They have a distinctive function in the care of patients through complex healthcare networks, guiding patients through specialist referrals and coordinating care to minimize the risk of care fragmentation. In light of expanding patient rolls and rising healthcare expenditure, family physicians' incorporation of preventive care practices is more meaningful today. With research showing that preventive interventions can convincingly reduce health disparities, family medicine complements public health programs and therefore effectively addresses public health issues (Bayley et al., 2023). Family medicine educationally entails comprehensive training in a broad field of medical specialties, including pediatrics, internal medicine, obstetrics, and geriatrics. Family medicine residents undergo rigorous training that not only develops clinical capabilities but also sharpens core communications and interpersonal abilities. Such training prepares them to manage diverse populations while being sensitive to cultural nuances and special patient needs. Moreover, the specialty encourages a lifetime of learning and flexibility, as family physicians must stay current with evolving medical guidelines and technology impacting patient care. Therefore, family medicine is an ever-evolving, dynamic medical specialty that plays a critical role in ensuring the quality of care across the healthcare system, facilitating whole-person management of individuals and populations (Singhal et al., 2023) (Figure 1.2).

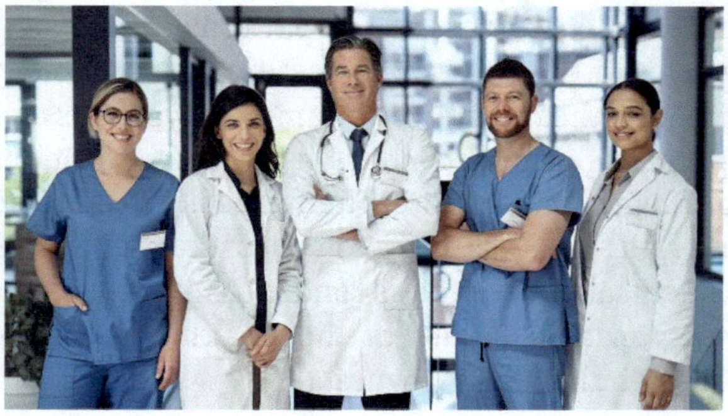

Figure 1.2. Family medicine subspecialties.

Source: https://www.mua.edu/uploads/sites/10/2023/03/family-medicine-subspecialties.webp.

Historical Development of Family Medicine

The history of family medicine can be traced back to the early 20th century, when it was created as a separate branch in medical practice. The specialty-based practice of medicine in those days often neglected the holistic treatment approach needed to cure a patient. The transition to family medicine began in the post-World War II era, when awareness of the community's health importance and the role of generalists increased. It was at this time that physicians and health systems began to focus on continuity of care, patient-centered models, and coordination across various health services. Specifically, the development of family practice residency programs in the 1960s and 70s helped cement family medicine as a key area of healthcare, focusing on its function to understand the complexities of patients' needs in the context of their families and society. Furthermore, various global movements and research have had a substantial impact on the development of family medicine. The World Health Organization and various national health authorities encouraged primary care as the keystone of health systems, endorsing the thesis that continuous, accessible care leads to better health. In countries like Cuba, a lot of importance has been placed on primary health care and specialist training in family medicine in the field of Natural and Traditional Medicine, as shown by recent studies aimed at improving professional training in this field. It aligns with the necessity to respond to diverse health requirements of the populations and to establish a link between traditional practice and modern medical practice.

The adaptability of family medicine across socioeconomic and cultural lines underscores its historic importance and its ongoing relevance in current healthcare. The legacy of great doctors and families in medicine, such as the Filatov dynasty, also appears in the history of family medicine. This medical clan not only established pioneering practices in pediatrics and ophthalmology but also set an example towards a commitment to the evolution of the general healthcare system. Their work highlighted the need to cater to the health needs of individuals and communities, establishing a model consistent with the values of family medicine. Since their work set a precedent for generations to come, the integration of personal health experiences and societal changes became clearly apparent. By way of historical record, the impact of figures like the Filatovs can be measured, as their contributions paved the way for the family medicine course and determined the present practice to enhance patient care in subtle ways.

1.1. Role of Family Physicians

Learning Outcome

1. Describe the comprehensive care across all ages
2. Understand the coordination of care with specialists
3. Emphasize the preventive care and health education

Family physicians play a key role in healthcare as the primary point of contact between doctors and patients for health problems. These physicians are trained to offer solutions across all aspects of health, from preventive care and diagnosis to the ongoing treatment of long-term illnesses. They possess a personal training that allows them to take into account the overall well-being of patients, families, and communities where they reside, instead of only treating disease. In more multicultural societies, family physicians need to adapt their practice to meet the varied health needs and to offer culturally sensitive care aligned with patients' values and beliefs, as suggested by the ongoing evolution of family medicine worldwide. As healthcare systems evolve, the role of family physicians will evolve as well, solidifying the foundation of their input on public health outcomes (Ohta et al., 2022). Among the most critical roles played by family physicians is establishing long-term patient relationships, which results in establishing trust and collaborative care. This continuity also enables family physicians to understand better their patients' medical history, social setting, and emotional issues, and thus provide more effective and tailored healthcare interventions. Through such relationships, family physicians can engage in preventive measures tailored to the unique needs of families, reducing the need for more costly interventions in the future. The promotion of preventive care emphasizes the importance of regular check-ups, immunizations, and health screenings to identify potential health issues before they become an issue. Not only do these initiatives add to the health of individuals but also to the larger area of health of populations, highlighting the essential role played by family doctors in public health intervention (Srivastava et al., 2020). The work of family physicians goes beyond clinical practice to encompass advocacy and education within their neighborhoods. They are teachers, educating patients on significant health facts and promoting healthy lifestyle habits. Family physicians also often serve as healthcare system leaders, providing access to essential resources and services for quality patient care. This multifaceted involvement positions family physicians as community health leaders, enabling them to identify system barriers to health outcomes. As the patterns in medicine evolve, for example, the integration of technology into healthcare delivery, family physicians are optimally positioned to leverage these innovations to enhance patient care. Their capacity to adapt to emerging health issues and the constant evolution of medical interventions render family physicians indispensable pillars of the healthcare system (Ohta et al., 2022) (Figure 1.3).

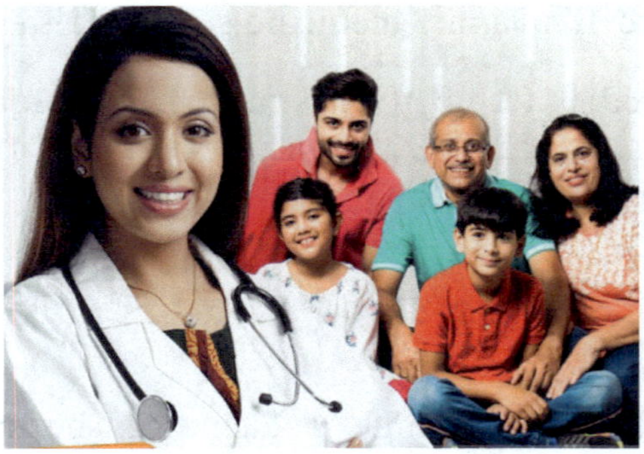

Figure 1.3. The Important role of a family physician.

Source: https://draravindan.com/images/blogs/17374346791787377681678f26371f27c.jpg.

1.1.1. Comprehensive Care Across all Ages

Family medicine is an expression of the philosophy of total care across all ages. It emphasizes a holistic approach to health delivery, recognizing the continuity of care needed at all life stages. Family physicians occupy a central place in this system in the delivery of medical care from child to geriatric care. This broad scope allows for the provision of preventive care, chronic disease management, and acute illness treatment, effectively addressing family and community health needs. Secondly, the strong doctor-patient relationship established through family medicine provides continuity of care, which is essential for developing trust, increasing patient engagement, and delivering public health outcomes. Consequently, family medicine is a foundational pillar to achieving comprehensive healthcare that is responsive to multi-age health concerns. Understanding the intricacies of comprehensive care involves understanding the prescriptive guidelines and methodologies that shape family physicians' actions. Literature indicates that family physicians demonstrate high levels of compliance with recommended treatment protocols, as illustrated in the management of common conditions such as ankle sprains. A study identified the need for continuing education, finding that while some physicians applied guidelines such as the Ottawa Ankle Rules effectively, many had knowledge deficits regarding follow-up and management choices (Alzahrani et al., 2025). This highlights the fact that repeated training and ongoing professional development of family doctors are necessary to ensure care that is holistic in all ages, not only is provided effectively, but also best practice-driven. Also, the length of training in family medicine significantly contributes to making graduates equipped to provide comprehensive care. Evidence shows that physicians who complete longer residency programs are better at delivering care across stages in life, with greater competency in prenatal and maternity care (Carney et al., 2025). This implies the importance of having proper training in readiness of family doctors to cater to the particular health needs arising at different ages. It follows that creating an educational system that emphasizes the interrelation of various factors in healthcare—ranging from prevention to care for chronic diseases—can significantly improve the quality of integrated care in family medicine. In other words, family physicians must be adequately trained and adhere to established guidelines to provide appropriate healthcare for any patient, regardless of age (Figure 1.4).

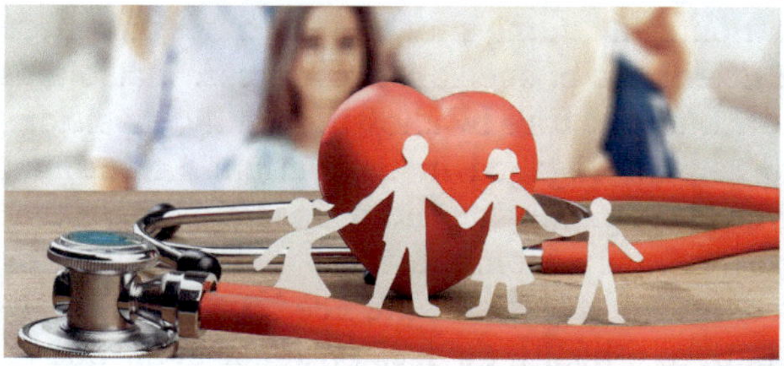

Figure 1.4. Preventive health check-ups for kids, adults, and elderly.

Source: https://www.kauveryhospital.com/blog/wp-content/uploads/2018/02/Preventive-Health-Check-Ups-for-Kids-Adults-Elderly-1200x545_c.jpg.

1.1.2. Coordination of Care with Specialists

In the case of family medicine, coordination with specialists is a critical component of patient care. The family physician is the primary caregiver who oversees patients' overall health and makes necessary referrals to specialists in cases beyond their scope of practice. Coordination of care requires effective communication among the family physician, the patient, and the specialist to ensure holistic, coordinated care. Successful strategies include regular follow-ups and community management plans that have a real potential to improve patient outcomes and satisfaction. Challenges in such coordination, however, because of problems such as the lack of an established communication procedure, tend to remind health providers that it is essential to constantly communicate and coordinate to obtain the best in patient care (O'Malley et al.,

2009). Another facilitation of care coordination is the implementation of e-consultation, which enhances communication among specialists and primary care professionals. The new approach enables clinicians to initiate specialist opinion without the need for face-to-face meetings, minimizing entry barriers and promoting timely interventions. The use of e-consultation within primary care clinics has been shown to benefit patients, including shorter wait times and more efficient use of specialist resources. It also aids continuity of care by allowing family physicians to remain engaged in the patient's treatment while still gaining access to specialist expertise. However, implementation is hampered by technical hurdles and the need for clinicians to adapt to e-health devices (Wagner et al., 2011). Ultimately, coordination of care with specialists in family medicine relies on a multifaceted approach that combines interpersonal factors and technological advancements.

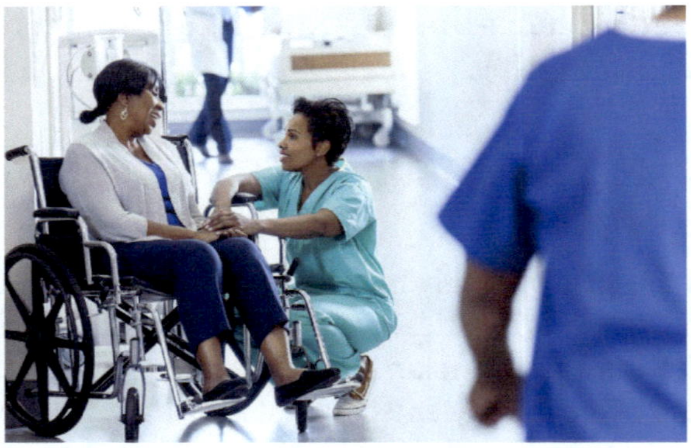

Figure 1.5. Patient care coordination.

Source: https://aihms.in/blog/wp-content/uploads/2021/01/pcc2.jpg.

Establishing a strong foundation of communication ensures clear roles for specialists and family doctors, enabling joint problem-solving in complex cases. The worth of this coordinated care model does not end at short-term health results; it also serves to enhance patient satisfaction and trust. As family medicine continues to evolve, recognizing the risks associated with specialist coordination and addressing them will play an essential role in delivering quality care. In doing so, the family practice not only enhances the patient experience but also becomes a vital building block of the overall healthcare system (O'Malley et al., 2009) (Figure 1.5).

1.1.3. Emphasis on Preventive Care and Health Education

In family medicine, preventive care and health education play a crucial role in enhancing patients' overall well-being. Preventive care encompasses a wide range of activities aimed at preventing health issues before they develop into more complex conditions. Through an active approach to determinants such as vaccinations, screenings, and lifestyle modification, family healthcare providers establish a culture in which disease prevention is a collective responsibility for practitioners and patients alike. Not only are the outcomes of health improved in this process, but also the economic burden imposed on healthcare systems. For instance, the requirements in the 2010 health care reform bill have been aimed at enhancing primary care by increasing reimbursement and improving financing for new methods of care delivery, enhancing the backstop function of preventive care in maintaining population health (Lawlor et al., 2011). Preventive care is further augmented by health education, which equips patients with the knowledge and skills needed to make informed health decisions. Family medicine doctors usually communicate with patients through educational interventions covering a variety of topics, such as diet, physical activity, and chronic disease management. Those educational interventions play a pivotal role in fostering a culture of health literacy, which has a causal effect on better health behaviors and outcomes. Besides, community-based health education initiatives, such as those shared in the Iowa Department of Public Health's monthly newsletter, assist in spreading essential health information to geographically defined populations. By educating patients and medical professionals, family medicine enables individuals to take greater responsibility for their health, ultimately leading to better preventive care and health promotion. Integration of prevention care and health education into family medicine not only produces healthier people but also helps make healthcare systems sustainable. Prevention can save healthcare resources from the strain of chronic diseases, which are extremely costly to treat and manage in the long term. Through early intervention, family practitioners can significantly contribute to reducing overall pressure on healthcare resources. Research has established that preventive care investments yield high economic returns because they reduce the need for more expensive medical interventions later on. Ongoing emphasis on expanding preventive services and increasing the value given to health education further reinforces the foundation of family medicine as a practice that is not just population-oriented but also population-aging. This emphasis represents a progressive shift towards a sustainable, integrated healthcare system (Figure 1.6).

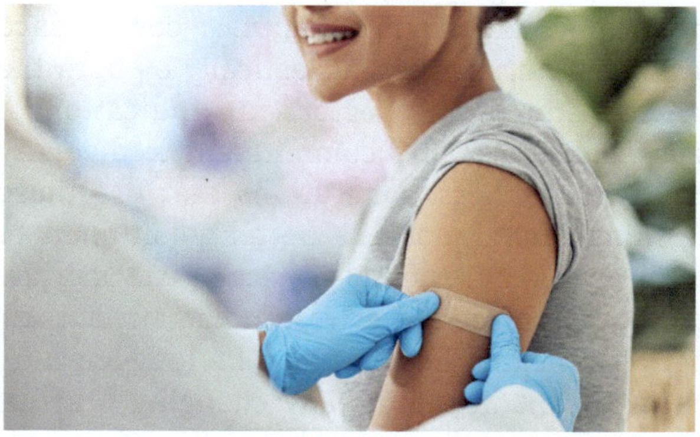

Figure 1.6. Preventive care.

Source: https://bloomfhw.com/wp-content/uploads/2024/06/Preventive-Care-Services.jpg.

Test Your Knowledge

1. What is the meaning of comprehensive care?
2. What is the preventive approach to health care?

1.2. Training and Education

Learning Outcome

1. Know the medical school requirements for Family Medicine
2. Describe the specifics of residency training in family medicine
3. Describe the continuing education and board certification

The foundation for family medicine is pegged mainly on the intensive schooling and training of its practitioners, who are required to be experts across a broad range of medical specialties. This schooling involves substantial coursework and clinical rotations that cover the gamut of diverse physiological, psychological, and social aspects of patient care. Family medicine training aims to acquire skills in the diagnosis and management of illnesses within the context of family relationships. As hinted at by future physician shortages in family practice, internal medicine, and pediatrics, there is a need to augment training pipelines to address growing healthcare needs in populations. Institutions increasingly recognize the importance of assigning value to creating dynamic learning environments that not only educate but also encourage empathetic, patient-centered practice. In conjunction with didactic medical training, cultural competence has become an essential component of family medicine education. With an increasingly diverse patient population, cultural awareness is imperative to maximize communication and provision of care. Programs that break down cultural and communication barriers have taken center stage in medicine, a testament to a desire to eliminate gaps in medical care. Education programs that promote cultural competence are being pursued enthusiastically by both the private and public sectors, an indication of the medical system's commitment to diversity and inclusiveness. Institutions that use these training techniques are better positioned to ensure that future family physicians can navigate the complex social networks that affect their patients' health. Emphasis on lifelong learning is important in the already changing practice of family medicine. Continuous professional development ensures that physicians keep up with evolving research, emerging therapeutic models, and new healthcare technologies.

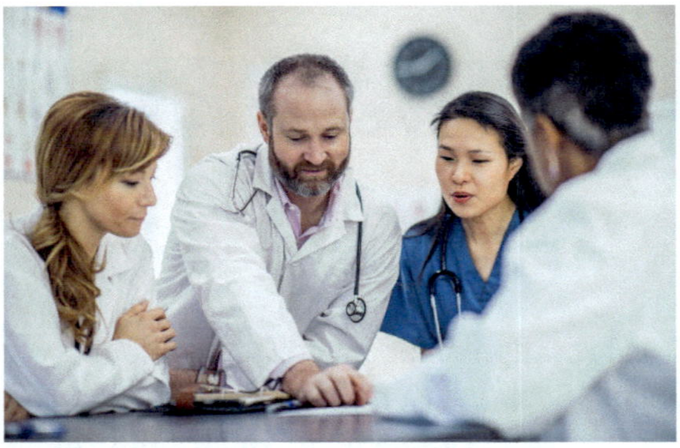

Figure 1.7. Training and education.

Source: https://www.cfpc.ca/CFPC/media/Images/Education%20and%20Professional%20Development%20Images/GettyImages-1007004502.jpg.

A number of institutions periodically update their curricula to reflect changes in medical practice and public health recommendations. Furthermore, cross-campus collaboration among family medicine residency programs can encourage the sharing of knowledge and best practices through conferences, webinars, and workshops. Not only does such cross-campus collaboration reinforce each provider's individual skill, but it also improves the quality of care provided overall within populations. With the constantly evolving nature of healthcare, the commitment to ongoing education is an essential prerequisite for creating effective and powerful family medicine doctors prepared to address the challenges of contemporary healthcare systems (Figure 1.7).

1.2.1. Medical School Requirements for Family Medicine

To become a Family Medicine doctor, future doctors need to take a challenging route that begins with a solid education in their undergraduate years. Most medical schools require applicants to hold a bachelor's degree, typically with an emphasis on science coursework, including biology, chemistry, and physics. Furthermore, institutions tend to encourage or require completion of certain pre-med courses, which not only prepare students for the Medical College Admission Test (MCAT) but also equip them with a comprehensive understanding of medical principles. Institutions also tend to seek applicants with strong communication and critical-thinking skills, as these are essential for effective patient engagement. Generally, a broad academic education and extracurricular activities that are relevant can prove very beneficial, enhancing an applicant's resume in the highly competitive process of medical school admissions. Once students are admitted to medical school, they tend to follow a four-year program that includes classroom instruction as well as hands-on clinical training. The program is designed to provide comprehensive education by integrating fundamental medical education with hands-on patient-care exposure. During the first two years, students are exposed to in-depth studies in anatomy, pharmacology, and pathology, as well as Family Medicine-specific courses. The latter are designed to generate an appreciation of the unique challenges and rewards of practicing in this branch. The final two years are spent primarily on clinical rotations, which allow students to gain hands-on experience in patient care across a variety of specialties, including Family Medicine. This widespread exposure ensures that future family physicians receive training to work with diverse populations and address a variety of health problems effectively. After medical school, graduates must complete a three-year residency in Family Medicine. During this period, residents are immersed in hands-on applications of the skills they have gained, progressing through a sequence of specialties to gain further insight into integrative patient care. Family Medicine residents become adept at treating a wide range of conditions and focus on preventive care, which is vital for reducing public health issues and promoting well-being among the population. Residency programs also provide residents with platforms for mentorship and guidance by practicing physicians, enabling them to develop their clinical skills and decision-making abilities. Not only does this intense training equip them to deal with board exams, but it also inculcates in them a firm commitment to the principles of Family Medicine, such as long-term patient relationships and continuity of care, fundamental principles of the specialty (Newman et al., 1955; University, 2018) (Figure 1.8).

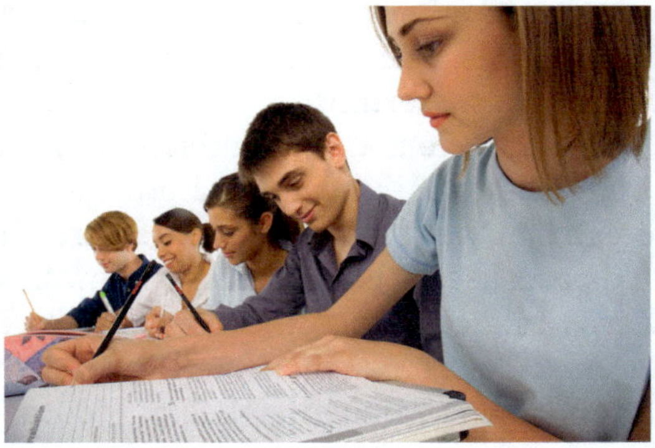

Figure 1.8. Medical college admission test (MCAT).

Source: https://www.mcreelearningcenter.com/wp-content/uploads/2016/12/act-sat-1024x683.jpg.

1.2.2. Residency Training Specifics

The specifics of the family medicine residency training are most critical to shaping effective healthcare providers who can address a range of varied patient needs. The residency programs are designed to develop Entrustable Professional Activities (EPAs), which constitute an official framework outlining the tasks residents must acquire to perform independently. In Brazil, the process has recently led to the creation of 14 country-specific EPAs tailored to the country's healthcare needs, considering the SUS practice routines. This is in accordance with the need to align residency training with local healthcare priorities to maximize family medicine physicians' competence. Their validation by consensus among experts shows an allegiance to improving training and educational outcomes and to standardizing training across programs, closing a gap that had been missing in Brazil's family medicine residency system (de Brito et al., 2025). Global health exposure is also a key component of family medicine residency training and an indicator of the increasing interconnectedness of health issues around the world. Family medicine residency programs are increasingly appreciating the value of incorporating global health curricula that align with ethical best practices for trainees seeking international experiences. Formal inclusion of a worldwide health curriculum considerably enhances training by exposing residents to required pretravel education on cultural competence and ethics. Residency programs whose faculty are specialized in global health are more likely to employ systematic pretravel education and mentoring, thus preparing residents for successful engagement in a variety of global environments. Not only does this enhance learning, but it also satisfies the Accreditation Council for Graduate Medical Education competency standards, thus ensuring the holistic growth of the future generation of physicians of family medicine (Chang et al., 2025). Furthermore, the relevance of such training should be tested periodically to assess its effectiveness. National health programs and residency schemes must work together to establish an ecosystem in which the competencies developed through EPAs and global health curricula are made dynamic to evolve with shifting healthcare settings. Through active engagement with stakeholders, including practicing family medicine physicians and public health experts, residency training can be attuned to emerging population health issues and new global health concerns. With preventive care and chronic disease management continuing to be priorities in family medicine, residency programs need to be vigilant about curricular changes to equip residents to handle not only clinical encounters but also health advocacy and community leadership. This combined effort will ultimately enhance the quality of family medicine care delivered and improve the healthcare system in general (Figure 1.9).

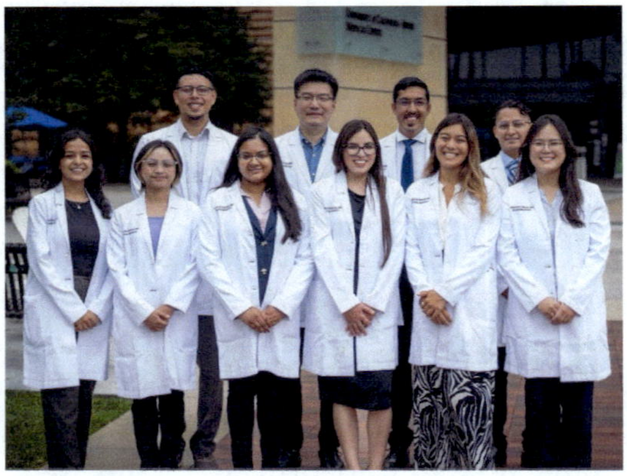

Figure 1.9. Family medicine residency program.

Source: https://medschool.uci.edu/sites/default/files/styles/callout_topic/public/media-images/family-medicine-residents_2027-class-photo.jpg?h=04b15cb4.

1.2.3. Continuing Education and Board Certification

Board certification and continuous education are critical components in family medicine that ensure the quality of care patients receive from practitioners. With the ever-evolving health landscape, continue to educate themselves throughout their lifespans to stay up to date with the latest research, guidelines, and best-practice protocols. Through ongoing education, skilled family physicians can improve patient outcomes. The emphasis on ongoing education is also supported by the requirements for board certification, which require ongoing attendance at educational programs to affirm competency. This process of education and certification not only improves the quality of care but also informs patients about their providers' competence and gives them confidence. While significant, the process of board certification has faced scrutiny in recent years regarding its value and effectiveness.

There have been allegations of growing financial surpluses held by medical boards, accumulated through billing physicians for recertification board procedures. As noted in recent reports, while some boards began moving assets, scores of others continue to amass money without considering actual improvement in the recertification process itself (Lieberman et al., 2020). This is an area of serious question as to whether current practice serves the ultimate goal of improving physician competency or evolves more about the financial safety of medical boards. Therefore, a discussion of the future of board certification is paramount in designing a system that genuinely addresses the concerns of both healthcare providers and their patients. Furthermore, education programs should be tasked with addressing specific health concerns related to specific populations, e.g., children. Recent recommendations call for the addition of environmental health education to the curricula of medicine and pediatric nursing. These curriculum additions can prepare healthcare professionals to diagnose and manage environmentally caused diseases more effectively (Dearry et al., 2004). By encouraging continuous education on these subjects, family medicine practitioners can achieve a three-dimensional view of the problems that confront different patient populations, developing a more holistic and responsive health care culture eventually. For this reason, the nexus between board certification and continuing education must be broadened in scope, incorporating not just conventional medical knowledge but also emerging fields relevant to diverse patient exigencies.

Test Your Knowledge

1. Describe the medical school requirements for family medicine.
2. What is family medicine residency?

1.3. Patient-Centered Care

Learning Outcome

1. Understand the importance of building patient-physician relationships
2. Learn about shared decision-making in treatment plans
3. Describe the cultural competence within the field of family medicine

In family medicine, the Patient-Centered Care (PCC) concept is a foundational principle that aims to enhance the quality of care. It emphasizes the value of patients' active participation in their treatment, rather than being merely passive recipients of medical care. By integrating patients' perspectives and agendas, health care professionals can deliver interventions that fulfill clinical needs while also addressing the emotional and psychological dimensions of well-being. The acknowledgment of patients as full partners creates an environment in which health outcomes can significantly improve. For example, it has been shown that more engaged patients are more satisfied and typically more adherent to care plans, underscoring the central role of PCC in modern family medicine. One of the most important aspects of Patient-Centered Care is engaging family members in the health process. Family-centered care (FCC) recognizes that family members contribute significantly to patients' health and well-being. In a variety of settings, but especially in pediatrics and palliative care, family engagement is one mechanism through which it can enhance patients' and loved ones' psychological safety, creating a vital support system amidst times of vulnerability. The shift in embracing family involvement has been extensive, with increasing recognition of its benefits across all healthcare professions. Recent research emphasizes that patients, in particular the older population, whose support systems are mobilized, are more likely to gain improved health literacy and treatment adherence, with a strong suggestion of the existence of a direct correlation between family involvement and health outcomes (Hribersek et al., 2024). As the healthcare environment itself continues to transform, with the inclusion of newer innovations such as machine learning and artificial intelligence, Patient-Centered Care remains invaluable to navigating complex decision-making in care. Sustaining genetic and genomic testing within patient-centered philosophies becomes ever more important; novel laboratory-developed tests (LDTs) must be validated to ensure they are analytically and clinically sound for quality, patient-centered healthcare delivery. Above all, in precision medicine, it is crucial that the models of regulation change and ensure these tests enable well-informed healthcare decisions for patients and families. A balance between technological innovation and patient engagement unlocks opportunities to develop responsive healthcare plans that recognize the intricate needs of individuals and, as such, embrace a holistic philosophy of healthcare in family medicine (Kurnat-Thoma, 2024) (Figure 1.10).

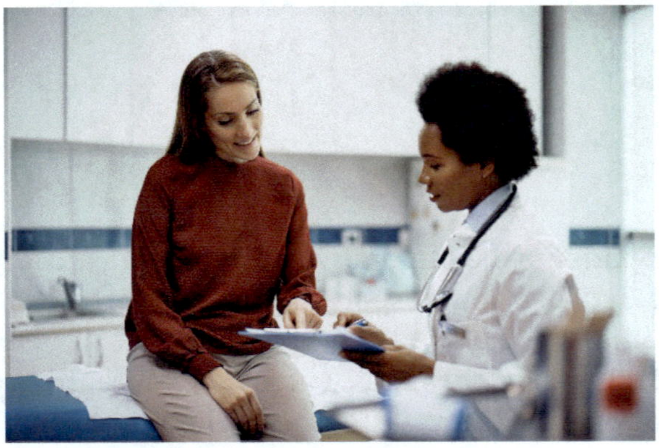

Figure 1.10. Patient-centered care.

Source: https://publichealth.tulane.edu/wp-content/uploads/sites/3/2024/04/patient-centered-care.jpg.

1.3.1. Importance of Building Patient-Physician Relationships

The physician-patient relationship forms the core of quality care delivery, particularly in family medicine. Establishing a good doctor-patient' relationship is an open communication channel that allows patients to air their worries and desires regarding their health. This trust is essential; without it, patients will only give limited information that might influence diagnosis and treatment. Research has shown that patient-centered care not only increases trust but also improves adherence to treatment regimes, improving long-term clinical outcomes. Family physicians' empathic communication has been shown to resonate strongly with patients, particularly those with multiple chronic conditions, supporting the notion that relational dynamics significantly affect patient experience and wellness (Alberto et al., 2019). Thus, building solid patient-physician relationships is a necessity for integrated care. In addition, subtleties of the patient-physician relationship extend beyond communication; they include cultural awareness and sensitivity. In increasingly diverse populations, physicians now encounter patients from diverse backgrounds with different health beliefs, values, and communication styles. Negotiating these differences is critical in achieving cooperation and understanding. Identification of cultural differences, in addition to expressing respect, enhances the therapeutic relationship. As becomes evident with the growing physician burnout and patient dissatisfaction around electronic health record systems and time pressures, healthcare systems must appreciate relational aspects as much as clinical pace (Lynch et al., 2019).

This dual focus can bridge gaps between physicians and patients, particularly those who are limited-English proficient or have different health literacies, ultimately leading to more balanced care. Given these considerations, strengthening the patient-physician relationship can lead to enormous improvement in healthcare effectiveness and patient outcomes. Legislative measures to counteract disparities in communication and access have begun to reshape the face of family medicine, but increased intensity is needed. Cultural competency education for healthcare workers can enhance understanding and compassion in patient interactions. Also, integrating patient feedback into practice can enable patients and encourage them to be more active in healthcare decision-making. Developing such frameworks not only fosters trust but also enhances community participation and health literacy across diverse populations, enabling family medicine to reach its full potential as a cornerstone of comprehensive healthcare (Lynch et al., 2019). How much more critical it is that strengthening patient-physician relationships must remain a priority in the changing practice of family medicine (Figure 1.11).

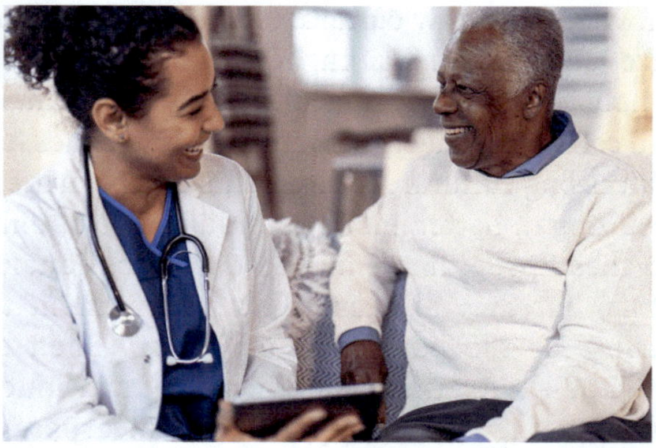

Figure 1.11. The importance of building trust in the physician-patient relationship.

Source: https://assets.contenthub.wolterskluwer.com/api/public/content/cd5144c4f85a424994cf76203042bb59?v=171ae119&t=w768l.

1.3.2. Shared Decision-Making in Treatment Plans

In family medicine, shared decision-making (SDM) represents the central component of patient-centered care. The process invites patient participation in significant decisions concerning their treatment plans. Compared to more traditional models that might focus on clinician dominance, SDM supports a relationship in which patients' values, priorities, and individual situations are taken into account. This open-ended approach not only increases patient satisfaction but also improves health outcomes by ensuring the treatment aligns with what the patient truly desires. Hence, the essence of communication between healthcare providers and patients comes into existence, where questions, concerns, and other possibilities are freely expressed. In most cases, family practice patient complexity necessitates a multicomponent treatment strategy, particularly in the context of chronic disease and palliative care. For instance, there are dementia patients requiring high-level care, which shows the importance of SDM in managing multiple and typically competing healthcare needs. The European Association for Palliative Care (EAPC) White Paper recommends that effective palliative care for individuals with dementia prioritize valuing shared decision-making so that interventions are truly aligned with the patient's desires and the facts of their case (Goodman et al., 2020). This structured approach not only increases compliance but is also essential for fostering mutual trust between providers and patients, leading to more personalized and efficient treatment plans.

Additionally, the incorporation of shared decision-making into treatment plans has some downsides, particularly for overall healthcare policies and systems. Health care reform developments emphasize the need for patient-participatory systems to facilitate patient empowerment and involvement by systematically measuring treatment outcomes and satisfaction (Macri et al., 2012). The recognition underpins the transition to an ethical and fair model of care, harmonizing treatment modalities with the patient's perspective. In practice, shared decision-making, while creating administrative challenges, is essential further to advance the effectiveness and quality of family medicine and, ultimately, toward a more comprehensive health care experience for patients (Figure 1.12).

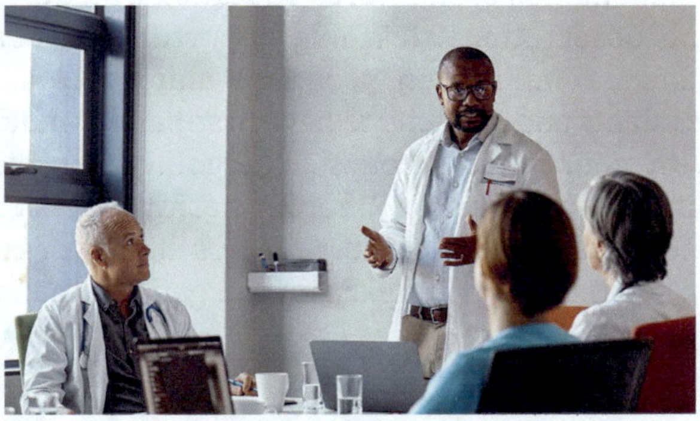

Figure 1.12. Shared decision-making for psoriasis treatment planning.

Source: https://www.zs.com/content/dam/images/stock/Medical-experts-in-a-meeting.jpg.

1.3.3. Cultural Competence in Family Medicine

Cultural competence in family medicine practice is critical for physicians who are tasked with caring for increasingly multicultural patient populations. As cultures become more multicultural, the family medicine practitioner needs to identify and integrate the unique cultural backgrounds of his or her patients into their practice. This necessitates an understanding of how cultural factors create different health values, behaviors, and communication styles. By engaging in culturally congruent activities, family medicine physicians are better positioned to establish patient trust and rapport, particularly for effective healthcare delivery. Hence, infusing cultural competence into the education of medical professionals is of paramount significance, enabling prospective caregivers to recognize the varied histories and identities of patients (Shopo et al., 2024). This root change is advantageous to both health outcomes and a healthcare environment that values diversity and inclusion, directly reflecting the demographic changes observed in patient populations. Cultural competence is built by fostering methods that promote understanding and respect for various cultural perspectives. This can be achieved in family medicine through a combination of structured educational modules and observational learning opportunities. For instance, immersion programs allow medical residents and students to have first-hand contact with other cultural groups, undergoing extensive direct experience of different health practices and attitudes. The learning process allows for an environment where learners can gain firsthand knowledge of how cultural issues affect patient care and outcomes. In addition, promoting collaboration between healthcare professionals and community agencies can provide avenues for addressing cultural requirements and priorities, resulting in better, more tailored care. Not only do these programs enhance the practitioners' skills, but they also exhibit a commitment to caring for the patient as an entity (Eden et al., 2024). As medical education continues to evolve, it is also important to incorporate cultural competence into the family medicine training curriculum. Institutional commitment to cultural competence is necessary to obtain systems-level change in family medicine. Policies at the medical school level that foster diversity and incentives for training in cultural competence are instrumental in the assurance of properly prepared future practitioners to engage with the complexities of patients. Leadership from healthcare organizations should also actively support programs that foster ongoing professional development in cultural sensitivity. Training sessions and workshops aimed at minimizing bias and increasing understanding of cultural context can greatly enhance clinical interactions between healthcare workers and patients. Yet education alone is not sufficient; creating a conducive, interactive setting for both staff and patients is critical. By prioritizing cultural competence, family medicine can create a more equitable healthcare setting in which individuals from every demographic feel heard and appreciated (Shopo et al., 2024). In the end, integrating cultural competence into family medicine will lead to a more effective and responsive healthcare system.

Test Your Knowledge

1. What is the importance of building patient-physician relationships?
2. Why is cultural competence important in family medicine?

1.4. Common Health Issues Addressed

Learning Outcome

1. Understand the chronic disease management
2. Recognize the mental health considerations within the framework of family medicine
3. Describe the pediatric and geriatric care

Family medicine is also crucial to addressing widespread health issues across populations. Patients typically first visit a family physician, who provides primary treatment for chronic conditions such as diabetes, high blood pressure, and obesity. These require ongoing care and close observation, which family medicine clinics can easily provide. Telehealth care, specifically, has proven a viable means of managing these chronic conditions, augmenting the availability of needed consultations and follow-ups for patients. Research shows greater efficiency in controlling diabetes and hypertension through telehealth interventions, providing evidence of how family medicine adapts to evolving healthcare (Bowman et al., 2024). These technologies not only streamline care but also have the potential to reduce health inequities that disproportionately burden underserved populations. In addition to chronic disease, family medicine also addresses a range of acute health issues, including respiratory illnesses, gastrointestinal disease, and mental illness. The comprehensive strategy of family practice allows physicians to diagnose and treat a broad variety of health conditions in the environment of the practice, limiting the incidence of specialist referrals and fostering continuity of care. For instance, family physicians can provide immediate treatment for uncomplicated respiratory infections, thereby reducing the workload in emergency departments. This willingness to care ensures that patients receive prompt interventions to prevent minor illnesses from becoming serious health crises. Moreover, the addition of health advocacy training in family medicine equips professionals to address the social determinants of health, which are critical to the management of both acute and chronic illnesses in their patient populations (Mören et al., 2024). Moreover, resolving excessive testing for common conditions shows evidence-based practice follow-through on the part of family medicine. Physicians must keep themselves updated about clinical practice guidelines so that they don't subject patients to unnecessary tests or procedures that will cause undue anxiety and expense. More and more pressure is being brought to bear to adhere to recommended standard practice for tests like Pulmonary Function Tests and screening for colon cancer, which have a direct impact on patient outcomes. Family practice, therefore, serves to treat ongoing illnesses while using preventive strategies to achieve better health outcomes. These are all integrated into teaching and training for family doctors, highlighting the importance of maintaining high standards of practice and enhancing the quality of patient care delivered in community practice (Bowman et al., 2024) (Figure 1.13).

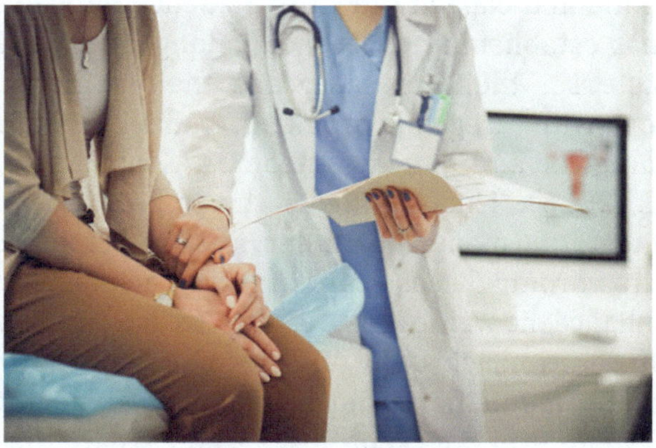

Figure 1.13. Uncovering the hidden causes and solutions of common health issues.

Source: https://healthcarebusinessclub.com/wp-content/uploads/2023/12/Uncovering-the-Hidden-Causes-Solutions-of-Common-Health-Issues.jpg.

1.4.1. Chronic Disease Management

Effective chronic disease management is a mainstay of family medicine, as it also aligns neatly with the specialty's thematic focus on holism. Chronic illnesses generally represent long-standing problems that require repeated support, education, and multidisciplinary management. Family physicians are ideally placed to monitor patients over time, making repeat assessments that can change with shifting clinical demand. This ongoing relationship allows for a better understanding of the patient's personal and family context, a consideration necessary for the patient's adherence to treatment. Additionally, health care intervention is feasible given the family processes influencing health behaviors, thereby enhancing a holistic management plan that focuses on both the individual and the family. The importance of understanding the psychosocial factors of chronic disease management cannot be overstated. Emotional and mental health can significantly affect a patient's capacity to adapt to their condition; therefore, family physicians must identify these factors. For instance, mothers managing children with chronic ailments experience higher levels of stress, which directly affects their quality of life and capacity to care. Evidence indicates that establishing coherence among caregivers increases their flexibility and their ability to cope with caregiving problems, leading to better caregiver and patient outcomes (Avaznejad et al., 2016). This highlights the importance of integrating mental health services and resources into chronic disease care in family medicine to enhance the well-being of caregivers and patients. In addition, chronic disease management in family medicine is more than just managing system-level interventions, a trend exemplified by initiatives such as Indonesia's "Program Rujuk Balik" (PRB). Such an initiative illustrates the potential role that family physicians can play in both accessing health care and controlling chronic conditions such as coronary heart disease (CHD) through integrated care. By adopting an interdisciplinary methodology incorporating risk factor modification and ongoing patient education, family practitioners are able to effectively manage the catastrophic costs of chronic conditions (Kuhon et al., 2022). The effectiveness of such efforts rests on family practices' ability to deliver integrative health care that meets unique patient needs, thereby validating the compelling overlap between community health services and effective chronic disease management in family medicine (Figure 1.14).

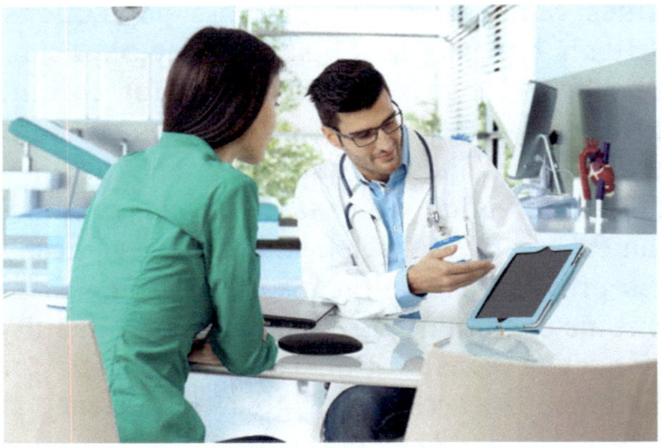

Figure 1.14. Chronic disease management.

Source: https://primarycarefriscotx.com/wp-content/uploads/chronic-disease-management-2107.jpg.

1.4.2. Mental Health Considerations

Recognition of mental health issues within family medicine is essential to comprehensive patient care. Family medicine providers will routinely meet with patients who have difficulty with mental health issues, which can frequently intersect with disease in the physical realm. The biopsychosocial model argues that mental health cannot be isolated from social and biological determinants of well-being. For example, social determinants such as socioeconomic status, education, and environment may influence a patient's mental state. Therefore, when family practitioners treat their patients, successful management of these determinants may lead to better treatment plans. The integration of mental health screens, particularly for health-related social needs (HRSN), is necessary to raise awareness and improve clinician-patient relationships, ultimately positively influencing outcomes and improving patient care (Porterfield et al., 2024). Training healthcare providers on the interaction between mental health and social determinants is key to effective family medicine practice. Medical education must place the highest priority on incorporating social accountability and mental health considerations into education. Students must be equipped with tools that allow them to recognize how social inequities can exacerbate mental health issues, rather than clinical symptoms in isolation. This perspective can be cultivated through projects such as the family medicine clerkship, which provide an opportunity to discuss the importance of mental health awareness and how it intersects with care provision for disadvantaged populations. By adopting a peer-teaching strategy that incorporates social accountability into clinical presentations, practicing physicians can develop a socially aware approach to patient care that reflects the complexity of mental health issues (Shah et al., 2023). Challenges to proper mental health care in family medicine require ongoing discussion and planning. Providers frequently indicate that they struggle due to time constraints, workload, and emotional demands that hinder their capacity to address mental health needs. Further, concerns regarding a lack of resources or skill in providing complete care may discourage providers from screening for mental health during routine visits. To avoid these barriers, workflow processes must be streamlined, teamwork enhanced, and technology used appropriately. An entirely integrated electronic medical record (EMR) system with mental health management tools can facilitate better identification and intervention for mental health problems. With a clear focus on team communication and the critical importance of HRSN screening, family medicine can be made into a more robust practice that exerts a profound impact on mental health outcomes and reduces health disparities (Porterfield et al., 2024).

1.4.3. Pediatric and Geriatric Care

The diversity of patients' needs across the lifespan necessitates individualized family practice, particularly in pediatrics and geriatrics. Pediatric practice addresses unique developmental and behavioral health demands in children in order to facilitate the realization of crucial growth milestones. Good pediatric practice, following today's recommendations, includes extensive surveillance and screening that are compatible with development milestones, thereby enabling early identification of potential disorders. The American Academy of Pediatrics underscores this holistic model, which includes not only medical evaluation but also psychological and behavioral evaluations to foster the child's overall health and development (Pamplin et al., 2013). The holistic approach is needed, as childhood is an optimal period for establishing long-term health habits. Conversely, geriatric care also takes into account the complexity of aging since older people acquire numerous comorbidities that complicate their ability to cope with their health. In family practice, geriatric care requires a high-level understanding of changes in physiology in old age, as well as social determinants of health, such as social isolation and cognitive impairment. In addition, intervention must be tailored to prioritize functional status and quality of life as much as medical care. For instance, careful management of drugs is necessary in a bid to minimize risks of polypharmacy as well as adverse drug interactions among older patients (Pamplin et al., 2013). Family doctors are tasked with the coordination of care between different healthcare settings to ensure continuity of care that is customized to meet the special needs of aging patients during the aging process. Merging both pediatric and geriatric care into the family medicine model promotes a general emphasis on patient health across the lifespan. The continuum enables anticipatory guidance and proactive intervention strategies tailored to address each stage's particular challenges. By establishing early intervention protocols in pediatrics and preventive care measures across the geriatric age range, family physicians can significantly enhance health outcomes. They are not only capable of identifying children's developing health issues but also of preserving the elderly's functional capacity and independence. Lastly, pediatric-geriatric care collaboration reflects the family medicine philosophy of treating the patient within his/her family and community environment, thereby providing comprehensive care for all ages (Section A on Developmental and Peditrics B, 2010) (Figure 1.15).

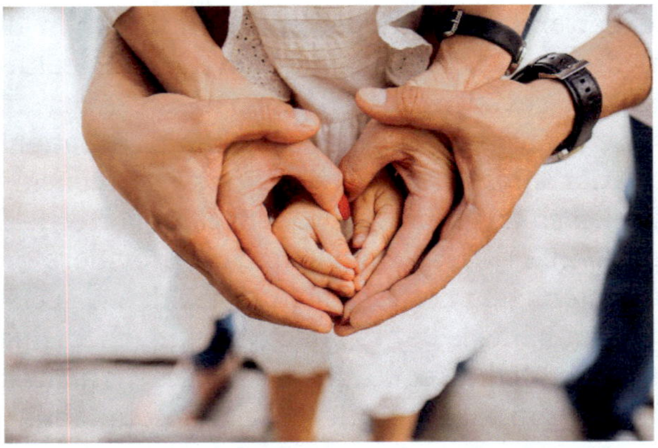

Figure 1.15. Pediatric to geriatric: the spectrum of care in family medicine.

Source: https://azprimaryclinic.com/wp-content/uploads/2024/08/AdobeStock_124870478-scaled.jpeg.

Test Your Knowledge

1. What is chronic disease management?
2. What is meant by geriatric care?

1.5. Family Medicine in Different Settings

Learning Outcome

1. Understand the urban vs. rural practice environments
2. Describe the family medicine in community health centers
3. Understand telemedicine and its impact on family medicine

Family practice plays a central role in many healthcare settings, providing holistic care to individuals across all demographics. Within inner-city settings, family doctors are routinely confronted with unique challenges, including socioeconomic disparity and prevalence rates for chronic disease among populations. These doctors must navigate complex social determinants of health deftly while creating equal access to services. Interventions for colorectal cancer screening, for instance, are particularly vital in these settings, as evidence indicates significant delays in detection due to poor health literacy and patient access barriers (Alsaqer et al., 2025). By adopting a responsive strategy that meets the specific needs of their groups, family doctors can optimize screening uptake and ultimately reduce illness. In rural areas, family doctors play a key role in addressing healthcare needs due to limited access to specialized services. Family practice flexibility allows such doctors to manage a wide range of health conditions, from preventive care to chronic disease management. Early diagnosis and management of illnesses like atrial fibrillation are particularly brought to the fore in such settings, in which patients do not often have the benefit of advanced treatment (Bulbul et al., 2024). Family doctors in rural community settings are also usually the initial contact point for most patients, and thus prioritizing screening tests and comprehensive management of prevalent ailments is essential. Their chronic patient relationships foster trust, enabling better treatment plan follow-up and overall community health. Family medicine flexibility is also present in varied healthcare systems, such as integrated models of care as well as community health programs. Such systems emphasize collaborative care, with family physicians working alongside specialists, behavioral health professionals, and social workers. Such an interdisciplinary approach is particularly helpful in managing complex cases in a way that comprehensive intervention can be rendered, covering many aspects of a patient's life.

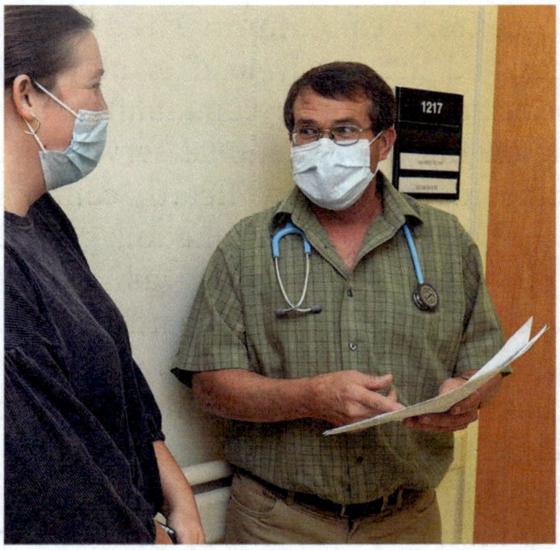

Figure 1.16. Family physician (right) reviewing a case with nurse (left) in clinic.

Source: https://upload.wikimedia.org/wikipedia/commons/b/b5/Family_Medicine_Clinic_at_Naval_Branch_Health_Clinic_Mayport.jpg.

For example, collaborative contributions to colorectal cancer screening programs have been shown to be effective in enhancing participation rates when there are robust support systems and sufficient resource reallocation (Alsaqer et al., 2025). By this collaborative framework, family medicine practitioners are able to reach out further, offering comprehensive care that is sensitive to the diverse needs of the patients, regardless of the healthcare setting in which they practice (Figure 1.16).

1.5.1. Urban vs. Rural Practice Environments

The varied life experience of family medicine practitioners in urban versus rural settings has a considerable impact on their working lives and determine their choices of practice location. Urban locations tend to provide more resources, including specialist backup, advanced medical technologies, and a more diverse patient population. These can foster job satisfaction and facilitate collaborative care models. Nevertheless, city practitioners often must contend with higher patient volumes, which can contribute to increased stress and burnout. Conversely, rural practice environments usually present unique challenges, including limited access to healthcare resources and a potential sense of professional isolation. Despite these difficulties, rural family medicine doctors report , intense feelings of community involvement and personal satisfaction due to working with their populations, which emphasizes the varied motivations for recruitment and retention between settings (Tort-Nasarre et al., 2023). Understanding the ins and outs of city and country practice settings requires a thorough analysis of special factors influencing recruitment and retention. In cities, the higher demand for family physicians can lead to a faster turnover rate, with the added complication of competing job markets that prefer specialists. Rural communities, on the other hand, face critical shortages of primary care physicians, exacerbated by poor living standards and lower compensation than their urban counterparts. Research indicates that completion of family and community medicine training programs can boost the attractiveness of rural practice by equipping potential providers with the skills and confidence to thrive in places beyond the urban core. In fact, successful recruitment and retention strategies primarily rely on addressing individual and structural determinants that are responsive to potential family physicians (Ward et al., 2020). While the sheer demands of practice can deplete family doctors, the effect is observed even in both urban and rural settings. In an extensive study, no actual disparity was observed between the two regarding burnout rates, and workload, job satisfaction, and personal characteristics were found to be more determining factors than the exceptional dynamics of urban or rural practice per se (Ward et al., 2020). This finding calls for reconsidering common presuppositions about practice environments and shifting the emphasis to systemic solutions that improve the overall experience of family medicine practitioners. Highlighting shared challenges rather than geographical segments enables stakeholders to develop specific interventions so that all family physicians' psychological well-being is supported, ultimately leading to better patient care in urban and rural settings as well.

1.5.2. Family Medicine in Community Health Centers

Integration of family medicine within community health centers is essential to addressing the diverse health care needs of often underserved populations. Family medicine emphasizes global and continuous care, which aligns with the primary mission of community health centers to provide accessible, preventive, and primary health care services. These clinics offer crucial points of entry for vulnerable populations, with integrated care that includes not only medical care but also prevention and education. Through established patient-physician relationships, family medicine facilitates team-based care that can significantly affect patient outcomes in these populations. This aligns with an increased value on the social determinants of health and on culturally relevant care. Thus, family medicine stands out as a vital part of the plan to improve health equity in community health centers. Besides, the evolving landscape of healthcare reform comes with challenges and prospects for family medicine within community health centers. As healthcare systems evolve, center administrators are called upon to transform into emerging models of care that aim for patient-centered results and aligned care teams. The intricacies of restructuring small primary care practices necessitate innovative solutions, enabling community health centers to tap resources such as Medicaid to catalyze and sustain care delivery transformations (Berenson et al., 2011). The transition usually involves receiving funding for training and operations support, enabling these centers to transition to a more efficient, coordinated care system voluntarily. With such investments, community health centers can improve the quality of services and ultimately lead to better access and health outcomes for communities that rely heavily on these foundational services. Family medicine in community health centers also entails proactive care coordination, particularly for vulnerable groups such as the elderly and those with complex health conditions. Evidence-based prevention policies are crucial for optimizing health outcomes (Morton et al., 2015). Family doctors have the ability to become central figures in developing care plans for their individual patients upon consideration of their own social contexts and conditions of illness. This high level of individualized care not only prevents chronic diseases but also reduces hospitalization and healthcare costs. Emphasize family caregivers' strengths. Within the system, one can plug some of those gaps in continuity of care. Ultimately, through a unified effort to infuse those practices, family medicine in community health centers can be a formidable pillar for boosting community health (Figure 1.17).

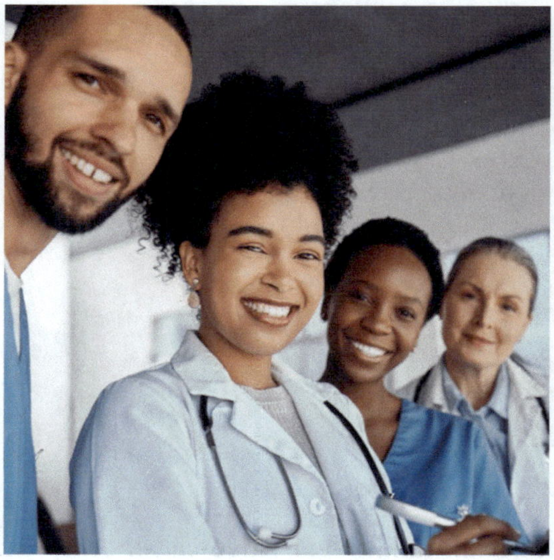

Figure 1.17. Family medicine in community health centers.

Source: https://www.durhamchc.ca/wp-content/uploads/2024/01/Family-Medicine_Website-Program-Images.png.

1.5.3 Telemedicine and Its Impact on Family Medicine

The integration of telemedicine in family medicine has transformed health care delivery, particularly following the COVID-19 pandemic. The rapid integration of telehealth services was driven by the need to curb disease spread, leading to the establishment of robust virtual health care systems. This shift not only provides access to healthcare while maintaining social distancing but also fosters a convenient environment for managing routine care and chronic illnesses. Furthermore, it enables patients to see healthcare professionals who might otherwise be geographically unavailable. The economic effect, if any, is equally enormous, with some estimates suggesting that as much as US$259 billion of healthcare spending could be shifted to virtual platforms, hence altering the dynamics of healthcare delivery in the United States (Yee et al., 2022). With greater access from afar, telemedicine can contribute significantly to care tailoring while curing health access gaps. However, telemedicine's potential benefits are preceded by challenges, namely concerns about health equity and patient trust. Inequity in access to broadband and technology can disproportionately affect marginalized populations, creating an amplification of already present inequity in accessing health care. In particular, evidence has shown that Black patients are highly resistant to engaging in telehealth services, and this is usually based on historical distrust of the healthcare system and lack of pre-existing relationships with caregivers (Yee et al., 2022).

The very basis of family medicine, such as establishing long-term patient-provider relationships, is directly incompatible in a virtual environment. Telemedicine, rather than just being viewed as a technology option, should be seen as a platform that requires establishing trust and rapport, a prerequisite for effective patient engagement and satisfaction. In primary care practice settings, the perceived appropriateness of telemedicine varies widely among healthcare providers.

Research has indicated that younger clinicians and clinicians in certain specialties are more open to telehealth as an acceptable option for future practice. For others, concerns about the adequacy of patient care and the limitations of physical examination deter them from embracing its implementation. Nevertheless, the majority of clinicians recognize the value of telemedicine for specific purposes, such as follow-up and medication management, particularly in low-resource settings. As telemedicine continues to evolve, there will be a need to promote awareness and education among clinicians to facilitate successful implementation in family medicine, particularly to maintain care quality and ensure access for diverse patient populations (Figure 1.18).

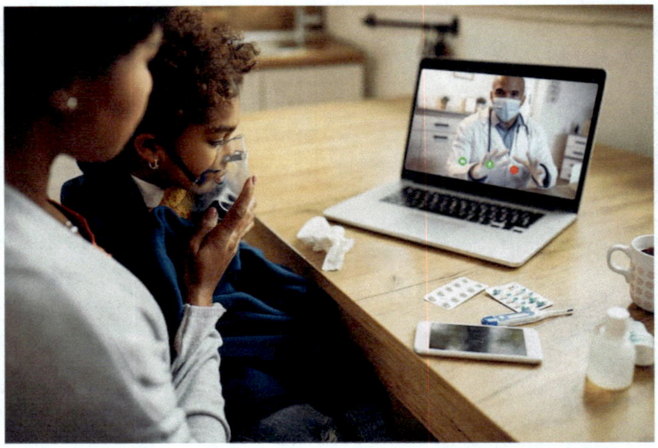

Figure 1.18. Telemedicine.

Source: https://img.freepik.com/free-photo/black-pediatrician-talking-via-video-call-mother-who-is-giving-her-daughter-inhaling-therapy-home_637285-11483.jpg?semt=ais_hybrid&w=740.

Test Your Knowledge

1. What is family medicine in community health centers?
2. What is the impact of telemedicine on family medicine?

1.6. Challenges in Family Medicine

Learning Outcome

1. Understand the burnout and work-life balance for family physicians
2. Navigate healthcare policies and insurance
3. Address health disparities in diverse populations

Family medicine is typically confronted by many problems that impact the delivery of healthcare. One of them is the insufficiency of healthcare professionals, particularly in rural areas. All regions are confronted with the unavailability of obstetricians and family physicians, leading to poor maternal and child healthcare. As identified in new studies, rural communities find it challenging to have suitable healthcare resources, which is usually compounded by the exodus of medical practitioners to urban areas, which compromises the conventional caregiving models in the communities (Ohta et al., 2024). This shortage of providers affects not just the availability of services but also contributes to wider health inequalities between urban and rural populations, presenting a significant gap to be bridged by family medicine in terms of delivering comprehensive and universal care for all patients. The second major challenge facing family medicine is the aging population and the increasing prevalence of chronic diseases. As the population profile evolves, family physicians are confronted with increasingly complex medical conditions that require ongoing assessment and individualized care. The integration of e-health tools is a plausible solution to this mounting dilemma; they can assist patients in managing their chronic diseases and enhance the efficiency of care delivery (Çöme et al., 2023). Nonetheless, the implementation of such technologies varies across regions and healthcare systems, reflecting different levels of adoption and infrastructure. Furthermore, scientific validation of the effectiveness of e-health applications continues to be important, as lack of proper scientific confirmation may hamper their practical application within family medicine practices. Furthermore, the dynamic nature of healthcare necessitates ongoing change among family medicine professionals. The need to remain abreast of developments in medical science, treatments, and health policy puts pressure on providers to be responsive and up-to-date. Demonstrating the outcomes of studies in maternal and child health, and overcoming obstacles such as insufficient training in specific domains and the unavailability of support systems within the community, can enhance the standard of care (Ohta et al., 2024). Family medicine must not only respond to immediate healthcare needs but also be proactive in future planning, such as developing integrated models of care and fostering interdisciplinary collaboration. These actions are important for creating resilience and sustainability in family medicine and ultimately improving health outcomes for increasingly diverse patient populations.

1.6.1. Burnout and Work-Life Balance for Family Physicians

The burnout epidemic among family physicians has come into the spotlight more and more in recent years, primarily due to its far-reaching impact on healthcare professionals as well as patient care. Burnout has been characterized by emotional exhaustion, depersonalization, and decreased feelings of personal accomplishment. These elements can be highly negative towards the effectiveness of family physicians in performing their roles. Contributing causes to burnout include high patient loads, administrative responsibilities, and the emotional toll of managing complex patient demands in a contentious healthcare environment. Research suggests that the growing trend towards telemedicine has further blurred the traditional work-life balance for family physicians. As noted in research, a measure of medical quality in teleconsultation is lower than in face-to-face meetings, highlighting the possibility of greater stress and burnout if physicians do not feel their work is meaningful or effective (Zacay et al., 2024). Maintaining work-life balance remains a crucial factor in mitigating burnout among family physicians, as it naturally influences their well-being and job satisfaction. The unpredictable and extended hours that are often required in family medicine induce severe stress, and with it, the phenomenon of burnout. Good work-life balance, in addition to enhancing physician satisfaction, also improves patient outcomes, as balanced physicians are more responsive and involved with their patients. Creating policies that eliminate unnecessary administrative tasks is essential. For instance, research has found that alleviating administrative burdens would significantly enhance work-life balance, reducing burnout rates and improving the quality of care provided by family physicians (Zacay et al., 2024). Efforts toward increasing scheduling flexibility and supportive systems can enable physicians to balance professional responsibilities and personal lives more effectively. Furthermore, the unpredictability of work settings has a significant impact on family physicians' work-life balance, causing burnout and job dissatisfaction. In particular, in intensive work environments such as emergency departments, physicians experience considerable work-life interference due to uncertain work schedules and heavy workloads. Facilitating a less stressful and more predictable work environment can eliminate some of these burdens and lead to improved mental health and physician retention. Rest and recovery, as well as approaches to developing supportive workplace cultures, are the key to preventing burnout among this cohort. As the healthcare landscape continues to evolve, organizational leaders and policymakers must prioritize these elements to create a sustainable practice environment that puts physician well-being and high-quality patient care first (Figure 1.19).

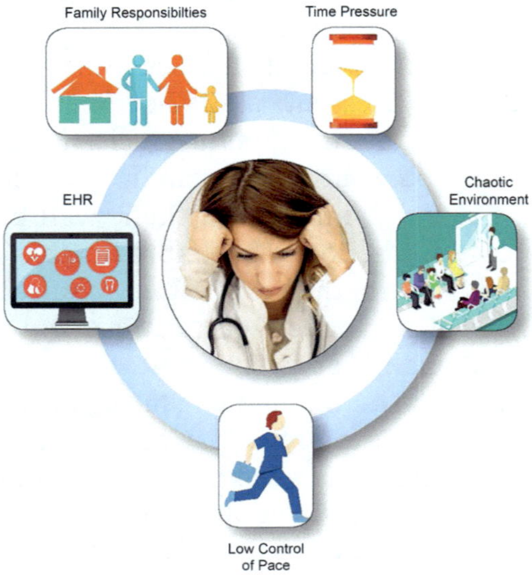

Figure 1.19. Causes of clinician burnout.

Source: https://www.ahrq.gov/sites/default/files/wysiwyg/professionals/clinicians-providers/ahrq-works/burnout_infographic_1.jpg.

1.6.2. Navigating Healthcare Policies and Insurance

Health insurance and healthcare policy are at the forefront of effective family medicine practice as they directly influence patient access to care and overall quality of services provided. In today's ever-evolving healthcare system, it becomes pivotal for family physicians to comprehend the intricacies of insurance programs, reimbursement systems, and regulatory requirements. With policy initiatives towards universal health coverage, such as the Affordable Care Act in the USA, healthcare providers must be adept at traversing various insurance schemes to obtain the services their patients require. Policies that manage reimbursement rates, benefit maximums, and documentation mandates can at times be obstacles for both patients and providers, affecting continuity and comprehensiveness of care. As healthcare systems are made more efficient and effective, family doctors are at the intersection of patient needs and administrative requirements. In particular, innovative models of care, such as the Patient-Centered Medical Home, emphasize the value of coordinated care amid insurance complexity. Mandates in policies favoring integrated care require family doctors to negotiate equitable payment rates with third-party payers. In addition, financial toxicity awareness—the imposition of high out-of-pocket costs among patients—that is faced by healthcare professionals requires the establishment of financial literacy among their patients in a bid to make informed decisions about their healthcare options (Cheng, 2024). Consequently, successful health policy and insurance navigation can enhance patient satisfaction and ultimately provide better health outcomes. In addition, healthcare policies play a significant role in shaping the context of rehabilitation services, which have been even more crucial in the context of family medicine. The World Health Organization highlights the significance of rehabilitation in universal health coverage, particularly as countries adjust to increasing demands for comprehensive health care (Carlos, 2024). Family physicians must be able to decipher these policies, particularly in light of legislative trends of the last few decades that have intermixed rehabilitation with core health packages. This intermixing provides an opportunity for family medicine to address unmet needs in a constructive manner, but places practitioners in the position of having to understand the limits established by insurance companies regarding coverage and access. Through the detailed knowledge of health policies surrounding rehabilitation, family doctors can serve their patients more effectively by ensuring that those requiring them get adequate resources and support for healing and enhanced quality of life (Figure 1.20).

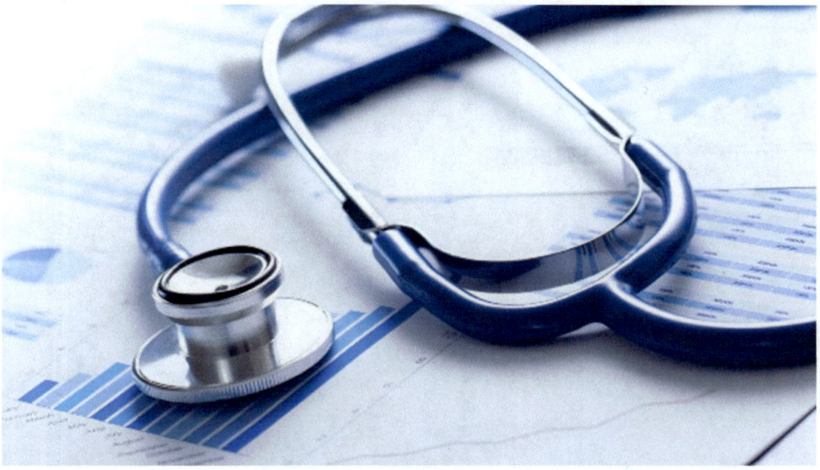

Figure 1.20. Navigating health insurance.

Source: https://images.goodreturns.in/img/2024/04/health6-1712481457.jpg.

1.6.3. Addressing Health Disparities in Diverse Populations

The pursuit of equitable health outcomes remains a core concern for family medicine, particularly in addressing disparities across diverse populations. Racial, linguistic, and socioeconomic differences often fuel inequalities in health by restricting access to preventive interventions and treatment. The evidence is that if health-seeking behavior is met with culturally appropriate educational strategies, it can have a profound impact. For example, in studies of Spanish-preferred patients, application of culturally responsive screening items led to a substantial reduction of non-adherence to breast cancer screening among such individuals (Strelow et al., 2025). This points towards the significance of embracing cultural competence in healthcare practice, as not only does it foster trust, but also ensures that information given to patients is meaningful to their respective cultures. Moreover, the broader context of family medicine is included within and facilitates holistic care with sensitivity to the social determinants of health. Family doctors have a special role in considering the numerous social, cultural, and environmental determinants that lead to health disparities. By offering a holistic approach to treatment plans, such healthcare providers are better situated to address illnesses that are prevalent in oppressed populations, like substance use disorder or chronic illness, disproportionately exacerbated by economic instability. By prioritizing robust rural family medicine and traditionally underrepresented groups, health equity is reinforced (Ventres et al., 2024). These initiatives show a commitment to understand and address the problems that accompany delivering health care in a multichanger world. Furthermore, closing health disparities goes beyond clinical interventions; systemic changes to healthcare delivery models, with a focus on accessibility and inclusivity, are required. Interventions such as community outreach, language assistance services, and policy advocacy are instrumental in guiding equitable healthcare models. In family medicine, understanding the specific needs of populations—LGBTQIA+ individuals or homeless ones—is what enables providers to decrease barriers that contribute to less-than-desirable health for those groups. As can be seen in many thematic analyses in the field, an integrative model of family medicine not only identifies but also seeks to dismantle the structural barriers that perpetuate health disparities (Ventres et al., 2024). By focusing on inclusivity and need-based care strategies, the profession can make significant contributions to health equity for all (Figure 1.21).

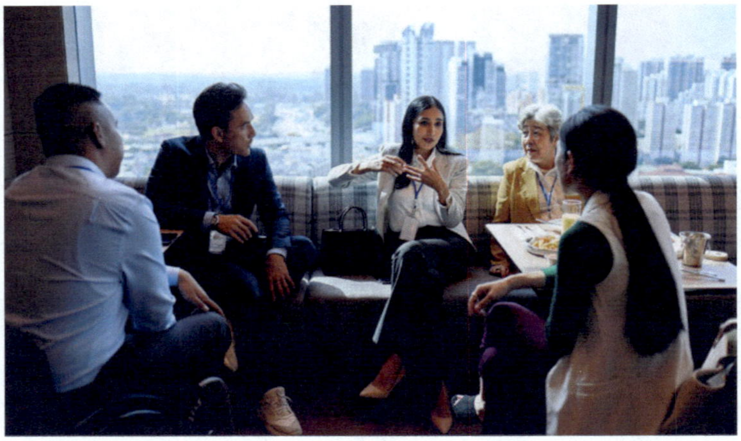

Figure 1.21. Addressing healthcare disparities.

Source: https://www.zs.com/content/dam/images/stock/Business-meet-senior-asian-businesswoman-and-her-diverse-team-of-colleagues-meeting-at-hotel-restaurant-insight.jpg.

Test Your Knowledge

1. What is the phenomenon of burnout for family physicians?
2. How do you address health disparities?

SUMMARY

Briefly, the contribution of family medicine to the broader healthcare landscape cannot be overstated. Family medicine is the cornerstone of coordinated patient care, with an emphasis on long-term relationships and holistic treatment that addresses physical and psychosocial dimensions. The continuity of care focus enables a deeper understanding of the individual patient's health complexities over time so that practitioners can deliver bespoke interventions. The central role of the family doctor is supported by their ability to bring care together across specialties, as supported by a number of studies emphasizing the beneficial outcomes of interdisciplinary work. Clinical observation interactions in palliative care, for instance, were reported to allow students to appreciate family and practitioner relationships, confirming communication at its best in practice (Breakwell et al., 2012). With the evolution of the art of healthcare, the incorporation of family medicine into the health systems is increasingly important. The patient-centered medical home model is the peak of incorporation, facilitated by active leadership and collaboration to deliver quality care optimized for patient needs. Practice transformation requires implementing change principles, with a focus on active participation and healing relationships between practitioners and patients. Increased availability of health care interventions and targeted interventions have the potential to dramatically improve health outcomes, particularly in disadvantaged communities. Thus, family medicine philosophy must be adapted and systematically translated into these new health care models to address the demands of a more sophisticated health care environment (Wagner et al., 2012). Finally, family medicine fate is connected inseparably with ongoing education and research that will create best practices. The clinical observation experiences of healthcare students help fill the experiential learning gap, allowing prospective medical professionals to grapple with the realities of patient care while building proficiency in palliative care. In a changing healthcare environment moving towards more collaborative models of care, an understanding of the intricacies of family dynamics in healthcare practice is a requirement. Continuing to facilitate interdisciplinary training and collaboration will equip healthcare professionals with the skill sets to practice in this field with sophistication. Therefore, reaffirming the fundamentals of family medicine and commitment to patient-centered care remains essential to continuing to build a healthier society and ensuring future healthcare initiatives' success.

Family medicine is a cornerstone of primary care, providing ongoing, comprehensive care to individuals and families of all ages and genders, across all illnesses. Its emphasis on preventive and whole-person care distinguishes it from other specialties, allowing family physicians to establish long-term relationships with their patients. This approach fosters continuity and trust, leading to improved health outcomes as patients are more likely to be treated, adhere to treatment regimens, and engage in preventive measures when they have a personal relationship with their physician. Family medicine is particularly relevant in the case of chronic disease care and in health education across population groups as these physicians typically act as the first point of referral in the medical system. Thus, their comprehensive perspective on things not only enhances patient care but also supports the community health structure, validating the inherent value of family medicine in fostering overall well-being. Moreover, the intrinsic value of family medicine lies not merely in the care of individual patients but in the continuum of health care. Family physicians are often coordinators of care, making specialist referrals and follow-up according to the unique health needs of a patient. This coordination is especially essential for managing intricate cases that require interdisciplinary approaches. Studies have proven that family medicine can lead to improved access to health care and reduced health spending, and is effective in managing population health more sustainably. Furthermore, as health systems worldwide face increasing pressure to deliver quality care at lower costs, the role of family medicine becomes even more important. It illuminates the extent to which primary care can reduce system stress by avoiding avoidable hospitalization and reducing the emergency care burden, a proactive rather than a reactive model of healthcare. In addition, promotion of family medicine as a core career choice for medical students is needed to ensure the future resilience of primary care systems. Literature indicates that future physicians value aspects of family medicine such as dedication to community and acceptable working hours, which correlate with a satisfactory work-life balance. Negative impressions that detract from its appeal—lower prestige as a specialist, for instance—are contradictory. Measures to enhance the promotion and appeal of family medicine within medical schools are pressing. This can be achieved through such perceptions and by providing a favorable environment that respects the contribution of family medicine to public and community health. Through this, medical schools would promote the future healthcare professionals. Thus, considering the contribution of family medicine is not only crucial in individual patient care but also in establishing a strong health care system capable of responding to evolving social needs (Bonowicz et al., 2025; Takeuchi et al., 2025).

KEY TERMS FROM THIS CHAPTER

Advocacy
Cultural competency
Health education
Healthcare delivery
Lifelong learning
Medicine
Pharmacology
Community health
Health disparities
Health equity
Healthcare system
Medical community
Patient care
Public health

CRITICAL THINKING QUESTIONS

1. **Which of the following is a key principle of family medicine?**
   a. Treating only chronic illnesses
   b. Providing care exclusively in hospitals
   c. Continuity of care over time
   d. Specializing in a single organ system
2. **Family medicine focuses on the care of which patient population?**
   a. Only elderly patients
   b. Only children and adolescents
   c. Individuals across all age groups and genders
   d. Only individuals with terminal illnesses
3. **What is the significant role of a family physician?**
   a. Performing complex surgeries
   b. Providing preventive care and health education
   c. Only referring patients to specialists
   d. Conducting only research activities
4. **Which of the following is a hallmark of patient-centered care in family medicine?**
   a. Decisions are solely made by the physician
   b. Patients are not involved in treatment plans
   c. Shared decision-making with patients
   d. Treatment focuses only on the disease
5. **What is the "biopsychosocial model" in family medicine?**
   a. A focus only on the biological aspects of a disease
   b. Considering biological, psychological, and social factors in health
   c. A treatment approach emphasizing expensive technology
   d. Ignoring psychological and social factors in diagnosis

Short Answer Questions

1. What is the meaning of family medicine?
2. Why is family medicine the best specialty?
3. Describe the role of a family physician.
4. What is patient-centered care?
5. What is the most common health issue?

Answer to Critical Thinking Questions

1. (c); 2. (c); 3. (b); 4. (c); 5. (b).

REFERENCES

1. Aap Section on Developmental and Behavioral Pediatrics. (2010). *AAP Developmental and Behavioral Pediatrics*. https://www.semanticscholar.org/paper/acfc8d4b64ff080087b2d82df430b226cfb10847 (accessed on 12th July 2025).
2. Simões, J., Alberto, K., Simões, P., Maurício, K., Rosendo, I., & Santiago, L. M. (2019). Communication and health: doctor-patient relationship in patients with multimorbidity, an exploratory study. *Family Medicine & Primary Care Review*, *21*(4), 377–380. https://doi.org/10.5114/fmpcr.2019.90169Alsaqer, R., Gosty, A., Faraj, S., Alobaisi, A., Alraddadi, S., Alharbi, M., Alshehri, N., et al. (2025). Strategies to enhance early detection of colorectal cancer in family medicine: A systematic review. *International Journal of Medicine in Developing Countries*. https://www.semanticscholar.org/paper/cedbb9b50d50bed2419b67a6ca6a751c166a966c (accessed on 12th July 2025).
3. Alzahrani, A. A., Alqarni, N. A., Alghamdi, F. S., & Alghamdi, T. A. (2025). Knowledge and attitude towards ankle sprain management among primary care physicians in the department of family medicine, King Fahad Armed Forces Hospital, Jeddah, Saudi Arabia. *Journal of Family Medicine and Primary Care*, *14*, 211–217. https://www.semanticscholar.org/paper/bc8d4529fa63061ec9a92801ca919a1a4b9a937f (accessed on 12th July 2025).
4. Avaznejad, N., Ravanipour, M., Bahreini, M., & Motamed, N. (2016). Comparison of the sense of coherence between mothers with healthy children and mothers of children with chronic disease in Kerman. https://core.ac.uk/download/77982085.pdf (accessed on 12th July 2025).
5. Bayley, M., Janzen, S., Harnett, A., Bragge, P., Togher, L., Kua, A., Patsakos, E., et al. (2023). INCOG 2.0 guidelines for cognitive rehabilitation following traumatic brain injury: What's changed from 2014 to now? *Journal of Head Trauma Rehabilitation*, *38*, 1–6. https://doi.org/10.1097/htr.0000000000000826 (accessed on 12th July 2025).
6. Berenson, J., & Highsmith, N. (2011). Driving value in Medicaid primary care: The role of shared support networks for physician practices. https://core.ac.uk/download/71358029.pdf (accessed on 12th July 2025).
7. Bonowicz, K., Jerka, D., Ławkowska, K., Łuniewska-Bury, J., Wrońska, I., Bai, Y., & Gagat, M. (2025). TGF-β: The molecular mechanisms of atherosclerosis—Insights into SMAD pathways and gene therapy prospects. *Current Medicinal Chemistry*. https://www.semanticscholar.org/paper/5808c9ccd91e6b94b2877f12446241113fc0320c (accessed on 12th July 2025).
8. Bowman, M. A., Seehusen, D., Britz, J., & Ledford, C. (2024). Research to improve clinical care in family medicine: big data, telehealth, artificial intelligence, and more. *The Journal of the American Board of Family Medicine*, *37*, 161–164. https://www.semanticscholar.org/paper/0e639bfdc663cfa68cae962704d390c3f0eac8d3 (accessed on 12th July 2025).
9. Breakwell, S., Callahan, M. F., Kim, M., et al. (2012). Clinical observation reflections from students in an interdisciplinary palliative care course. https://core.ac.uk/download/213079311.pdf (accessed on 12th July 2025).
10. Brito, L. A. R., Caramori, U., D'Abreu, N. B., Cardoso Filho, C., Cunha, L. O., & Bragança, J. F. (2025). Entrustable professional activities for family and community medicine residency in the Brazilian context. *Revita Brasileira de Educação Médica*. https://www.semanticscholar.org/paper/339b14888c1bdbaeeb1fae0541cdf1b151081f00 (accessed on 12th July 2025).

11. Bulbul, E., Simsek, E., & Kizmaz, M. (2024). Evaluation of physicians' screening practices and knowledge levels regarding atrial fibrillation in patients over 65 years of age: A prospective study. *Medicine Science | International Medical Journal*. https://www.semanticscholar.org/paper/2f51512d9c6f044c90a54ec559468e062a0505cd (accessed on 12th July 2025).

12. Carlos, F. A. B. (2024). Health systems approach to strengthen rehabilitation. *Acta Medica Philippina, 58*, 6–8. https://www.semanticscholar.org/paper/eb4994fbde6a15ae791ef02a3f71690478496a3f (accessed on 12th July 2025).

13. Carney, P. A., Valenzuela, S., Ericson, A., Dinh, D. H., Conry, C., Peterson, L. E., Douglass, A. B., et al. (2025). The impact of length of training on clinical preparedness among new graduates: A report from the length of training pilot study in family medicine. *Family Medicine*. https://www.semanticscholar.org/paper/fb1f2fafeaf794378e7a3c27022e12c08198d0a2 (accessed on 12th July 2025).

14. Chang, K. Z., Bull, L., Hernandez, R. H., Aldulaimi, S., Kratz, N., Myers, O., & Johnston, E. M. (2025). Global health curriculum in US family medicine residencies. *PRiMER, 9*, 21. https://www.semanticscholar.org/paper/11bcdc02fffaa2433254282f4d920c471d9778ff (accessed on 12th July 2025).

15. Cheng, F. (2024). The comprehensive cancer center: Development, integration, and implementation. *Annals of Innovation in Medicine*. https://www.semanticscholar.org/paper/4faf514449ae39ab40d09a113ec15377a99148be (accessed on 12th July 2025).

16. Çöme, O., & Mevsim, V. (2023). E-health solutions in primary health care. *The Journal of Turkish Family Physician*. https://www.semanticscholar.org/paper/a8d6deab6f48481a2aece78054005b484fccaaf1 (accessed on 12th July 2025).

17. de la Cruz, M. D. L., Chou, A., Edberg, D., Leach, W. T., Guariglia, C., Schultz, J. T., & Flattau, A. (2025). Value-based care education in family medicine residency programs: A CERA study of program directors. *Family Medicine, 57*(4), 298–302. https://www.semanticscholar.org/paper/08f5ea7f071d524d224a8f9a571ebbacdc38cd79 (accessed on 12th July 2025).

18. Dearry, A., Rogers, B., Roberts, J., Paulson, J., McCurdy, L. E., Lindberg, M. A., Witherspoon, N. O., et al. (2004). Incorporating environmental health into pediatric medical and nursing education. https://core.ac.uk/download/pdf/3775759.pdf (accessed on 12th July 2025).

19. Demirören, M., & Başer, D. A. (2024). Educational needs assessment for health advocate role in family medicine residency training in Turkey: A Delphi study. *The European Journal of General Practice, 30*. https://www.semanticscholar.org/paper/005a9f9fe3ee6cdb495ab204b5877ab284e72f20 (accessed on 12th July 2025).

20. Dreher, A. C., Ko, J., Becker, C., Bischoff, M., Förster, C., Jähnig, T., Stengel, S., et al. (2025). Core values and principles of general practice and family medicine: Perspectives of German GP residents—a cross-sectional study. *Frontiers in Medicine, 12*. https://www.semanticscholar.org/paper/f4bb3c5fa646b535cce945a8942996304cebebfa (accessed on 12th July 2025).

21. Eden, C. A., Chisom, O. N., & Adeniyi, I. S. (2024). Cultural competence in education: Strategies for fostering inclusivity and diversity awareness. *International Journal of Applied Research in Social Sciences*. https://www.semanticscholar.org/paper/b264e994d417980ca557965b5127ceb013f208fe (accessed on 12th July 2025).

22. Feldker, N., Ferrazzi, F., Schuhwerk, H., Widholz, S. A., Guenther, K., Frisch, I., Jakob, K., et al. (2020). Genome-wide cooperation of *EMT* transcription factor *ZEB* 1 with *YAP* and *AP*-1 in

breast cancer. *The EMBO Journal, 39*. https://doi.org/10.15252/embj.2019103209 (accessed on 12th July 2025).

23. Fuentes, R. M. B., Vives, M. R., Padilla, K. R., Pérez, M. G., & Rodríguez, L. S. (2024). Strategy of professional superacion on natural and traditional medicine in the primary attention of health. *Health Leadership and Quality of Life*. https://www.semanticscholar.org/paper/832d931fa74f9c11595a2acd09bf04d915a23a1e (accessed on 12th July 2025).
24. Goodman, C., Parker, D., Sampson, E. L., Bunn, F., Froggatt, K., Phillips, J. L., van der Steen, J. T., et al. (2020). Components of palliative care interventions addressing the needs of people with dementia living in long term care: A systematic review. https://core.ac.uk/download/323056264.pdf (accessed on 12th July 2025).
25. Hribersek, M., Eibensteiner, F., Bukowski, N., Yeung, A., Atanasov, A. G., & Schaden, E. (2024). Research areas and trends in family-centered care in the 21st century: A bibliometric review. *Frontiers in Medicine, 11*. https://www.semanticscholar.org/paper/627ee856fae4018423a8aad1e6c393e86291883b (accessed on 12th July 2025).
26. Kuhon, F. V., Naamin, J., & Ottay, R. I. (2022). Gambaran penanganan penyakit kronis: Program rujuk balik penyakit jantung koroner pada dokter keluarga di Kota Manado. https://core.ac.uk/download/554263917.pdf (accessed on 12th July 2025).
27. Kurnat-Thoma, E. L. (2024). Patient safety and healthcare quality of U.S. laboratory developed tests (LDTs) in the AI/ML era of precision medicine. *Frontiers in Molecular Biosciences, 11*. https://www.semanticscholar.org/paper/05c95ed60d023e96fda42078503db965152ebdaf (accessed on 12th July 2025).
28. Lawlor, G., Abrams, M., Nuzum, R., & Mika, S. (2011). Realizing health reform's potential: How the Affordable Care Act will strengthen primary care and benefit patients, providers, and payers. https://core.ac.uk/download/71354230.pdf (accessed on 12th July 2025).
29. Lieberman, M. R., Schwartz, Z., & Siegel, D. M. (2020). The evolving maintenance of certification process: Update on the financial status of the medical boards. https://core.ac.uk/download/287622748.pdf (accessed on 12th July 2025).
30. Lynch, C. (2019). The patient-physician relationship: Overcoming language and cultural barriers. https://core.ac.uk/download/213463696.pdf (accessed on 12th July 2025).
31. Macri, J., & Millenson, M. L. (2012). Will the Affordable Care Act move patient-centeredness to center stage? https://core.ac.uk/download/71357580.pdf (accessed on 12th July 2025).
32. Morton, S., & Dunn, W. (2015). Addressing the health needs of an aging America: New opportunities for evidence-based policy solutions. https://core.ac.uk/download/75783019.pdf (accessed on 12th July 2025).
33. Newman, N. E. (1955). A study of the understanding and use of social agencies by physicians in a given community. https://open.bu.edu/bitstream/2144/7895/1/Newman_Nancy_1955_web.pdf (accessed on 12th July 2025).
34. Nies, S., Patel, S., Shafer, M., Longman, L., Sharif, I., & Pina, P. (2021). Understanding physicians' preferences for telemedicine during the COVID-19 pandemic: Cross-sectional study. *JMIR Formative Research, 5*, e26565–e26565. https://doi.org/10.2196/26565 (accessed on 12th July 2025).
35. Ohta, R., & Sano, C. (2022). Family physicians as system-specific specialists in Japan's aging

society. *Cureus*. https://doi.org/10.7759/cureus.30811 (accessed on 12th July 2025).

36. Ohta, R., & Sano, C. (2024). Family medicine implementation to maternal and child health in rural Japan: A narrative review. *Cureus, 16*. https://www.semanticscholar.org/paper/87f90dedded64f2bec60a3132428eb5bf972c728 (accessed on 12th July 2025).

37. O'Malley, A. S., Tynan, A., Cohen, G. R., Davis, M. M., & Kemper, N. M. (2009). Coordination of care by primary care practices: Strategies, lessons and implications. https://core.ac.uk/download/71350438.pdf (accessed on 12th July 2025).

38. Pamplin, J. C., Anders, S., Brown, J., Crandall, B., Grome, A., Chung, K., Mann-Salinas, E., et al. (2013). 5: Discovering complexities in critical care and their challenges to health IT design in a burn ICU. *Critical Care Medicine, 41*. https://www.semanticscholar.org/paper/e3161e580bc6f52610922002877280c663884c86 (accessed on 12th July 2025).

39. Porterfield, L., Jan, Q. H., Jones, F., Cao, T., Davis, L., Guillot-Wright, S., & Walcher, C. (2024). Family medicine team perspectives on screening for health-related social needs. *The Journal of the American Board of Family Medicine, 37*, 180–186. https://www.semanticscholar.org/paper/e3b6ac5035300bc89f47d322c28ef771f5961f93 (accessed on 12th July 2025).

40. Pudasaini, S., Schenk, L., Möckel, M., & Schneider, A. (2022). Work-life balance in physicians working in two emergency departments of a university hospital: Results of a qualitative focus group study. *PLOS ONE, 17*. https://www.semanticscholar.org/paper/731d8c53e828962a49cdddbbff191562b28237e2 (accessed on 12th July 2025).

41. Shah, P., Ross, S., Konkin, J., Au, L., & Lee, A. S. (2023). Rubric invites discussions of social determinants of health. *Medical Education, 57*, 487. https://www.semanticscholar.org/paper/6bfdae9fc5b1a5fda52b1f9093e9e4b267019f38 (accessed on 12th July 2025).

42. Shopo, K. D., Nuuyoma, V., & Chihururu, L. (2024). Enhancing cultural competence in undergraduate nursing students: An integrative literature review of strategies for institutions of higher education. *Journal of Transcultural Nursing: Official Journal of the Transcultural Nursing Society*. https://www.semanticscholar.org/paper/7ebe227fab129c3af40b5138e396b522eb75d9ae (accessed on 12th July 2025).

43. Singhal, K., Azizi, S., Tu, T., Mahdavi, S. S., Lee, J., Chung, H. W., Scales, N., et al. (2023). Large language models encode clinical knowledge. *Nature, 620*, 172–180. https://doi.org/10.1038/s41586-023-06291-2 (accessed on 12th July 2025).

44. Srivastava, A., Santagostino, E., Dougall, A., Kitchen, S., Sutherland, M. L., Pipe, S. W., Carção, M., et al. (2020). WFH Guidelines for the management of hemophilia, 3rd edition. *Hemophilia, 26*, 1–158. https://doi.org/10.1111/hae.14046 (accessed on 12th July 2025).

45. Strelow, B., Carmean, A., Fuentes-Camacho, S., Gilliland, A., Moysis, A., Weston, R., Herndon, J., et al. (2025). Previniendo el Cáncer de las Mamas: Addressing breast cancer screening disparities in Spanish-preferred populations. *Archives of Breast Cancer*. https://www.semanticscholar.org/paper/5f7f1b89e5d9365c9f31c2099b077e775877cddb (accessed on 12th July 2025).

46. Takeuchi, Y., Chen, Q., & Fetters, M. D. (2025). Medical students' views on family medicine in Japan: Insights from an international comparison. *PRiMER, 9*, 10. https://www.semanticscholar.org/paper/14ce94f420a9edfe0f6eaab9c9238bdb3241c941 (accessed on 12th July 2025).

47. Tort-Nasarre, G., Vidal-Alaball, J., Pedrosa, M. J. F., Abanades, L. V., Arcarons, A. F., & Rosanas, J. (2023). Factors associated with the attraction and retention of family and community

medicine and nursing residents in rural settings: A qualitative study. *BMC Medical Education, 23*. https://www.semanticscholar.org/paper/08d1583ffd118f1559216b27bcbfd8bd0cb210ac (accessed on 12th July 2025).

48. Ventres, W., Stone, L. A., Abou-Arab, E. R., Meza, J., Buck, D. S., Crowder, J. W., Edgoose, J., et al. (2024). Storylines of family medicine IX: People and places—Diverse populations and locations of care. *Family Medicine and Community Health, 12*. https://www.semanticscholar.org/paper/825df39048b5cfa8bdac519bfd75cd88e45abc9a (accessed on 12th July 2025).

49. Virginia Commonwealth University. (2018). *Virginia Commonwealth University Professional Bulletin*. https://core.ac.uk/download/215485746.pdf (accessed on 12th July 2025).

50. Wagner, E., Sugarman, J. R., Phillips, K., Coleman, K., & Reid, R. J. (2012). Guiding transformation: How medical practices can become patient-centered medical homes. https://core.ac.uk/download/71358341.pdf (accessed on 12th July 2025).

51. Wagner, E., Tufano, J., & Horner, K. (2011). Electronic consultations between primary and specialty care clinicians: Early insights. https://core.ac.uk/download/71358065.pdf (accessed on 12th July 2025).

52. Ward, Z. D., Morgan, Z. J., & Peterson, L. E. (2020). Family physician burnout does not differ with rurality. *The Journal of Rural Health: Official Journal of the American Rural Health Association and the National Rural Health Care Association*. https://www.semanticscholar.org/paper/1349a74a374bbfdede2a2a18e89884e2a4812e06 (accessed on 12th July 2025).

53. Yee, V., Bajaj, S. S., & Stanford, F. C. (2022). Paradox of telemedicine: Building or neglecting trust and equity. *The Lancet Digital Health, 4*, e480–e481. https://doi.org/10.1016/s2589-7500(22)00100-5 (accessed on 12th July 2025).

54. Zacay, G., Adler, L., Schonmann, Y., Azuri, J., Yehoshua, I., Vinker, S., Heymann, A. D., et al. (2024). "A day in the life"–telemedicine in family medicine and its relationship with practicing physicians' satisfaction: A cross-sectional study. *Israel Journal of Health Policy Research, 13*. https://www.semanticscholar.org/paper/be51b488e51988b6118e58595ff08999f8d291a7 (accessed on 12th July 2025).

55. Zaitseva, K. I., Lukyanova, T. V., & Semeleva, E. V. (2024). The Filatov medical dynasty. *SCIENCE SPACE*. https://www.semanticscholar.org/paper/6b6064d9fd09c07bfc1caf28da4ba24236f0043b (accessed on 12th July 2025).

ROLES AND RESPONSIBILITIES OF A FAMILY PHYSICIAN

2

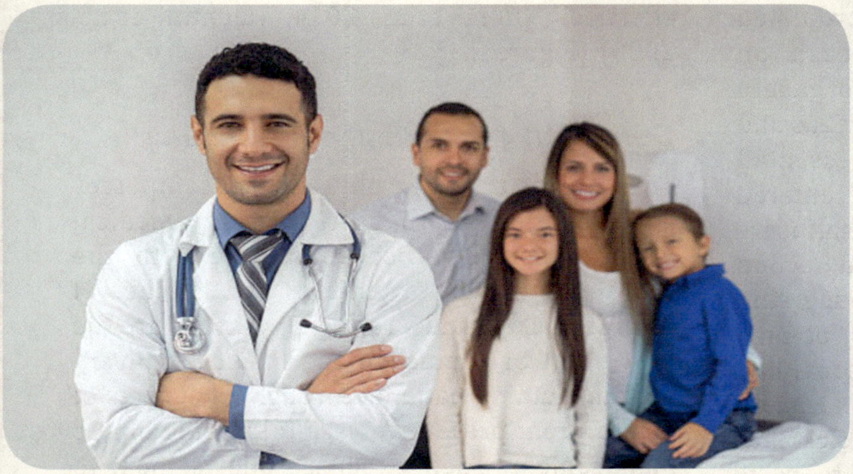

LEARNING OBJECTIVES

After studying this chapter, you will be able to:

1. Describe the patient care
2. Understand the role of preventive medicine in the practice of family physicians
3. Describe the effective coordination of care
4. Understand the ethical responsibilities of family physicians

Introduction

In contemporary healthcare, the role of the family physician is pivotal in determining the overall health and well-being of the populations they serve. As the point of entry into the healthcare system, family physicians have broad-ranging responsibilities that encompass prevention, disease management, and health education. This multifaceted role necessitates a deep understanding of a patient's medical and psychosocial history so that physicians can make informed decisions that account for the patient's unique needs. Moreover, family physicians often operate within complex healthcare systems, representing patients and arranging care for a diverse array of healthcare providers. This particular role highlights the importance of their contribution to individual patient outcomes and to public health policies more broadly, and it underscores the need for a solid framework to define their roles and responsibilities in the evolving environment of medicine. Family physicians are most productive when they collaborate with other medical professionals, such as physician assistants and nurses. Such interprofessional collaboration is fundamental to delivering comprehensive, patient-centered care because it ensures that a patient's overall health is properly attended to. Communication and trust between family physicians and their complementary team members are key to effective healthcare delivery. Understanding this factor, current research emphasizes that better collaboration and communication can improve patient outcomes and increase healthcare practitioners' satisfaction. The results of these studies indicate the need for a well-coordinated system of team care, with an emphasis on continuous education and training to ensure proper communication between physicians and their teammates. These measures are essential in providing a peaceful healthcare unit centered on patient care. As the intricacies of healthcare change, family physicians' roles extend beyond direct clinical duties to encompass leadership and advocacy in their communities. Not only are family physicians focal points for providing health services, but they are also opinion leaders in public health, advocating for policies that increase health equity and access to care. This advocacy sometimes requires an intimate understanding of the determinants of health and a commitment to reducing disparities affecting at-risk populations.

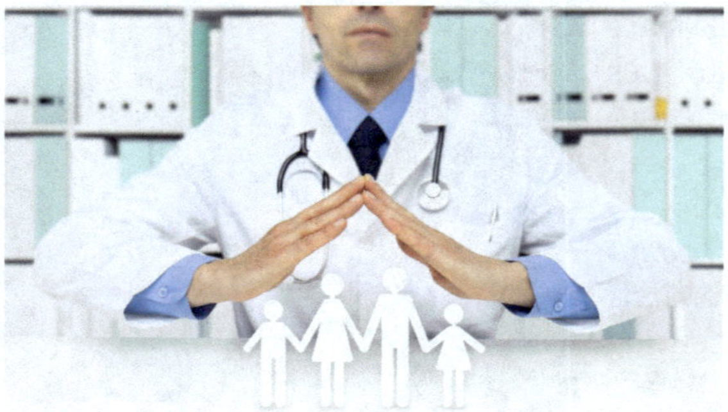

Figure 2.1. Essential roles of a family physician.

Source: https://wp02-media.cdn.ihealthspot.com/wp-content/uploads/sites/456/2020/12/iStock-649856154.jpg.

Furthermore, since the healthcare environment continues to shift, family physicians must stay up-to-date with emerging technology and treatment guidelines so that their practice is aligned with best practices today. The growing consensus on the importance of inter-professionalism highlights that family physicians must not only excel in their clinical roles but also play active roles in shaping policies and systems that govern the delivery of healthcare in an effort to fulfill their multifaceted roles effectively (Bond et al., 2014; Valentini et al., 2020) (Figure 2.1).

Definition of a Family Physician

The role of a family physician encompasses an integrated approach to primary medical care, a high level of commitment to the overall well-being of patients and families of diverse backgrounds. Family physicians are the first point of contact in the medical delivery system, guiding patients through all aspects of health, from preventive care to chronic illness management. Their expertise allows them to provide continuous care, which is essential when monitoring their patients' long-term wellbeing. Besides, family physicians are trained to treat not only physical ailments but also mental health problems, thereby caring for the whole person rather than just the symptoms of a disease. This systems philosophy is critical to building patient trust and achieving optimal health outcomes, allowing family physicians to become part of an individual's life, as reflected in the most basic of patient-centered care principles. Family physicians' roles also extend beyond the one-on-one patient relationship to reach into large public health initiatives and into community roles. They play a key role in educating patients about prevention and healthy lifestyle choices that can have a profound impact on population health. Family doctors are usually leaders in organizing health care resources for families and communities, coordinating with specialists and other health care professionals to deliver comprehensive treatment plans. This interprofessional practice is now more and more recognized as the route to improving the quality of delivery of primary care; family physicians must develop teamworking approaches to enhance their practice, as highlighted by new evidence on effective inter-professional working (Bond et al., 2014). Through developing trusting partnerships, family physicians can improve patient outcomes and satisfaction and thus become key stakeholders in the healthcare system. Aside from their clinical responsibilities, family physicians also navigate the intricacies of healthcare policy and patient advocacy to ensure their patients receive the right assistance and resources. Together with the latest research, as discussed in current evidence, family physicians have indicated a wish to increase their role in dealing with long-term health issues, including coordinating treatment for cancer survivors through shared-care programs with oncologists (Chan et al., 2020). This emphasizes the importance of adequate training and well-defined roles in maximizing family physicians' potential to address complex health problems. Ultimately, the term family physician describes a broad range of tasks that combine clinical skill, community engagement, and policy advocacy into a dynamic yet critical function of brokering equal access to healthcare and promoting community health outcomes (Figure 2.2).

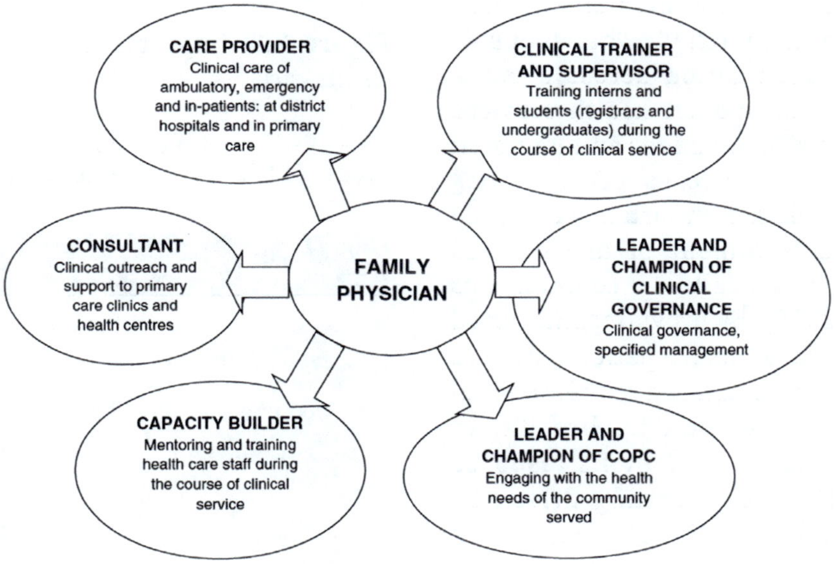

Figure 2.2. Roles and competencies expected of a family physician.

Source: https://www.researchgate.net/profile/Tracey-Naledi/publication/269720353/figure/fig1/AS:271745504509997@1441800585988/Roles-and-competencies-expected-of-a-family-physician.png.

Importance of Family Medicine in Healthcare

Family medicine is a vital part of the health care system, with its wide, patient-centered approach to care, treating the entire person and all of the elements of a family. Family doctors are in the best position to provide continuity of care over time by forming long-term relationships with patients, with more trust and communication. Continuity not only enables a better understanding of patients' medical history and way of life, but also leads to better health outcomes. As the first port of call for most with the health service, family doctors possess the skills to address a variety of health concerns, guiding patients through consultation, treatment, and prevention. The practice is appreciated given the necessity of good teamwork within primary care settings; more inter-professional work is required to allow effective healthcare provision and lead towards improved patient satisfaction and outcomes (Bond et al., 2014). In addition to promoting comprehensive care, family medicine emphasizes preventive health practices that help limit chronic disease. Family physicians engage in anticipatory patient education, teaching individuals about the risk of illness and prevention for their unique conditions. The addition of wellness screenings, immunizations, and lifestyle counseling to routine check-ups demonstrates how family medicine works to reduce health disparities. This focus is evident in care coordination across sectors, for example, between mental health services and the community. The need for an integrated model in the delivery of care, especially among children, underscores the importance of family physicians in the treatment of disease and in promoting overall health in communities (McAllister et al., 2009). By providing integrated care, family physicians ensure patients receive comprehensive support tailored to their overall health needs. Additionally, the applicability of family medicine is aggravated by its response to the evolving healthcare setting driven by sociocultural forces. Family physicians need to deal with mixed patient populations while also responding with appropriate care that is sensitive to cultural values and personal choices. This adaptability is crucial in a more multicultural world, where understanding and managing diverse health beliefs can significantly influence treatment adherence and patient satisfaction. Family medicine clinics tend to extend beyond typical clinical settings, incorporating advocacy that addresses the social determinants of health. These roles underscore the dual function of family physicians, who not only need to provide clinical care but also to be engaged in community health promotion and policymaking efforts. Lastly, family medicine's place in healthcare is more than isolated patient encounters; it is a higher level of commitment to improving public health through comprehensive, culturally sensitive care (Figure 2.3).

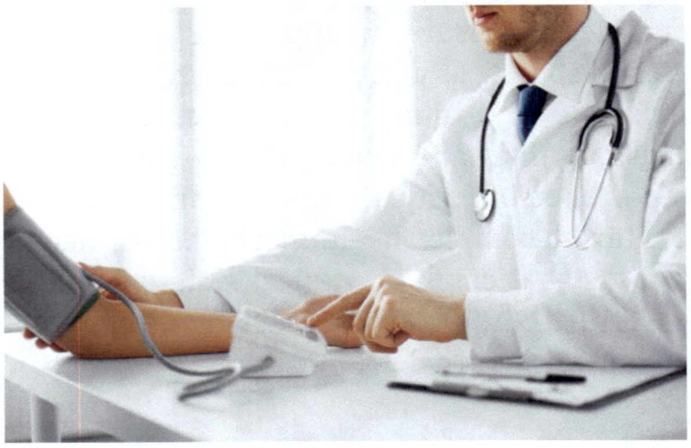

Figure 2.3. Importance of family medicine in healthcare.

Source: https://www.aucmed.edu/media/11521/family-medicine.jpg.

2.1. Patient Care

Learning Outcome

1. Describe the comprehensive health assessments
2. Understand the development of personalized treatment plans
3. Learn about management of chronic diseases

Care of patients constitutes the core of the family physician's work, and it entails a holistic response that takes into account both the patient's physical and mental health. Family physicians develop ongoing relationships with patients, in which they come to know patients' health histories, lifestyles, and family structures. Armed with such extensive information, physicians can tailor care plans to suit individual patient requirements best. The role played by communication in the formation of such relationships is extremely crucial; good talk enhances patient adherence and trust, which in turn results in healthier outcomes. Research indicates that improved communication among healthcare teams plays a significant role in influencing the quality of patient care and hence requires the acquisition of communication skills by family physicians along with other healthcare professionals, i.e., physician assistants and specialists (Valentini et al., 2020). Through the establishment of clear and understandable pathways of communication, family doctors are able to more effectively navigate the complexities of patient care across diverse settings of medicine. The effectiveness of patient-centered practice by family doctors is also directly tied to working in team-based healthcare systems. As integral leaders in such systems, family doctors work with a range of medical specialists to optimize the delivery of care. This collaborative approach taps into the strengths of different healthcare providers, as best seen in practice models that emphasize paying for performance to enhance quality and reduce costs, particularly for patient groups such as Medicare beneficiaries (Pope et al., 2008). Through the combining of different expertise, family doctors can guarantee that the patient is given complete care covering all aspects of his or her health. The dynamics of teamwork in healthcare necessitate family physicians investing time in establishing professional relationships among peers, enhancing communication and cooperation to maximize quality patient care. Teamwork thus becomes an essential component of effective family medicine practices. In addition to establishing communication and cooperation, family physicians play a key role in addressing social determinants of health that significantly impact patient care. These determinants include socioeconomic status, education, and access to resources, all of which can affect health. Family physicians are ideally positioned to identify these problems through day-to-day interactions with patients, thereby providing a means of instituting necessary interventions within the healthcare system. For instance, in addressing treatment barriers, family physicians can team up with local institutions to facilitate access to services addressing housing, nutrition, and mental health—determinants essential to maximizing overall well-being. By proactively addressing those determinants, family physicians not only enhance individual patient care but also push for systemic change that can extend to populations. This multidimensional analytical approach underscores the importance of the family doctor's role in negotiating and addressing the challenges of patient care (Figure 2.4).

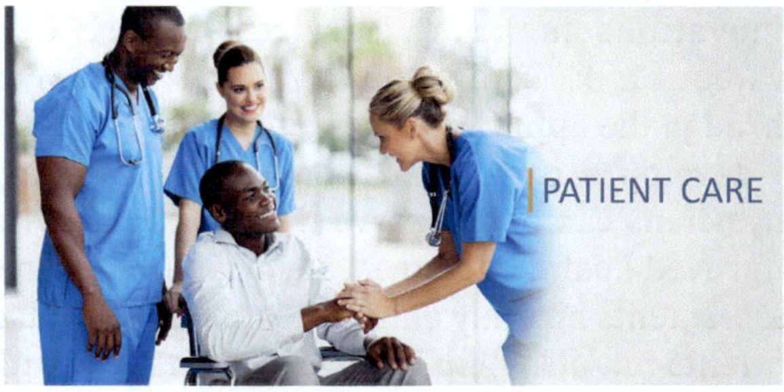

Figure 2.4. Patient care.

Source: https://www.physioline.in/wp-content/uploads/2017/07/Patient-Care.jpg.

2.1.1. Comprehensive Health Assessments

A thorough health assessment is an utmost important charge for family physicians, as it provides a foundation for effective diagnosis and treatment planning. This system assessment includes a vigilant review of a patient's history, medication list, and lifestyle, and physical examinations tailored to the patient's requirements. By integrating medical knowledge with an understanding of personal and family history, doctors can identify risk factors and comorbidities that may not be readily apparent. Furthermore, this allows doctors to establish a trusting relationship with patients, which is key to promoting adherence to medical advice and treatment strategies. Engaging the patient in the evaluation enhances communication openness, as they tend to voice sensitive issues that can affect their health, thereby improving the overall quality of care provided. Furthermore, comprehensive health evaluations have an essential role in the management of the diverse health needs of multi-patient populations. Family doctors are likely to treat patients from diverse cultural and linguistic backgrounds, and therefore must have a keen awareness of how these factors shape definitions of health and care-seeking behavior. Applying models that maximize cultural competence is crucial here. For instance, practical strategies for coping with language limitations, as strategized in innovations in health services, ensure that evaluation is comprehensive and inclusive. Through the application of an eight-step process to develop a communications strategy, family physicians can better serve their patients, with improved health outcomes. Such comprehensive assessments not only enhance care for individual patients but also help resolve systematic health inequities in communities, so that all patients receive the care that they require.

Finally, the role of comprehensive health assessment extends far beyond to encompass public health issues. By recognizing population health status trends, family physicians are well-positioned to advocate for community health programs and policy change. These assessments not only provide information about individual patient care but also collect information that can determine racial and ethnic health disparities and, therefore, inform interventions to minimize them. The appropriate application of assessment tools that address cultural and linguistic competency will also enable physicians to navigate disparities more effectively. Hence, not only do family doctors play a crucial role in delivering direct care through whole-person assessments but they also play an active part in advocating overall health transformations that will promote the overall health of the community (Figure 2.5).

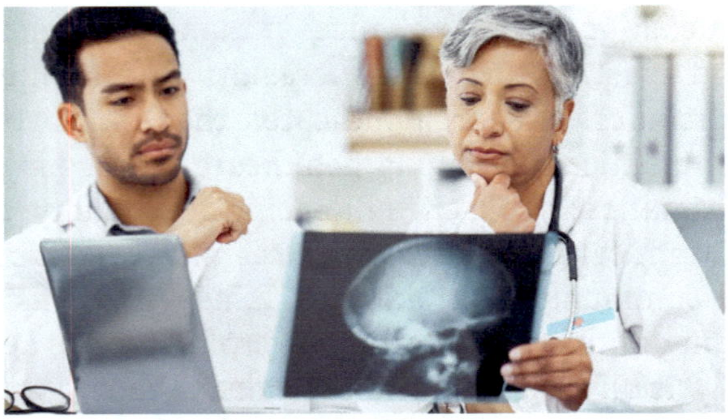

Figure 2.5. Comprehensive health assessments.

Source: https://bloom.insure/wp-content/uploads/2023/08/What-is-a-comprehensive-healthcare-assessment.webp.

2.1.2. Development of Personalized Treatment Plans

Individualized treatment planning is a cornerstone of the family physician's specialty because it delivers personalized care tailored to each patient's unique needs. A family physician must consider numerous variables, such as genetic predispositions, environmental influences, and individual lifestyle habits, when formulating treatment plans. With the adoption of a comprehensive approach, family physicians are then in the position to utilize such tools as comprehensive patient histories and data-driven health assessments to establish individualized plans. This method, in addition to making the treatments more effective, promotes a healthier physician-patient relationship built on trust and understanding. Evidence indicates that customized healthcare plans can lead to improved patient outcomes and adherence to treatment regimens, thereby strengthening the central role family physicians play in their patients' health care (Bonica et al., 2017). Besides, ongoing advancements in medical technology also significantly impact the customization of treatment plans. Increasingly, family doctors use electronic health records (EHRs) and health information technology systems to examine patient information, which allows real-time adjustment of treatment protocols. Using these technologies, doctors can track patients' progress more effectively while applying evidence-based practices in their care models. These kinds of programs, such as those in complex care management programs, including the Aetna Medicare Advantage Embedded Case Management Program and Intermountain Healthcare's Care Management Plus, demonstrate the potential benefits of tailored treatment strategies in a collaborative care model. Whereas family doctors encourage the use of these advanced methods, they not only enhance the specificity of care but also aid in more effective chronic disease management. Moreover, patient involvement in treatment planning is vital to ensuring tailored care succeeds. Family doctors have the responsibility of informing their patients about potential treatments and making them active players in the decision-making process for their healthcare.

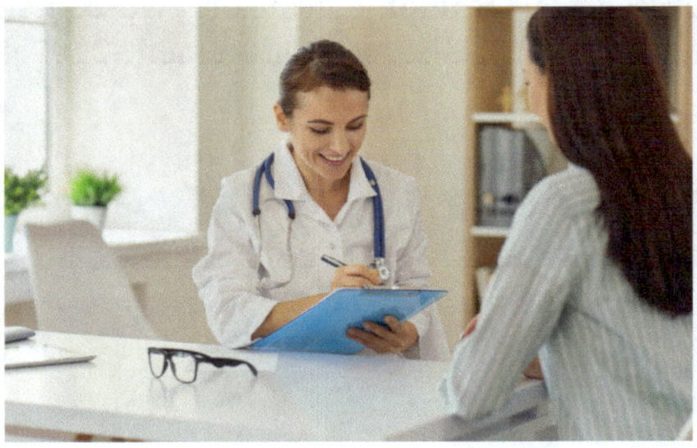

Figure 2.6. Personalized treatment plans.

Source: https://kineticrehabspine.com/wp-content/uploads/2023/07/personalized-treatment-1080x675.png.

This collaborative design not only enables patients but also responds to their values, preferences, and concerns, aligning treatment plans with their individual lifestyles and beliefs. When patients are co-creators of their health, adherence to prescribed interventions is greatly enhanced. Ultimately, the production of tailored treatment plans is a testament to the family physician's dedication to offering whole and empathetic care, combining clinical acumen with the inherent nature of patients, and delivering care that is both effective and patient-centric (Figure 2.6).

2.1.3. Management of Chronic Diseases

A key component of the family physician's role is the proper management of chronic diseases, which has become increasingly important in healthcare today. Chronic diseases like diabetes, hypertension, and osteoporosis necessitate constant monitoring and multi-component treatment modalities to regulate the progression of the disease and enhance the quality of life of patients. Family physicians are best positioned to coordinate continuity of care for patients with complex disorders because of their comprehensive understanding of individual health histories and family backgrounds. Through coordinated care, they can tailor interventions that address both medical and psychosocial factors, thereby enhancing patient compliance with treatment regimens and lifestyle modifications. This multidisciplinary approach is not only important for enhancing patient outcomes, but also necessary to alleviate the strain on the health system at a systemic level. Policies that promote family practices to deliver high-quality, cost-effective care further highlight the utility of this multidisciplinary model in managing chronic disease (Pope et al., 2008). Beyond treatment, family physicians' involvement in managing chronic diseases also includes prevention and patient education. With patient education that empowers patients about their conditions, family physicians help them acquire the necessary skills to manage their health appropriately. It is particularly crucial within chronic disease settings, where lifestyle factors often have a vital role in disease progression. Instituting educational workshops and providing access to resources enable family physicians to address common myths and misconceptions about chronic diseases. Offering instruction on how to overcome them fosters a nurturing relationship that empowers patients to be active participants in their own care. Such a proactive stance is imperative, as studies have proven that well-educated patients are likely to follow treatment protocols, thereby increasing compliance and ultimately improving overall health outcomes (Chan et al., 2020). In addition, as the healthcare landscape evolves further, family physicians' roles in managing chronic disease are being translated into care models that prioritize collaboration, where strategic partnerships with specialists are imperative. Family doctors also like to work together with oncologists, cardiologists, and other specialists to provide coordinated care, particularly to those with complex, interdependent medical needs. Such shared care enables family doctors to monitor not only patients with chronic illnesses but also the potential complications associated with other therapies. For instance, in breast cancer survivor care, family physicians are best placed to play a central role in addressing both the psychological aspects of survivorship and the management of comorbidities that arise secondary to cancer treatment (Chan et al., 2020). Hence, through robust clinician communication networks, patients are guaranteed to receive comprehensive, well-coordinated care that is responsive to their evolving needs in long-term disease management (Figure 2.7).

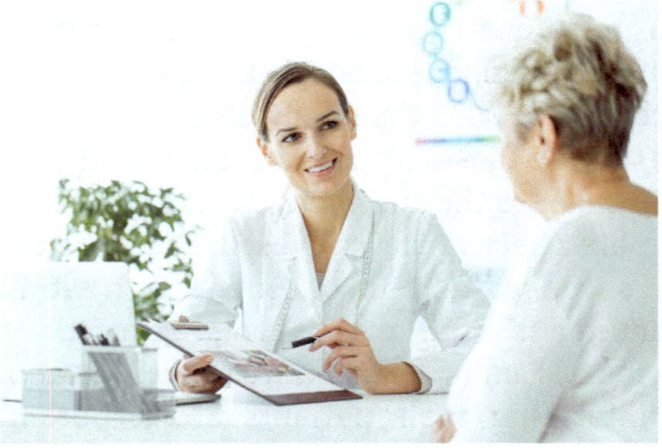

Figure 2.7. Management of chronic diseases.

Source: https://campmedicine.org/wp-content/uploads/chronic-disease-management-2107.jpg.

Test Your Knowledge

1. What is a comprehensive health assessment?
2. What is the management of chronic disease?

2.2. Preventive Medicine

Learning Outcome

1. Understand the importance of vaccinations and screenings
2. Know the health education and promotion
3. Describe the lifestyle counseling for patients

The role of preventive medicine in the practice of family physicians is invaluable towards enhancing patient health outcomes and boosting the well-being of communities. Preventive medicine focuses on early detection and intervention, which can effectively reduce the incidence of chronic diseases. Family physicians play a key role in conducting repeated screening and examination to identify the onset of probable health complications before they become full-blown conditions. This approach not only renders patients more independent in their health but also reduces the overall cost of health care by reducing the need for extensive treatment. In addition to their fundamental duties, family doctors must be knowledgeable about the latest preventive health guidelines and recommendations so they can provide evidence-based care that effectively addresses diverse patient needs. Integration of preventive health services into primary care also significantly enhances the patient health handling strategy. Family physicians are typically the first point of entry into the healthcare system and, as such, are in the most effective position to coordinate preventive care strategies. For instance, the implementation of medical home programs allows doctors to personalize care by tailoring interventions to patients' specific needs and preferences (O'Malley et al., 2008). These programs have the potential to facilitate the delivery of preventive services for an individual, ranging from immunizations to life-style counseling. Such coordination improves health outcomes and strengthens patient-physician relationships through greater trust and cooperation. As family physicians embrace preventive medicine, they can help build healthier communities and reduce disparities in health access and outcomes.

An integral component of prevention medicine embraced by family physicians is addressing oral health, and particularly within high-risk populations. Research outlines innovative efforts to integrate oral health care into primary medical settings, thereby providing preventive oral health care to those who might otherwise be excluded from access (Krol et al., 2013). Family physicians and their multidisciplinary practice teams can deliver critical education and screenings with emphasis on the relationships between oral health and overall health. Family physicians can extend preventive care services and bridge gaps for high-risk populations, with the help of dental hygienists and community organizations. These efforts not only improve the practice of health care more effectively but also highlight the appropriateness of an integrated model of care, further emphasizing the pivotal role of family physicians in preventive care and general health management (Figure 2.8).

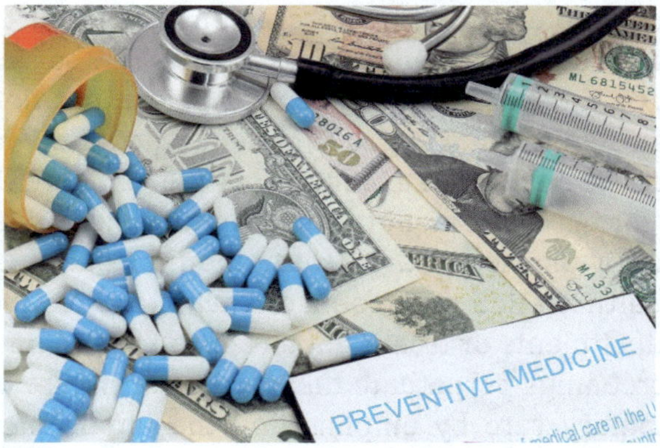

Figure 2.8. Preventive medicine.

Source: https://pix4free.org/assets/library/2021-07-12/originals/preventive-medicine.jpg.

2.2.1. Importance of Vaccinations and Screenings

Screening and vaccination have an important effect on the quality of care in family practice, reflecting family physicians' preventive orientation toward patients' health. Vaccination is essential for preventing infectious diseases, reducing their morbidity and mortality rates. Vaccination programs allow healthcare professionals to recommend to families the importance of immunizations, often accompanied by evidence-based recommendations from health agencies. By ensuring vaccines are administered on time, family physicians can help achieve community herd immunity, which protects not just individual patients but also immunocompromised individuals who are unable to be vaccinated due to health conditions. Therefore, vaccines are an integral component of preventive care that secures long-term health outcomes for patients and the population overall, thereby underscoring the role of the family physician in promoting public health. Screenings complement vaccinations by enabling early identification and treatment of a variety of health conditions, including chronic diseases such as diabetes and high blood pressure. Family physicians are uniquely positioned to encourage and implement regular screenings tailored to each patient's individual risk profile. This serves to promote health equity, as prompt identification can significantly improve patient outcomes and reduce healthcare expenditures over time. With rigorous assessment through routine check-ups, family physicians are able to monitor patients' health trends and counsel them on lifestyle adjustments or treatment as appropriate. Thus, screenings perpetuate the integrative nature of primary care by emphasizing the importance of integrating preventive measures into the fabric of family practice. Essentially, these screenings not only identify disease early but also bolster the patient-physician relationship, encouraging preventive health behavior that transcends generations (Bonica et al., 2017). In addition, the interlinked roles of screenings and vaccinations extend beyond care at the patient level; they also promote the family physician as an educator within communities.

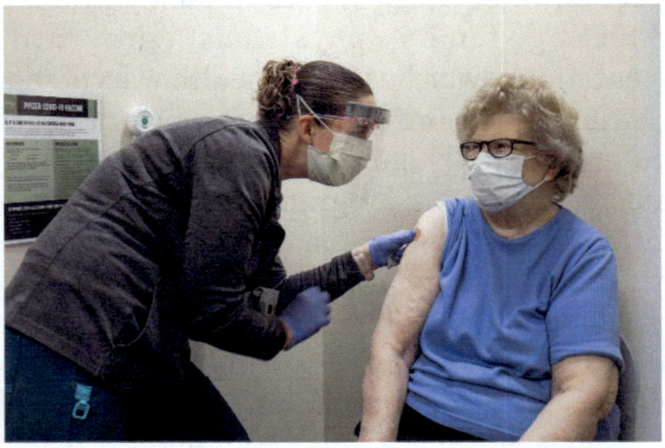

Figure 2.9. Importance of vaccinations and screenings.

Source: https://www.granditasca.org/-/jssmedia/MHealthFairview/Project/GrandItascaOrg/Images/Blog-Images/COVID-Vaccination_Dorthy-Pollard-4.ashx?hash=8310C182835CF5C302C74580A004989D&w=1100.

Through health promotion and community outreach, family physicians can combat vaccine misinformation and reluctance, fostering a culture of informed decision-making in health matters. The education process may involve community seminars, educational leaflets, and collaborative efforts with public health organizations to make accurate information accessible. By educating families regarding the safety and benefit of vaccines and the importance of regular screening, family physicians are performing a critical public health function. Such commitment enhances community health literacy and resilience, ultimately resulting in healthier populations and reduced disease burden in society, and concurs with the overall objectives of family medicine (Figure 2.9).

2.2.2. Health Education and Promotion

Health education and promotion are essential aspects of what family physicians bring to the health care system. Physicians directly influence health outcomes and behavior by providing proper information and resources to patients. This is a multi-component activity that integrates clinical practice with community health programs. Family physicians are well-positioned to address health inequalities by educating patients on prevention, nutrition, and the importance of regular exercise. Interventions of this kind, if applied systematically, can bring about long-term improvements in public health and reduce the burden of chronic disease. Thus, family physicians should remain abreast of new health education techniques to effectively advise patients in making well-informed lifestyle choices that will enhance their overall well-being. Moreover, incorporating health education into family practice is not only an additional undertaking in patient care but also a core responsibility. Patient engagement through participatory decision-making encourages them to be more aware and actively engaged in health management. This process holds particular promise when family doctors offer individualized advice attuned to a patient's specific needs and circumstances. An example is a survey of primary care physicians in which most indicated a willingness to become more active in managing cancer survivor comorbidity, underscoring the need for education and training to facilitate the successful implementation of health promotion interventions. These findings underscore the importance of family doctors having extensive knowledge of up-to-date evidence-based guidelines to inform patients better and promote healthier populations through collaboration with other healthcare professionals (Chan et al., 2020). Finally, as medical care continues to evolve, the family doctor must adapt to new challenges such as the resulting increased demand for integrated care due to changes in population and increases in levels of non-communicable diseases. Innovative methods must be adopted to maximize the use of resources, such as efficient deployment of nursing and allied health professionals in practice to boost health education activities. By developing strong partnerships with patients and improving their communication skills, family physicians can foster a culture of health literacy that empowers individuals to take charge of their own health. With the anticipated deficit in primary care physicians within healthcare systems, family physicians' role in educating and promoting health is more critical to provide equitable access to quality care and ultimately enhance population health (Ormond et al., 2011) (Figure 2.10).

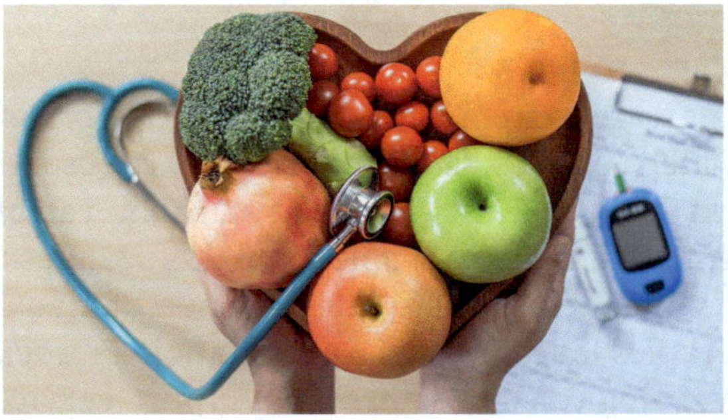

Figure 2.10. Health education and promotion.

Source: https://www.waldenu.edu/media/5021/seo-1568-bs-222353704-1200x675.

2.2.3. Lifestyle Counseling for Patients

The function of family physicians extends beyond the treatment of immediate health problems; it entails a fundamental obligation in the guidance of lifestyles that lead to enduring good health and well-being for the patients. Family physicians are best suited to provide integrated care because they recognize that lifestyle determinants of nutrition, physical conditioning, and stress management have a pivotal role in shaping health outcomes. Engaging in lifestyle counseling requires physicians to assess the unique situation of their patients, e.g., socioeconomic status and personal wants, which can affect how they will make better decisions. This holistic approach not only strengthens patient-physician relationships but also encourages patients to become participants in their own health. Thus, by integrating lifestyle counseling into their practice, family physicians are a part of preventive medicine, and this is crucial in avoiding the spread of chronic diseases that overwhelm today's world. Besides, effective lifestyle counseling not only involves the transmission of information but also the application of motivational skills, as this is personalized to patients. General practitioners must identify barriers preventing a patient from acquiring better practices, such as a lack of knowledge, resources, or motivation. This involves the understanding of psychological and social determinants of behavior change. For instance, a workshop on tackling men's health identified societal attitudes and denial as significant barriers to adopting healthy lifestyles (McHugh et al., 2004). With the removal of these barriers, family physicians can customize interventions that resonate with their patients. Such patient-specific intervention can increase the likelihood of successful behavioral change, leading to better long-term health. Moreover, including exercise in lifestyle counseling is most crucial, especially because most of chronic disease can be avoided through regular exercise.

Current guidelines recommend that patients do at least 30 minutes of exercise on most weekdays to derive health benefits. Although this information is vital, evidence indicates that medical professionals, such as nurses and family physicians, often rank physical activity advice lower than other activities for patients (Bayles et al., 2012). This may reflect a greater demand for more intensive training and a shift in attitude towards the role of physical activity in patient management. By making lifestyle counselling, including physical activity, a priority, family physicians not only help with overall patient well-being but also help to lower overall healthcare costs associated with preventable disease (Figure 2.11).

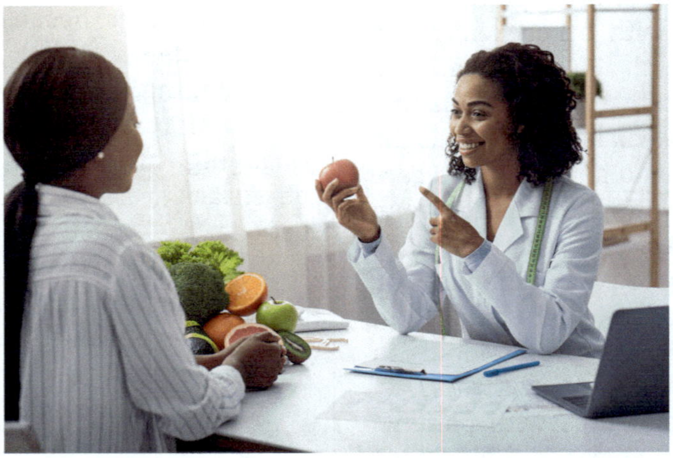

Figure 2.11. Lifestyle consulting

Source: https://www.sanatanwellness.com/uploads/images/service/1671537319.png.

Test Your Knowledge

1. What is meant by health education and promotion?
2. What is lifestyle counselling for patients?

2.3. Coordination of Care

Learning Outcome

1. Collaborate with specialists
2. Understand the referral processes and follow-ups
3. Integrate the healthcare services

Coordination of care is a fundamental part of a family physician's duties and roles. In a healthcare system with multiple providers and isolated services, family physicians are essential patient navigators between care in various settings, and they are able to do this seamlessly. This includes not only the provision of medical therapies but also the coordination of social, psychological, and spiritual support services, which might be required by the patient. For instance, the Community-Oriented Palliative Care Initiative (COPCI) advocates that there is strong demand for integrative networks of health care and social service agencies to address the overall needs of seriously ill patients and their carers in an effective and timely manner (Hopper, 2003). This type of coordinated care allows family physicians to advocate for their patients, providing access to the appropriate resources and establishing a sense of continuity in care that is paramount to both patient satisfaction and outcomes. One of the most important functions family physicians perform in care coordination is having robust networks of communication with other healthcare professionals, specialists, and support services. These stakeholders can dramatically reduce the risk of duplication and oversight with open communication. Sharing protocols for information and patient referrals are key to creating a unified care experience. By adopting a medical home model, which is based on coordinated care and puts the patient's needs first, family physicians can align their practices with an integrated approach to health management. This model establishes a culture of collaboration where both providers and patients are proactively involved in care decision-making, resulting in care plans derived from tailored responses to each patient's unique situation (O'Malley et al., 2008).

The activity of family physicians also includes health systems navigation education for families and even patients, which is naturally coupled with care coordination. Informed patients regarding their treatment options, potential referrals, and social services available for them enhances their ability to communicate needs and preferences throughout the healthcare encounter. Empowerment of this sort guarantees that patients are not passive recipients but active participants who help improve adherence to and follow-up on prescribed treatments. Within the COPCI tradition, integrating diverse community resources into care plans is one illustration of how family physicians can address the complexity of illness by extending services beyond medical care (Hopper, 2003). Through coordination, in this way, family physicians become integral in improving overall health outcomes and quality of life for patients (Figure 2.12).

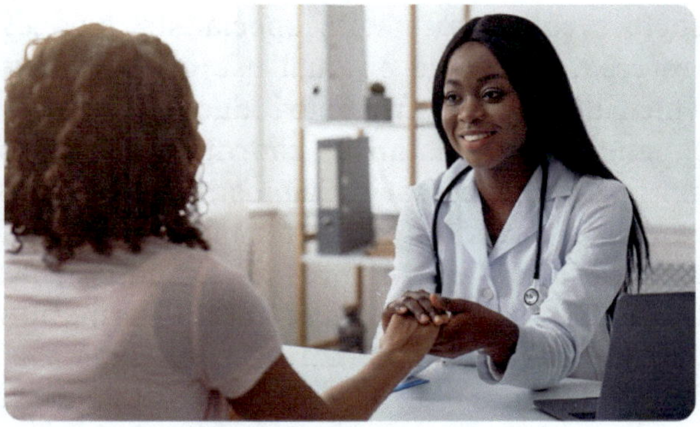

Figure 2.12. Care coordination.

Source: https://www.clearwaterhealth.com/hs-fs/hubfs/Clearwater%20New%20Website/Images/img-care-coordination-we-are-here-to-help-you.jpg?width=1106&height=665&name=img-care-coordination-we-are-here-to-help-you.jpg.

2.3.1. Collaboration with Specialists

Family physicians occupy a pivotal place in the care continuum as the first point of contact for patients. They have one of their primary functions being to work with specialists so that they can offer comprehensive care. This coordination is particularly vital when a family physician presents with complex medical problems that require specialized expertise and interventions. By partnering with specialists such as cardiologists and endocrinologists, family physicians can help improve the accuracy of diagnoses and treatment strategies. Integrative efforts of this nature not only facilitate streamlined care for patients but also improve overall health outcomes by helping ensure patients receive individualized interventions that are uniquely suited to address particular health requirements. With the transforming healthcare environment towards more patient-centric models of care, the ability to collaborate becomes a very important asset for family doctors who wish to provide integrated, comprehensive care. The benefits of collaboration not only apply in the direct care of patients but also extend to the more effective healthcare systems. When family doctors collaborate with specialists, bridges are created for the optimal use of resources, which ultimately translate to reduced healthcare expenses. For instance, coordination helps minimize unnecessary diagnostic testing and duplicate care that often stem from a lack of communication among providers. Additionally, specialists can offer important information that directs preventive care actions such that family doctors can use interventions best suited to their patients unique circumstances. As the evidence supports, in the event that health professionals work in collaboration as has been evidenced in some of the models of health policy, for instance, in resolving market forces in healthcare organizations, the patients enjoy seamless transitions between various levels of care. The processes underscore the necessity of effective collaborative practice to enhance patient outcomes and satisfaction. One coordinated approach to collaboration also calls for focus on continuity of care, particularly for the patient who is chronically ill or has a complicated health history. Family physicians will have to organize ongoing management with specialists, ensuring that care plans are coordinated and implemented efficiently. Consistent communication among providers is essential, such as reporting progress for the patient, adjusting medicines, and addressing any issues in relation to treatment efficacy. For example, in the treatment of children with disabilities, effective coordination between school specialists and family physicians is key to developing customized care plans tailored to a child's individual special needs (Dennis et al., 1999). Not only do collaborative interventions build a common perception of treatment goals, but they also empower patients by involving them in their care process. By prioritizing work with specialists, family physicians can preserve their leadership role in promoting inclusive, patient-centered care that recognizes the multidimensional nature of health and well-being (Figure 2.13).

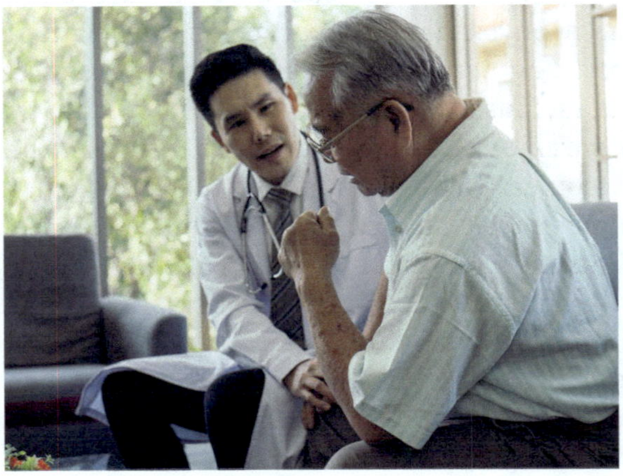

Figure 2.13. Family physicians collaborate on behavioral health.

Source: https://www.aafp.org/dam/brand/aafp/news/2023-may/bhp800.jpg.

2.3.2. Referral Processes and Follow-Ups

The referral process and follow-up are a part of the core responsibilities of a family physician's role, as they ensure continuity of treatment for acutely or chronically ill patients. Once the family physician identifies an illness that requires specialist intervention, the physician must initiate a lengthy referral process. It includes selecting the appropriate specialist, good communication with the patient and the specialist, and the transfer of all relevant medical information. Furthermore, timely follow-ups are essential as they enable tracking of the patient's progress and clarification of any problems that may have developed. Through smooth transitions of care, family physicians ensure they are at the epicenter of the health system and thereby enhance patient outcomes as well as adherence to treatment. Effective follow-up protocols also play a significant role in improving patient activation and reducing the likelihood of fragmented care. Once referred, the general practitioner is responsible for ensuring that patients have been informed of their follow-up consultations, the expected treatment, and the necessity of ongoing monitoring of their condition. This anticipatory care is critical, especially in chronic disease management or complicated cases, as it underscores the physician's commitment to comprehensive patient care. Secondly, the inclusion of follow-up data in a patient's electronic medical record allows the family physician to monitor treatment outcomes and make informed decisions regarding future referrals or interventions. As a result, this communication loop not only empowers patients but also enhances health literacy and self-care. The significance of effective referral processes is even more pressing given the long-term impacts on health outcomes in vulnerable populations. Research has indicated that well-planned referral systems can significantly enhance care efficiency and health outcomes for patients, especially in safety-net health centers seeking to become patient-centered medical homes (Phillips et al., 2010). In addition, interventions that target a range of healthcare services, rather than focusing on a few specific health conditions, have been found to be more effective at reducing health risks among marginalized communities (Aupont et al., 2012). Family physicians, therefore, must perceive their role as being key to fostering not only individual patient health but also the health landscape more broadly through the establishment of strong networks of care and the delivery of well-coordinated follow-up care that tackles comprehensive health needs.

2.3.3. Integration of Healthcare Services

The integration of health services plays a central role in enhancing family physicians' effectiveness. Family physicians serve as the core providers of healthcare, delivering continuous, integrated care. By integrating health services, practitioners can collaborate with various specialists and ancillary providers, making it easier to manage patients. This model of cooperation allows family doctors to deal with not only immediate medical problems but also chronic care and prevention more efficiently. Consequently, patients receive more integrated treatment plans tailored to their needs, which improve health outcomes. The interdependence of family physicians with other health professionals highlights the necessity of effective communication and shared resources to maximize efficiency and prevent duplication of effort, which becomes crucial in a healthcare system increasingly controlled by market forces and consumerism. The inclusion of services also addresses the growing shortages of primary care physicians. As the demand for healthcare continues to increase, the need for greater cooperation is increasingly evident. Family physicians can learn to embrace this by reconfiguring their practices to make effective use of nurses' and other healthcare professionals' professional expertise. For instance, they can implement team-based approaches that allow physician assistants and nurse practitioners to assume patient management roles to complement family physicians' capacity to treat more patients (Ormond et al., 2011). This strategic deployment of health personnel not only relieves pressure on primary care physicians but also ensures that patients receive appropriate and timely care, upholding the significant role of family physicians within an integrated healthcare system. In addition, incorporating health services facilitates continuity of care, a fundamental concept within the practice of family medicine. Through collaboration with other healthcare professionals and coordination of care across multiple settings, family physicians can ensure patients experience smooth transitions between inpatient and outpatient care. Continuity is vital in ensuring the long-term well-being of the patients, particularly those with complex or chronic diseases who require constant supervision and management. To that end, integrated services also enable family physicians to gather and assess comprehensive patient data, thereby making better clinical decisions. As healthcare evolves, family physicians' ability to deliver integrated care will be crucial to achieving optimal health outcomes and enhancing the patient experience, underscoring their pivotal role in contemporary healthcare delivery (Figure 2.14).

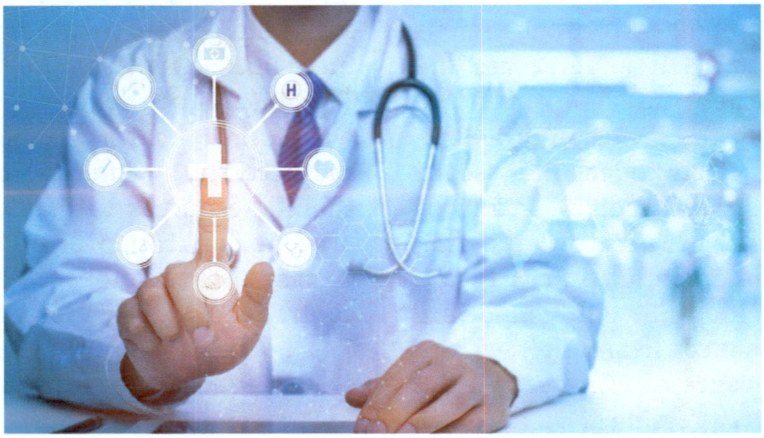

Figure 2.14. Healthcare integration services.

Source: https://images.prismic.io/cabot/ZfPqgbTwE6aM1KtH_Healthcare-Integration-Services.jpg?auto=format%2Ccompress&fit=max&w=3840.

Test Your Knowledge

1. What are the referral processes and follow-ups?
2. What is the integration of health services?

2.4. Ethical Responsibilities

Learning Outcome

1. Maintain patient confidentiality
2. Understand the informed consent and patient autonomy
3. Address ethical dilemmas in practice

The ethical responsibilities of family physicians encompass a broad range of concerns that extend far beyond mere clinical skills. Central to this ethical framework is the obligation of beneficence, which requires physicians to act in the best interests of their patients. Family physicians are often tasked not only with diagnosing and treating disease; they are also tasked with understanding the general circumstances of their patients' lives. This mandate requires them to navigate complex social and cultural determinants that drive health outcomes. Reports emphasize the need to bolster medical education by incorporating ethics and social responsibility, encouraging future physicians to practice integrated problem-solving that considers diverse patient needs (Tyler et al., 2008). Thus, family doctors must create a strong ethical foundation that dictates their clinical choices so that they advance and prioritize the health of their patients in a manner that ensures trust and responsibility. No less crucial is the ethical role of family doctors in unprecedented circumstances, like the COVID-19 pandemic. Doctors are compelled to act ethically when dealing with resource management and their own safety. The idea of a duty to treat is controversial against the backdrop of a reality of suboptimal protective practices and emotional distress among healthcare professionals. Physicians must weigh their commitment to the care of patients against their personal and familial health risks, being forced to make difficult decisions on whether to continue practicing among their communities (Iserson et al., 2020).

This is an example of the necessity of open communication from institution leaders about resources present and risks that can permit a more informed reaction to the ethical challenges that face clinicians. The performance of these duties is not only clinical competence but also a strong ethical sensitivity in order to deal with the complex problems of contemporary medicine. Moreover, integrating ethical considerations into family medicine can strengthen the relationship between doctors and patients by fostering a shared understanding of health and well-being. Ethical responsibility requires family physicians to speak on behalf of marginalized populations and adjust structural imbalances in access to healthcare. By adopting the medical-legal partnership paradigm, as espoused by more recent educational initiatives, family physicians can collaborate with legal professionals to address the social determinants of health affecting marginalized families (Tyler et al., 2008). This interdisciplinary paradigm underscored the interconnectedness of health and social justice, enabling physicians to effectively advocate for patients who might otherwise not receive the requisite care. As family physicians navigate their ethical tightrope, they enhance the quality of care they provide and also assist in making the healthcare system more equitable with its emphasis on whole-person, patient-centric care.

2.4.1. Maintaining Patient Confidentiality

Patient confidentiality is an ethical foundation of the practice of family medicine. Family doctors establish trusting relationships with their patients, and confidentiality is crucial to trust building. Patients must feel secure enough to share sensitive information without fear, and confidentiality is vital to proper diagnosis and effective treatment. Violations of privacy can lead not only to a loss of the patient-physician relationship but also to severe emotional and psychological harm to the patient. It is therefore incumbent on family physicians to implement robust privacy policies and procedures to ensure that patient information is kept secure against unauthorized access and dissemination. Through vigilant adherence to confidentiality practices, family physicians not only uphold professional standards but also contribute to overall integrity within the health system. Given the emergence of medical technologies, the dilemma of patient confidentiality is even more complex. The use of electronic medical records (EMRs) and telemedicine holds great promise for improving patient care, but it also poses threats to data privacy. Family physicians will have to accommodate these technologies while staying in sync with regulations such as the Health Insurance Portability and Accountability Act (HIPAA). Also, as (Assist. Adina Bălan Ph. D) would note, health data fragmentation poses a threat to maintaining intact and confidential patient records. The importance of interoperable and standardized electronic medical records cannot be overstated, as such systems allow for safer communication among healthcare providers while safeguarding patient data. Investment in technology and training is therefore paramount for family physicians to manage and secure patients' information effectively. Interprofessional collaboration between healthcare practitioners is essential in ensuring patient confidentiality. As revealed in (Bond et al., 2014), efficient inter-professional collaboration is able to boost the provision of primary care while building a culture of respect for patients' privacy. Where family doctors practice alongside nurses, specialists, and administrative personnel, it is in such an environment that everyone will have a stake in ensuring confidentiality levels. Training sessions and discussions concerning privacy procedures on a regular basis are capable of instilling a commitment from all parties towards safeguarding patient information. In addition, creating an open culture enables team members to raise any issues with confidentiality preemptively. By incorporating confidentiality into the yarn of team functioning, family doctors can ensure that privacy for their patients is an unwavering part of care, ultimately resulting in improved health outcomes and strengthened patient trust (Figure 2.15).

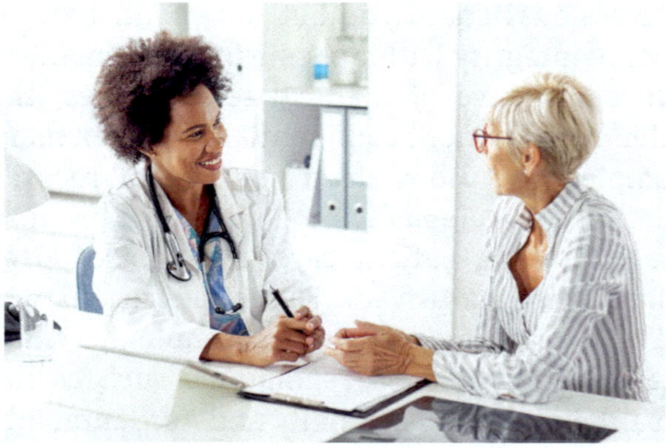

Figure 2.15. Maintaining patient confidentiality.

Source: https://online.maryville.edu/wp-content/uploads/sites/97/2020/10/caregiver-patient.jpg?w=1024.

2.4.2. Informed Consent and Patient Autonomy

The doctrine of informed consent is a hallmark of patient autonomy, particularly in the context of a family doctor's obligation. Informed consent requires doctors to ensure that patients are properly informed about their illness, treatment options, risks, and benefits before making decisions about their care. This system not only empowers the patient but also fosters a respectful physician-patient relationship. General practitioners must navigate this tricky terrain by providing clear, transparent information tailored to each patient's unique context so the patient feels empowered. On top of that, good communication methods, such as those taught by courses like Team STEPPS, can serve to facilitate the process of informed consent more effectively because they emphasize teamwork and patient engagement in decision-making (Jones et al., 2016). Principles of patient autonomy go far beyond merely obtaining the patient's signature on consent documents. Autonomy mandates that patients can be in control of the decision-making process for their own health, supported by adequate information from their own physicians. Shared decision-making practice is essential in this matter; it is a shared process in which physicians and patients discuss therapeutic choices, taking into account potential outcomes and personal beliefs. This approach not only respects patient autonomy but also improves care satisfaction and treatment adherence. Thus, by adhering to patient autonomy and informed consent before anything else, family physicians play a key role in developing a healthcare culture in which patients feel valued and respected, and, as such, achieve improved overall healthcare outcomes. Moreover, challenges often arise regarding informed consent, particularly among multicultural patient groups. Differences in health literacy, patient-specific needs, and culture can significantly influence patients' ability to comprehend medical information. Family doctors should therefore adopt culturally sensitive practices that recognize and respond to these differences that guarantees all patients are empowered to play active roles in their healthcare decisions. For instance, using plain language or visual aids can help those with low health literacy understand. By surmounting these hurdles, family physicians not only fulfill their ethical obligations but also demonstrate an unyielding commitment to principles of patient autonomy. By doing so, enhancing informed consent processes aligns with broader agendas of patient-centered care, arguing that each patient's voice matters significantly in health management (Sage et al., 2003) (Figure 2.16).

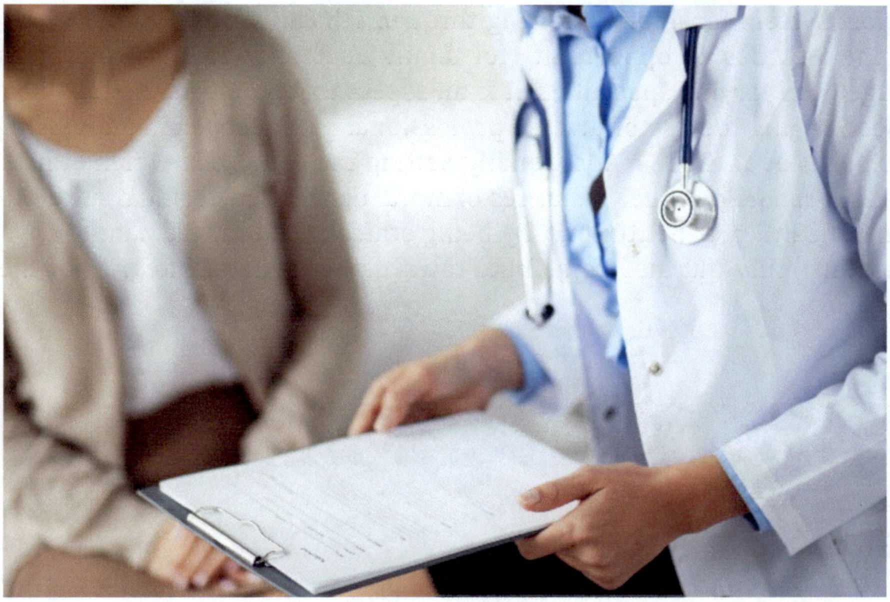

Figure 2.16. Informed consent.

Source: https://www.news-medical.net/images/Article_Images/ImageForArticle_24607_17086988947716561.jpg.

2.4.3. Addressing Ethical Dilemmas in Practice

In the multifaceted role of a family physician, the capability to manage ethical issues is a critical aspect of effective practice. They tend to arise in varied situations, for example, when patient autonomy and medical recommendations come into conflict, or when resource management raises ethical issues. GoodWork Project identifies that ethical challenges arise in multifaceted forms, entailing attention to detail and classification, indicating the dynamic nature of professional duties (Mucinskas et al., 2013). As healthcare providers face these challenges, the ability to exercise prolonged reasonableness and reflective practice is paramount. Family physicians must facilitate conversation that respects patients' autonomy without compromising health outcomes. By cultivating an ethical awareness of the stakes in everyday clinical decisions, doctors can enhance their commitment to providing quality care grounded in moral integrity. Additionally, the existence of moral distress underscores the complexity family physicians experience in situations involving ethical conflict. It is defined as the feeling of anxiety or frustration that occurs when one is unable to do what they feel is ethically correct, moral distress has the potential to influence physician decision-making and well-being significantly (Matchett et al., 2018). Family physicians may face situations in which institutional or systemic constraints limit their ability to provide the best possible care, leading to ethical tension. Knowledge of these problems is essential because it can guide personal and professional development. Overcoming moral distress by training interventions and support systems is necessary so that physicians can reflect on their experience and practice resilience. By considering the ethical dimension of their profession, family physicians gain a greater sense of professional identity and responsibility, and ultimately of patients' well-being. In resolving ethical issues, family doctors can utilize an interdisciplinary team process. This not only expands the scope of opinion that can be tapped to resolve complex clinical issues, but also provides a support system for doctors sorting through ethical issues. Resolution of dilemmas in a team environment provides an opportunity for family doctors to learn from others and to utilize others' knowledge with varying specialties. It is an aspect that supports the ideology posited by the GoodWork Project, urging the use of diverse professional perspectives in addressing ethical issues effectively (Mucinskas et al., 2013). Additionally, setting the context in which ethical conversations become mainstream can help reduce instances of moral distress, fostering a culture of transparency and compassion in healthcare institutions. By being ethically committed, family physicians not only uphold their responsibility but also contribute towards the general integrity of the medical field.

Test Your Knowledge

1. How do you maintain patient confidentiality?
2. What is informed consent?

SUMMARY

An examination of the quest for the roles and duties of a family physician reveals that the role far exceeds clinical activities. Family physicians are very much at the center of the healthcare system, weaving their practices through preventive care, chronic disease management, and patient education. Family physicians are optimally suited to address the uniqueness of individual health matters within familial and communal contexts. By establishing long-term relationships with patients, these physicians can supply personalized care that is not only treatment but also overall well-being. This multifaceted role underscores family physicians' commitment to helping patients through key health choices and across varied phases of life, underscoring the need for prolonged professional development to improve care planning and develop effective communication methods. Also, family physicians' practice relies on interdisciplinary collaboration to achieve optimal patient outcomes. Multidisciplinary collaboration with specialists and other practitioners is critical, especially in the management of chronic diseases and multidisciplinary health issues. In the context of transforming health systems, family physicians' practice involves advocating for their patients and securing access to needed services. This not only enhances the quality of care but also solidifies the family-centered principle of care, where the complexity of patient backgrounds and values is known and accepted. Upon experiencing transition care and resource use challenges, flexible family physicians must use available community resources and engage in ongoing education to best address such challenges in an equitable manner across their diverse patient populations. Lastly, taking on the dynamic nature of their profession equips family physicians to address the evolving demands of healthcare systems. Through an emphasis on holistic care practices and being informed on guidelines and best practices, family physicians have the opportunity to lead in building patient and community resilience. The significance of screening and preventive care, highlighted by studies on healthcare interventions, underscores their role in promoting early detection and health gains (Deliens et al., 2019; Lindsay et al., 2018). Thus, in playing the role of patient champions and navigating the complexities of healthcare provision, family doctors solidify their role as foundation providers in healthcare, delivering care respectful to patients, culturally competent to their needs, and tailored to the specific circumstances of their lives.

A family doctor's practice encompasses a broad range of duties extending beyond physical treatment and disease diagnosis. At its core, their work involves the creation of a trusting and continuous relationship with patients, which serves to encourage good communication and facilitate a holistic approach to healthcare. Family physicians serve as first-line providers of healthcare, caring for acute and chronic medical conditions and promoting prevention through regular screening and education. This comprehensive approach aims to enhance the patient's independence and engagement in their health care, ultimately leading to improved health outcomes and overall well-being. The extensive understanding of patients' medical histories and family patterns allows family physicians to develop customized care plans tailored to specific needs, further solidifying their position as an integral part of the health care system. In the current model of health care, family physicians are increasingly being asked to adapt to evolving modes of care focused on quality and cost-effectiveness. The majority of these practices have also begun to receive payment for performance for improving these aspects of healthcare provision, so far as Medicare fee-for-service beneficiaries are concerned. Such financial incentives complement the responsibility of family physicians to not only provide quality medical care but also to be a part of innovative practice strategies that maximize care coordination and patient satisfaction. Through active participation in quality improvement activities, family physicians are the pillars of continuous development of healthcare practice, reducing processes but emphasizing patient-centered care, such that they are well equipped to deal with the myriad needs of their patients in a constantly changing environment (Pope et al., 2008). Further, the impending shortage of primary care physicians is a significant issue in meeting the growing demands on family medicine. With more individuals gaining access to health care through expanded insurance coverage, there is a need to develop policy and practical solutions to ensure the quality and accessibility of care. Finding strategies, such as restructuring practice infrastructure to maximize nurses' and other health care personnel's roles, can effectively address this issue. Family physicians are not only tasked with providing direct patient care but are also responsible for systemic improvements that can enhance their ability to serve more populations. In this manner, they will be in a position to ensure that comprehensive and timely health care remains available, thus affirming their significant role in the overall public health context (Ormond et al., 2011).

KEY TERMS FROM THIS CHAPTER

- Chronic illnesses
- Communication
- Community resources
- Healthcare policy
- Leadership
- Mental health
- Patient advocacy
- Collaboration
- Community engagement
- Disease management
- Holistic care
- Medical information
- Nutrition
- Patient-centered care

CRITICAL THINKING QUESTIONS

1. **Which of the following is a primary responsibility of a family physician?**
   a. Conducting highly specialized surgeries
   b. Providing comprehensive and continuous care to patients
   c. Treating only chronic diseases
   d. Limiting practice to inpatient hospital care
2. **What is the role of a family physician in preventive care?**
   a. Ignoring preventive strategies and focusing on treatment
   b. Screening for diseases, providing vaccinations, and promoting healthy lifestyles
   c. Referring all patients to specialists for preventive care
   d. Focusing solely on the treatment of infectious diseases
3. **Family physicians are often referred to as:**
   a. Specialists in acute diseases
   b. First-contact care providers
   c. Emergency care specialists
   d. Hospital-based care providers
4. **One of the key roles of a family physician is to:**
   a. Provide care for a specific age group only
   b. Manage only medical conditions that require hospitalization
   c. Coordinate care among specialists for the patient
   d. Avoid involving the patient in care decisions
5. **Family physicians play an integral role in:**
   a. Treating advanced-stage cancers exclusively
   b. Managing health issues within the context of the family and community
   c. Performing heart and brain surgeries
   d. Limiting their services to rural areas only

Short Answer Questions

1. What is the main role of a family physician?
2. Why is family medicine important in healthcare?
3. What is meant by patient care?
4. Describe the role of preventive medicine in the practice of family physicians.
5. What is the meaning of coordination of care?

Answer to Critical Thinking Questions

1. (b); 2. (b); 3. (b); 4. (c); 5. (b).

REFERENCES

1. Henny, K. D., Crepaz, N., Lyles, C. M., Marshall, K. J., Aupont, L. W., Jacobs, E. D., Liau, A., Rama, S., Kay, L. S., Willis, L. A., & Charania, M. R. (2012). Efficacy of HIV/STI behavioral interventions for heterosexual African American men in the United States: A Meta-Analysis. *AIDS and Behavior, 16*(5), 1092–1114. https://doi.org/10.1007/s10461-011-0100-2
2. Bălan, A. (2025). *Electronic Medical Record–Success or Failure in the Medical Decision from the Romanian Health System?* https://core.ac.uk/download/pdf/6239954.pdf (accessed on 12th July 2025).
3. Bayles, C., Hoffman, L., Jakicic, J., et al. (2012). Examination of acute care nurses' ability to engage in patient education related to physical activity as a health behavior. https://core.ac.uk/download/12212129.pdf (accessed on 12th July 2025).
4. Bond, A., O'Malley, A. S., Draper, K., Tirodkar, M., & Gourevitch, R. (2014). Overcoming challenges to teamwork in patient-centered medical homes: A qualitative study. https://core.ac.uk/download/75780924.pdf (accessed on 12th July 2025).
5. Bonica, M. (2017). *Healthcare Management Primer*. Students of Health Management 721.01, University of New Hampshire. https://core.ac.uk/download/215509297.pdf (accessed on 12th July 2025).
6. Chan, A., Fok, R. W. Y., Ke, Y., et al. (2020). Roles and recommendations from primary care physicians towards managing low-risk breast cancer survivors in a shared-care model with specialists in Singapore—a qualitative study. https://core.ac.uk/download/305124440.pdf (accessed on 12th July 2025).
7. Deliens, L., Gastmans, C., Gilissen, J., et al. (2019). Implementing advance care planning in routine nursing home care: The development of the theory-based ACP+ program. https://core.ac.uk/download/237011878.pdf (accessed on 12th July 2025).
8. Dennis, R. E., Edelman, S. W., Giangreco, M. F., et al. (1999). Related services for Vermont's students with disabilities. https://core.ac.uk/download/51067326.pdf (accessed on 12th July 2025).
9. Hopper, S. S. (2003). Crossing organizational boundaries in palliative care: The promise and reality of community partnerships. https://core.ac.uk/download/71365063.pdf (accessed on 12th July 2025).
10. Iserson, K. V. (2020). Healthcare ethics during a pandemic. https://core.ac.uk/download/305124104.pdf (accessed on 12th July 2025).
11. Jones, T. S. (2016). Implementation of TeamSTEPPS. https://core.ac.uk/download/129592699.pdf (accessed on 12th July 2025).
12. Krol, D., Cheung, K., Cruz, K., Carver, L., & Revels, M. (2013). Providing preventive oral health care to infants and young children in Women, Infants, and Children (WIC), Early Head Start, and primary care settings. https://core.ac.uk/download/71362896.pdf (accessed on 12th July 2025).
13. Lindsay, S. (2018). Understanding facilitators and barriers to contraception screening and referral in young women with cancer. https://open.bu.edu/bitstream/2144/32681/7/Lindsay_bu_0017N_14014.pdf (accessed on 12th July 2025).

14. Mason, M. A. (2007). *Equality in Health: An Annotated Bibliography with Resources on Health Disparities and Cultural and Linguistic Competency*. https://core.ac.uk/download/71346571.pdf (accessed on 12th July 2025).

15. Matchett, N. J. (2018). What's philosophical about moral distress? https://core.ac.uk/download/186330341.pdf (accessed on 12th July 2025).

16. McAllister, J. W., Popp, J., & Antonelli, R. (2009). Making care coordination a critical component of the pediatric health system: A multidisciplinary framework. https://core.ac.uk/download/71352885.pdf (accessed on 12th July 2025).

17. McHugh, B., Estrine, J., & Moran, R. (2004). Promoting men's health: Addressing barriers to healthy lifestyle and preventive health care. https://core.ac.uk/download/71356600.pdf (accessed on 12th July 2025).

18. Mucinskas, D., & Gardner, H. (2013). Educating for good work: From research to practice. https://core.ac.uk/download/75779869.pdf (accessed on 12th July 2025).

19. O'Malley, A. S., Peikes, D., Pham, H. H., Maxfield, M., & Ginsburg, P. B. (2008). Making medical homes work: Moving from concept to practice. https://core.ac.uk/download/71352896.pdf (accessed on 12th July 2025).

20. Ormond, B. A., & Bovbjerg, R. R. (2011). Assuring access to care under health reform: The key role of workforce policy. https://core.ac.uk/download/71356903.pdf (accessed on 12th July 2025).

21. Perkins, J., & Youdelman, M. (2005). Providing language services in small health care provider settings: Examples from the field. https://core.ac.uk/download/71354088.pdf (accessed on 12th July 2025).

22. Phillips, K., & Coleman, K. (2010). Providing underserved patients with medical homes: Assessing the readiness of safety-net health centers. https://core.ac.uk/download/71354090.pdf (accessed on 12th July 2025).

23. Pope, G., Kautter, J., Aggarwal, J., Trisolini, M., & Leung, M. (2008). The Medicare physician group practice demonstration: Lessons learned on improving quality and efficiency in health care. https://core.ac.uk/download/71353237.pdf (accessed on 12th July 2025).

24. Robiner, W. N., Tompkins, T., & Tumlin, T. R. (2013). Psychologists and medications in the era of interprofessional care: Collaboration is less problematic and costly than prescribing. https://core.ac.uk/download/143958393.pdf (accessed on 12th July 2025).

25. Sage, W. M. (2003). Managed care's Crimea: Medical necessity, therapeutic benefit, and the goals of administrative process in health insurance. https://core.ac.uk/download/62548773.pdf (accessed on 12th July 2025).

26. Tobin, E. T. (2008). Allies not adversaries: Teaching collaboration to the next generation of doctors and lawyers to address social inequality. https://core.ac.uk/download/56703780.pdf (accessed on 12th July 2025).

27. Valentini, J. (2020). Communication patterns between physicians and physician assistants. https://core.ac.uk/download/322851171.pdf (accessed on 12th July 2025).

RESPIRATORY DISORDERS

3

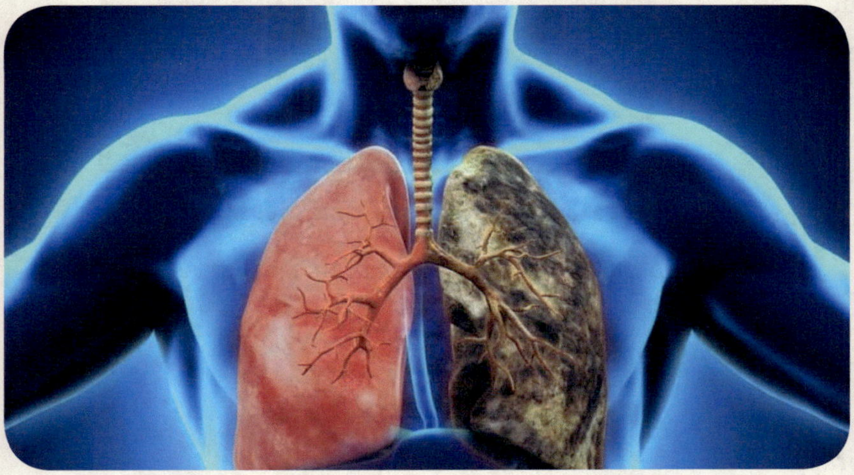

Introduction

Respiratory diseases encompass a broad spectrum of conditions that affect lung function and the overall respiratory system. They range from long-term conditions such as asthma and chronic obstructive pulmonary disease (COPD) to acute disease, for instance, pneumonia and pulmonary embolism. The significance of learning about respiratory diseases is underscored by their high incidence in the population and their impact on public health. Identification of these conditions is particularly important in that respiratory disease ranks among the leading causes of morbidity and mortality worldwide. Early identification and optimal management are paramount for improving patient outcomes, and environmental factors and genetic influences are implicated in the pathogenesis of such disorders, underscoring the importance of extensive education on the complexities of respiratory health. In the last few years, medical research and treatment strategies have transformed the management of respiratory disorders. Advances in pharmacotherapy and novel therapeutic mechanisms have improved the management

LEARNING OBJECTIVES

After studying this chapter, you will be able to:

1. Describe the anatomy of the respiratory system
2. Learn about common respiratory disorders
3. Describe the causes and risk factors of respiratory disorders
4. Understand the symptoms and diagnosis of respiratory disorders
5. Know the treatment options for respiratory disorders
6. Learn about prevention and management for respiratory disorders

of once-chronic or previously untreatable diseases. For instance, understanding the pathophysiology of respiratory disorders has led to the development of targeted therapies directed against the underlying pathophysiology rather than symptomatic control alone.

Also, interdisciplinary collaboration among healthcare professionals, including doctors, respiratory therapists, and rehabilitation professionals, has led to a more comprehensive model of care for patients. Not only does this change in thinking aim to improve respiratory function, but it also addresses the overall quality of life for patients with these debilitating illnesses, making it imperative to continue to develop trends in respiratory medicine. Furthermore, the role of diagnostics in the management of respiratory disease cannot be overstated. The ability to accurately diagnose and classify these diseases provides more specific treatment protocols and better outcomes. Diagnostic interventions, ranging from imaging tests to advanced molecular techniques, are now an integral component of respiratory therapy.

For example, in cases of non-specific symptoms like high-grade fever and inflammatory signs, a broad range of tests, including imaging studies and lab findings, can prove to be quite helpful in providing valuable information regarding underlying respiratory compromise, further supplemented by pulmonary congestion evaluation in similar clinical presentations (Żaczek et al., 2025).

Similarly, the implications of respiratory function in neuromuscular conditions such as spinal muscular atrophy underscore the evolving notion of the bridge between neurobiology and respiratory well-being (Rastegina et al., 2024). Ongoing research will be essential to establish these diagnostic tools further and offer comprehensive care to subjects of respiratory disorders as this field continues to evolve (Figure 3.1).

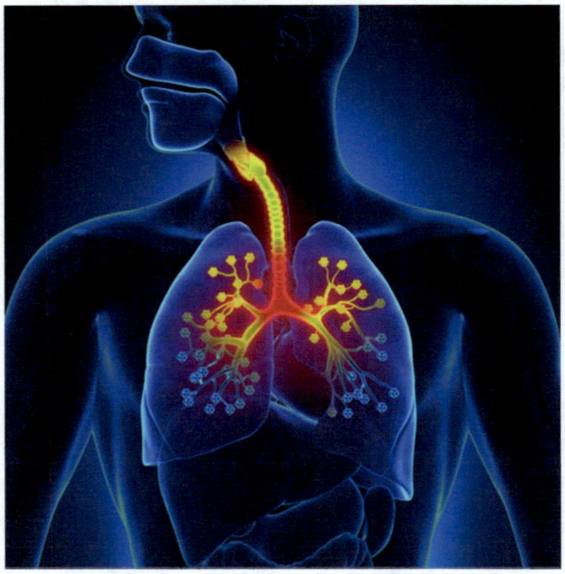

Figure 3.1. Respiratory disorders.

Source: https://www.chandigarhayurvedcentre.com/wp-content/uploads/2021/06/RESPIRATORY-DISORDERS-.jpg.

3.1. Anatomy of the Respiratory System

Learning Outcome

1. Describe the structure of the lungs
2. Know the function of the airways
3. Understand the role of the diaphragm and respiratory muscles

The anatomy of the respiratory system is intricate, allowing efficient gas exchange and protecting the body from external damage. The system consists of several structures, including the nasal cavity, pharynx, larynx, trachea, bronchi, and lungs. Each of these plays an important role in the process of breathing. The nasal cavity, lined with thin hairs and mucus, traps particles and germs, and they are not permitted to travel down to the lower respiratory passages. The larynx, also referred to as the voice box, is an airway but also guards against aspiration of food. The trachea also divides into bronchi, which further branch into smaller bronchioles deep within the lungs. This branching formation maximizes the surface area for gas exchange within the alveoli, small sacs where oxygen and carbon dioxide are transferred. This complex structure is the foundation for the respiratory system's function and its ability to adapt to various disorders. Knowledge of respiratory system anatomy is required for diagnosis and successful treatment of respiratory disorders. Asthma, chronic obstructive pulmonary disease (COPD), and pneumonia illustrate the significance of such anatomical knowledge. Asthma, with features of airway inflammation and bronchoconstriction, is caused directly by structural changes of the bronchi and bronchioles. COPD, however, leads to destruction of alveolar walls, reducing surface area and impairing gas exchange. Pneumonia, an infection of the lungs, may lead to a buildup of fluid in the alveoli, further obstructing airflow. The connectivity of these structures requires an interdisciplinary understanding of what they do and how they might be weak. Clinicians' ability to treat and evaluate such disorders lies in their of the intricacies of respiratory anatomy, so that interventions can be customized for the patient's particular situation. Advances in understanding the respiratory system's anatomy have taken on greater importance in recent years, particularly in light of respiratory diseases such as COVID-19. The emergence of this novel coronavirus, transmitted primarily through respiratory droplets, underscored the importance of understanding how respiratory anatomy could dictate disease transmission and outcomes. The virus binds to the angiotensin-converting enzyme 2 (ACE2) receptor, expressed predominantly in respiratory tissue, suggesting structural susceptibilities to extreme presentations such as acute respiratory distress syndrome (ARDS) in vulnerable populations. Furthermore, pre-existing respiratory diseases like clinical conditions increase the risk of severe complications in patients with COVID-19, linking anatomical vulnerability to clinical presentation. As treatment modalities and prevention measures, such as potential antiviral therapy, are being explored by scientists, understanding the underlying anatomy of the respiratory system remains critical in averting the impact of such respiratory ailments as well as enhancing patient care (Guo et al., 2020; Ponikowski et al., 2016) (Figure 3.2).

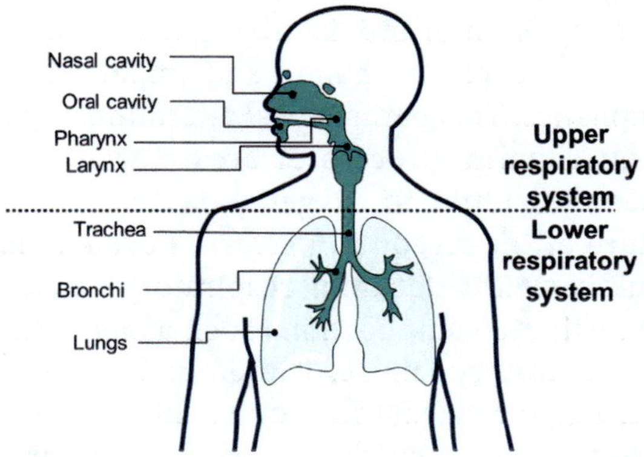

Figure 3.2. Anatomy of the respiratory system.

Source: https://www.researchgate.net/profile/Jesus-Lujan-Montelongo/publication/357470377/figure/fig1/AS:1121095860142082@1644301490964/Anatomy-of-respiratory-system.png.

3.1.1. Structure of the Lungs

The lungs are the primary organs of the respiratory system, with a gas-exchange function necessary to maintain life. Their anatomy comprises the bronchi, bronchioles, alveoli, and pleurae. The trachea branches into the primary bronchi, which then descend into the lungs and further subdivide into smaller bronchi and bronchioles, ultimately terminating in alveolar sacs. Within the alveoli, a network of minute air sacs, the exchange of oxygen and carbon dioxide takes place. This highly evolved structure not only maximizes surface area for gas exchange but also provides for adequate perfusion and ventilation, which are essential for homeostasis. The structural sophistication of the lungs underscores their involvement in numerous respiratory diseases that can impair function, thereby making it challenging to maintain the balance of gas exchange and potentially leading to severe health consequences. When examining the lungs, one must consider how their structure affects specific respiratory diseases. The acute respiratory distress syndrome (ARDS) is a prime example of the impact of structural change on lung function. In ARDS, the alveolar-capillary membrane is disrupted, resulting in impaired gas exchange and impaired lung compliance. This pathological alteration impairs the mechanical process of breathing and also poses difficulties to oxygenation of the blood. Failure of the alveoli to perform normally may result in swiftly declining respiratory efficiency and facilitate complications such as hypoxemia and respiratory failure. Therefore, information regarding the normal structure of lungs provides a critical background for comparing how various disorders contribute to respiratory morbidity and overall patient outcomes, such as how interventions, as observed in studies that compared PaO2/FiO2 ratios in ARDS (Villar et al., 2022), help. Furthermore, the use of biomarkers to assess lung structural integrity and as prognostic factors has also become more prominent in recent literature. Among them, soluble receptor for advanced glycation end-products (sRAGE) has been employed as a potential marker of lung epithelial injury. Plasma sRAGE alterations in ARDS patients may reflect ongoing injury and can serve as a prognostic indicator for clinical treatment. Studies have demonstrated that higher baseline sRAGE levels and increases over time are also correlated with 90-day mortality, so monitoring sRAGE can help in the risk stratification of respiratory patients (Jabaudon et al., 2021). By integrating biomarker assessment with structural measurements, physicians can better understand the importance of lung pathophysiology and tailor treatment strategies more specifically in critically ill respiratory patients (Figure 3.3).

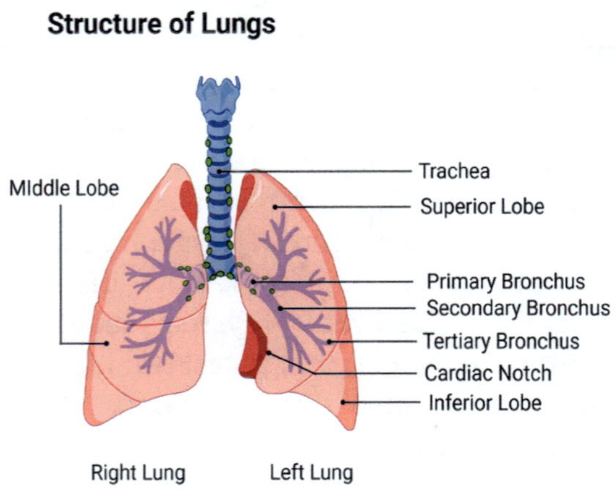

Figure 3.3. Structure of lungs.

Source: https://microbenotes.com/wp-content/uploads/2022/06/Structure-of-Lungs.jpeg.

3.1.2. Function of the Airways

The airways are the vital channels for the passage of air to and from the lungs, making possible the exchange of gases, including oxygen and carbon dioxide. The structure of the airways, including the trachea, bronchi, and bronchioles, plays a significant role in successful respiratory function. The bronchial tree, which is a series of increasingly smaller airways, is lined with a mucous membrane that produces mucus, which acts as a filter for pathogens and particulate matter in the outside environment. This defense mechanism is important for preventing respiratory illness, as it keeps harmful chemicals away from the delicate alveolar sacs where gas exchange occurs. When airway function becomes compromised, as in asthma or chronic obstructive pulmonary disease (COPD), the implications for overall health are unfavorable, resulting in respiratory distress and impaired gas exchange. Furthermore, the dynamic nature of the airways is emphasized through their sensitivity to stimuli. In healthy individuals, airway smooth muscle can contract and relax, thereby controlling airflow appropriately during exercise or in response to allergens. This can be abnormal with illnesses of airway inflammation and obstruction. For example, in bronchiolitis obliterans, the fibrotic process involves small conducting airways and is imitated by other respiratory illnesses such as COPD, which complicates diagnosis and management (King et al., 1989). These modifications in airway function—neither structural only, but also environmental—demonstrate the complex role of the respiratory system in disease and health. Forming an understanding of the multifaceted role of the airways is essential for effective treatment of respiratory disease. Age also brings with it significant physiological changes to airway function, germane to treatment and management of respiratory disease (Ebejer et al., 1999). As one grows older, the structure of the airway may weaken, reducing elasticity and altering airway resistance. Such alterations can produce lower pulmonary reserve, and older people are especially vulnerable to respiratory disease such as COPD, which is both age- and environment-induced. The presence of chronic inflammation and enhanced airway reactivity can also make this environment more difficult, so it is important to understand the interactions between airway function and physiologic changes that occur in aging. As populations age, respiratory status deteriorates and the burden of airway-related disease increases, necessitating that medical providers stay closely focused on these trends (Figure 3.4).

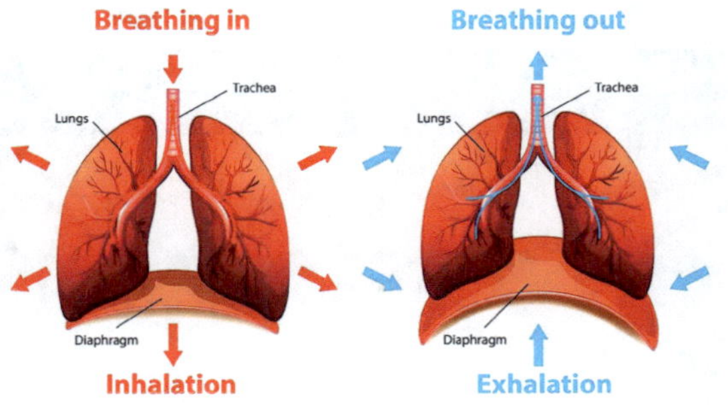

Figure 3.4. Mechanism of breathing.

Source: https://microbenotes.com/wp-content/uploads/2022/06/Mechanism-of-Breathing.jpg.

3.1.3. Role of the Diaphragm and Respiratory Muscles

The diaphragm, which is a dome-shaped muscle situated at the base of the thoracic cavity, is at the heart of the breathing mechanism. It is the primary respiration muscle that facilitates the inhalation process by contracting and expanding, thereby enlarging the thoracic cavity's volume and opening the air passage to enter the lungs. The diaphragm is also very important in patients with respiratory disease, where its function can be compromised. Chronic obstructive pulmonary disease (COPD), for example, can result in structural and functional alterations of respiratory muscles, such as the diaphragm. With time, the alterations compromise the muscle contractility and hence the contractile performance of the diaphragm, resulting in increased work of breathing and reduced exercise capacity. Ultrasound scan, for instance, quantification of the amplitude and velocity of diaphragmatic contraction, has begun to separate the extent of diaphragmatic dysfunction and its correlation with disease severity and symptomatology in patients with COPD (Meridj et al., 2024). In addition to the diaphragm, other muscles of the chest, the intercostal, and the abdominal muscles also contribute importantly to respiratory work. These muscles help with both inhalation and exhalation, enhancing the efficiency of ventilation and respiratory mechanics overall. In systemic lupus erythematosus (SLE) conditions, patients may develop complications such as shrinking lung syndrome (SLS), which can affect the strength and mobility of respiratory muscles. Evidence shows that inspiratory muscle training (IMT) can increase diaphragm thickness and mobility in SLE patients, thereby enhancing respiratory muscle strength and functional exercise capacity. These developments underscore the interdependence of peripheral and respiratory muscle performance in patients with asthma. These findings underscore that, in addition to lung function, muscle training interventions should be considered a significant area for treating respiratory disorders as a whole (Sari et al., 2024). The respiratory muscle and diaphragm function is not merely mechanical, but it profoundly influences a patient's quality of life in the presence of respiratory disease. Increasing respiratory muscle weakness and fatigue will lead to decreased physical endurance and worsened dyspnea, once again degrading a person's capacity to perform activities of daily living. Interventions aimed at enhancing respiratory muscle function, such as IMT, have effects and help rehabilitate affected individuals. Additional studies are needed to explore the complex interplay between quality of life and respiratory muscle performance. Understanding these dynamics can lead to optimized treatments that not only alleviate symptoms but also improve the overall health and well-being of patients with chronic respiratory diseases, paving the way for long-term gains in their health status (Figure 3.5).

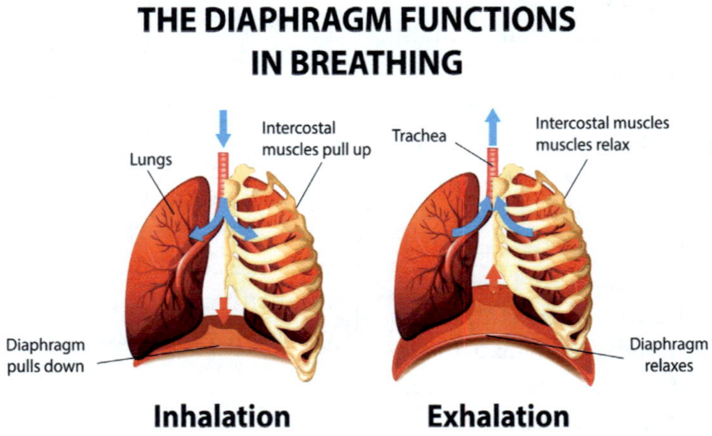

Figure 3.5. The diaphragm functions in breathing illustration.

Source: https://blackburnahg.com.au/wp-content/uploads/2023/12/Diaphragm-functions-1536x962.jpg.

Test Your Knowledge

1. What is the structure of the lungs?
2. What are the airways functions?

3.2. Common Respiratory Disorders

Learning Outcome

1. Learn about asthma
2. Describe the chronic obstructive pulmonary disease (COPD)
3. Understand the pneumonia

The geography of respiratory diseases encompasses a vast array of diseases with a significant impact on global health. The most common among these diseases are asthma, chronic obstructive pulmonary disease (COPD), and pneumonia, each with its pathophysiological mechanisms, risk factors, and treatment approaches. Asthma, characterized by airway inflammation and hyperreactivity, is a very challenging issue for patients because it is episodic and can be triggered by many environmental stimuli, such as allergens and irritants. COPD, often due to long-term exposure to noxious particulates, is characterized by progressive airflow limitation and includes chronic bronchitis and emphysema. Meanwhile, pneumonia, an inflammation of lung tissue most often caused by infection, remains a leading cause of morbidity and mortality, particularly in vulnerable populations, which emphasizes the necessity for stringent public health interventions to manage such prevalent ailments (Murray et al., 2022). The rising incidence of respiratory disease has been accompanied by growing concern about antimicrobial resistance (AMR), particularly in the treatment of pneumonia. The toll of over 1.5 million deaths attributable to resistance associated with lower respiratory infections in 2019 indicates the severity of the consequences of neglecting to target AMR in managing respiratory disease. Bacteria such as Streptococcus pneumoniae and Escherichia coli are at the core of this crisis, with some strains resistant to multiple antibiotics causing infections that make therapy challenging (Wichmann, 2020). Healthcare facilities worldwide must accord close attention to efficient infection control and prevention methods that can reduce the transmission of resistance. More monitoring and data collection within resource-limited settings will play a critical role in informing policy interventions aimed at slowing the development of AMR and its impact on respiratory disease.

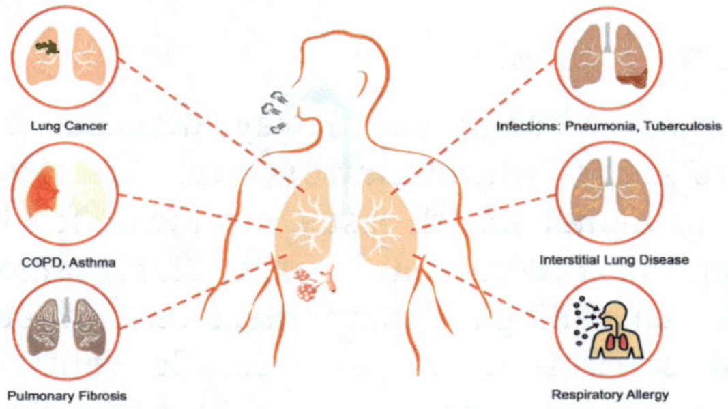

Figure 3.6. Common respiratory diseases: respiratory diseases are among the leading causes of death worldwide. Chronic respiratory conditions, including COPD and asthma, affect most people. All respiratory diseases have symptoms varying from mild to severe and can also be life-threatening.

Source: https://www.researchgate.net/profile/Jesus-Shrestha/publication/338429576/figure/fig1/AS:847043081797634@1578962216226/Common-respiratory-diseases-respiratory-diseases-are-among-the-leading-cause-of-deaths.png.

Moreover, the interaction between environmental factors, including healthcare access and socioeconomic status, and respiratory disease is a key element of management strategies. Those with comorbid respiratory illnesses such as asthma and COPD are likely to experience deteriorating health outcomes due to inappropriate health services, particularly in low-income environments. Correction of inequalities through public health interventions by education, smoking cessation, and increased access to medication can significantly alter the disease course. Measures to empower communities to access healthcare, raise awareness about respiratory disease, and promote healthy environments can substantially contain the burden of respiratory diseases. In light of the evolving global health landscape, it is imperative to adopt measures across multiple fronts to reduce their incidence and severity (Murray et al., 2022) (Figure 3.6).

3.2.1. Asthma

Asthma, a complex airway disease with persistent inflammation, is a critical international health issue. Its incidence has been on the increase, particularly among children, calling for comprehensive knowledge and control of the disease. Conventional treatments primarily rely on bronchodilators and corticosteroids to treat acute symptoms and inflammation. However, these medications are not without their disadvantages, including potential side effects that could compromise patient adherence to treatment protocols. The growing concern about the long-term safety of conventional pharmacotherapy necessitates exploring alternative approaches, particularly those derived from natural compounds. This is underscored by studies showing the therapeutic promise of molecules such as curcumin and tulsi, which offer a new vision for controlling asthma, aimed at minimizing side effects and maximizing efficacy (Babu et al., 2023). Asthma management is multifaceted and must be addressed on an individual basis, considering the various factors influencing the condition. A representative case is that of an 11-year-old boy who had a marked asthma attack in the midst of a routine inhaler regimen. His symptoms did not resolve, indicating that standard treatment alone was insufficient. After thorough evaluation, he was found to have not only asthma, but also vocal cord dysfunction and psychological conditions, which contributed to his respiratory complaints. This case demonstrates the necessity of thoroughgoing evaluations that extend beyond physiological parameters. In his scenario, resolution of his dyspnea and cough was finally aided by the resolution of underlying psychological etiologies through psychiatric intervention, illustrating that treatment of asthma must be holistic and, in many cases, may require interdisciplinary collaboration between medical specialties (Khazaei et al., 2023).

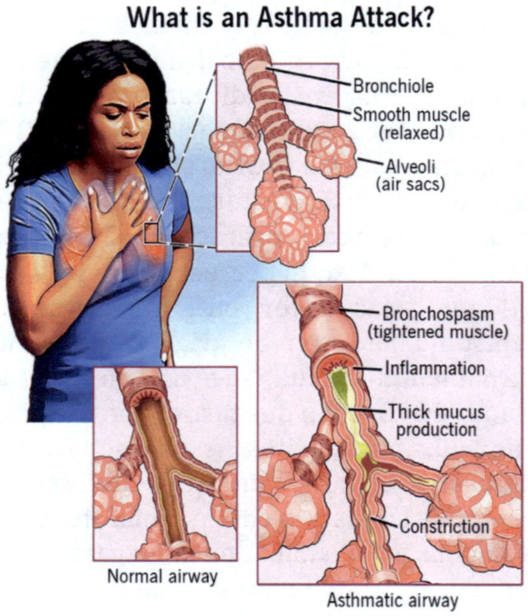

Figure 3.7. Asthma causes bronchospasms, inflammation, thick mucus and constriction in the airways.

Source: https://my.clevelandclinic.org/-/scassets/images/org/health/articles/6424-asthma.

With continued research into the complexities of the interaction among the genetic, environmental, and psychological variables that lead to asthma, it is becoming clearer that traditional treatment paradigms may be insufficient. The potential of incorporating natural products such as curcumin and tulsi in the treatment of asthma is huge. In addition to offering an alternative therapeutic approach, these drugs underscore the importance of safety in the therapeutic regimen. Given the limitations and side effects of conventional drugs, more research is needed to identify and demonstrate the efficacy of these natural treatments in larger numbers. With practitioners moving towards more integrative models of care, understanding more about the bigger picture of patients' lives, like the psychological state, is important. This integrated approach could redefine asthma management, ultimately improving patient outcomes and quality of life (Babu et al., 2023) (Figure 3.7).

3.2.2. Chronic Obstructive Pulmonary Disease (COPD)

Chronic Obstructive Pulmonary Disease (COPD) is now a significant global health concern, with high mortality rates and widespread prevalence requiring acknowledgment. As chronic airflow limitation and persistent respiratory symptoms, such as dyspnea and cough, COPD fundamentally alters the quality of the patient's life. The condition is initiated almost exclusively by chronic exposure to damaging particles or gases, the significant proportion of cases being caused by cigarette smoke. In addition, environmental toxic exposures and workplace hazards are foundational to disease development. The Global Initiative for Chronic Obstructive Lung Disease (GOLD) provides comprehensive guidelines on COPD knowledge and management, addressing the nature and necessity of personalized therapeutic interventions.

Management of this multifaceted disorder includes a holistic strategy that encompasses symptom relief and the control of acute exacerbations, whose impact can significantly affect patient outcomes and healthcare expenditure (Manochithra et al., 2025). In addition to its pulmonary implications, COPD is often associated with various extrapulmonary comorbidities that complicate patient management. Research indicates that psychiatric disorders, like depression and anxiety, frequently co-occur in patients with COPD, aggravating the physical and mental health conditions (Moretta et al., 2024). Two-way interaction between the psychiatric disorders and COPD raises the disease burden on well-being since social isolation and bodily incapacity always cause more psychological distress. Early recognition and management of comorbidities are critical components of high-quality COPD management because they can significantly influence the disease course and quality of life. Multidisciplinary team involvement, including pulmonologists and psychologists, is necessary to address the psychological components of COPD comprehensively, enabling appropriate interventions (Moretta et al., 2024).

Ideal therapeutic strategies for COPD include not only controlling respiratory symptoms but also promoting overall patient well-being, encompassing the physical and psychological dimensions of treatment. There are a variety of pharmacologic therapies in use, ranging from bronchodilators to inhaled corticosteroids and novel drug delivery systems to optimize therapeutic effects while reducing side effects (Manochithra et al., 2025). Recent advances in targeted drug delivery, for instance, the use of nanoparticles, have been hopeful in enhancing drug bioavailability and reducing systemic toxicity. Further, non-pharmacologic strategies, including pulmonary rehabilitation, patient education, and psychological counseling, have been shown to improve overall health outcomes and reduce exacerbation rates. As research continues to advance our understanding of COPD, it is crucial that future studies investigate new treatment modalities, particularly those that integrate mental health evaluation with traditional respiratory care models, providing a clearer picture of how to improve patients' lives (Manochithra et al., 2025) (Figure 3.8).

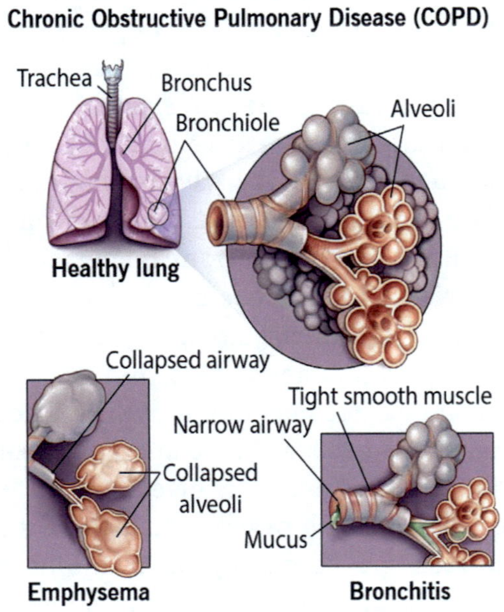

Figure 3.8. Features of COPD include loss of elasticity, inflamed and narrowed airways, enlarged and damaged alveoli, and thick mucus.

Source: https://my.clevelandclinic.org/-/scassets/images/org/health/articles/8709-copd.jpg.

3.2.3. Pneumonia

Pneumonia is a serious respiratory infection that afflicts all age groups of individuals and often leads to high morbidity and mortality. An inflammation of the lung air sacs is a hallmark feature of pneumonia and can be caused by various pathogens, including bacteria, viruses, and fungi. Symptoms of the disease can be mild or severe and range from fever, cough, and dyspnea. Of specific importance are community-acquired pneumonia (CAP), which is a frequent health concern, particularly in vulnerable subjects such as the elderly and children. Another respiratory infection, which is a complication of respiratory infection such as CAP, is aspiration pneumonia (AP), occurring as a result of inhalation of oropharyngeal contents. The state is frequently underdiagnosed in elderly patients who may also have dysphagia, which indicates an extended relationship between respiratory status and swallowing disorders (Ortega et al., 2024). Diagnosis of pneumonia relies on the correlation of clinical and imaging findings. Clinicians prefer using chest X-rays and lab tests to assess the presence of infection and inflammation. Among children, pneumonia remains the primary cause of hospitalization, with public health concerns. A recent retrospective study in the GKMC Swabi Department of Pediatrics documented that out of children who came in with respiratory illness, 40% had pneumonia, indicating the importance of early detection and treatment to prevent complications (Ahmad et al., 2023).

Effective management typically involves a multimodal approach including antibiotic therapy for bacterial pneumonia, supportive care, and in some cases, hospitalization. Knowledge of pneumonia's prevalence, particularly in children under the age of five, underscores the need for increased research into the effectiveness of treatment and prevention measures. Prevention is essential to the relief of pneumonia's burden on public health. Immunization against common pathogens such as Streptococcus pneumoniae and influenza is essential to the prevention of occurrence, especially in high-risk populations, including infants and the elderly. Promotion of good oral hygiene and dysphagia treatment is also a significant step toward the prevention of aspiration pneumonia, as suggested in the new guidelines with an emphasis on the inclusion of artificial intelligence tools in risk stratification (Ortega et al., 2024). Moreover, fostering greater awareness of pneumonia-related risk factors, such as frailty and malnutrition, can encourage preventive interventions in healthcare settings. In sum, prevention of pneumonia, a severe respiratory disease, requires an interdisciplinary approach through efficient treatment regimes and preventative strategies to improve outcomes and reduce the disease burden globally (Figure 3.9).

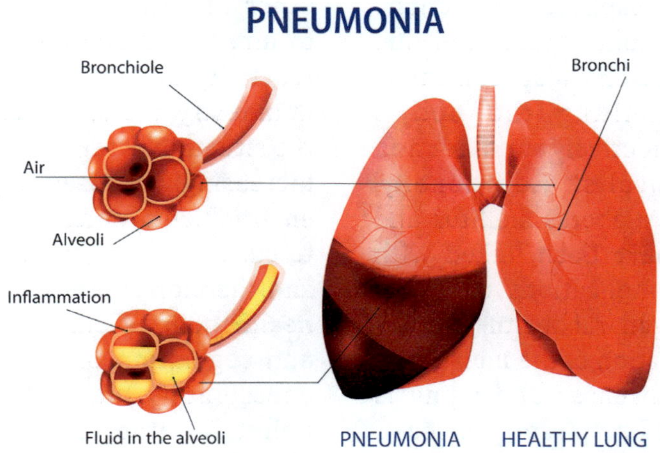

Figure 3.9. Pneumonia.

Source: https://ssbhealthcare.com/wp-content/uploads/2022/11/Pneumonia-1.png.

Test Your Knowledge

1. What is chronic obstructive pulmonary disease (COPD)?
2. What is pneumonia?

3.3. Causes and Risk Factors

Learning Outcome

1. Know the impact of environmental factors on respiratory disorders
2. Understand the genetic predisposition
3. Know the influence of lifestyle choices on respiratory health

The pathogenesis of respiratory conditions is attributable in the majority of instances to an intersection of environmental, biological, and lifestyle factors. The most significant risk determinants are exposure to air pollutants, including tobacco smoke, industrial emissions, and automobile exhaust. Long-term exposure to such pollutants could lead to chronic illness through chronic obstructive pulmonary disease (COPD) and lung carcinoma. Besides, genetics also plays a significant role in determining a person's susceptibility to respiratory illnesses. For instance, patients with a history of asthma or other respiratory diseases in the family are at a higher risk, which means genetic factors can actually make a person highly susceptible to external stimuli. As their interaction grows, it is all the more necessary to understand how they function in harmony to impact respiratory well-being. Old age has been recognized as a significant risk factor for respiratory disease, as physiological changes associated with aging may weaken lung function and resistance. Older individuals have decreased lung elasticity, respiratory muscle strength, and pulmonary secretion clearance, all of which result in an increased prevalence of respiratory infections and chronic disease. Immunosuppression due to age or chronic conditions also continues this downtrend by limiting the body's capacity to respond effectively to infection and environmental insults. Additionally, chronic diseases such as diabetes mellitus and cardiovascular disease have been linked with amplified respiratory complications based on their systemic impact on general health (Oleszko et al., 2025). The identification of the interaction between such chronic diseases and aging is vital in the prevention of respiratory disease. There are certain occupational and behavioral factors that, with significant effects, can elevate the risk of respiratory disease, particularly among high-risk populations. For instance, individuals who are involved in industries with high exposure to dust, chemicals, and irritants, such as manufacturing or construction work, are more likely to develop respiratory diseases such as pneumoconiosis or chemical-induced lung disease. Aside from that, smoking remains among the most important causes of preventable respiratory illness; not only does it directly contribute to lung cancer, but it also makes chronic conditions such as asthma and COPD worse. Developing respiratory illness during operation further underscores how anesthetic and procedural methods can affect outcomes, with respiratory and hemodynamic issues as the leading causes of mortality in these operations (Лебединский et al., 2024). Prevention of these risks through policy action and awareness will be essential to reducing the disease burden of respiratory diseases across various populations.

3.3.1. Environmental Factors

Environmental determinants of respiratory diseases are a crucial area of research, as they play a significant role in their etiology and severity. Air pollution is one of the most critical environmental determinants of the pathogenesis of respiratory diseases like asthma and COPD. Contact with delicate particulate matter and other airborne toxins, as studies show, can lead to airway inflammation, heightened bronchial reactivity, and impaired lung function. The rise in industry and urbanization has also worsened the situation, with larger populations becoming increasingly exposed to poor air quality. These environmental determinants need to be managed to curb the rising rates of respiratory diseases and, therefore, the need for comprehensive public health policies ensuring improved air quality and regulation of automobile and industrial emissions (Jalilova et al., 2024). Besides air pollution, other environmental determinants also play a significant role in the causation and exacerbation of respiratory diseases. Indoor air quality is also underappreciated but extremely crucial to respiratory well-being. Common indoor pollutants such as tobacco smoke, mold, and volatile organic compounds in household cleansers are all well known to exacerbate asthma and induce chronic bronchitis. Additionally, socio-economic status can lead to health inequalities, with poorer communities likely to have more substandard housing and higher levels of indoor air pollution. These conditions exacerbate pre-existing respiratory ailments, creating a cycle of health inequities that is hard to break. Reducing both indoor and outdoor pollution through targeted interventions can curb these risks and improve public health outcomes (Ibrahim, 2024). Climate change poses a multi-dimensional threat to respiratory health because it affects both outdoor air quality and pollen production. Weather pattern changes lead to higher levels of ground-level ozone, which further exacerbate respiratory diseases, particularly in the summer. In addition, warmer temperatures are associated with longer and more intense pollen seasons, hence increased instances of allergic respiratory illnesses. The link between climate change and respiratory diseases calls for an integrated approach to managing health and the environment. Public health interventions must aim at climate interventions targeting greenhouse gas reductions and promoting practices that ensure the most resilient ecosystems, culminating in improved air quality and public health (Ibrahim, 2024; Jalilova et al., 2024) (Figure 3.10).

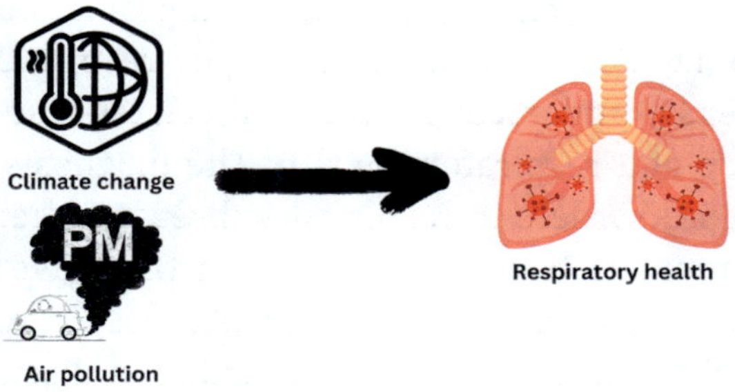

Figure 3.10. The impact of air pollution on respiratory diseases in an era of climate change.

Source: https://ars.els-cdn.com/content/image/1-s2.0-S0048969723049653-ga1_lrg.jpg.

3.3.2. Genetic Predisposition

Genetic susceptibility investigation has a prominent position in determining the etiology of most respiratory ailments, particularly asthma. Asthma is increasingly considered to result from the interaction between environmental and genetic factors. Investigations show that individuals with a family history of asthma have a higher likelihood of being at risk, thus underlining the role of heritability in asthma. Genetic studies have mapped numerous loci associated with asthma susceptibility and identified major pathways implicated in airway inflammation and hyperreactivity. The genetic architecture not only determines the mechanism of asthma initiation but also directs therapeutic targets, paving the way for precision medicine approaches based on genetic underpinnings. Consequently, understanding the genetic underpinnings of asthma can provide better prevention and treatment strategies that address individual susceptibility based on genetic makeup. Furthermore, interaction between obesity and respiratory illness, in particular asthma, sheds light on the multidimensional nature of genetic predispositions. Obesity impacts the severity and prevalence of asthma via numerous mechanisms, including systemic inflammation and lung mechanical changes. Research has shown that genetic factors that contribute to higher body mass index (BMI) can predispose to respiratory conditions such as asthma. For instance, from extensive cohort studies, evidence indicates a high association between genetic susceptibility to increased BMI and increased risk for lower respiratory tract infections and severe wheezing among children, irrespective of their current BMI (Jensen et al., 2024).

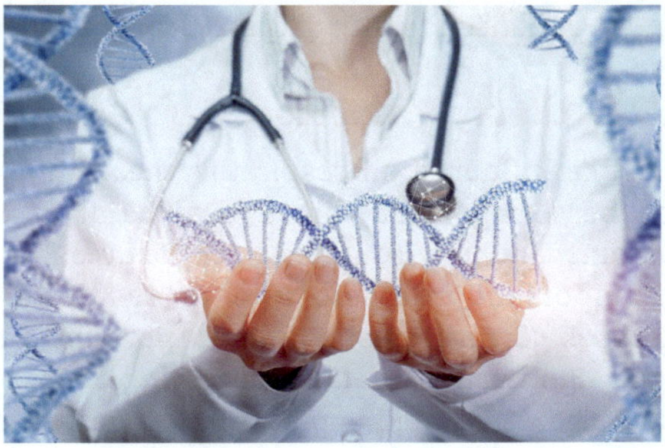

Figure 3.11. Genetic predisposition.

Source: https://centerforfamilymedicine.com/wp-content/uploads/2021/02/center-for-family-medicine-What-Does-It-Mean-To-Have-A-Genetic-Predisposition-Family-History-And-Your-Health.jpg.

This would mean that genetic predisposition to obesity may expose people not just to metabolic diseases but also to respiratory diseases, implying overlapping biological mechanisms that need to be investigated further. Moreover, genetic predisposition is not limited to asthma and obesity and explains the connection between other respiratory disorders and psychiatric disorders. The heritability of eating disorders is heavily entwined with respiratory well-being, revealing a complex neurobiological setting in which genetics plays an important role. Genetic research has identified specific genes associated with eating disorders that may affect respiratory health through mechanisms of inflammation and neurobehavioral factors (Rashid et al., 2025). The relationship between eating behavior, genetic predisposition, and the respiratory system reinforces the need for an integrated health concept involving both physical and mental status. The recognition of genetic predisposition of multifactorial origin can thus direct more holistic therapeutic interventions in the management of the interaction between psychiatric and respiratory disorders with the aim of enhanced health (Figure 3.11).

3.3.3. Lifestyle Choices

Lifestyle influence on respiratory health must not be exaggerated, since the majority of customs and environmental exposures have an important etiologic role in respiratory diseases. Cigarette smoking is perhaps the most significant risk factor for lung function since cigarette smoking places injurious factors on lung tissue and aggravates conditions like COPD and asthma. Moreover, being exposed to secondhand smoke is highly perilous to non-smokers, and particularly children, and they can develop various breathing conditions. Alongside smoking, physical inactivity and diet are also contributory factors towards respiratory health. Involvement in regular physical activity has been shown to improve lung function and respiratory capacity, and antioxidant-rich diets may mitigate oxidative stress and inflammation, thereby supporting better overall lung health, as indicated by sleep health studies and their impact on chronic illness, including respiratory disease (Porcacchia et al., 2025).

Moreover, sleeping patterns are increasingly viewed as a vital element of life habits that influences respiratory health. Sleep disorder patients, such as those with sleep apnea, usually experience disturbed breathing during sleep, which may render them more prone to illnesses such as cardiovascular disease and respiratory disease. Research has established that sleep-breathing disorder symptomatology is linked to an increased risk of respiratory disease, underscoring the interrelatedness of sleep and respiratory health. The diagnosis of sleep disorders in respiratory disease patients exemplifies two-way causality in that adverse sleep outcomes can exacerbate respiratory ailments, initiating a chain reaction of disease. Therefore, sleep health consciousness and its relevance in the context of respiratory diseases are instrumental in creating comprehensive treatment methods to improve sleep quality and reduce the incidence of respiratory illnesses among populations (Porcacchia et al., 2025).

In addition, other allied lifestyle measures, such as diet and physical exercise, can significantly affect respiratory diseases, rendering lifestyle selection an intimate association with an individual's well-being. A bad diet, such as high salt and sugar intake, raises the risk of hypertension, an illness with a close association with lung function. Evidence from research points toward eating a nutritious diet low in processed food but rich in whole grains, fruits, and vegetables to enhance lung function and reduce inflammation-related respiratory illness. In parallel with dietary modification, the addition of routine exercise—emphasized for its capacity to strengthen the immune system and shield against chronic stress—can likewise be the deciding element in the management of risk factors for respiratory conditions. Concentration on such lifestyle modification cannot only avert symptoms of already established respiratory disease but also potentially offer preventive therapy against the development of respiratory complications in the future (Figure 3.12).

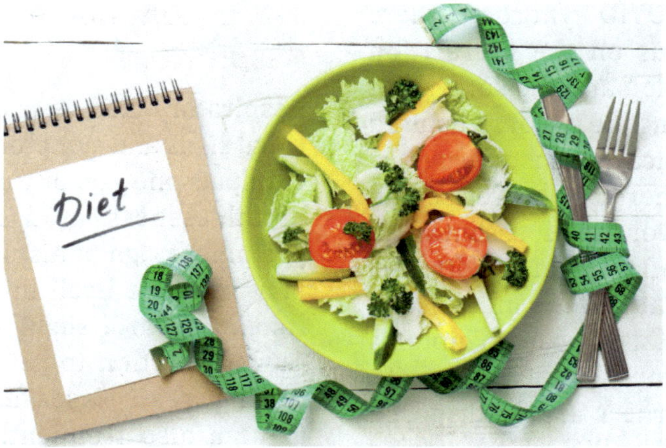

Figure 3.12. Role of diet and lifestyle in respiratory diseases.

Source: https://bibo.health/cdn/shop/articles/blog_75.png?v=1682069575.

Test Your Knowledge

1. What is the impact of environmental factors on respiratory disorders?
2. What is the meaning of genetic predisposition?

3.4. Symptoms and Diagnosis

Learning Outcome

1. Understand the common symptoms of respiratory disorders
2. Describe the diagnostic tests and procedures of respiratory disorders
3. Understand the importance of early detection of respiratory disorders

Accurate recognition of symptoms is of central importance for the diagnosis of respiratory illnesses, as these manifestations typically play the first role in signaling the presence of underlying pathologies. The most frequently met symptoms are chronic cough, wheezing, shortness of breath, and chest pain. All of them can vary considerably in severity and duration based on the specific disease and the patient's medical history. For instance, a chronic cough may point towards anything ranging from asthma to severe conditions such as COPD. Moreover, detailed history-taking, including assessment of environmental and occupational exposure, is essential for determining the precise nature of the disorder. The consciousness of situational history of these symptoms enables medical professionals to formulate targeted diagnostic investigations and guide subsequent treatment regimens accordingly. Diagnosis of respiratory disorders is usually a multi-step process that includes clinical evaluation, radiological studies, and laboratory studies. Physical examination usually begins with auscultation to detect abnormal breath sounds, which can provide crucial pointers to pathology. This is followed by imaging techniques such as chest X-rays or CT scans to visualize the lung parenchyma and detect abnormalities, such as inflammation or fluid accumulation. Furthermore, laboratory testing, for instance, complete blood counts and sputum cultures, are also part of infectious etiology or inflammatory process identification.

In the context of post-COVID syndrome, there has been a greater focus on the correlation between symptom duration and the severity of past infections, highlighting the use of structured patient histories to enhance diagnostic accuracy (Greissel et al., 2024). Therefore, a precise and systematic diagnostic workup is essential to effective management of respiratory disease. Recent literature has identified the influence of comorbidities on respiratory disease symptoms and diagnoses. For example, individuals with histories of mental disorders are predisposed to develop illnesses such as PCS, characterized by chronic systemic and respiratory symptoms ranging from malaise to fatigue (Greissel et al., 2024). Such a connection underscores the reality that healthcare providers need to consider a broad spectrum of factors when diagnosing respiratory conditions, especially post-infection sequelae. The effects of these comorbidities extend beyond symptom management as they can significantly affect patients' quality of life and mortality risk, particularly in older adults who have severe respiratory diseases (Bilichenko, 2022). These results highlight the importance of treatment plans that address not only respiratory symptoms but also psychosocial concerns, with the ultimate goal of improving patient outcomes (Figure 3.13).

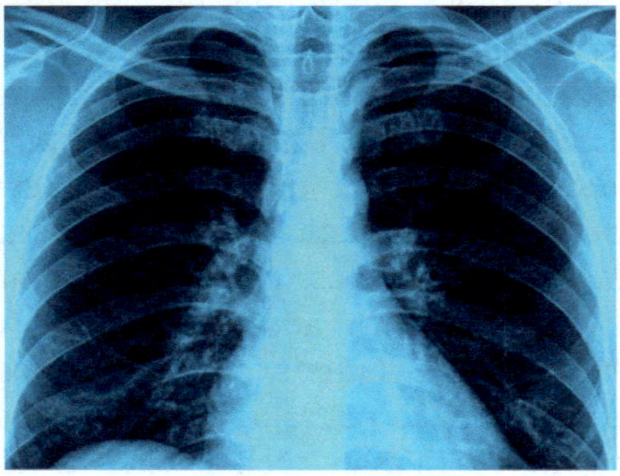

Figure 3.13. COPD X-ray.

Source: https://media.post.rvohealth.io/wp-content/uploads/sites/3/2018/10/COPD_X-ray_GettyImages92988886_Thumb-732x549.jpg.

3.4.1. Common Symptoms of Respiratory Disorders

Respiratory disease is characterized by a set of usual signs and symptoms that have the capacity to impact one's quality of life negatively. Of these, breathlessness, or dyspnea, is a particularly prominent sign of respiratory distress. Dyspnea may manifest itself in a wide variety of ways, ranging from a slight sense of breathlessness during exertion to severe shortness of breath during rest. Diseases such as COPD and asthma also frequently occur with dyspnea, which is suggestive of airway obstruction or inflammation beneath. Wheezing, a whistling sound on the breath, is also frequently present in diseases such as bronchitis and asthma. Together, these symptoms not only impinge on everyday functioning but also constitute significant clinical signs for the diagnosis and management of respiratory disease, suggesting the need for prompt medical evaluation at the time of presentation. In addition to wheezing and dyspnea, patients with respiratory illness often present with chronic cough, productive or non-productive. This is a major feature of many respiratory diseases, including pneumonia, bronchitis, and even allergies. A productive cough, which includes the production of phlegm or mucus, is a sign of a chronic infection or chronic airway inflammation. But a dry or non-productive cough may be a sign of asthma or environmental irritation. These diverse features are critical tips for clinicians in assessing the underlying pathology of respiratory conditions. Specifically, in evaluating cough as a symptom, doctors analyze its duration, frequency, and related signs to make the correct diagnosis and treatment plan, highlighting the significance of thorough symptom analysis in respiratory health. Chest pain is a notable other symptom of diverse respiratory conditions. This symptom can range from mild discomfort to a severe acute pain that can mimic cardiac attacks. Chest pain in respiratory diseases is typically due to pleuritic inflammation or muscle strain induced by relentless coughing. Pneumonia, pulmonary embolism, and pleurisy frequently present with a manifesting symptom of chest pain and require careful diagnostic examination. In addition, the coexistence of fever with other systemic presentations can indicate infections that compromise respiratory function and must be managed urgently. Awareness of the etiology and clinical presentation of chest pain in respiratory illness not only aids diagnosis but also highlights the intricate interdependence of respiratory and systemic health. Secondly, it emphasizes the need for prompt clinical assessment to avoid complications, particularly in susceptible populations such as those with impaired immune response or comorbid conditions, as in the use of bacterial infections referenced among studies in patients with hematologic disorders (Shimada et al., 2024) (Figure 3.14).

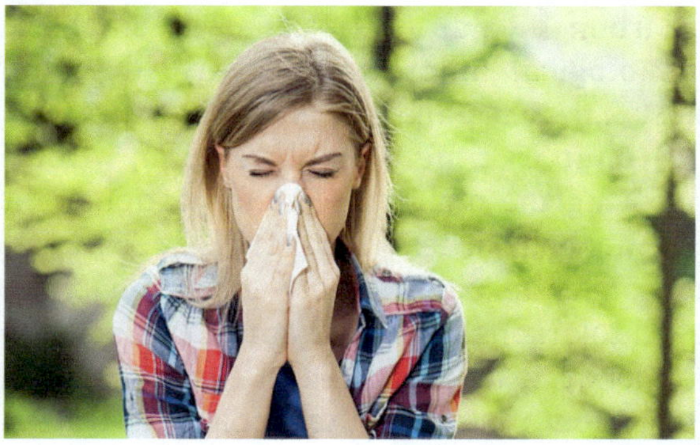

Figure 3.14. Common respiratory disease symptoms.

Source: https://www.unitedconcordia.com/content/dam/ucd/en/commercial/website/images/wp-content/uploads/2018/04/allergy_547181.jpg.

3.4.2. Diagnostic Tests and Procedures

In respiratory disease, diagnostic testing and examinations are necessary for diagnosing and treating various conditions effectively. These examinations are necessary for determining the existence of the disease, the severity of the condition, and the management of treatment. Standard tests such as chest X-rays and pulmonary function tests (PFTs) are important in the diagnostic process. A chest X-ray can visualize lung structures and reveal signs of infection, tumors, or pleural effusions. PFTs like spirometry assess lung function by measuring the volume and rate of airflow during inhalation and exhalation, which is helpful in diagnosing conditions like asthma and COPD. These preliminary tests help clinicians make informed decisions about further specialized testing and treatment, optimizing patient safety and quality of care. Greater specificity in diagnosing respiratory disease frequently necessitates advanced imaging techniques. Computed tomography (CT) scanning, particularly high-resolution thoracic CT (HRCT), provides detailed visualization of lung parenchyma that may be below the level of detection on routine X-rays. This technique is particularly important for identifying interstitial lung diseases (ILDs) with fibrosis, as advanced imaging can distinguish fibrosis patterns and abnormalities that are not visible on standard scans. CT scan results play an important role in treatment and therapeutic management of diseases such as idiopathic pulmonary fibrosis. In addition, invasive procedures, such as bronchoscopy and transbronchial biopsies, allow for direct visualization and biopsy of lung tissue, aiding in the diagnosis of malignancy or idiopathic lung disease. These sophisticated methods strengthen the methodological basis for expanding the knowledge base of a patient's respiratory health. In addition, the requirement for successful diagnostic assessment extends beyond the limited determination of respiratory diseases; it encompasses a panoramic vision of patient care. As illustrated by research, ILD prevalence underscores the need for meticulous diagnostic evaluation, with many patients receiving a range of tests, such as bronchoalveolar lavage and tissue biopsies, to ensure proper diagnoses (Fenech et al., 2012). The data acquired with these tests tell clinicians not only the type of respiratory disorder but also the appropriate management pathways—ranging from corticosteroid regimens to more aggressive immunosuppressive therapy. The incorporation of diverse diagnostic modalities thus ensures that patients receive tailored management, improving health-related quality of life and clinical outcome in general. This emphasis on those specific patient assessments is paramount, since the relationship between diagnostic findings and therapeutic choices can significantly affect long-term respiratory health and recovery strategies (Bilzer et al., 2002) (Figure 3.15).

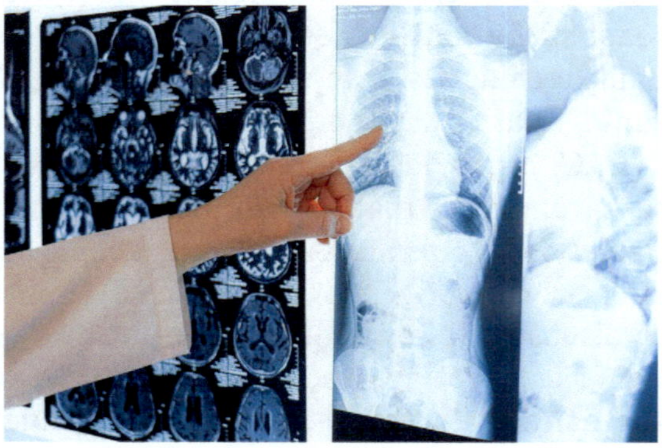

Figure 3.15. Diagnostic tests for respiratory disorders.

Source: https://coughpro.com/wp-content/uploads/2022/09/diagnostic-tests-.jpg.

3.4.3. Importance of Early Detection

Early diagnosis of respiratory disease is crucial for optimizing patient outcomes and enhancing the effectiveness of treatment strategies. If respiratory diseases like COPD or asthma are diagnosed early, there is a greater opportunity to apply measures that can prevent the disease from advancing. This preventive approach not only relieves symptoms but also curtails the likelihood of developing life-threatening complications associated with advanced stages of such diseases. By using advanced diagnostic equipment and technologies, medical professionals can detect abnormal breathing patterns and airway constriction at earlier stages. For instance, recent developments in applying machine learning methods to monitor respiratory dynamics using Photoplethysmography (PPG) signals highlight this need, indicating that early detection can form the foundation for effective management of respiratory well-being (Manochithra et al., 2025). Apart from improving treatment success, early detection contributes to the more comprehensive optimization of healthcare resources. By early identification of respiratory disorders, health practitioners can tailor interventions to be less traumatic and less expensive. This not only saves healthcare systems but also minimizes the economic impact on patients and their families. Besides, machine learning models, such as those based on the Chi2 Probability Density Function and the Cuckoo Search model, for Partial Pressure of Carbon Dioxide (PCO_2) analysis emphasize technological innovation in early detection. These models enhance diagnostic precision and enable timely intervention, greatly improving the quality of life for patients with respiratory disorders (Afsal et al., 2025). Lastly, the consequences of early detection extend beyond personal health to societal effects on a grander scale in public health. Additionally, the integration of advanced technology in tracking respiratory health promotes the importance of early detection through greater availability. Technological advancements in low-cost, non-invasive diagnosis, such as the use of LASSO regression to identify significant respiratory signals, can be applied across settings, including primary care and telemonitoring environments. This allows anyone, particularly individuals from marginalized populations, to be able to access early diagnosis and treatment. Consequently, health systems are particularly well-situated to deal with the burden of respiratory disease, an ongoing chief source of morbidity and mortality worldwide. Therefore, the importance of early detection in the arena of respiratory disease cannot be overestimated; it is a critical component that facilitates improved health results, optimal utilization of resources, and equitable access to health intervention, thus transforming the environment of respiratory health care (Manochithra et al., 2025) (Figure 3.16).

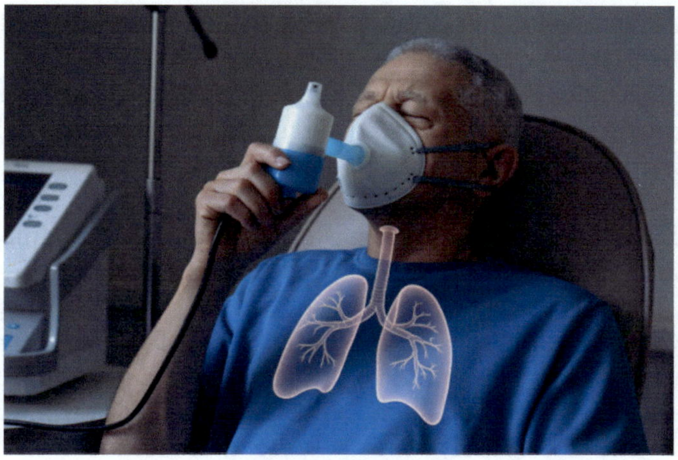

Figure 3.16. The role of spirometry in early detection of respiratory diseases.

Source: https://www.coherentmarketinsights.com/blogimg/1739964339.jpg.

Test Your Knowledge

1. What is the diagnostic test for respiratory disease?
2. Why is early detection important in the treatment of respiratory disorders?

3.5. Treatment Options

Learning Outcome

1. Learn about medications and inhalers in the management of respiratory disorders
2. Know the lifestyle modifications in the management of respiratory disorders
3. Describe the surgical interventions in the management of various respiratory disorders

Treatment modalities for respiratory disease include a broad range of interventions focused on symptom relief, lung function improvement, and quality-of-life improvement. The cornerstone of the treatment of diseases such as asthma and chronic obstructive pulmonary disease (COPD) is bronchodilators, corticosteroids, and other medications. Bronchodilators, for instance, relax bronchial smooth muscle and thereby dilate the airways and improve airflow, a key for those with acute exacerbation. Corticosteroids, on the other hand, address inflammation deep within the airways, reducing the frequency and severity of asthma attacks. Newer therapies, such as biologics targeting specific inflammatory mechanisms, offer alternative avenues for patients with severe or chronic forms of these diseases, underscoring the need for individualized regimens tailored to the patient's needs. Other than the pharmacological interventions, non-pharmacological strategies are also essential in the general management of respiratory disorders. Pulmonary rehabilitation facilities have been discovered to encourage physical functioning and healthier lifestyles among patients with chronic respiratory illness. Pulmonary rehabilitation programs most commonly combine exercise training, dietary counseling, and educationally oriented components to empower patients to manage their condition more effectively. Furthermore, smoking cessation treatments remain an essential component of therapy for tobacco-induced respiratory conditions based on the well-documented impact of tobacco on the lungs. As multidisciplinary treatments, they not only contribute to the benefit of the patient but also to improved understanding of how changes in behavior can reverse respiratory disease. In more complex situations, such as respiratory disease due to obesity, the application of targeted therapies might offer new avenues to improve the patient's quality of life. Research indicates that obesity strongly increases the risk of respiratory disease from associated disorders of obstructive sleep apnea and lung dysfunction (Varra et al., 2024). Thus, weight management, exercise, and dietary modifications are significant components of the treatment regimen of these patients. Moreover, new therapies for the treatment of chronic inflammation that characterizes obesity are being developed, emphasizing the need for individualized treatment addressing the interface between respiratory and metabolic disease. This interdisciplinary approach provides a framework for improved management of respiratory disease, opening promising avenues for future investigation into treatment methods tailored to the complexity of each patient's condition (Mroczek et al., 2023).

3.5.1. Medications and Inhalers

In the management of respiratory disease, medication and inhalers are critical components that facilitate effective therapy and adherence. Medications such as bronchodilators, corticosteroids, and leukotriene modifiers all play distinct roles in alleviating symptoms and controlling inflammation in asthma and chronic obstructive pulmonary disease (COPD). Each of these classes of drugs operates through distinct mechanisms within the respiratory system to improve airflow and reduce exacerbations. For example, beta-agonists, a common feature of inhalers, provide quick relief by relaxing smooth muscle in the bronchial passages. Knowledge of the pharmacodynamics and pharmacokinetics of these drugs will help healthcare professionals tailor treatment regimens, thereby increasing patient compliance and maximizing therapeutic outcomes. Inhalers, especially metered-dose inhalers (MDIs) and dry powder inhalers (DPIs), play a central role in delivering these drugs directly to the lungs. MDIs employ pressurized cans that deliver a metered dose of drug in the shape of an aerosol, while DPIs rely on the patient's breathing to activate the device. The choice between MDI and DPI is typically based on patient preference, specific physiological conditions, and aerosol transmission risk factors, particularly observed during the COVID-19 pandemic. Current studies indicate that, although nebulization is still a common method of drug delivery, it is challenging in terms of viral spread due to aerosol formation. This has prompted clinicians to debate the safety of nebulizers compared with inhalers, which requires comparing their functionality with clinical evidence where available (Sengupta, 2024). Moreover, inhalers contain a dose of medication that effectively manages chronic respiratory disease, yet proper technique and patient education must be used when using them as well. Inappropriate use of inhalers will lead to ineffective drug delivery and control of symptoms, eventually causing increased risk of exacerbations and hospitalizations. Regular training and re-evaluation of inhaler technique are crucial for patients with respiratory diseases, particularly those with conditions such as Down Syndrome, where anatomical variations and hypotonia may pose challenges to medication adherence (Everard et al., 2025). As healthcare professionals adapt to a shifting landscape of respiratory care, the incorporation of patient-centered care practices with technological innovation will continue to improve asthma and COPD management results. Therefore, an integrated approach that focuses on medication and inhaler education is crucial in promoting patient empowerment and improving overall respiratory well-being (Figure 3.17).

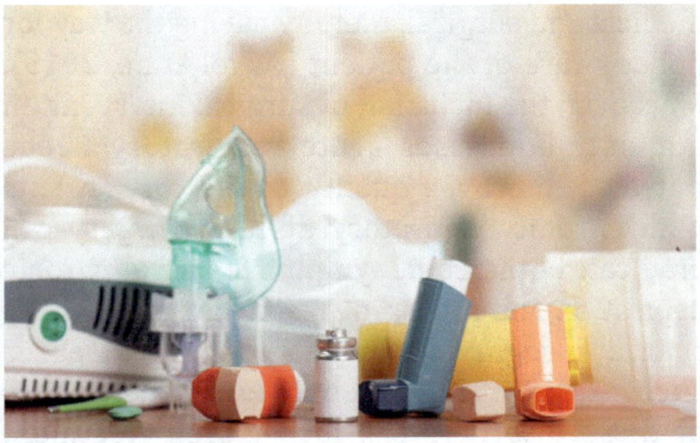

Figure 3.17. Inhaler devices for respiratory medicines.

Source: https://www.nps.org.au/assets/_750x468_crop_center-center_75_none/GettyImages-868815768.jpg.

3.5.2. Lifestyle Modifications

Lifestyle modification is an integral part of respiratory disorder treatment, significantly affecting symptom relief and overall disease prognosis. Cessation of smoking is one of the most essential among these modifications in patients with chronic obstructive pulmonary disease (COPD) or asthma. Smoking increases airway inflammation and is a cause of chronic bronchitis and emphysema, two conditions that severely compromise respiratory function. Smoking cessation sessions that expose people to behavioral therapy and medication to relieve cravings have yielded promising results. In addition, a smoke-free home environment improves the lung health of both patients and their household members, thereby reducing the occurrence of respiratory-related complications among non-smoking family members. Emphasizing these habits is crucial in improving an integrated approach to the management of respiratory disorders and the overall well-being of the patients. Exercise as part of daily habits is another highly significant lifestyle modification that can greatly benefit people with respiratory issues. Exercise makes the lungs larger and the respiratory muscles more powerful, leading to greater oxygen use and greater endurance. Recommended exercises are typically aerobic, such as walking, swimming, or cycling, for at least 150 minutes per week at moderate intensity. Besides, attending respiratory rehabilitation sessions can also teach patients appropriate breathing skills and exercises tailored to their conditions to help maintain symptom control and improve quality of life. It has been revealed that exercise regularly can also reduce the acceleration of asthma attacks as well as enhance the respiratory function of chronic disease patients. Thus, incorporating exercise into one's life is a powerful medicine for effectively managing respiratory disorders. Nutrition is also another important factor in lifestyle modifications that can be applied to respiratory function. A well-balanced diet rich in fruits, vegetables, whole grains, and omega-3 fatty acids can help individuals manage inflammation and support overall immunity. For example, specific nutrients like vitamin C and antioxidants in certain foods can regulate oxidative stress in lung tissue and improve pulmonary function. Additionally, maintaining a healthy weight through proper diet is essential because obesity is a key factor that can hinder lung function and increase the severity of respiratory diseases. The integration of these dietary changes offers a basis for improved respiratory health, ultimately enabling patients to maintain their own health. Enhancement of lifestyle changes in an integrated form not only allays the symptoms of respiratory diseases but also instills long-term immunity against potential complications, thereby improving the quality of life of patients (Figure 3.18).

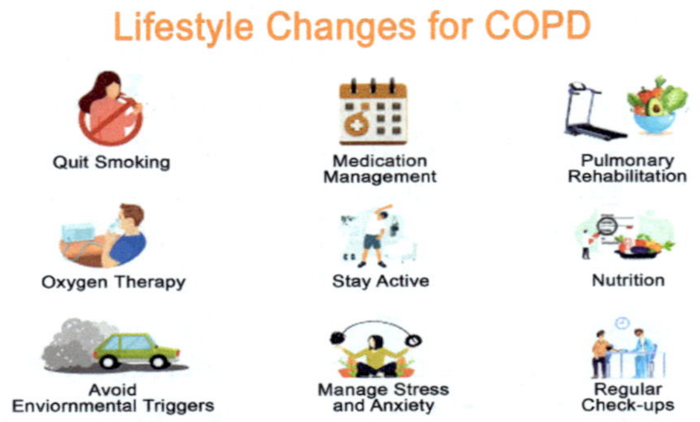

Figure 3.18. Lifestyle changes for COPD.

Source: https://d1qoubmzbxxtfm.cloudfront.net/wp-content/uploads/Living-with-COPD3.jpg.

3.5.3. Surgical Interventions

Surgery plays a vital role in the treatment of most respiratory diseases when conventional medical interventions prove to be ineffective. Surgery is able to cure anatomical defects that lead to obstructive effects, thereby improving airflow alongside overall respiratory function. Septoplasty and turbinate reduction are common operations to correct defects in nasal passage structures, enabling unobstructed breathing. In addition, in those with very severe COPD or asthma, surgical lung volume reduction may be an option to remove non-functioning lung tissue to enhance pulmonary function. Whether or not to undergo any surgery is a multifaceted decision requiring careful consideration of the unique individual patient factors, including the severity of the disorder and co-morbid illnesses that may complicate the risk of surgery. In some cases, e.g., mucopolysaccharidosis (MPS), surgery is particularly complicated. There has been evidence-based practice foregrounding the need to address not only the immediate respiratory complications but also their concomitant complications because the disorders are systemic in nature. Surgical treatment in the guise of tracheostomy is an option for complicated respiratory failure with adequate ventilation and oxygenation that fails non-invasive means. Apart from this, the involvement of a multidisciplinary team of physicians in such a scenario is important for ensuring desired results. The recommendations and guidelines formulated through the collective work of various healthcare professionals provide significant avenues for the treatment of respiratory manifestations of MPS, both medical and surgical, thereby paving the way for holistic care of the patient (Akyol et al., 2019). Moreover, the inclusion of surgical intervention not only addresses acute respiratory needs but also improves quality of life for patients with chronic respiratory disease. Surgery can eradicate bothersome symptoms, such as chronic aspiration and recurrent respiratory infections, that are regularly encountered in diseases such as MPS VI. The specific characteristics of these disorders call for tailored treatment where surgical procedures can be employed alongside other forms of therapy, such as enzyme replacement or hematopoietic stem cell transplantation. Taking a broad treatment approach that includes surgery can help health care professionals optimize patient outcomes and make a greater overall impact on health and wellness. Therefore, existing research and consensus among doctors emphasize operative intervention as a critical component in treating respiratory disease (Akyol et al., 2019) (Figure 3.19).

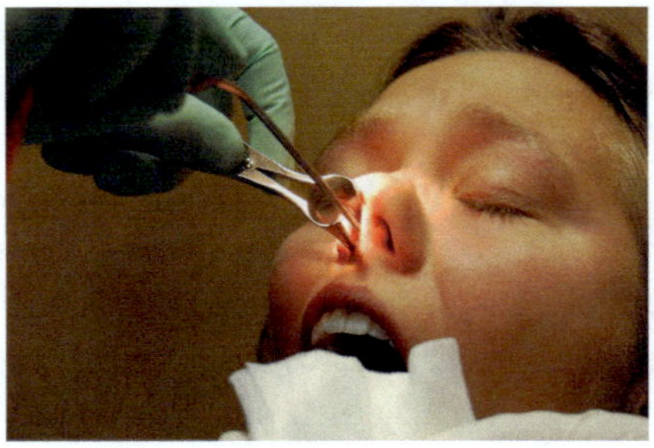

Figure 3.19. Septoplasty and turbinate surgery.

Source: https://www.belsareenthospital.com/wp-content/uploads/2016/11/5906967326_424a921b4e_b.jpg.

Test Your Knowledge

1. What medication is used for respiratory disease?
2. How can maintaining a healthy lifestyle help us to prevent respiratory disorders?

3.6. Prevention and Management

Learning Outcome

1. Describe the prevention strategies for respiratory disorders
2. Understand the importance of regular check-ups in managing respiratory disorders
3. Understand the role of education and awareness in addressing respiratory disorders

Effective prevention and control are crucial in respiratory disease, as early action can make a dramatic difference in patient outcomes. Awareness of risk factors such as smoking, environmental pollutants, and work-related exposures is a key strategy. Public information campaigns can equip people with the knowledge needed to prevent exposure to these risks. Furthermore, public health initiatives that address air quality control and smoking cessation make a notable contribution towards the prevention of respiratory disease. The CDC's Building Resilience Against Climate Effects (BRACE) framework highlights community resilience as vital to public health by demonstrating how effective strategies can make communities prepared for cleaner air and better respiratory disease outcomes (Aytur et al., 2014). By uniting education and regulation, we can establish the environments that foster lung health and minimize the incidence of respiratory illness. From prevention onwards, effective management of existing respiratory illnesses requires a multi-faceted approach involving both treatment and lifestyle changes. The plan of treatment should also be specific to the nature of the respiratory disorder diagnosed, ranging from bronchodilators for asthma to corticosteroids for inflammatory disorders. There is also a need for continued monitoring to detect disease progression, as in the management of pulmonary hypertension, where it guides treatment changes (Abbott et al., 2020). The patients must be made to participate actively in the process of care, be able to recognize signs of exacerbation, and remain adherent to therapy. Merging clinical management with patient education has been shown to enhance self-efficacy and help people become independent in managing their own health, eventually leading to improved respiratory health. It also necessitates integrating interdisciplinary care teams, including physicians, nurses, respiratory therapists, and social workers. These health care workers can collaborate to deliver integrated care that addresses not only the physical dimensions of respiratory diseases but also the psychological and social ones, which can determine patient compliance with therapy. Furthermore, intersectoral collaboration, for instance, between Public Health and community organizations, can enhance access to resources, such as pulmonary rehabilitation and smoking cessation services. According to the BRACE framework, addressing social determinants of health is essential to formulating effective strategies that resonate with heterogeneous populations (Aytur et al., 2014). By establishing a climate of teamwork and diversity, prevention and management efforts may become both inclusive and dynamic, and ultimately enhance the well-being and health of those affected by respiratory diseases (Figure 3.20).

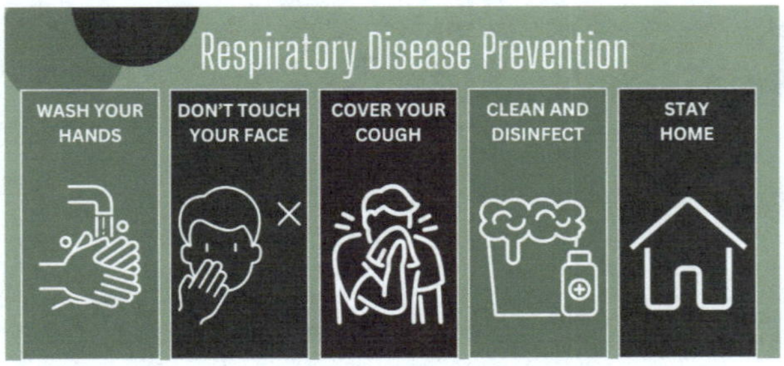

Figure 3.20. Respiratory diseases prevention.

Source: https://www.lbphd.ne.gov/vimages/shared/vnews/stories/64c0151ddbc84/Add%20a%20subheading%20(29).png.

3.6.1. Strategies for Prevention

Successful prevention interventions for respiratory disease involve a multi-pronged approach that reduces risk factors and promotes healthier settings. Education plays a key role in prevention interventions, particularly educating individuals about the dangers of tobacco smoking and exposure to air pollution. Prevention interventions that teach awareness of the significance of tobacco avoidance and inhalation of noxious agents can go a long way in impacting lung health. Additionally, focused awareness campaigns targeted at groups of individuals, such as employees in the industrial sector exposed to volatile organic compounds, can instill protective practices and the wearing of personal protective equipment. The enforcement of overall workplace safety standards, especially in petroleum-based industries, also helps reduce health hazards associated with long-term exposure to fuel pollutants (Al-Barnawi, 2025). By creating an informed populace and offering environmental health protection, we can feasibly decrease the incidence of respiratory illness. Another main prevention technique is promoting pulmonary rehabilitation centers, particularly for those already diagnosed with chronic respiratory disease. Not only do these programs focus on symptom control, but also on the importance of exercise and overall health. There is evidence that, with structured pulmonary rehabilitation, patients' lung function and quality of life can be enhanced, reducing the use of drugs (Krzykawski et al., 2024). Such rehabilitation programs, involving nutritional counseling and psychotherapy, aim to meet every need of an individual, thereby promoting healthier self-management of disease. Physical exercise also promotes regular physical activity, thereby reducing the risk of lung cancer and pneumonia and serving as an inhibiting factor in other respiratory complications. Inclusion of overall rehabilitation in medical practice can thus adequately cater to prevention and treatment of respiratory disorders. Furthermore, considering environmental factors is important for preventing respiratory disorders. Strict controls over air quality, particularly in cities, can actually reduce exposure to noxious pollutants known to exacerbate respiratory diseases. Campaigning for cleaner-burning fuels and more stringent emission standards can achieve tangible gains in public health. Public policy interventions that lower air pollution not only safeguard vulnerable populations, but they also yield long-term health dividends for the lungs. Similarly, initiatives that encourage the reduction of indoor air pollutants, such as cooking or heating, should be given priority. Encouraging practices such as improved indoor ventilation and the use of non-toxic materials can help prevent respiratory diseases. Through policy interventions, community engagement, and individual practices, we can construct a strong foundation for preventing respiratory diseases (Krzykawski et al., 2024).

3.6.2. Importance of Regular Check-Ups

Follow-ups on a routine basis are a staple of respiratory disease treatment because they enable early detection and treatment, significantly improving patient outcomes. By visiting patients periodically, physicians can monitor lung function and detect changes in conditions such as asthma, COPD, and lesser-known conditions such as Potter's syndrome. For instance, the prompt identification of infant respiratory distress due to congenital causes can lead to essential preemptive care that maximizes survival. For example, in a reported case of Potter's syndrome, early antenatal management might have altered the neonate's treatment pathway, highlighting the importance of frequent medical follow-up and evaluation (Agrawal et al., 2025). This vigil underscores how proactive health care can avoid acute crises by promoting early intervention and tailored treatment regimens. In addition to early diagnosis, regular check-ups also assist with patient education and adherence to the therapy regimen. The visits provide an excellent opportunity for healthcare providers to discuss prevention and the risk factors for respiratory illness. For high-risk patients for developing illness such as oral submucous fibrosis (OSF), it is impossible to overstate the importance of knowing because knowledge empowers them to make informed decisions that can potentially avert their risk. Serial visits enable one to continuously assess the efficacy of the interventions and make necessary changes as guided by the treatment providers. The risk of malignant change in OSF underscores the utmost significance of follow-up (Gondivkar et al., 2020). Through frequent follow-ups, healthcare providers are able to encourage adherence to lifestyle modification recommendations and keep patients cognizant of changes in their health condition. Furthermore, frequent check-ups serve to provide leverage for the doctor-patient relationship, which enhances the overall effectiveness of care for respiratory disease. A healthy relationship facilitates open communication, allowing patients to air concerns and difficulties with their health that might otherwise go unnoticed. This relationship is essential for conditions that must be managed over time and lifestyle modifications, as the intricacies of respiratory disease frequently cause patient frustration and discontentment. Frequent interaction during health evaluations fosters a partnership atmosphere, enabling patients to become active participants in their health plans. These collaborations of patients and providers not only create more positive health results but also guide towards an overall higher quality of life because patients feel more supported and engaged in their medical treatment (Figure 3.21).

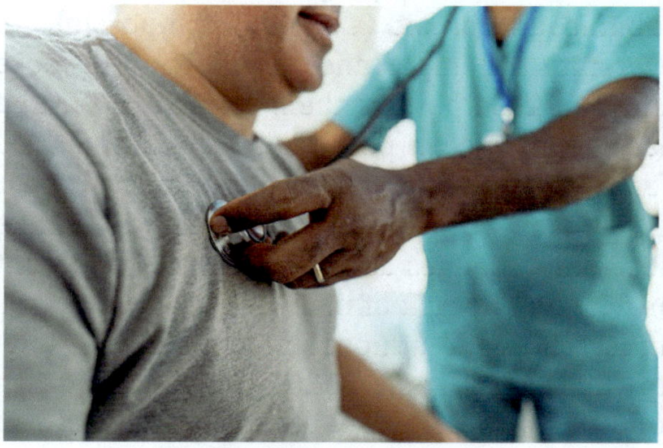

Figure 3.21. The importance of regular check-ups.

Source: https://www.sjpp.org/wp-content/uploads/2024/02/check-ups.jpg.

3.6.3. Role of Education and Awareness

Follow-ups on a routine basis are a staple of respiratory disease treatment because they enable early detection and treatment, significantly improving patient outcomes. By visiting patients periodically, physicians can monitor lung function and detect changes in conditions such as asthma, COPD, and lesser-known conditions such as Potter's syndrome. For instance, the prompt identification of infant respiratory distress due to congenital causes can lead to essential preemptive care that maximizes survival. For example, in a reported case of Potter's syndrome, early antenatal management might have altered the neonate's treatment pathway, highlighting the importance of frequent medical follow-up and evaluation (Agrawal et al., 2025). This vigil underscores how proactive health care can avoid acute crises by promoting early intervention and tailored treatment regimens. In addition to early diagnosis, regular check-ups also assist with patient education and adherence to therapy regimens. The visits provide an excellent opportunity for healthcare providers to discuss prevention and the risk factors for respiratory illness. For high-risk patients for developing illness such as oral submucous fibrosis (OSF), it is impossible to overstate the importance of knowing because knowledge empowers them to make informed decisions that can potentially avert their risk. Serial visits enable one to continuously assess the efficacy of the interventions and make necessary changes as guided by the treatment providers. The risk of malignant change in OSF underscores the utmost significance of follow-up (Gondivkar et al., 2020). Through frequent follow-ups, healthcare providers are able to encourage adherence to lifestyle modification recommendations and keep patients cognizant of changes in their health condition. Furthermore, frequent check-ups provide leverage in the doctor-patient relationship, enhancing the overall effectiveness of care for respiratory disease. A healthy relationship facilitates open communication, allowing patients to air concerns and difficulties with their health that might otherwise go unnoticed. This relationship is essential for conditions that must be managed over time and lifestyle modifications, as the intricacies of respiratory disease frequently cause patient frustration and discontentment. Frequent interaction during health evaluations fosters a partnership atmosphere, enabling patients to become active participants in their health plans. These collaborations of patients and providers not only create more positive health results but also guide towards an overall higher quality of life because patients feel more supported and engaged in their medical treatment (Figure 3.22).

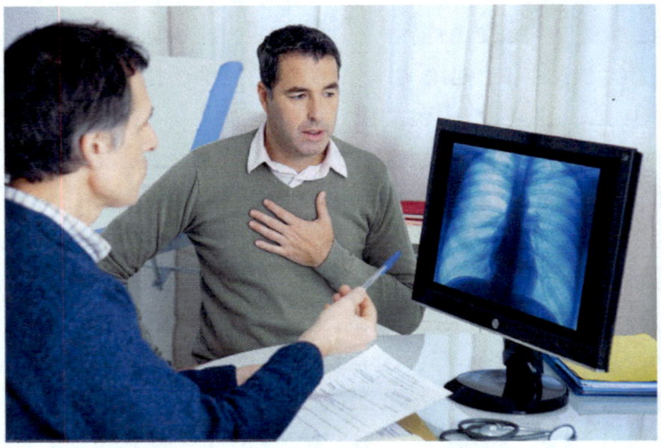

Figure 3.22. The crucial role of education in respiratory disease management.

Source: https://cdn.prod.website-files.com/642b120c6f2bf024f54b03dc/66267cd4e2fb55476a7eeb40_BC_Blog_LungPatient.jpg.

Test Your Knowledge

1. What are the prevention strategies of respiratory disease?
2. What is the importance of regular check-ups in managing respiratory disorders?

SUMMARY

In short, the extensive reach of respiratory illnesses on public health should not be underestimated. The pandemic of COVID-19 is a grim reminder of the virulence and intricacy of viral infections of the respiratory tract. As with the high prevalence of depression and post-traumatic stress disorder during previous outbreaks such as SARS and MERS, the psychological effect of respiratory disease may have an extent that goes beyond somatic manifestations. It should be highlighted that recent evidence indicates that the prevalence of depression during the COVID-19 pandemic was up to 27.0%, which means that mental health is now a key element in managing respiratory disorders. This overlap between psychological distress and physical health demands an integrated treatment strategy that addresses both fields; thus, patients are not only treated for their respiratory conditions but also seen for their emotional and mental well-being (Fan et al., 2021). Moreover, the qualitative patient experiences of COVID-19 reveal the complex interplay between physical and psychological health. Reports by patients show generalized mental stresses comprising fear, anxiety, and loneliness during their disease. These psychological responses were usually in tandem with the physical manifestations of the disease, which suggests that an integrated response is required when managing respiratory illness. The coping mechanisms employed by most patients, including religiosity and self-medication, show the vast array of ways people adapt to what they go through. These findings accentuate the importance of having medical professionals capable of providing psychological and spiritual support alongside physical treatments for facilitating complete recovery and resistance in patients coping with the complexities of respiratory disease (Jesmi et al., 2021). Lastly, holistic health modalities that address both mental and physical health in the context of respiratory disease. While the population struggles with the effects of the COVID-19 pandemic, successful intervention will need to address mental health care as well as standard respiratory therapy. Treating the immediate health problems that afflict infected individuals is only one advantage of pursuing such a dual strategy. The long-term psychological harm that may result from having to suffer through such debilitating diseases is also provided for. Thus, public health policy and clinical practice will need to be altered to support these necessary components so that patients with respiratory disorders receive integrated care that respects and meets their multifaceted experiences and needs. With a holistic approach in mind, it can pave the way to healthier outcomes and improved quality of life for patients with respiratory disorders.

The prevalence of respiratory disorders has become an invaluable public health problem, and effective preventive measures and control interventions must be implemented. The understanding of the role of external factors, such as environmental health and infectious diseases, is a key element in addressing such disorders. Emerging evidence indicates that, given their popularity for health benefits, probiotics may reduce the severity and prevalence of respiratory tract infections. A systematic review found that probiotics can reduce antibiotic use in children and infants with acute respiratory infection and offer a promising line of research for preventing antibiotic resistance and promoting intestinal health (Connors et al., 2019). These findings underscore the need to investigate other treatment modalities to enhance respiratory health, especially among vulnerable populations. Second, climate change is another threat to respiratory health through poor air quality and increased greenhouse gas emissions, leading to more respiratory illness. The Centers for Disease Control and Prevention (CDC) offers guidelines that states can use to develop strategies to respond to the health impacts of climate trends, with a focus on public health system resilience (Aytur et al., 2014). Engaging in adaptation measures for climate is essential in the backdrop of avoiding the expense of respiratory infections, particularly among residents of areas exposed to extreme weather or lower air quality due to pollutants. By addressing the intersection of respiratory health and climate change, public health interventions may work to minimize adverse health effects and foster community resilience against environmental threats. Increasing empirical evidence for respiratory disorder essentially demands an interdisciplinary solution that entails preventive as well as adaptive actions. Introducing probiotics into health care practice can reduce antibiotic use and lower rates of childhood infections, thereby improving overall respiratory health outcomes (Connors et al., 2019). While doing so, responding to the effects of climate change is required to counter respiratory issues and build public health resilience (Aytur et al., 2014). By combining new therapeutic interventions with aggressive climate strategies, stakeholders can better prepare communities to adapt to rising respiratory illness cases and ultimately safeguard population health in a changing world.

KEY TERMS FROM THIS CHAPTER

Allergens
Chronic ailments
Medical research
Neurobiology
Pharmacotherapy
Pollutants
Respiratory medicine
Asthma
Chronic obstructive pulmonary disease
Nasal cavity
Neuromuscular disorders
Pneumonia
Pulmonary embolism
Respiratory system

CRITICAL THINKING QUESTIONS

1. **Which of the following is the most common cause of chronic obstructive pulmonary disease (COPD)?**
   a. Allergic reactions
   b. Tobacco smoking
   c. Viral infections
   d. Genetic mutations
2. **What is the hallmark symptom of asthma?**
   a. Constant chest pain
   b. Progressive weight loss
   c. Recurrent episodes of wheezing, breathlessness, and chest tightness
   d. Persistent high fever
3. **Which of the following is NOT a characteristic feature of restrictive lung diseases?**
   a. Decreased lung compliance
   b. Reduced total lung capacity (TLC)
   c. Normal or elevated forced expiratory volume in 1 second (FEV1)/forced vital capacity (FVC) ratio
   d. Airway obstruction
4. **Which of the following diagnostic tests is used to confirm asthma?**
   a. Chest X-ray
   b. Spirometry with bronchodilator reversibility testing
   c. Arterial blood gas analysis
   d. CT scan of the chest
5. **Which respiratory condition is often triggered by allergens, exercise, or cold air?**
   a. COPD
   b. Asthma
   c. Pulmonary fibrosis
   d. Pulmonary edema

Short Answer Questions

1. What is the respiratory system?
2. What are the most common respiratory disorders?
3. What are the causes and risk factors of respiratory diseases?
4. How do you diagnose a respiratory disease?
5. What are the treatment options for respiratory disorder?

Answer to Critical Thinking Questions

1. (b); 2. (c); 3. (d); 4. (b); 5. (b).

REFERENCES

1. Reinero, C., Visser, L. C., Kellihan, H. B., Masseau, I., Rozanski, E., Clercx, C., Williams, K., Abbott, J., Borgarelli, M., & Scansen, B. A. (2020). ACVIM consensus statement guidelines for the diagnosis, classification, treatment, and monitoring of pulmonary hypertension in dogs. *Journal of Veterinary Internal Medicine, 34*(2), 549–573. https://doi.org/10.1111/jvim.15725Abd-Elrazek, M. N. (2025). Holistic care among patients with chronic illness in Saudi Arabia. *Journal of Holistic Nursing Science.* https://www.semanticscholar.org/paper/329484528abd03248515b3e9956fb3d3d2cedfef (accessed on 12th July 2025).
2. Afsal, M. J., Dhamodharan, B., Hariharan, C., Chellappan, D., & Rajaguru, H. (2025). Machine learning-driven early detection and monitoring of respiratory disorder using PCO2 analysis. *2025 Fourth International Conference on Smart Technologies, Communication and Robotics (STCR).* https://www.semanticscholar.org/paper/8787ae9a3465a5f08b4c0e25300d5ceaf21f84e7 (accessed on 12th July 2025).
3. Agrawal, G., Agarwal, B., Gupta, A., & Sao, A. (2025). A case report of fatal Potter's syndrome/sequence. *International Journal of Science and Research (IJSR).* https://www.semanticscholar.org/paper/fa0afbf83c6ece8605f3f50f710b2160701841da (accessed on 12th July 2025).
4. Ahmad, K., Khan, M. Q., Ali, A., Jabar, A., Anus, H., & Suleman, M. (2023). Prevalence, symptoms, and treatment of bronchiolitis and pneumonia in pediatric patients. *Journal of Health and Rehabilitation Research.* https://www.semanticscholar.org/paper/f72f1a7f776e164142e29f1ad1e2336a0ac5a722 (accessed on 12th July 2025).
5. Akyol, M. U., Alden, T. D., Amartino, H., et al. (2019). Recommendations for the management of MPS IVA: Systematic evidence- and consensus-based guidance. https://core.ac.uk/download/323075225.pdf (accessed on 12th July 2025).
6. Al-Barnawi, I. B. M. (2025). The health risks associated with long-term fuel exposure on Saudi Arabian workers: Prevention strategies and best practices. *International Journal of Science and Research Archive.* https://www.semanticscholar.org/paper/216f797e53586a5c410a80712ee2717e641ecc3b (accessed on 12th July 2025).
7. Aytur, S., Bucci, J., & Wake, C. P. (2014). An assessment of the impact of climate change on human health in New Hampshire. https://core.ac.uk/download/84123597.pdf (accessed on 12th July 2025).
8. Babu, A. K., Rosdi, N. A., Tan, C. S., Menon, B. V. V., & Paneerselvam, G. S. (2023). Curcumin and Tulsi for pulmonary disorders in the pandemic century. *Progress in Drug Discovery & Biomedical Science.* https://www.semanticscholar.org/paper/ef9620c1cb020ffcf3998a10f8af5c3dcc4eb158 (accessed on 12th July 2025).
9. Bhaskar, A., Goyal, M., & Panara, K. (2024). Understanding chronic obstructive pulmonary disease and its management—Ayurvedic point of view: A scoping review. *AYU (An International Quarterly Journal of Research in Ayurveda).* https://www.semanticscholar.org/paper/d2b592cd64b9f78f4d1e5fdabc2d5a1a264c3842 (accessed on 12th July 2025).
10. Bilichenko, T. (2022). Post-COVID syndrome: Risk factors, pathogenesis, diagnosis, and treatment of patients with respiratory damage after COVID-19 (overview). *Russian Medical Inquiry.* https://www.semanticscholar.org/paper/d03df51cda885cce49bce227a9d2317e2317a29b (accessed on 12th July 2025).

11. Bilzer, M., Ehrentraut, S., Gerbes, A. L., et al. (2002). Psychiatric and psychosocial outcome of orthotopic liver transplantation. https://core.ac.uk/download/16432271.pdf (accessed on 12th July 2025).

12. Cheng, S., Schumann, M., & Bloch, W. (2021). Translational medicine and exercise prescription (TMEP): Advancing the era of exercise medicine. *Translational Medicine and Exercise Prescription*. https://www.semanticscholar.org/paper/f17111c540081880ef6cc37d4c5d348fd80af874 (accessed on 12th July 2025).

13. Connors, G., Gould, K., King, S., et al. (2019). Does probiotic consumption reduce antibiotic utilization for common acute infections? A systematic review and meta-analysis. https://core.ac.uk/download/323070509.pdf (accessed on 12th July 2025).

14. Ebejer, M. J., & Lesauskaite, V. (1999). Age-related changes in the respiratory system. https://core.ac.uk/download/46601782.pdf (accessed on 12th July 2025).

15. Everard, M. L., Hsieh, K. S., Lethbridge, R., Craven, V. E., Daw, W. J., Wan, J. W. Y., & Elphick, H. E. (2025). Respiratory and airway disorders in children with Down syndrome: A review of the clinical challenges and management. *Frontiers in Pediatrics, 13*. https://www.semanticscholar.org/paper/efa7704214ed4d4c58887c9c4de0c8b994e66fe7 (accessed on 12th July 2025).

16. Fan, F., Zhang, S., & Cheng, Y. (2021). Incidence of psychological illness after coronavirus outbreak: A meta-analysis study. *Journal of Epidemiology and Community Health*. https://www.semanticscholar.org/paper/eef5dabba707422e34d9e151dfb504928f292c04 (accessed on 12th July 2025).

17. Fenech, M., Gouder, C., & Montefort, S. (2012). Interstitial lung disease in Malta. https://core.ac.uk/download/46602323.pdf (accessed on 12th July 2025).

18. Gondivkar, S., Sarode, S., Gadbail, A., Chole, R. H., Sarode, G., Gondivkar, R. S., & Yuwanati, M. (2020). Telemedicine approach for oral submucous fibrosis in coronavirus disease-2019 hot spots. *World Journal of Dentistry, 11*, 253–254. https://www.semanticscholar.org/paper/4e9528ff4acc4476c001599a6763495822acaa2a (accessed on 12th July 2025).

19. Greissel, A., Schneider, A., Donnachie, E., Gerlach, R., Tauscher, M., & Hapfelmeier, A. (2024). Impact of pre-existing mental health diagnoses on the development of post-COVID and related symptoms: A claims data-based cohort study. *Scientific Reports, 14*. https://www.semanticscholar.org/paper/08e7749a2a1d3217b54fcf91737975f168e2d63a (accessed on 12th July 2025).

20. Gundawar, S. A., Painginkar, T., Ligade, G. K., Pai, K. R. R., & Sg, V. (2025). An overview of COPD: Its advanced therapeutic management and challenges for drug release at the targeted site. *International Journal of Applied Pharmaceutics*. https://www.semanticscholar.org/paper/1a39a43c1dd040a1fbf464692afa99200e212f3b (accessed on 12th July 2025).

21. Guo, Y. R., Cao, Q. D., Hong, Z. S., Tan, Y. Y., Chen, S. D., Jin, H. J., Tan, K. S., et al. (2020). The origin, transmission, and clinical therapies on coronavirus disease 2019 (COVID-19) outbreak–an update on the status. *Military Medical Research, 7*. https://doi.org/10.1186/s40779-020-00240-0 (accessed on 12th July 2025).

22. Hasan, A., Saboo, N., & Kacker, S. (2025). Effect of yoga and diet on cognitive functions among hypertensives: A review. *MGM Journal of Medical Sciences*. https://www.semanticscholar.org/paper/74a7bb0d3965f6142f50718f79239dd4a9213e75 (accessed on 12th July 2025).

23. Ibrahim, M. (2024). The role of environmental factors in the development of chronic diseases: A comprehensive systematic review. *Egyptian Journal of Health Care*. https://www.semanticscholar.org/paper/a16b2d6e052aa51a456be3ef23389e1c156abdcf (accessed on 12th July 2025).

24. Jabaudon, M., Pereira, B., Laroche, E., Roszyk, L., Blondonnet, R., Audard, J., Godet, T., et al. (2021). Changes in plasma soluble receptor for advanced glycation end-products are associated with survival in patients with acute respiratory distress syndrome. *Journal of Clinical Medicine, 10*. https://www.semanticscholar.org/paper/74ed5aa98b892b1d7f4a25deddd445737f3ff8d7 (accessed on 12th July 2025).

25. Jalilova, G., Rasulova, N., Mukhamedova, N., & Kravchenko, L. (2024). Impact of environmental factors in current industrial development. *BIO Web of Conferences*. https://www.semanticscholar.org/paper/40982d3dc62f8a06c50548ae8101e8685994edd2 (accessed on 12th July 2025).

26. James, S. L., Abate, D., Abate, K. H., Abay, S. M., Abbafati, C., Abbasi, N., Abbastabar, H., et al. (2018). Global, regional, and national incidence, prevalence, and years lived with disability for 354 diseases and injuries for 195 countries and territories, 1990–2017: A systematic analysis for the Global Burden of Disease Study 2017. *The Lancet, 392*, 1789–1858. https://doi.org/10.1016/s0140-6736(18)32279-7 (accessed on 12th July 2025).

27. Jensen, S., Pedersen, C., Fischer-Rasmussen, K., Melgaard, M. E., Brustad, N., Kyvsgaard, J., Vahman, N., et al. (2024). Genetic predisposition to high BMI increases risk of early life respiratory infections and episodes of severe wheeze and asthma. *European Respiratory Journal, 64*. https://www.semanticscholar.org/paper/de4e5fd4e83902a9878fac23dd98d0021e7d2f87 (accessed on 12th July 2025).

28. Jesmi, A., Mohammadzade-Tabrizi, Z., Rad, M., Hosseinzadeh-Younesi, E., & Pourhabib, A. (2021). Lived experiences of patients with COVID-19 infection: A phenomenology study. *Medicinski Glasnik: Official Publication of the Medical Association of Zenica-Doboj Canton, Bosnia and Herzegovina, 18*(1). https://www.semanticscholar.org/paper/dfdc26b2edea4b97e6c5302489cc5d1282f7b016 (accessed on 12th July 2025).

29. Khazaei, N., Shariat, M., Effatpanah, M., Pourmirzaiee, M. A., Olfat, M., & Mirlohi, S. H. (2023). An 11-year-old boy with dry cough and respiratory distress (from Children's Medical Center Grand Rand). *Iranian Journal of Pediatrics*. https://www.semanticscholar.org/paper/f2c77fbd6171666ef16ad9d4a9ce53daf9258c59 (accessed on 12th July 2025).

30. King, T. E. (1989). Bronchiolitis obliterans. https://core.ac.uk/download/323073306.pdf (accessed on 12th July 2025).

31. Krzykawski, K., Maciejczyk, T., Mól, P., Sadowski, J., Zabawa, B., Dołęga, J., Papież, Ł., et al. (2024). The role of pulmonary rehabilitation and physical activity in the prevention, treatment, and management of respiratory diseases: A comprehensive review. *Quality in Sport*. https://www.semanticscholar.org/paper/b60bfa7657484fd72e5e6c38fdda57d0b9b86cd8 (accessed on 12th July 2025).

32. Labib, A. (2019). Sepsis care pathway 2019. *Qatar Medical Journal, 2019*. https://www.semanticscholar.org/paper/0650c1232f4389c7941706c874b1cdb91abb17b2 (accessed on 12th July 2025).

33. Meridj, A. B. R., & D. Y. (2024). Influence of COPD on the diaphragm and muscles of the lower limbs. *Journal of Pulmonology and Respiratory Research*. https://www.semanticscholar.org/

paper/cfe49e02efd0cdece225000e6a261a1f81c4a304 (accessed on 12th July 2025).

34. Moretta, P., Cavallo, N. D., Candia, C., Lanzillo, A., Marcuccio, G., Santangelo, G., Marcuccio, L., et al. (2024). Psychiatric disorders in patients with chronic obstructive pulmonary disease: Clinical significance and treatment strategies. *Journal of Clinical Medicine, 13*. https://www.semanticscholar.org/paper/5b95391ecc29d1dcbf8b2424b80899fb9f63cc5c (accessed on 12th July 2025).

35. Mroczek, M., & Iyadurai, S. (2023). Neuromuscular and neuromuscular junction manifestations of the PURA-NDD: A systematic review of the reported symptoms and potential treatment options. *International Journal of Molecular Sciences, 24*. https://www.semanticscholar.org/paper/f17f8716862c898e5848e41ce3063a2c1ba74946 (accessed on 12th July 2025).

36. Murray, C. J. L., Ikuta, K. S., Sharara, F., Swetschinski, L. R., Robles Aguilar, G., Gray, A. P., Han, C., et al. (2022). Global burden of bacterial antimicrobial resistance in 2019: A systematic analysis. *The Lancet, 399*, 629–655. https://doi.org/10.1016/s0140-6736(21)02724-0 (accessed on 12th July 2025).

37. Oleszko, M., Zapolnik, P., Kmiecik, W., & Czajka, H. (2025). Herpes zoster: Risk factors for occurrence, complications, and recurrence with a focus on immunocompromised patients. *Diseases, 13*. https://www.semanticscholar.org/paper/96e2489bc5118b23d180917ba619154b133e755b (accessed on 12th July 2025).

38. Ortega, O., Guidotti, L., Yoshimatsu, Y., Sitges, C., Martos, J., Miró, J., Martin, A., et al. (2024). Swallowing and aspiration: How to evaluate and treat swallowing disorders associated with aspiration pneumonia in older persons. *Seminars in Respiratory and Critical Care Medicine, 45*, 678–693. https://www.semanticscholar.org/paper/45de788d399f0430637520e1fa52d19e9a00cb13 (accessed on 12th July 2025).

39. Ponikowski, P., Voors, A. A., Anker, S. D., Bueno, H., Cleland, J. G. F., Coats, A. J. S., Falk, V., et al. (2016). 2016 ESC guidelines for the diagnosis and treatment of acute and chronic heart failure. *European Heart Journal, 37*, 2129–2200. https://doi.org/10.1093/eurheartj/ehw128 (accessed on 12th July 2025).

40. Porcacchia, A., Vallim, J., D'Almeida, V., Andersen, M., & Tufik, S. (2025). Associations between sleep health and chronic conditions: A cross-sectional study of NHANES 2017–2020. *SLEEP*. https://www.semanticscholar.org/paper/560997f2ffbe2aad61d2551d5cc6babaff5b313d (accessed on 12th July 2025).

41. Rashid, M. H., Deora, N., Kolur, S. R., Malini, S. S., & Sen, P. (2025). Genetic predisposition and severity of eating disorders: A review. *CNS & Neurological Disorders Drug Targets*. https://www.semanticscholar.org/paper/ff407b48430bff7006c730d209bf1ee00a9a8d75 (accessed on 12th July 2025).

42. Rastegina, S. E., Vlodavets, D., & Mizernitskiy, Y. (2024). The functional state of the respiratory system of patients with proximal spinal muscular atrophy 5q (SMA 5q): From the natural history of the disease to the era of pathogenetic therapy. *Rossiyskiy Vestnik Perinatologii i Pediatrii (Russian Bulletin of Perinatology and Pediatrics)*. https://www.semanticscholar.org/paper/2c0f96c6e694b0fbac3a2a18fdf2ff9b67d24e32 (accessed on 12th July 2025).

43. S. Manochithra, A., Rajaguru, H., et al. (2025). Early detection and monitoring of respiratory disorders using LASSO regression on PPG signals with elephant search optimization. *Journal*

of Innovative Image Processing. https://www.semanticscholar.org/paper/83af21336bf18f56 1a8b6285c29e40cb60c28269 (accessed on 12th July 2025).

44. Sari, F., Oskay, D., & Tufan, A. (2024). The effect of respiratory muscle training on respiratory muscle strength, diaphragm thickness/mobility, and exercise capacity in patients with systemic lupus erythematosus and associated shrinking lung syndrome. *Lupus*, *33*, 289–292. https://www.semanticscholar.org/paper/f6306825fb0784ea77202216fde686a91f75c47d (accessed on 12th July 2025).
45. Sengupta, A. M. (2024). Important takeaway from COVID-19 trial on nebulization and inhaler use to direct future developments in respiratory disorders. *International Journal of Scientific Research*. https://www.semanticscholar.org/paper/8bb728a1f1231aa47160295c25b66cef82 eabbc5 (accessed on 12th July 2025).
46. Shilpa, P. N., & Shanmugaloga, S. (2025). Lifestyle modifications in anorectal disorders: A review. *Journal of Ayurveda and Integrated Medical Sciences*. https://www.semanticscholar.org/paper/91a628a85c7a756e3976e459d701df547a0ed4ad (accessed on 12th July 2025).
47. Shimada, T., Ishikawa, K., Kawai, F., & Mori, N. (2024). Corynebacterium bacteremia in patients with hematologic disorders: A case series and systematic literature review. *Leukemia & Lymphoma*, *65*, 997–1002. https://www.semanticscholar.org/paper/db9d17c7dcb1d9d029495bc85f11f40cc537ed61 (accessed on 12th July 2025).
48. Smith, G. D., Ng, F., & Li, W. (2020). COVID-19: Emerging compassion, courage, and resilience in the face of misinformation and adversity. *Journal of Clinical Nursing*, *29*, 1425–1428. https://doi.org/10.1111/jocn.15231 (accessed on 12th July 2025).
49. Souza, M., Moysés-Oliveira, M., Porcacchia, A., Rosa, D., Tufik, S., & Andersen, M. (2024). Exploring common genetic factors between obstructive sleep apnea and asthma: Insights into inflammatory pathways. *SLEEP*. https://www.semanticscholar.org/paper/698c0c3a77b 88101090c25fbff604ad13591f086 (accessed on 12th July 2025).
50. Varra, F., Varras, M., Varra, V., & Theodosis-Nobelos, P. (2024). Molecular and pathophysiological relationship between obesity and chronic inflammation in the manifestation of metabolic dysfunctions and their inflammation-mediating treatment options (Review). *Molecular Medicine Reports*, *29*. https://www.semanticscholar.org/paper/278c41556edeec2e0975c1afab9cd5c4 1bfc0e31 (accessed on 12th July 2025).
51. Villar, J., Fernández, C., González-Martín, J., Ferrando, C., Añon, J. M., del Saz-Ortíz, A. M., Díaz-Lamas, A., et al. (2022). Respiratory subsets in patients with moderate to severe acute respiratory distress syndrome for early prediction of death. *Journal of Clinical Medicine*, *11*. https://www.semanticscholar.org/paper/b729f9e9c6664f4c80ccc7c506078359ec87a28b (accessed on 12th July 2025).
52. Wichmann, D. (2020). Autopsy findings and venous thromboembolism in patients with COVID-19. *Annals of Internal Medicine*, *173*, 1030–1030. https://doi.org/10.7326/l20-1206 (accessed on 12th July 2025).
53. Żaczek, B., Kozłowski, J., Kamińska, A., Kupczak, W., Bujak, K., Kocjan, A., Alsoubie, I., et al. (2025). Diagnosis and treatment of sepsis in a fourteen-year-old patient: A case study of pulmonary inflammatory discharge without typical features of respiratory tract infection. *Journal of Education, Health and Sport*. https://www.semanticscholar.org/paper/de4216081412399d056236dd96dfd5d64891addc (accessed on 12th July 2025).

CARDIOVASCULAR DISORDERS

4

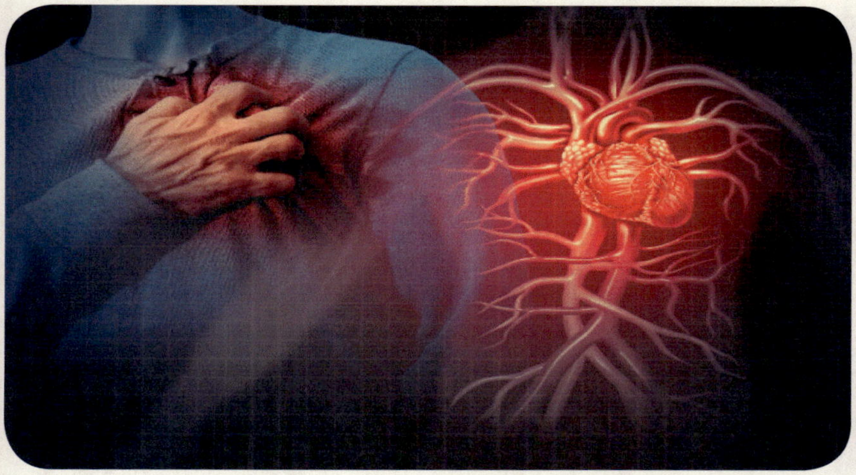

LEARNING OBJECTIVES

After studying this chapter, you will be able to:

1. Describe the types of cardiovascular disorders
2. Know the risk factors contributing to cardiovascular disorders
3. Understand the symptoms and diagnosis of cardiovascular disorders
4. Describe the treatment options for cardiovascular disorders
5. Describe the prevention strategies for cardiovascular disorders

Introduction

Cardiovascular disorders in man constitute an important public health concern, affecting millions of individuals across different demographic populations. The conditions encompass a wide range of disease states, including coronary artery disease, hypertension, heart failure, and arrhythmias, which account for the high incidence of morbidity and mortality among the world's population. The multifactorial nature of cardiovascular diseases necessitates an intimate understanding of their etiological mechanisms and risk factors. Lifestyle, genetics, and the environment are all paramount in the etiology and exacerbation of such disorders. The interactions between these factors and how they are conducive to resiliency or vulnerability towards such disease come into play, particularly when faced with environmental stressors that can potentially exacerbate their cardiovascular status. New research has made the contribution of resilience to stress-related disorder reaction more explicit, especially how individual differences may act as a determinant of cardiovascular disease susceptibility. Stressful life events can elicit a range of adverse health reactions, yet not everyone with such stressors will develop cardiovascular disorders. This highlights that the resilience theory—capacity to respond favorably to adversity—corresponds to an immediate need for objective markers to assess mechanisms. Research has begun to correlate biological markers, including heart rate variability (HRV), with resilience levels, suggesting that the body's response to stress affects cardiovascular health. Referring to (Carnevali et al., 2018), understanding the physiological markers related to resilience and cardiovascular disease can highlight the question of why some are more vulnerable than others, thus guiding preventive interventions tailored to needs. Moreover, food constituents, particularly flavanols in food and beverages, have been investigated for their cardioprotective effect.

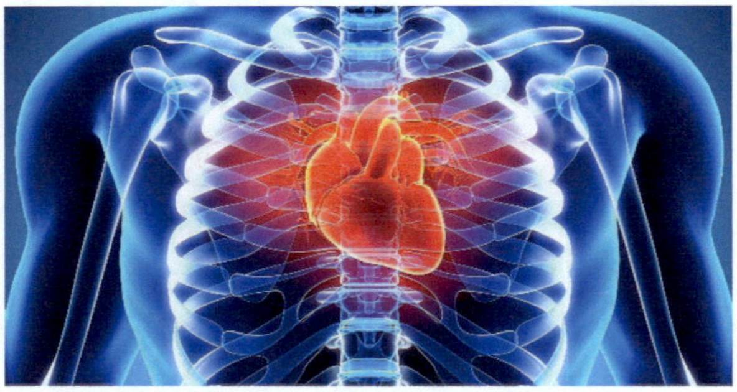

Figure 4.1. Cardiovascular disease.

Source: https://www.endocrine.org/-/media/endocrine/images/patient-engagement-webpage/condition-page-images/cardiovascular-disease/cardio_disease_t2d_pe_1796x943.jpg.

A number of randomized controlled trials demonstrate that diets rich in flavanols may lead to significant reductions in cardiometabolic risk factors, such as LDL cholesterol and body mass index. However, best integration of such dietary interventions into public programs is based on understanding the determinants of individual responses, such as initial health and lifestyle. Variability in responses of individuals to flavanol intake, as discussed in (Combet et al., 2017), confirms that others will benefit more than others, and therefore, there is a need for individualization in diet management for the avoidance of cardiovascular diseases. This underscores the enormous potential of diet to serve as a pillar of cardiovascular health promotion, particularly when combined with other lifestyle and stress-reduction interventions (Figure 4.1).

Importance of Studying Cardiovascular Health

Understanding cardiovascular health is imperative in developing effective prevention and treatment strategies against various cardiovascular conditions. Cardiovascular health is influenced by a combination of genetic, environmental, and behavioral factors, thereby making the study a complex subject in medical science. By analyzing these determinants, researchers can identify modifiable risk factors, such as diet, physical activity, and stress management, that exert substantial effects on cardiovascular outcomes. This holistic method acknowledges the interconnectedness of physical and psychosocial dimensions, which is especially critical with the growing prevalence of cardiovascular illness globally. A holistic concept of cardiovascular well-being not only helps address acute medical problems but also enables preventive measures that can enhance quality of life. Furthermore, studies underpin the multifaceted relationship between mental well-being and cardiovascular disease. Depression and anxiety have also been linked with increased risk for ischemic heart disease and other cardiovascular disorders, suggesting that mental health is at the heart of cardiovascular health. In this sense, studies on the psychology of cardiovascular illness can offer pointers to effective treatments. Major depressive disorder (MDD) and coronary heart disease pathophysiology are noted for a multifactorial interaction where systemic factors such as vascular dysfunction and obesity determine the heart's health, as well as the heart's intrinsic protective mechanisms being overwhelmed by mental conditions (Budiono et al., 2017). Elaborative examination of these interactions can direct more holistic treatment strategies that take into account both the mental and cardiovascular state, thereby improving patient outcomes. Secondly, the role of stress throughout an individual's life is also a critical factor in cardiovascular health. Chronic stress will lead to direct physiological changes that negatively affect the heart's performance, and therefore, there needs to be an integrated approach to healthcare that involves mental as well as physical well-being (Estrine et al., 2006). This realization of stress as a fundamental driver drives research into resilience mechanisms that will enhance cardiovascular health. With the incorporation of stress coping skills and mental health knowledge, health care professionals are able to minimize the effect of cardiovascular disease. Thus, the study of cardiovascular health is imperative not only to understand heart diseases but also to drive health practices as a whole towards enhancing quality of life and reducing the likelihood of developing cardiovascular diseases (Figure 4.2).

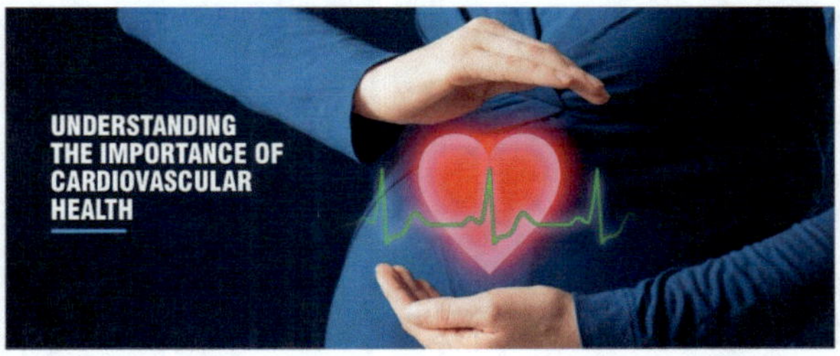

Figure 4.2. Understand the importance of cardiovascular health.

Source: https://healinghospital.co.in/wp-content/uploads/2024/04/WhatsApp-Image-2024-04-29-at-4.07.37-PM-1-1024x415.jpeg.

4.1. Types of Cardiovascular Disorders

Learning Outcome

1. Describe the coronary artery disease
2. Understand the heart failure
3. Learn about arrhythmias

There are many cardiovascular diseases, which have significant impacts on human health, with each of them possessing its own individual clinical presentations and complexities. Two of the most frequent are coronary artery disease (CAD) and heart failure, and both may be brought about by a myriad of risk factors, including hypertension and hyperlipidemia. CAD is caused by the deposition of atheromatous plaques in coronary arteries, which leads to reduced blood flow to the cardiac muscle, and subsequently angina or myocardial infarction. Conversely, heart failure is a spectrum of diseases where the heart is unable to circulate blood efficiently and, in its presentation, may be either systolic or diastolic dysfunction. The relationship among these diseases is that they all have shared risk factors, so that prevention and treatment of one variant is pivotal to decreasing the load of cardiovascular disease as a whole. Arrhythmias are another emergent category of cardiovascular conditions, characterized by abnormal heart rhythms that can result from electrical or structural dysfunction in the heart. Common examples are atrial fibrillation, bradycardia, and tachycardia. Atrial fibrillation is particularly risky as it increases the chance of stroke due to blood clotting within the atria. These arrhythmias that disrupt the heart's normal rhythm can lead to hemodynamic instability and decreased cardiac output, necessitating immediate intervention. Although multiple pharmacologic interventions, including antiarrhythmics and anticoagulants, are commonly employed, psychological factors in arrhythmias cannot be overlooked. As stated, stress can impact cardiovascular health, highlighting the potential role mental health could play in the etiology and management of such disorders (Estrine et al., 2006). Further, psychological factors, such as major depressive disorder (MDD), may even influence cardiovascular health considerably, particularly in the context of ischemic heart disease. Current studies have pinpointed the direct effects of MDD on the intrinsic processes of the heart, depicting how depression may compromise coronary health as well as function as a causative agent for high morbidity and mortality rates associated with coronary heart disease (Budiono et al., 2017). Biological changes, such as hypothalamic-pituitary-adrenal axis dysregulation and inflammation processes, further interweave this interaction. Clarification of these links could inform more effective management by adding both psychological and physiological treatments to enhance the overall treatment of cardiovascular disorder patients. As research in this field advances, it increasingly shows that addressing this set of problems through a holistic process is essential to mitigate the systemic effects on both cardiovascular and mental health (Figure 4.3).

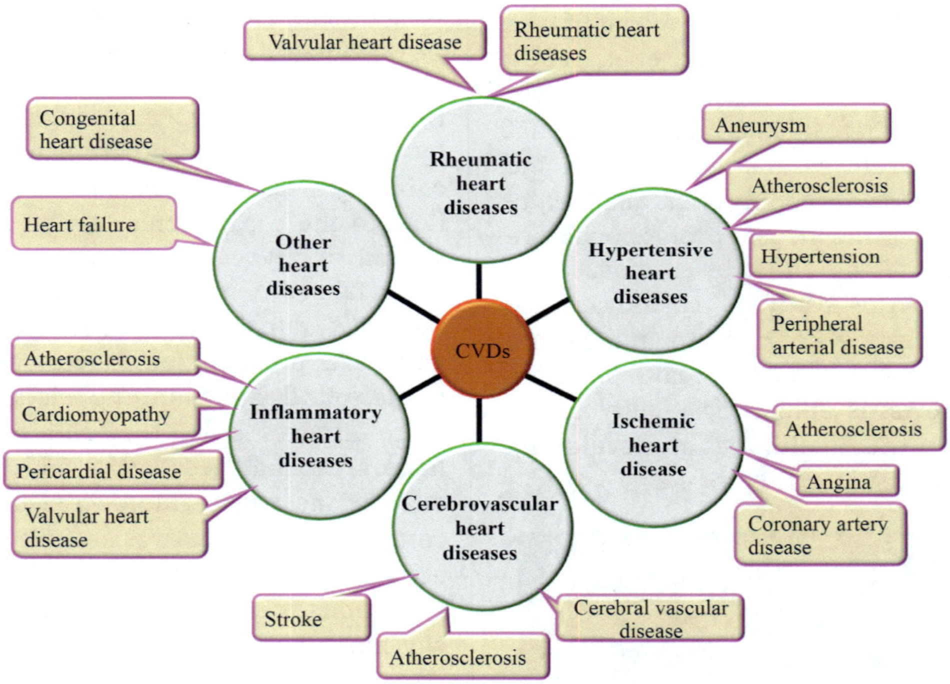

Figure 4.3. Summary of common cardiovascular conditions.

Source: https://www.researchgate.net/profile/Prashant-Kesharwani/publication/280630317/figure/fig1/AS:391490237943808@1470349954014/Fig-1-Summary-of-common-cardiovascular-conditions.png.

4.1.1. Coronary Artery Disease

Coronary artery disease (CAD) is one of the most prevalent cardiovascular diseases, significantly impacting world health. CAD occurs when the coronary arteries that supply blood to the heart muscle become narrowed or blocked by plaque, a buildup of cholesterol, fat, and other substances. This process of pathology, atherosclerosis, can lead to oxygen insufficiency in the heart muscle, creating angina or myocardial infarction. Risk factors for CAD include lifestyle risk factors of smoking, dietary excess, and physical inactivity, combined with genetic predisposition and comorbid risk factors of hypertension and diabetes. The rising incidence of obesity contributes to the risk, and CAD becomes not merely a clinical condition but a public health concern necessitating multidisciplinary regulatory as well as preventive measures. The physiological impact of CAD is profound, reaching far beyond the heart and being severely dangerous outside of it to the body as a whole. The compromised blood flow can lead to a variety of complications, from failure of the heart to arrhythmias and increased vulnerability to cardiac events. Moreover, research has also placed center stage the correlation between chronic inflammation and CAD, as systemic inflammatory conditions propagate atherosclerotic processes and thus create correlations between diseases such as rheumatoid arthritis and heightened cardiovascular risk. Significantly, studies have revealed that the occurrence of anti-carbamylated protein antibodies (anti-CarP) in rheumatoid arthritis patients is linked to endothelial dysfunction and subclinical atherosclerosis, illustrating the manner in which systemic disease affects coronary disease directly. Consequently, by identifying these complex interdependencies, health practitioners are better able to refine risk stratification and management protocols for CAD, particularly in the context of coincident populations (Alessandri et al., 2017). Over the last few years, advances in diagnostic imaging modalities have enabled early detection and stratification of coronary artery disease, yielding improved therapeutic outcomes. Diagnostic modalities such as coronary angiography, CT coronary angiography, and stress testing provide valuable information about the extent of coronary occlusion and myocardial perfusion. Pharmacologic therapies such as antiplatelet therapy, statins, and lifestyle changes play a significant role in managing CAD as well as preventing recurrent cardiovascular events. Also, newly suggested findings indicate that lifestyle interventions, especially those promoting increased physical activity and healthier diets, significantly influence the development of CAD. Specifically, caffeine's dual role in cardiovascular action, where it increases as well as raises the threat of toxicity, necessitates a cautious strategy in its administration among CAD patients (Aromatario et al., 2015). In summary, a deep understanding of coronary artery disease is crucial to improve the results of patients and develop improved models of treatment in the specialty of cardiovascular diseases (Figure 4.4).

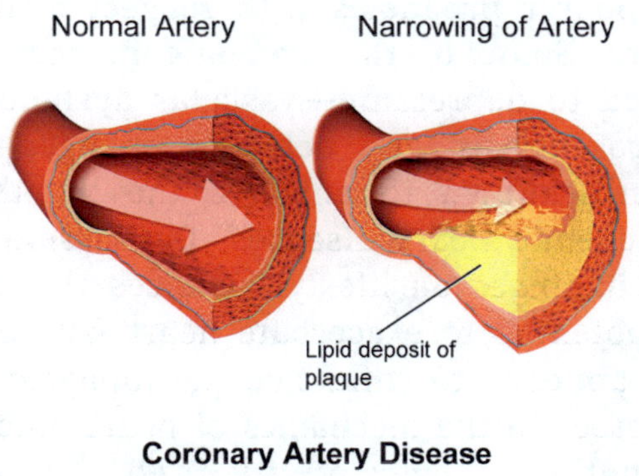

Figure 4.4. Coronary artery disease.

Source: https://upload.wikimedia.org/wikipedia/commons/6/6d/Blausen_0259_CoronaryArteryDisease_02.png.

4.1.2. Heart Failure

Heart failure is a significant global health issue, being a multifactorial syndrome resulting from various underlying cardiovascular diseases. It is characterized as the inability of the heart to circulate sufficient blood to meet the body's needs, leading to symptoms such as fatigue, shortness of breath, and swelling. Heart failure pathophysiology is a combination of functional and structural cardiac derangements typically initiated by such diseases as valvular disease, ischemic heart disease, or hypertension. These are the causes of decreased cardiac output, initiating neurohormonal activation that facilitates worsening of heart dysfunction. Understanding the multifaceted pathophysiology of heart failure is crucial for effective diagnosis and treatment, and ongoing research aims to decipher the molecular mechanisms of this debilitating disease and how it cross-talks with other psychosocial diseases, such as psychiatric disorders, such as major depressive disorder (Budiono et al., 2017). The interaction between psychiatric disorders and heart failure also adds another level of complexity to its management. Studies have confirmed that major depressive disorder patients have a greater prevalence and poorer prognosis with respect to heart failure. Some of the systemic mechanisms related to depression—vascular dysfunction, atherosclerosis, and behavior changes—are directly known to enhance the likelihood of ischemic heart diseases. Depression not only impinges on lifestyle choices that have the potential to exacerbate heart failure but also appears to influence pathophysiologic processes in the mechanics of heart function. Sympathetic overactivity and immune-inflammatory processes have been cited as mediators of the psycho-cardiac interaction in this regard. Mental health treatment is therefore important in conjunction with heart failure therapy in order to maximally enhance cardiac function and overall quality of life (Budiono et al., 2017). Research on novel therapeutic modalities continues to be an emerging area for the management of heart failure. Recent studies have also identified melatonin, a hormone naturally synthesized in the body, as a potential therapeutic for the pathophysiologic impact of cardiovascular diseases. Melatonin has been shown to promote improved cardiovascular parameters, including blood pressure regulation and platelet function, and decreased hormone levels are associated with coronary artery disease and heart failure. Its antioxidative effect may contribute to cardioprotective advantages by potentially preventing oxidative damage to the myocardium. Based on these findings, the use of melatonin in clinical trials could be a significant breakthrough in heart failure and its associated diseases. Knowledge of the interaction between melatonin and heart failure could not only improve patients' outcomes but also expand the paradigm for understanding and treating cardiovascular health in the clinic (Figure 4.5).

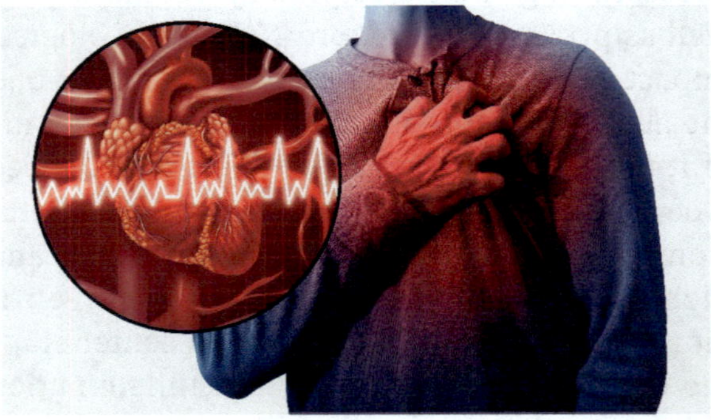

Figure 4.5. Heart failure.

Source: https://hinduja-prod-assets.s3.ap-south-1.amazonaws.com/s3fs-public/2024-03/Heart%20Failure%20and%20Symptoms.jpg.

4.1.3. Arrhythmias

Arrhythmias are a widespread category of cardiovascular diseases, characterized by irregular heart rhythms with important impacts on human health. These disturbances of cardiac rhythms can be caused by a wide range of etiopathogenetic reasons such as genetic predispositions, primary heart diseases, or external causes such as stress and drug consumption. The arrhythmias are also generally divided by their site of origin (atrial or ventricular) and their rate (bradycardia or tachycardia). When the heart beats either faster or slower than usual, it results in inefficient circulation of blood, which may result in severe consequences such as stroke, heart failure, or sudden cardiac death. Understanding the variability and complexity of arrhythmias is most critical for both diagnosis and management, and thus arrhythmias are a focus of attention in the study of cardiovascular disease in humans. Recent advances in arrhythmia treatment have highlighted the scope of genetic therapies. Gene therapy developments came forward with the suggestion that genetic changes could offer new hope for the treatment of atrial fibrillation and congenital long QT syndromes. Researchers have explored the use of biological pacemakers built from viral vectors and mesenchymal cells to induce a permanent heart rate by altering the heart's conduction pathways, particularly the left bundle branch. Genetic interventions that address the atrioventricular (AV) node seek to mimic the beta-blocker effects, opening up new therapeutic avenues. Also, manipulating pathological calcium cycling in heart failure with genetics is believed to improve ventricular function and reduce arrhythmic events, underscoring the convergence of technological advancement and clinical treatment in the successful management of arrhythmias (Francis et al., 2006). A good understanding of the interplay between cardiovascular disease and mental illness is also essential in the context of arrhythmias. Recent research has established an association between major depressive disorder (MDD) and risk for coronary heart disease (CHD), with the implications that systemic processes linked with MDD, such as diabetes, obesity, and inflammation, may be underlying contributors to the prevalence and incidence of arrhythmias. Also, the physiological effects of MDD, including impaired stress response pathways and impaired cardiac protection, can even add to myocardial vulnerability. Vulnerable myocardial cells may demonstrate heightened sensitivity to ischemic injury, rendering the clinical presentation even more complicated in patients with both psychiatric disorders and arrhythmias. Detection of these correlations not only aids in comprehensive patient planning and management but also highlights the significance of an interdisciplinary model in the treatment of cardiovascular diseases (Budiono et al., 2017) (Figure 4.6).

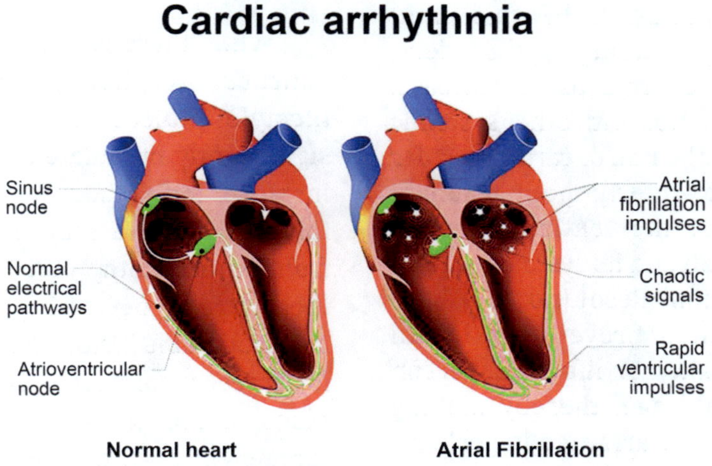

Figure 4.6. Arrhythmias.

Source: https://cdn-ilbdkgn.nitrocdn.com/KyPgQQQAVfBmOoLeBzkzAekksAGOgYiS/assets/images/optimized/rev-754064b/www.modernheartandvascular.com/wp-content/uploads/2022/10/arrythmia.png.

Test Your Knowledge

1. What is coronary artery disease?
2. What are arrhythmias?

4.2. Risk Factors

Learning Outcome

1. Understand the genetic predisposition in the development of cardiovascular disorders
2. Describe the lifestyle choices in determining cardiovascular health
3. Describe the environmental influences of cardiovascular disorders in humans

Among the myriad risk factors for cardiovascular disease, age remains a top contender. As age advances, so does the prevalence of chronic ailments and physiological changes that increase susceptibility to cardiovascular disease. This is compounded by a process called inflammaging, in which chronic inflammation occurs without an apparent cause. Evidence indicates that inflammation of this kind has been linked to various aging disorders, including atherosclerotic cardiovascular disease. Inflammation, in conjunction with other systemic influences, potentiates the risk of cardiovascular complications in the elderly population, a compelling rationale for interventions aimed at controlling inflammation and its systemic effects in this aging population. Resolution of these factors not only might improve heart health but also optimize quality of life as a person progresses through old age, thereby making preventive interventions warranted in geriatric medicine. Lifestyle is similarly significant in influencing cardiovascular health, and nutritional intake plays an important role. Malnutrition leads to obesity, hypertension, and dyslipidemia, all of which are well-established precursors to cardiovascular disease. Epidemiological studies indicate the potential benefits of dietary flavanols, particularly from foods such as tea, cocoa, and apples, in the regulation of cardiometabolic risk factors. Meta-analyses have indicated that these flavanol-dense foods can lead to significant reductions in body mass index and total cholesterol levels, thereby decreasing the risks associated with unwholesome dietary patterns. The variable response to such nutrition manipulation underscores the necessity of custom-fit nutrition. In particular, those with higher baseline values, such as higher BMI, may derive greater benefits, suggesting that tailored dieting strategies might be crucial for the successful management of cardiovascular risk across diverse populations. Additionally, the synergistic interaction between genetic susceptibility and environmental inputs makes the cardiovascular risk factor landscape even more challenging.

While there is indeed a genetic factor in a patient's susceptibility to cardiovascular disease, lifestyle choices and environmental trauma significantly modulate such inherent risks. For instance, individuals with genetic risk factors for dyslipidemia may have magnified effects from an unhealthy diet. Thus, a knowledge of the interplay between genetic predispositions and modifiable factors, such as diet and exercise, is necessary for developing effective prevention plans. Moreover, as described in many reports, targeted interventions on these overlapping risk factors would also enhance health outcomes. The urgency of such comprehensive care explains the need for ongoing studies into how multifactorial influences converge on cardiovascular disease and how better prevention can be achieved in the clinical setting (Figure 4.7).

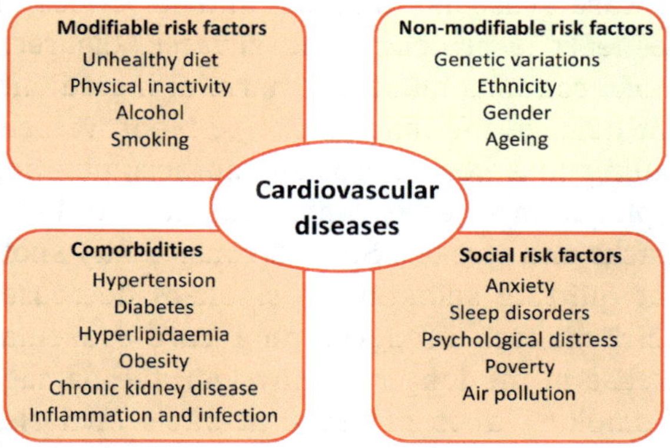

Figure 4.7. Main risk factors for cardiovascular diseases (CVDs).

Source: https://www.mdpi.com/biomolecules/biomolecules-14-01032/article_deploy/html/images/biomolecules-14-01032-g001.png.

4.2.1. Genetic Predisposition

Genetic susceptibility is a significant etiological factor for cardiovascular disease, with implications for susceptibility and disease progression. This underlying vulnerability can manifest in a wide variety of ways through biological processes, e.g., by the presence of specific genes and epigenetic modifiers interacting with the environment. There have been recent reports of a number of genetic variants for myocardial infarction and other cardiovascular diseases, which suggest that people who carry specific combinations of genes are at greater risk. These predispositions are not isolated; life factors such as diet and exercise tend to worsen them, leading to complex interactions between genetic and environmental factors. Genetic predisposition plays an important role in the development of targeted prevention and treatment approaches that can potentially reduce the incidence of cardiovascular disease in high-risk populations. Research has highlighted the role of sexual dimorphism in genetic predisposition to cardiovascular disease. Gender disparity in the expression of genes between males and females can influence the incidence and severity of such disorders, whose presentation tends to be variable in clinical terms. Hormonal variations, particularly sex steroid hormone-induced variations, play a role in regulating genes responsible for cardiovascular function. Aside from this, microRNAs have also been found to play a role in the process, via sex-specific regulation of gene expression, which is responsible for the variation in cardiovascular disease impact. Researching the reasons behind these variations in mechanisms will enable scientists to develop more effective therapeutic approaches tailored to gender-based requirements. The literature emphasizes the importance of comprehensive studies that consider sexual differences in genetic vulnerability to improve the prognosis of patients with cardiovascular health, as evidenced by recent findings on the role of microRNAs as pathogenic entities (Eghbali et al., 2014). Additionally, diabetes mellitus is most significantly associated with genetic factors that highly sensitize the individual towards cardiovascular complications, particularly ischemic heart disease (IHD). Pathophysiologic background of IHD in diabetes is multifaceted, sometimes with manifestations of both macro- and microvascular complications. Gene variants of ion channels, such as those regulating ATP-dependent potassium channels, are presently considered to be principal protagonists linking metabolic derangement to altered regulation of coronary blood flow. This genetic background complicates the clinical treatment of diabetic patients and requires individually tailored strategies based on individual gene profiles. Targeting these genetic predispositions is not only key to explaining the heightened risk of cardiovascular complications in patients with diabetes but also key to creating interventions that can mitigate such risks significantly (Marchis et al., 2018). Thus, studying genetic predispositions to cardiovascular disease provides useful information to enhance prevention and treatment strategies tailored to specific at-risk populations.

4.2.2. Lifestyle Choices (Diet, Exercise, Smoking)

Dietary lifestyle factors are most significant in determining cardiovascular health and the occurrence of cardiovascular disease disorders. Among the lifestyle factors, dietary intake is most distinctive: a fruit, vegetable, whole-grain, and protein-based diet has proven effective in lowering the risk of cardiovascular disorders. Conversely, consumption of foods containing saturated fat, sodium, and sugar can strongly contribute to heart disease. There is good evidence supporting the view that greater adherence to a healthy diet not only lowers low-density lipoprotein (LDL) cholesterol but also achieves improved cardiovascular well-being, with a greater likelihood of preventing obesity and hypertension—two conditions highly linked with cardiovascular disease. In addition, targeted health promotion strategies that encourage healthy eating can positively influence stress levels and, by extension, cardiovascular health outcomes, as observed in research with college students (Badger et al., 2019). Physical exercise is yet another central lifestyle choice with direct implications for cardiovascular health. Exercise has been associated with a range of health benefits, including improved heart function, increased blood flow, and better weight control. Participation in moderate to high-intensity aerobic exercises for at least 150 minutes per week can significantly reduce the complications of heart disease. Exercise is beneficial for cardiovascular health by maintaining an ideal body weight and improving cholesterol levels, thereby reducing the risk of cardiovascular disease. Additionally, the effects of physical exercise extend beyond mere physical condition; regular exercise has been shown to lower anxiety and stress levels, with psychological relief intrinsic to the well-being (Estrine et al., 2006). Hence, promoting an active lifestyle is intrinsic to avoiding the disease burden of cardiovascular diseases. Smoking is a significant and variable risk factor for cardiovascular disease, and its effect on the heart is profound and adverse. Cigarette smoke contains numerous harmful ingredients that damage the inner lining of blood vessels, leading to atherosclerosis—the accumulation of plaque in arteries, which may lead to heart attacks and strokes. Studies consistently show that quitting smoking by smokers decreases their chances of developing cardiovascular disease in the long run. However, the damage of smoking does not stop at one's own risk but extends to loved ones through secondhand exposure. Public campaigns encouraging quitting smoking can also help individuals adopt a better lifestyle, thereby decreasing occurrences of cardiovascular disorders. By integrating smoking cessation programs with broader lifestyle health campaigns, health care professionals can promote holistic strategies that improve heart health and overall wellness within the population (Figure 4.8).

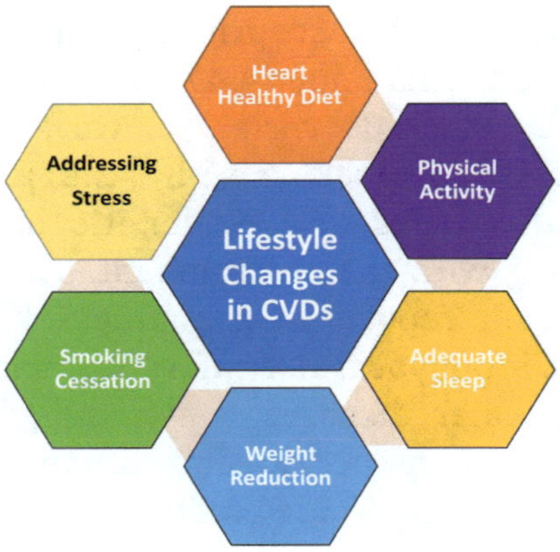

Figure 4.8. Lifestyle changes in cardiovascular disease.

Source: https://assets.cureus.com/uploads/figure/file/688742/lightbox_49d74ce022d111ee9a792dbb7719cd14-Lifestyle.png.

4.2.3. Environmental Influences

Several environmental determinants are involved in the etiology and development of cardiovascular disease in humans. These include socio-economic status, up to lifestyle choices and exposure to chronic stress. Individuals with poor socio-economic status have limited access to healthcare services, nutritious food, and secure living conditions that result in elevated risks of cardiovascular disease. Additionally, lifestyle components such as lack of exercise, poor diets, and drug use further compound the cardiovascular condition of these populations. These environmental determinants collectively create a multifaceted landscape, and through it, shape health outcomes; therefore, there is an equally strong argument for targeted interventions in high-risk populations to attempt to reverse the occurrence of cardiovascular disease. Another key environmental determinant of cardiovascular health is exposure to chronic stress. Stressors such as job insecurity, financial adversity, and interpersonal conflicts have been evidenced to induce physiological changes leading to predisposition to heart disease.

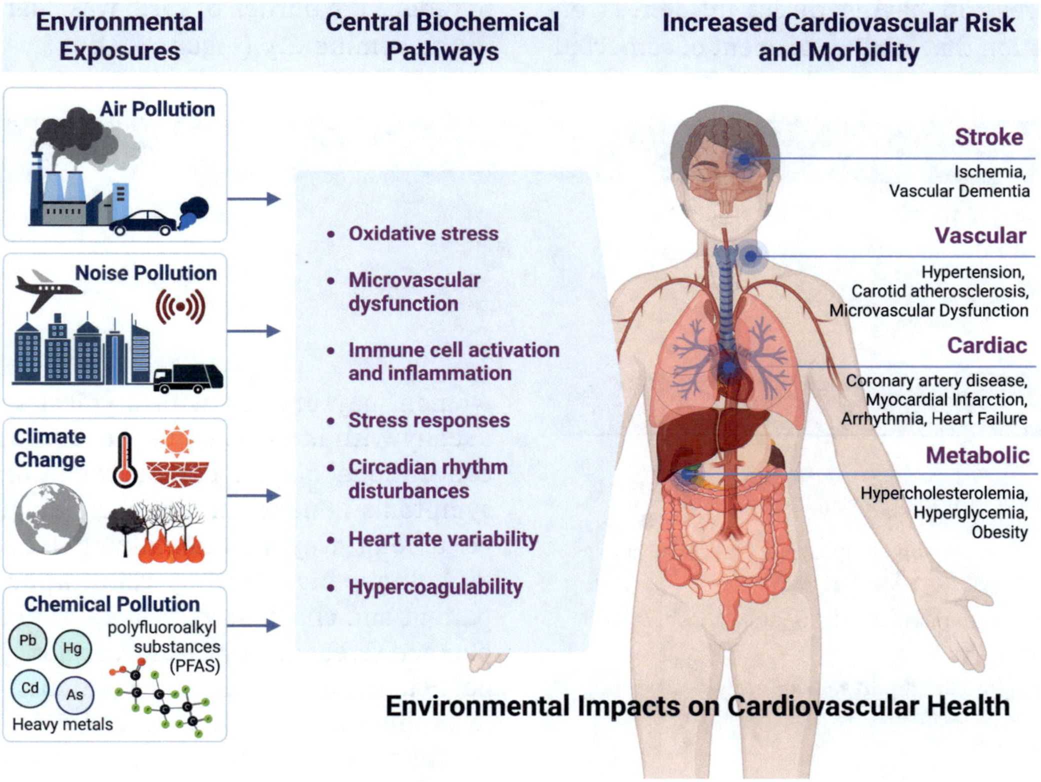

Figure 4.9. Environmental exposures and cardiovascular health.

Source: https://www.ahajournals.org/cms/10.1161/CIRCRESAHA.123.323613/asset/e4f932cc-cd95-4124-a755-3d0e5a055c2e/assets/graphic/circresaha.123.323613.fig01.jpg.

The body's response to stress tends to activate the sympathetic nervous system, leading to increased blood pressure and heart rate. In the long term, these physiological changes may lead to vascular dysfunction and heightened susceptibility to ischemic heart disease. Furthermore, evidence shows that stress hinders resilience, thereby complicating recovery from adverse cardiovascular events (Carnevali et al., 2018). Proof in the relationship between stress and psychological response hints at the need for holistic interventions considering physical and mental well-being to promote cardiovascular health among individuals (Carnevali et al., 2018). Nevertheless, more evidence in the psycho-cardiac relationship suggests that mental illness has significant associations with poor cardiovascular outcomes. Major depressive disorder (MDD), for instance, is associated with a host of systemic risk factors that are predictive of heart disease, including obesity and impaired vascular function. Notably, however, the association between MDD and cardiovascular health is complex, with depression having direct influences on heart function that are independent of comorbid conditions. Enhanced sympathetic function and dysregulation of hormonal responses, including HPA axis dysfunction, are among the factors that underlie the association between the two (Budiono et al., 2017). Therefore, understanding these psychosocial and environmental factors provides a hopeful agenda for developing effective prevention and intervention strategies. Dual treatment of mental and cardiovascular disorders improves the outcomes at the individual level as well as public health efforts to reduce the burden of cardiovascular diseases in the community (Figure 4.9).

Test Your Knowledge

1. What is the meaning of genetic predisposition?
2. What are the lifestyle choices for cardiovascular health?

4.3. Symptoms and Diagnosis

Learning Outcome

1. Know the common symptoms of cardiovascular disorders
2. Describe the diagnostic tests of cardiovascular disorders
3. Understand the importance of early detection of cardiovascular disorders

Detection of cardiovascular diseases typically begins with the evaluation of a patient's symptoms, which can present in many ways. Some typical symptoms include chest pain, shortness of breath, palpitations, and fatigue, and can be indicative of conditions such as coronary artery disease or heart failure. The varied presentation of these symptoms is one reason it can be challenging to make an accurate diagnosis, as the symptoms often overlap with those of other diseases. In some patients, women may present with atypical symptoms, usually with indigestion or anxiety rather than conventional angina. Early recognition of these symptoms is necessary, as early diagnosis can go a long way in maximizing management outcomes, highlighting the importance of patient and clinician awareness. In this regard, planned screening for cardiovascular symptoms, particularly among high-risk patients, is crucial to enable early intervention and avert potential complications. Following the observation of symptoms, numerous diagnostic modalities are employed by healthcare workers to establish the existence of cardiovascular disease. The initial assessment typically includes a complete history and physical exam, followed by non-invasive tests such as electrocardiograms (ECGs) and echocardiograms. These devices are essential for diagnosing heart rhythms, structural anomalies, and overall cardiac function. More sophisticated imaging techniques, such as magnetic resonance imaging (MRI) and computed tomography (CT) scans, can be applied, if necessary in complex cases, to give more anatomical details. Blood tests can also be used to detect markers of cardiac stress or damage. All these diagnostic techniques, combined, enable the general health of the cardiovascular system to be understood, allowing clinicians to make appropriate treatment recommendations based on the patient's. The incorporation of genetic testing into the diagnostic process has become increasingly important, especially for certain hereditary cardiovascular diseases. For example, familial hypercholesterolemia or Marfan syndrome can only be confirmed by genetic testing and should inform the management plan.

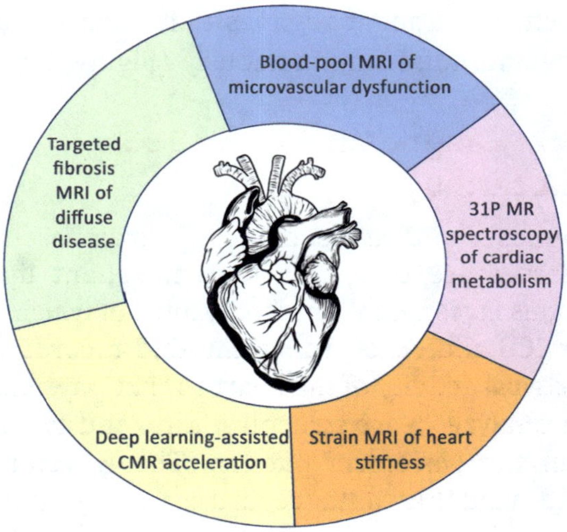

Figure 4.10. Emerging cardiac MRI (CMR) techniques for molecular and functional characterization of the diseased heart.

Source: https://images-provider.frontiersin.org/api/ipx/w=410&f=webp/https://www.frontiersin.org/files/Articles/1072828/fcvm-09-1072828-HTML/image_m/fcvm-09-1072828-g001.jpg.

These tests not only help identify specific disorders but also evaluate possible risk factors in family members. Furthermore, genetic knowledge is the key to the care of complex syndromes with complex presentations, including 22q11.2 deletion syndrome, which presents with congenital heart malformations and other systemic disorders (Bassett et al., 2015). With the implementation of a multidisciplinary model that integrates genetic counseling with more conventional diagnostic procedures, medical professionals can improve the precision of diagnoses and cultivate an understanding of cardiovascular diseases that reaches beyond isolated patients to include their broader familial contexts (Figure 4.10).

4.3.1. Common Symptoms of Cardiovascular Disorders

Symptoms of cardiovascular disorders can be rather varied, with a tendency to present special challenges in diagnosing them correctly and taking necessary action in a timely fashion. Classic symptoms are pain in the chest, dyspnea, and exhaustion, which can indicate lurking pathologies like coronary artery disease or congestive heart failure. patients as pressure or squeezing and may radiate to the arms, neck, or back. This kind of pain can be an important warning signal, warranting immediate medical care. Additionally, shortness of breath can make everyday activities more difficult, suggesting the possible development of cardiovascular disease. Early identification of such symptoms is important as they can directly influence the success of treatment and overall quality of life. Recognition of such symptoms not only enables timely treatment but also informs public health interventions for cardiovascular disease prevention. In addition to the classic symptoms, cardiovascular disease may present with comparatively mild symptoms that are usually not appreciated by patients and doctors. Symptoms like palpitations, dizziness, or spontaneous swelling of the feet and ankles can be signs of arrhythmias or heart failure. Palpitations, which typically feel like a racing or fluttering in the chest, are often a sign of an abnormal heart rhythm that should be further investigated. Dizziness, particularly when accompanied by extreme fatigue, can be a sign of compromised blood flow, especially with exertion. Also, swelling of the lower extremities can result from fluid accumulation due to cardiac failure. Identification of such other symptoms bears significant influence on early diagnosis and intervention as they could be antecedent to more complicated cardiovascular events, citing population health plans' significance in cardiovascular disease education in general.

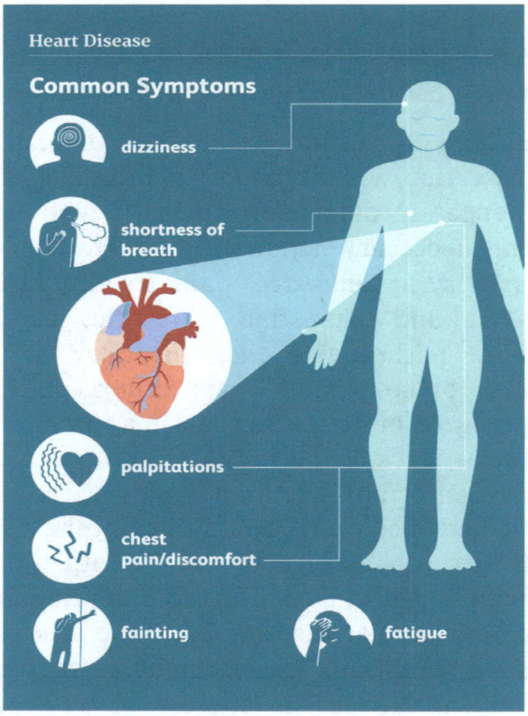

Figure 4.11. Symptoms of heart disease.

Source: https://www.verywellhealth.com/thmb/dLBLVSgvB1IrR71qP6N7wQo9lhg=/1500x0/filters:no_upscale():max_bytes(150000):strip_icc()/heart-disease-symptoms-5b0d5b648e1b6e003e6a3347.png.

Last but not least, lifestyle and psychological problems can manifest in the cardiovascular form, emphasizing the body-mind connection. As an illustration, excessive stress has been found to affect cardiovascular function, which may subsequently lead to a heightened heart rate and elevated blood pressure. The resilience model of stress coping is also related to physiological responses, which further exacerbate cardiovascular problems, and thus symptom assessment should consider the psychological as well as the biological component (Carnevali et al., 2018). Furthermore, substances such as caffeine also worsen the clinical presentation by palpitations or tachycardia, particularly when they are consumed in excess (Aromatario et al., 2015). Therefore, there is a need for an integrated approach that addresses lifestyle and mental health in the diagnosis and management of cardiovascular disease, and espouses more effective treatment regimes that address both body and mind simultaneously (Figure 4.11).

4.3.2. Diagnostic Tests (ECG, Echocardiogram)

Diagnosis and assessment of cardiovascular illnesses are to a great extent reliant upon various investigative methods, some of which are the ECG and echocardiogram. ECG records the electrical activity of the heart so that physicians can analyze heart structure, rate, and rhythm from the waveform pattern. The waveforms yield valuable data regarding arrhythmias, myocardial infarction, and abnormalities. The ECG not only serves diagnostic purposes but also plays a vital role in monitoring patients both during and after treatment. As cardiac diseases may manifest as abnormal heart rhythms, the ECG's ability to detect autonomic dysfunction is particularly valuable for revealing homeostatic failures and predicting adverse cardiac outcomes (Baumert et al., 2021). Thus, the integration of ECG findings into clinical practice is increasingly recognized as essential to effective patient management and targeted therapeutic interventions. Complementing the ECG, echocardiography uses ultrasonic waves to generate real-time images of the heart's chambers, valves, and blood flow patterns. This noninvasive test offers rich information on cardiac structure and function. Clinicians employ echocardiography to evaluate conditions such as valve disorders of the heart, cardiomyopathies, and congenital heart disease, thus making diagnoses accordingly. Echocardiograms also help identify changes in heart function over time, indicating whether the current treatment is effective. In addition, modalities such as Doppler echocardiography facilitate thorough analysis of blood flow and pressure gradients, which are crucial in heart failure and pulmonary hypertension. These skills render echocardiography an essential modality in the overall assessment of cardiovascular disease, leading to better patient outcomes through early diagnosis and therapy. As diagnostic equipment continues to improve, the interaction between ECG and echocardiography is increasing. New signal processing advancements have enabled more robust interpretation of ECG data, including nonlinear methods that reveal subtleties in heart rate variability (HRV) indicative of underlying conditions (Maji et al., 2020). As with the intricacy of echocardiographic images obtained by ultrasound, with dimensional and functional data aiding in understanding cardiac well-being. A combination of the above tests not only maximizes diagnostic sensitivity and specificity but also yields a more integrated understanding of cardiovascular health. Thus, integrating ECG and echocardiographic measurements into a comprehensive diagnostic approach can maximize the detection of cardiovascular disease, ultimately guiding targeted therapies and improving patient treatment protocols. Multidisciplinary application in this fashion underscores the benefits of using state-of-the-art diagnostic techniques to inform clinical decision-making in cardiovascular medicine (Figure 4.12).

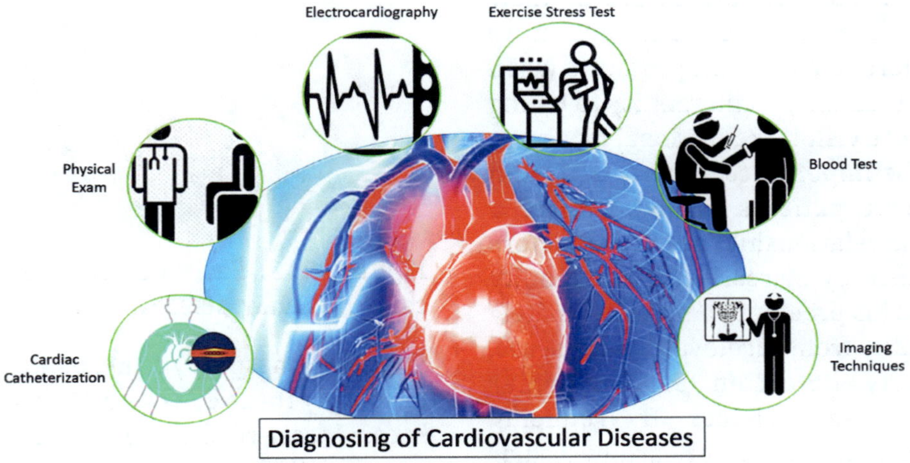

Figure 4.12. Current diagnosis techniques for CVDs.

Source: https://www.mdpi.com/chemosensors/chemosensors-09-00067/article_deploy/html/images/chemosensors-09-00067-g002.png.

4.3.3. Importance of Early Detection

Early detection of cardiovascular diseases is a significant consideration that directly affects patient outcomes and treatment success. Detection of these conditions followed by early intervention plays an essential role in the prevention of complications such as heart failure, stroke, or cardiac arrest. Cardiovascular diseases usually arise silently, without clear symptoms; hence, chronic screening and knowledge about risk factors among patients are significant. Advances in medical and screening technologies allow for improved diagnostic precision. It is important to note that the application of genetic testing for conditions such as 22q11.2 deletion syndrome, which is associated with congenital heart disease, illustrates how diagnosis can alter treatment strategy and enhance patient care. By appropriately treating cardiovascular disease at an early stage, healthcare systems can effectively allocate resources, thereby improving individual health outcomes and overall public health measures. Not only does early detection matter, but it's also a central component of lifestyle modification and patient education. When patients are aware of their risk status for conditions such as hypertension, diabetes, and hyperlipidemia, they are in charge. They can make sound decisions about their health once their risk status is identified. Preventive measures such as diet and exercise can be promoted more effectively when patients are aware of their risk status. Furthermore, patients are more inclined to adhere to treatment protocols when diagnosed early, as their vulnerability to falling sick is made more visible. Educational measures emphasizing the importance of early detection not only educate patients but also foster a communication relationship between doctors and patients, thereby increasing accountability in health care. This preemptive move ultimately reduces morbidity from cardiovascular disease. Moreover, early detection carries wider socioeconomic consequences. By reducing the occurrence and severity of cardiovascular illnesses through early intervention, health systems can mitigate the cost impact of advanced treatment, extended lengths of stay in hospitals, and chronic care. Preventive care, such as routine screening, can reduce overall healthcare expenditure by minimizing the need for intensive medical interventions. Promotion efforts that advocate for routine cardiovascular screening highlight the necessity for embedding such practice in regular health assessments. This well-oriented diversion of healthcare resources may improve the quality of life in risk-prone populations. Due to the increasing prevalence of cardiovascular diseases, developing an early diagnosis culture is not only beneficial but also necessary to secure long-term healthcare systems and improved outcomes in communities (Figure 4.13).

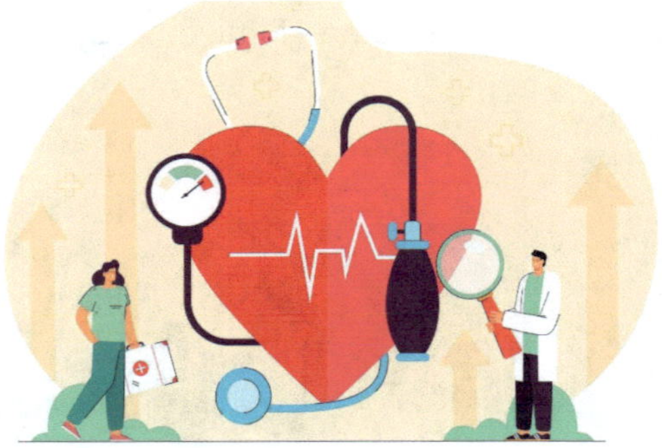

Figure 4.13. Early detection key to reducing cardiovascular disease.

Source: https://cdn-res.keymedia.com/cdn-cgi/image/w=1000,h=600,f=auto/https://cdn-res.keymedia.com/cms/images/ca/159/0379_638648588226268942.jpg.

Test Your Knowledge

1. What is the diagnostic test for cardiovascular disease?
2. Why is early detection of cardiovascular disease important?

4.4. Treatment Options

Learning Outcome

1. Know the lifestyle modifications in the prevention and management of cardiovascular disorders
2. Describe the medications in the management of cardiovascular disorders
3. Understand the surgical interventions in the management of cardiovascular disorders

Adequate control of cardiovascular conditions involves sufficient understanding of the available treatment options, which are broadly classified into pharmacological interventions, lifestyle modification, and surgical procedures. Pharmacologic therapies generally involve the use of drugs to manage symptoms, reduce the risk of complications, and address the underlying causes. For instance, antithrombotic agents are critical in preventing thromboembolic events in individuals with atrial fibrillation. A review of treatment variation revealed that hospitals with specialized anticoagulation and heart failure clinics achieved better outcomes, and the significance of targeted therapies has been highlighted (Camm et al., 2012). Furthermore, beta-blockers and ACE inhibitors are effective in treating heart failure as well as hypertension, and they have a direct impact on morbidity and mortality rates among cardiovascular disease patients. In addition to pharmacological management, lifestyle modifications are an essential part of the management of cardiovascular disorders. Dietary modifications, increased exercise, and smoking cessation are some of the salient elements of lifestyle modifications that all contribute to maximum heart health. A regular routine and dietary regimen designed for heart health have been shown to lower blood pressure and improve cardiovascular well-being. The correlation between lifestyle interventions and clinical outcomes also indicates the role of patient education for self-management of cardiovascular disease. Research has also shown that behavior change programs can be as effective as medication in some cases (Babic et al., 2020). These integrated approaches are instrumental not only for preventing the progression of cardiovascular diseases but also for enhancing the quality of life of individuals suffering from such conditions. Surgical options also play a crucial part in the management model of cardiovascular disease. Angioplasty, stenting, and CABG are often needed for patients with severe obstructive illness or who are unable to tolerate medical treatment. The decision to go ahead with surgical intervention would consider the general condition of the patients, the severity of the illness, and the prognosis. For instance, the RHYTHM-AF trial identifies variability in practice patterns across nations and suggests that accessibility of newer surgical technologies significantly influences treatment outcomes for individuals with atrial fibrillation (Camm et al., 2012). Overall, an interdisciplinary approach through pharmacological, lifestyle, and surgical treatments has a significant role in reducing the issues created by cardiovascular disease in humans (Figure 4.14).

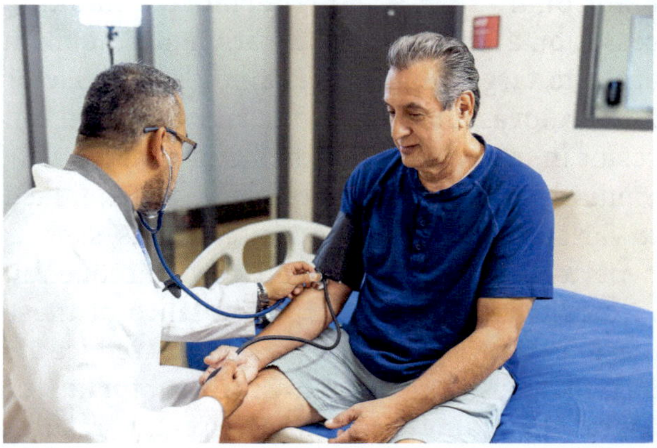

Figure 4.14. Treatment options for cardiovascular disorders.

Source: https://www.woosterhospital.org/wp-content/uploads/sites/229/2024/10/Cardiovascular-Disease-1.jpg.

4.4.1. Lifestyle Modifications

Lifestyle modifications are at the heart of the prevention and control of cardiovascular disease, as they directly influence risk factors such as obesity, hypertension, and diabetes. Research consistently underscores the importance of a balanced diet, physical activity, and a healthy weight. The Mediterranean diet, with high intakes of fruit, vegetables, whole grains, and healthy fats, is particularly well-researched for its cardiovascular benefits. Also, exercise has been shown to lower blood pressure, improve lipid levels, and generally improve cardiovascular health. By employing these alterations in lifestyle, individuals can create a healthier environment for their heart conditions, preferably lowering the risks of obtaining serious conditions like coronary artery disease and heart failure, most linked to cardiovascular disorders. Besides the lifestyle changes in dietary consumption and physical activity, psychological and behavioral changes are part of an entire lifestyle regimen. Interventions in stress management, such as mindfulness meditation and yoga, have yielded significant findings for cardiovascular health, including reduced cortisol levels and improved emotional status. Furthermore, smoking cessation and alcohol moderation are the main areas to target. Smoking is a potent risk factor for cardiovascular disorders, and cessation can result in instant improvements in heart health. Similarly, excessive alcohol use has been linked to various cardiovascular complications, such as hypertension and cardiomyopathy. Consequently, in cardiovascular disease, acceptance of these lifestyle interventions can significantly reduce the aggregate risks associated with harmful habits, thereby yielding healthier aggregate results. Environmental and social health determinants also play a critical role in determining the success of lifestyle changes. Access to resources such as healthful foods, safe opportunities for physical activity, and facilitating social relationships has a significant bearing on one's capacity to initiate and maintain lifestyle change. Community-based interventions that promote healthy living and active eating can create an environment conducive to heart health. Moreover, health practitioners can assist in improving patient outcomes by introducing education programs that emphasize the positioning of preconception diet and lifestyle components, given their long-term implications for future cardiovascular well-being. Through these complex themes, it is easier to adopt and sustain health-promoting behaviors, eventually leading to a significant reduction in the incidence of cardiovascular disease and an improvement in quality of life, as supported by lifestyle interventions in chronic disease (Bernier et al., 2012; Holleran et al., 2017).

4.4.2. Medications (Antihypertensives, Anticoagulants)

Treatment of cardiovascular disease often necessitates antihypertensive therapy, which accounts for the prevention of acute cardiac events. The most important drug groups are angiotensin-converting enzyme inhibitors (ACEIs), angiotensin II receptor blockers (ARBs), beta-blockers (BBs), calcium channel blockers (CCBs), and thiazides. Experience has shown that the effectiveness of these drugs may vary astonishingly with respect to patient individuality and adherence to medication therapy. Of specific note, a recent longitudinal study reported that long-term monotherapy using thiazides or ARBs indicated a lower prevalence of acute cardiac drug therapy compared to BBs, particularly in high-risk individuals with diabetes. This underscores the importance of tailored treatment regimens in optimizing outcomes for individuals with hypertension and related cardiovascular diseases (Li et al., 2024). Anticoagulants form an integral component of managing cardiovascular disease, particularly in individuals with a high risk for developing a thromboembolic episode. Anticoagulants like warfarin, direct oral anticoagulants (DOACs), and heparins are administered to prevent clot development, leading to severe consequences like stroke or myocardial infarction. The choice of anticoagulant is usually based on the specific clinical syndrome, i.e., the patient's renal function, other drugs, and factors that increase bleeding risk. A comparative effectiveness review found that certain anticoagulants, particularly DOACs, may offer good safety profiles and improved patient compliance compared with traditional therapies, and suggested a paradigm shift in selecting anticoagulants for cardiovascular disease patients. These advancements highlight the evolving dynamics of cardiovascular pharmacotherapy and require continuous monitoring of drug efficacy and safety across diverse patient populations (Li et al., 2023).

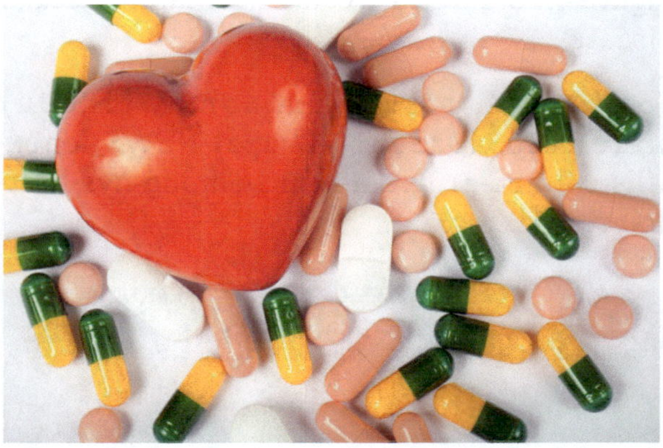

Figure 4.15. Oral antihypertensive drugs.

Source: https://www.drugoffice.gov.hk/eps/do/en/images/subtitle/consumer/news_informations/Product5.jpg.

A combination of antihypertensives and anticoagulants in the management of cardiovascular diseases is a comprehensive approach towards patient therapy. The combined impact of such drugs can lead to dramatic alterations in patient outcomes, including enhanced morbidity and mortality. However, judicious assessment of drug interactions, side effects, and individual patient profiles should be carried out to maximize gains and minimize risks. Continuous observation of patient responses to such medication is also critical, as adjustments are made to accommodate shifts in health or adherence patterns. Coordination among healthcare providers, patients, and caregivers is ultimately responsible for the enhanced effectiveness and safety of treatment programs for cardiovascular disease, thereby reducing the overall burden of cardiovascular disease (Li et al., 2024) (Figure 4.15).

4.4.3. Surgical Interventions (Bypass surgery, Stenting)

The presence of cardiovascular disease necessitates a variety of operations, with stenting and bypass surgery becoming core procedures in contemporary medicine. Bypass surgery involves creating an alternate channel for blood flow when there is arterial blockage, typically using veins or arteries from other parts of the body. The operation is necessary for patients who have coronary artery disease, where atherosclerosis weakens the heart's circulatory system. The effectiveness of these therapies has been substantiated by numerous clinical trials, resulting in dramatic improvements in outcomes for postoperative patients. In addition to reperfusion of ischemic territories, bypass surgery continues to exert a beneficial, long-term effect on quality of life and exercise capacity, underscoring its role as an anchor treatment for complex cardiovascular disease. Stenting, which is less extreme than bypass surgery, also plays an important role in the management of cardiovascular disease, particularly in patients with not-so-extensive arterial blockages. The procedure involves placing a small mesh tube, or stent, in narrowed arteries to maintain patency and facilitate unobstructed blood flow. Drug-eluting stents have also revolutionized this area by reducing the rate of restenosis, or re-narrowing of the artery. Studies have revealed that stenting not only symptomatically improves symptoms such as angina but also cardiovascular outcomes in both acute and chronic states. The relative ease and lower recovery period with stenting, compared to bypass surgery, make it particularly attractive to those who may be at higher risk for complications from surgery, thereby making more patients treatable. The dual approach of these surgical interventions, both stenting and bypass surgery, is a multifocused therapy meant to treat cardiovascular diseases. Both treatments focus on the pathophysiological process underlying coronary artery disease and are appropriate for various patient needs and situations. Also, recent research verifies that patients undergoing metabolic surgical treatments, such as gastric bypass, exhibit positive outcomes in terms of obesity and its comorbid conditions, which are leading risk factors for cardiovascular disease. By emphasizing the connection between weight loss surgical procedures and cardiovascular health, health care professionals can develop more comprehensive treatment plans for high-risk populations. This integrated approach is crucial for reducing the burden of cardiovascular disease and strengthening the role of surgery in contemporary cardiology (Labashova et al., 2024; Bhanja et al., 2025) (Figure 4.16).

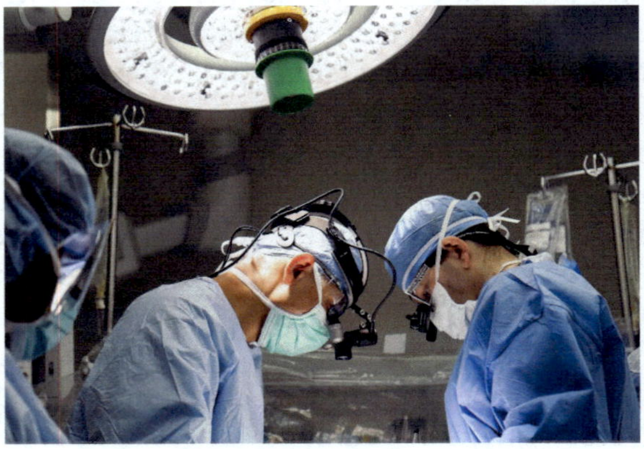

Figure 4.16. Surgical treatment of cardiovascular diseases.

Source: https://dam.northwell.edu/m/1e1fce6349aa6b1f/Drupal-NEWS_lenox-hills-cardiac-program-ranks-among-nys-best-doh-reports.jpg.

Test Your Knowledge

1. What is the medication for cardiovascular disease?
2. What is the surgical treatment for cardiovascular disease?

4.5. Prevention Strategies

Learning Outcome

1. Understand the importance of regular health screenings
2. Understand the role of diet and exercise in the prevention of cardiovascular disorders
3. Describe the public health initiatives and education of addressing cardiovascular disorders

Effective prevention strategies for cardiovascular disease are based on a multifaceted approach that combines lifestyle modification, public health interventions, and clinical care. The starting point is promoting a healthy lifestyle, with diet, exercise, and smoking cessation being key to avoiding risk factors such as hypertension, hyperlipidemia, and obesity. For instance, the addition of a high-fruit and vegetable diet, whole grains, and lean protein supports cardiovascular well-being through reduced systemic inflammation and blood pressure regulation. In addition, routine physical exercise, even at minimal levels, significantly enhances cardiovascular resilience. Public health measures, such as community exercise programs and diet education, play a key role in engaging populations toward a healthier way of life and, again, underscore the need for interdisciplinary collaboration to stem the tide of cardiovascular diseases. Prevention of cardiovascular disease also includes proactive management of risk factors by therapeutic interventions. Utilization of screening programs that target the selection of individuals at high risk has also grown increasingly crucial in contemporary healthcare protocols. Such programs are inclined to use tools such as blood pressure screening, lipid profile, and blood glucose to enable early detection of cardiovascular disease in candidates. Besides, direct interventions such as drug therapy for hypertension and hyperlipidemia and lifestyle change counseling have demonstrated efficacy in avoiding the onset of cardiovascular events. Combining technological advancements, such as telemedicine visits for remote observation and learning, presents promising methods to aid patients in cardiovascular disease management. Such a program ensures that vulnerable patients receive timely intervention, thereby preventing progression to more complex complications. Lastly, the role of resilience in public health cannot be stressed too much in interventions towards cardiovascular disorder prevention. Community resilience, as encapsulated under the Centers for Disease Control and Prevention's BRACE framework, enables communities to develop the capacity to anticipate as well as respond to health challenges. Building resilience involves tackling social determinants of health, such as access to health care, socioeconomic resources, and the environment. (Aytur et al., 2014) emphasizes how effective communities are in establishing resilience, enabling them to survive health risks without causing deleterious health effects. Not only is this composite notion of resilience empowering people to be health-informed agents of their own determinants, but it also fosters intersectoral collaboration in working towards developing enabling environments. Besides this, recent evidence identifies the antioxidant function in combating oxidative stress—a fundamental cause of cardiovascular disease—that further underscores the importance of ongoing research into new innovative advanced therapeutic nutritional interventions to support cardiovascular health and prevent disease progression (Conti et al., 2016) (Figure 4.17).

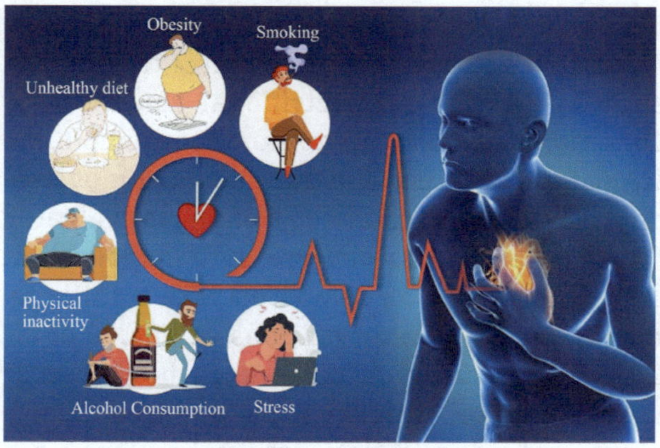

Figure 4.17. Prevention strategies for cardiovascular disorders.

Source: https://blog.thyrocare.com/wp-content/uploads/2021/11/prevent-cardiovascular-diseases.jpg.

4.5.1. Importance of Regular Health Screenings

Routine health screening is most critical for early diagnosis and control of cardiovascular disease, greatly affecting patient outcomes. By performing routine exams, clinicians can identify risk factors such as hypertension, elevated cholesterol levels, and diabetes, which play a central role in the development of heart disease. For instance, a screening program that includes the measurement of blood pressure and lipid profiles not only facilitates the early detection but also allows preventive interventions to be initiated. These preventive interventions can decrease the occurrence of significant cardiovascular events such as heart attacks and strokes, thus enhancing the quality of life. In addition, educating the patient about their state of health encourages lifestyle changes that reduce cardiovascular risk, demonstrating that screenings are not merely diagnostic instruments but are integral to the package of promoting overall well-being and good health. Adding cardiovascular screenings to routine healthcare practices underscores the significance of lifestyle as a determinant of disease prevention. Recent studies highlight the importance of nonpharmacological treatments, such as exercise and nutritional guidance, for conditions such as hypertension. For example, the HAEL Study is great illustration of an innovative approach in which exercise training is evaluated for its potential in blood pressure management among older adults, compared with traditional health education interventions (Alberton et al., 2019). This research centers on how regular screenings will inform individualized health plans and educate patients on how they can adopt healthier lifestyles. These interventions may include planned exercise routines and dietary changes based on established health profiles, all supported by data gathered from regular checkups. Herein, screenings serve as staging grounds that enable integrated health management. Moreover, the efficiency of early intervention by repeated health screening is reinforced by medical progress addressing cardiovascular ailments. The evolving therapeutic environment underscores the imperative for active case-finding among those at risk. For instance, current guidelines demand heterogeneous screening strategies tailored to a wide range of demographic parameters, thereby ensuring patient-profile-specific interventions. As scientific studies of microbial health reveal complex interdependencies between the gut microbiota and cardiovascular health, such information can redefine screening protocols to embrace more comprehensive concepts of health (Hage et al., 2017). Incorporating these factors illustrates an awareness that cardiovascular health is not an independent entity; it is a set of competing factors that screenings can help identify. Consequently, regular screening not only facilitates early diagnosis but also provides an overall perspective of health, relieving the population burden of cardiovascular conditions (Figure 4.18).

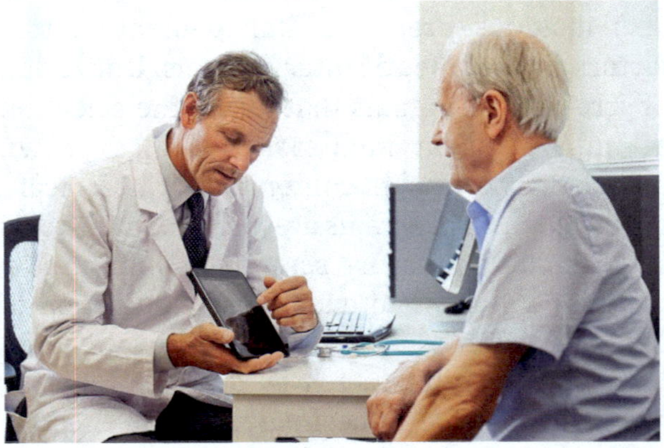

Figure 4.18. Importance of regular heart health checkups.

Source: https://www.harleystreet.sg/img/regular-checkup-4.jpg.

4.5.2. Role of Diet and Exercise in Prevention

The role of diet and physical exercise in the prevention of cardiovascular disease is a critical component of public health measures aimed at reducing the cases of such disorders. A healthy diet that incorporates plenty of fruits, vegetables, whole foods, and healthy fats has been shown to reduce cardiovascular risk factors, including hypertension and hyperlipidemia. Moreover, regular physical exercise plays a crucial role in maintaining a healthy weight, endothelial function, and blood pressure regulation. The combined effects of dietary modification and physical exercise lead to improved metabolic health, which is important for minimizing the risk of cardiovascular disease. The adoption of such lifestyle changes, however, requires sustained effort and education, particularly in groups identified as being at risk, such as women who have experienced hypertensive disorders of pregnancy (HDP) (Giorgione et al., 2020). Utilization of community programs for physical activity and nutrition can also support these preventive interventions. Successful behavior change strategies are also important in the promotion of healthier lifestyles and the prevention of cardiovascular diseases. Individual-level interventions, such as counseling from health professionals, have also been shown in research to increase smoking cessation rates, improve dietary habits, and increase physical activity among patients (Hillsdon et al., 2006). For example, in high-risk groups like those with a history of HDP, these interventions enable the patients to acquire lifestyle modifications that are beneficial in future cardiovascular risk reduction. Individualized counseling to address the individual's specific needs increases the likelihood of compliance, supporting sustained behavior that benefits long-term cardiovascular health. Passive interventions such as community initiatives and education can also help create supportive environments that promote healthier diets and more active lifestyles, underscoring the importance of including lifestyle change techniques in public health policy on a systemwide basis. In a nutshell, the combination of dietary change and exercise is of foremost importance in the prevention of cardiovascular disorders.

By focusing on appropriate lifestyle choices, medical professionals not only provide people with enough information to make the right decisions but also foster a prevention culture. Prevention is particularly vital following pregnancy complications such as HDP, where women undergoing them are at increased risk of developing cardiovascular diseases in the future (Giorgione et al., 2020). Nutrition and physical activity-based health promotion, complemented by community-based interventions, can be a mighty pillar in the fight against cardiovascular disease. As the evidence base for protective benefits of healthy living continues to grow, it becomes more clearly apparent that there must be sustained efforts at dietary improvement and physical exercise in the quest for cardiovascular health and lifespan (Figure 4.19).

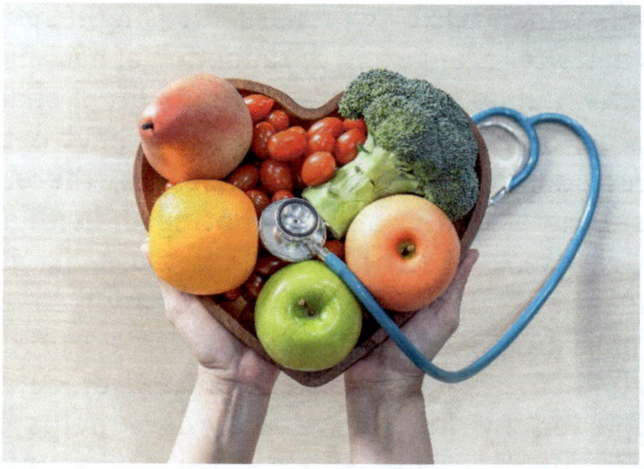

Figure 4.19. The role of diet in preventing cardiovascular disease.

Source: https://www.news-medical.net/images/news/ImageForNews_738336_16759119197148855.jpg.

4.5.3. Public Health Initiatives and Education

Under intervention of cardiovascular disease, education and public health interventions are key to playing a role in the decrease of risk factors as well as improving the general outcome of health. These interventions primarily focus on lifestyle modifications, such as consuming a balanced diet and ensuring physical activity, which are essential for preventing cardiovascular disease. Schools, community centers, and health centers collaborate frequently to educate the population about heart health, enabling them to make informed choices about their health. Social marketing campaigns, leveraging persuasive messages, as well as community involvement, have been successful in educating the public about the dangers of inactive living and unhealthy diets. Interventions that prioritize integrating cardiovascular health education into existing health programs can significantly reduce the prevalence of cardiovascular disease across various populations and thereby help build healthier communities. Education in cardiovascular health, nonetheless, extends further than basic awareness, focusing instead on behavior change and the adoption of healthier habits. Public health interventions often share the personal stories of patients who have been affected by cardiovascular diseases, thereby fostering empathy and prompting individuals to reassess their health behaviors. These educational interventions are supported by clinical interventions, in which awareness of risk factors, including hypertension and diabetes, imparted by healthcare providers helps in early identification and control. Community workshops have demonstrated a notable increase in knowledge acquisition, revealing that tailored educational interventions can be effective in addressing diverse demographic needs. The workshops acknowledge the imperative role of continuing education in the cardiovascular disorders war, identifying proactive healthcare management as a means to reduce incidence rates across various populations. Furthermore, the use of technology in public health efforts has increased access to and the impact of educational activities on cardiovascular diseases. Social networks, mobile applications, and online lectures are all available resources for individuals who want to learn about cardiovascular health. Such technologies provide user-based health education with content that targets the individual's particular health interests and needs. Furthermore, the widespread accessibility afforded by technology ensures that significant information about cardiovascular health reaches numerous groups, some of whom might otherwise have remained unknown. Organizations have now begun to take advantage of these assets to provide instant data and educational materials, ultimately contributing to an informed population. By this modern approach, public health initiatives not only disseminate valuable information but also create an environment where individuals are empowered to place greater significance on cardiovascular well-being, thereby being instrumental in contributing significantly towards a notable reduction in the incidence of such disorders in society.

Test Your Knowledge

1. What is the importance of regular health screenings?
2. What is the role of diet and exercise in the prevention of cardiovascular disorders?

SUMMARY

In summary, the intricacies of cardiovascular diseases in man require a multidisciplinary comprehension of their etiology and treatment. The relationship between physiological factors such as heart rate variability (HRV) and psychological resilience is a significant topic of research. Individual variations in HRV have been used in recent studies to propose varying degrees of resistance against stress-related illness, which influence the onset of cardiovascular disease. This finding highlights the need to incorporate psychological models into cardiovascular health assessments, which could lead to novel therapeutic interventions tailored to the patient's personal profile, thereby mitigating the impact of psychological stressors on cardiac well-being. Such integrated approaches may ultimately contribute to better treatment protocols that not only treat the physiological covariates of cardiovascular disease but also the psychological variables that influence patient outcomes (Carnevali et al., 2018). Furthermore, oxidative stress plays a role in aging and cardiovascular disease. Older individuals are at higher risk for oxidative damage, primarily due to lowered antioxidant defenses. The recognition of the disproportion between pro-oxidants and antioxidants has profound implications for understanding cardiovascular pathologies. While antioxidant supplementation has been proposed as a preventive strategy, clinical trials have yielded mixed results, underscoring the complexity of this topic. Such inconsistency may stem from variations in individuals' metabolic demands and genetic predispositions, suggesting an erroneous one-size-fits-all approach to antioxidant treatment. Future studies must be capable of refining their methodology in order to better capture the heterogeneous response to oxidative stress, so interventions are specific and effective at managing age-related cardiovascular diseases (Conti et al., 2016). Finally, cardiovascular diseases will need to be managed through an integrated strategy that incorporates both biological and psychological factors. As studies continue to elucidate the interactions among cardiovascular well-being, stress resistance, and oxidative stress, practitioners will need to adapt their practices to reflect these discoveries. Through supporting a holistic understanding of cardiovascular health, one that takes into account physical, psychological, and environmental factors—healthcare providers can better aid their patients. This comprehensive approach not only favors effective treatment protocols but also emphasizes the merit of preventive measures, encouraging lifestyle modification that enhances resilience while reducing oxidative stress. In this way, the field of cardiovascular health can advance toward more robust, resilient health outcomes for individuals across all age groups, ultimately improving quality of life for an aging population.

While learning about cardiovascular disease in humans, it is essential to understand the complexity of the diseases, which encompass a wide variety of disease conditions affecting the heart and blood vessels. They are serious health conditions that can lead to severe morbidity and mortality. Risk factors like high blood pressure, elevated cholesterol levels, obesity, and diabetes are all established causes of cardiovascular disease, which makes understanding how these interact with overall health critical. It is also important to acknowledge the influence of psychosocial determinants, since psychological distress and mental illness can have a significant effect on cardiovascular health. As indicated in a study, throughout the life course, stress is an important determinant of disease and health, emphasizing that there is a need for an interdisciplinary treatment strategy considering physical as well as psychological well-being to treat cardiovascular diseases to the best and improve patient outcomes (Estrine et al., 2006). The role of environmental causes of cardiovascular health has also gained attention recently. Climate change itself is a critical health risk to human populations, including cardiovascular health. Increased temperature, air pollution, and the occurrence of extreme weather events can exacerbate existing diseases and bring on new problems in managing cardiovascular diseases. The recommendations of the Centers for Disease Control and Prevention include calling for establishing measures to address health issues related to climate change. These strategies are necessary because they aim to build community resilience to environmental changes that could adversely affect heart health (Aytur et al., 2014). This intersection between the environment and cardiovascular diseases demands ongoing research and interventions that integrate public health and environmental science. Ultimately, prevention and control of cardiovascular diseases require a cross-sectoral, collaborative response. Caregivers, policymakers, and community organizations must cooperate to address the social and environmental determinants of cardiovascular health. By establishing interventions to foster healthier ways of living, increased access to care, and community resilience, stakeholders can effectively stem the burden of cardiovascular diseases. Community engagement is crucial in identifying local health needs and framing relevant interventions that address them. This holistic strategy not only addresses immediate health concerns but also ensures improved cardiovascular health outcomes in the long term, in line with overall public health goals. The union of these elements can yield effective strategies to address cardiovascular disease in a rapidly evolving world.

KEY TERMS FROM THIS CHAPTER

- Arrhythmias
- Atrial fibrillation
- Bradycardia
- Cardiovascular health
- Coronary artery disease
- Diet
- Exercise
- Heart failure
- Heart rate variability
- Hypertension
- Major depressive disorder
- Myocardial infarction
- Physical health
- Stress management

CRITICAL THINKING QUESTIONS

1. **Which of the following is the leading risk factor for coronary artery disease (CAD)?**
   a. Hypertension
   b. Low cholesterol levels
   c. High physical activity
   d. Anemia
2. **What is the most common symptom of myocardial infarction (heart attack)?**
   a. Abdominal pain
   b. Crushing chest pain radiating to the left arm or jaw
   c. High-grade fever
   d. Persistent headache
3. **Which of the following is a non-modifiable risk factor for cardiovascular disease?**
   a. Smoking
   b. Physical inactivity
   c. Family history of cardiovascular disease
   d. Obesity
4. **Which test is the gold standard for diagnosing coronary artery disease?**
   a. Chest X-ray
   b. Coronary angiography
   c. Electrocardiogram (ECG)
   d. Echocardiography
5. **What is the most common type of arrhythmia?**
   a. Atrial fibrillation
   b. Ventricular tachycardia
   c. Complete heart block
   d. Torsades de Pointes

Short Answer Questions

1. What is meant by cardiovascular disorder?
2. List the types of cardiovascular disorders.
3. What is an arrhythmia?
4. What are the treatments for cardiovascular disease?
5. What are the strategies to prevent cardiovascular disease?

Answer to Critical Thinking Questions

1. (a); 2. (b); 3. (c); 4. (b); 5. (a).

REFERENCES

1. Pandi-Perumal, S. R., BaHammam, A. S., Ojike, N. I., Akinseye, O. A., Kendzerska, T., Buttoo, K., Dhandapany, P. S., Brown, G. M., & Cardinali, D. P. (2016). Melatonin and human cardiovascular disease. *Journal of Cardiovascular Pharmacology and Therapeutics*, *22*(2), 122–132. https://doi.org/10.1177/1074248416660622Alberton, C. L., Alves, L., Bock, P. M., et al. (2019). The "Hypertension Approaches in the Elderly: A Lifestyle Study" multicenter, randomized trial (HAEL Study): Rationale and methodological protocol. https://core.ac.uk/download/305121369.pdf (accessed on 12th July 2025).
2. Alessandri, C., Ciciarello, F. L., Colasanti, T., et al. (2017). Association between antibodies to carbamylated proteins and subclinical atherosclerosis in rheumatoid arthritis patients. https://core.ac.uk/download/98347599.pdf (accessed on 12th July 2025).
3. Anderson, B., Bechara, B., Bechara, B., Boubela, C., Cannon, J., et al. (2015). Interactions between visceral afferent signaling and stimulus processing. https://core.ac.uk/download/30612909.pdf (accessed on 12th July 2025).
4. Aromatario, M., Cappelletti, S., Piacentino, D., et al. (2015). Caffeine: Cognitive and physical performance enhancer or psychoactive drug? https://core.ac.uk/download/54528776.pdf (accessed on 12th July 2025).
5. Aytur, S., Bucci, J., & Wake, C. P. (2014). An assessment of the impact of climate change on human health in New Hampshire. https://core.ac.uk/download/84123597.pdf (accessed on 12th July 2025).
6. Babić, M., van der Giet, M., Herrmann, J., et al. (2020). Research models for studying vascular calcification. https://core.ac.uk/download/323258131.pdf (accessed on 12th July 2025).
7. Badger, J., Morrell, J. S., & Quatromoni, P. A. (2019). Relationship between stress and healthy lifestyle factors of college students. https://core.ac.uk/download/322973288.pdf (accessed on 12th July 2025).
8. Bassett, A. S., Emanuel, B. S., Marino, B., et al. (2015). 22q11.2 deletion syndrome. https://core.ac.uk/download/188828218.pdf (accessed on 12th July 2025).
9. Baumert, M., & Stein, P. (2021). Comment on 'The effect of persistent U-shaped patterns in RR night-time series on the heart rate variability complexity in healthy humans. *Physiological Measurement*, *42*. https://www.semanticscholar.org/paper/64e42b8719a5fe0b6fea0f432da1f8da0776e004 (accessed on 12th July 2025).
10. Behjati, M. (2016). Orthopedic problems: An underestimated hidden risk factor for development and progression of atherosclerosis; An inconspicuous joint link. *ARYA Atherosclerosis*, *12*, 115–117. https://www.semanticscholar.org/paper/c911fdb86647c73983e56069fc62337ee0cff397 (accessed on 12th July 2025).
11. Bernier, D. (2012). Polycystic ovary syndrome: Pathogenesis, health consequences, and treatment of PCOS in relation to insulin resistance. https://core.ac.uk/download/72048051.pdf (accessed on 12th July 2025).
12. Bhanja, M., & Vaishnaw, A. (2025). Evaluating the long-term outcomes of metabolic surgery in obesity management: Effects on weight loss, comorbidities, quality of life, and sustainability of surgical interventions. *Journal of Neonatal Surgery*. https://www.semanticscholar.org/paper/9276e5108adae30b53ba5141c9b8f629eeb4288e (accessed on 12th July 2025).

13. Brankovic, A., & Jukić, S. (2024). The financial toll of BMI on health services: A comparative cost assessment using big data. https://core.ac.uk/download/657027661.pdf (accessed on 12th July 2025).

14. Budiono, B. P., Headrick, J. P., Neumann, D. L., et al. (2017). The heartbreak of depression: 'Psycho-cardiac' coupling in myocardial infarction. https://core.ac.uk/download/196605092.pdf (accessed on 12th July 2025).

15. Camm, A. J., Maggioni, A. P., Bernhardt, A. A., Martín, A., Gitt, A. K., Go, A. S., Lown, B., et al. (2012). RHYTHM-AF: Design of an international registry on cardioversion of atrial fibrillation and characteristics of participating centers. https://core.ac.uk/download/12797722.pdf (accessed on 12th July 2025).

16. Cammisotto, V., Carnevale, R., Castellani, V., et al. (2017). Extra virgin olive oil and cardiovascular diseases: Benefits for human health. https://core.ac.uk/download/141695177.pdf (accessed on 12th July 2025).

17. Canova, C., Ludvigsson, J. F., Pitter, G., et al. (2016). Risks of hospitalization and drug consumption in children and young adults with diagnosed celiac disease and the role of maternal education: A population-based matched birth cohort study. https://core.ac.uk/download/53531106.pdf (accessed on 12th July 2025).

18. Carnevali, L., Koenig, J., Ottaviani, C., et al. (2018). Autonomic and brain morphological predictors of stress resilience. https://core.ac.uk/download/157570373.pdf (accessed on 12th July 2025).

19. Combet, E., Dall'Asta, M., Dumont, J., et al. (2017). A systematic review and meta-analysis of the effects of flavanol-containing tea, cocoa, and apple products on body composition and blood lipids: Exploring the factors responsible for variability in their efficacy. https://core.ac.uk/download/84148912.pdf (accessed on 12th July 2025).

20. Conti, V., Corbi, G., De Lise, F., et al. (2016). Antioxidant supplementation in the treatment of aging-associated diseases. https://core.ac.uk/download/77014107.pdf (accessed on 12th July 2025).

21. De Marchis, M., D'Amato, A., Fedele, F., et al. (2018). Diabetes mellitus and ischemic heart disease: The role of ion channels. https://core.ac.uk/download/159269109.pdf (accessed on 12th July 2025).

22. Eghbali, M., & Sharma, S. (2014). Influence of sex differences on microRNA gene regulation in disease. https://core.ac.uk/download/323079075.pdf (accessed on 12th July 2025).

23. El Hage, R., Hernandez Sanabria, E., & Van de Wiele, T. (2017). Emerging trends in 'smart probiotics': Functional consideration for the development of novel health and industrial applications. https://core.ac.uk/download/147045642.pdf (accessed on 12th July 2025).

24. Elias, P. M., & Man, M. Q. (2019). Could inflammaging and its sequelae be prevented or mitigated? https://core.ac.uk/download/323062598.pdf (accessed on 12th July 2025).

25. Estrine, J., & DeLisle, L. (2006). Stress: Putting the brain back into medicine. https://core.ac.uk/download/71356692.pdf (accessed on 12th July 2025).

26. Estrine, J., & O'Brien, N. (2003). Sleep, health, and aging. https://core.ac.uk/download/71356671.pdf (accessed on 12th July 2025).

27. Francis, J., Johnson, P., Praveen, S. V., & Venugopal, K. (2006). Gene therapy in cardiac arrhythmias. https://core.ac.uk/download/pdf/86511.pdf (accessed on 12th July 2025).
28. Galea, C., Galea, M., & Sciberras, C. (2014). Attention deficit hyperactivity disorder: An overview. https://core.ac.uk/download/46603082.pdf (accessed on 12th July 2025).
29. Giorgione, V., Khalil, A., Melchiorre, K., et al. (2020). Hypertensive disorders of pregnancy and future cardiovascular health. https://core.ac.uk/download/322832242.pdf (accessed on 12th July 2025).
30. Hillsdon, M., Summerbell, C., & Thorogood, M. (2006). Changing behavior. https://core.ac.uk/download/46332.pdf (accessed on 12th July 2025).
31. Holleran, A. R. (2017). The impacts of preconception nutrition on pregnancy: An educational module promoting preconception care. https://core.ac.uk/download/84397645.pdf (accessed on 12th July 2025).
32. Hummig, W., & Cruz, M. M. E. (2021). Bruxism as a clinical indicator of mental illness: Lessons from the COVID-19 to the future! *Revita De Psiquiatria Clinica, 48*, 127. https://www.semanticscholar.org/paper/50bd5abb02f987e60b0a70d63cdcaa060a174297 (accessed on 12th July 2025).
33. Labashova, V., Pateyuk, I., Dydyshko, Y., Stebunov, S., Kachan, A., Yelesina, M., Zarqua, A., et al. (2024). Cardiovascular risk in comorbid patients after metabolic surgery. *Emergency Cardiology and Cardiovascular Risks*. https://www.semanticscholar.org/paper/bd5b163fcfb354f1d83337587edd3b20a65317f6 (accessed on 12th July 2025).
34. Li, X., Bijlsma, M., Bos, J., Schuiling-Veninga, C., & Hak, E. (2023). Long-term comparative effectiveness of antihypertensive monotherapies in primary prevention of cardiovascular events: A population-based retrospective inception cohort study in the Netherlands. *BMJ Open, 13*. https://www.semanticscholar.org/paper/5817aae8ef42be6668ab9e82df9e741a124cd3fb (accessed on 12th July 2025).
35. Li, X., Bijlsma, M., de Vos, S., Bos, J. H. J., Mubarik, S., Schuiling-Veninga, C., & Hak, E. (2024). Comparative effectiveness of antihypertensive monotherapies in primary prevention of cardiovascular events—a real-world longitudinal inception cohort study. *Frontiers in Pharmacology, 15*. https://www.semanticscholar.org/paper/cf71397ccd2c6ae17511fe06d1db5a2509bf13bb (accessed on 12th July 2025).
36. Livingston, G., Huntley, J., Sommerlad, A., Ames, D., Ballard, C., Banerjee, S., Brayne, C., et al. (2020). Dementia prevention, intervention, and care: 2020 report of the Lancet Commission. *The Lancet, 396*, 413–446. https://doi.org/10.1016/s0140-6736(20)30367-6 (accessed on 12th July 2025).
37. Maji, C., Sengupta, P., Batabyal, A., & Chaudhuri, H. (2020). Nonlinear and statistical analysis of ECG signals from arrhythmia-affected cardiac system through the EMD process. *arXiv: Signal Processing*. https://www.semanticscholar.org/paper/b4df96e57e33b45dde84e0e53e81029100a4f8b5 (accessed on 12th July 2025).
38. Ventriglio, A., Sancassiani, F., Contu, M. P., Latorre, M., Di Slavatore, M., Fornaro, M., & Bhugra, D. (2020). Mediterranean diet and its benefits on health and mental health: A literature review. *Clinical Practice and Epidemiology in Mental Health, 16*, 156–164. https://doi.org/10.2174/1745017902016010156 (accessed on 12th July 2025).

ENDOCRINOLOGY DISORDERS

5

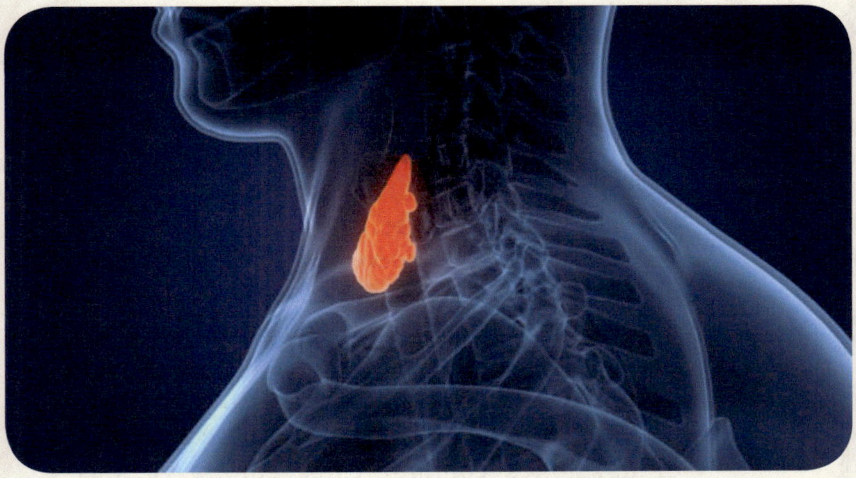

LEARNING OBJECTIVES

After studying this chapter, you will be able to:

1. Describe the types of endocrinology disorders
2. Understand the causes of endocrine disorders
3. Describe the symptoms of endocrine disorders
4. Learn about the diagnosis of endocrine disorders
5. Know the treatment options for endocrinology disorders
6. Describe the current research and advances in endocrinology

Introduction

The discipline of endocrinology encompasses the science of hormones, their functions, and the various endocrine diseases that arise from hormonal imbalances. Human endocrine disorders significantly affect the body's physiological systems, generating disease states that can affect growth, metabolism, and reproductive processes. Examples of such widely prevalent disorders are diabetes mellitus, thyroid disorders, and adrenal insufficiency, which all reflect the critical regulation of health by hormones. They are often characterized by multifactorial etiologies involving genetic, environmental, and lifestyle factors, which complicate diagnosis and management. As more is discovered about the mechanisms of such conditions, accurate identification of genetic mutations, such as those associated with steroidogenic factor 1 (SF-1), becomes imperative; these mutations are key to understanding specific disorders of sex development and emerging endocrine challenges in populations (Achermann et al., 2009). Recent research in endocrinology has underscored the need to bridge laboratory findings to real-world implications for human health. Workshops on the impact of, for instance, sleep disturbance on metabolic health demonstrate the intricate interdependencies between endocrine function and other biological processes. Disturbances of circadian rhythms, for example, have been shown to impact the sensitivity of glucose metabolism and insulin, thus underlining the importance of integrated approaches in endocrine research (Arble et al., 2015). Such an integrative framework has been proposed to create an immediate need for cross-disciplinary studies that can lead to new approaches aiming not just to understand endocrinology disorders better but also to enhance public health interventions to lower their incidence and impact.

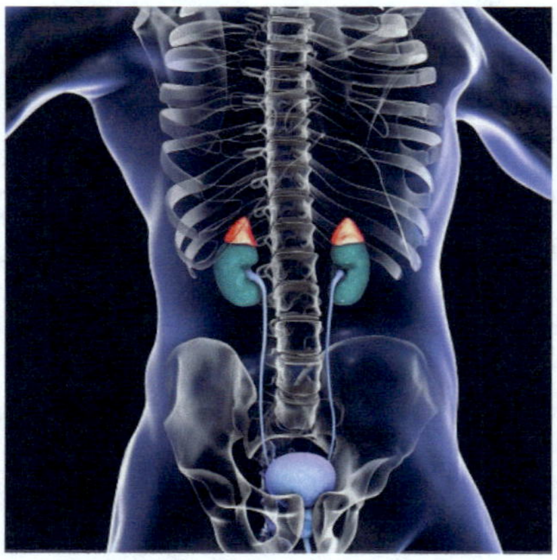

Figure 5.1. Endocrinology disorders.

Source: https://www.integratedspecialistmedicalcare.com.au/wp-content/uploads/2023/10/900-x-900-1-min.jpg.

As we further advance in our understanding and management of endocrine diseases, it is imperative that we consider the whole system of hormonal health across life's stages. The management of endocrine disease requires a three-faceted approach that integrates genetic research, lifestyle factors, and environmental determinants in prevention and treatment. Moreover, awareness that some disorders, such as severe hypospadias, have an early onset and are associated with genetic mutations justifies the need for early diagnosis and intervention (Achermann et al., 2009). Current and future research must also complement what is already known by exploring the contributions of endocrine disruptions, such as those caused by sleep and circadian disruptions, to general health issues such as obesity and type 2 diabetes. Addressing these needs in an interconnected manner is crucial for progress toward improved outcomes in endocrinology (Figure 5.1).

Definition of Endocrinology

Endocrinology is a significant field within the vast medical field that specializes in the study of glands and hormones that govern numerous physiological processes. The scope of biological processes is extensive, covering growth, metabolism, reproduction, and stress reactions. Endocrinologists diagnose and treat hormonal imbalance disorders, thereby resulting in severe health conditions such as diabetes, thyroid, and adrenal insufficiency. The intricate network of hormones communicates among various segments of the body, highlighting the endocrine system's role in regulating homeostasis. Understanding endocrinology's definition is fundamental to learning about its relevance to human health, particularly endocrine disorders resulting from hormonal dysregulation, which strongly affect a person's overall health. Surprisingly, endocrinology extends to the study of lifestyle factors and environmental influences that affect hormonal balance and overall health. For instance, research has established that lifestyle, such as drug abuse and diet, is closely related to fertility and other endocrine diseases. Literature that reviews the impact of tobacco smoking, alcohol consumption, and drug addiction on reproductive potential highlights the relationship between risky behavior and low fertility in both genders (Angelis et al., 2018). These findings emphasize the need for preventive interventions to mitigate the risk of endocrine diseases, highlighting the role of the endocrinologist in treatment and education. Promoting healthier lifestyles, endocrinologists aim to address the root causes of hormonal disturbances prior to their progression into more complex health conditions or chronic disease. Furthermore, understanding the underlying physiology of endocrine disorders and how they engage with other systems, such as the renal system, enhances our knowledge of these conditions. Chronic kidney disease (CKD), for example, is defined by many hormonal modifications that have a direct effect on patient outcomes and quality of life. High concentrations of pro-inflammatory cytokines and dysregulation of hormonal pathways can exacerbate conditions such as hypertension and insulin resistance, reflecting the interconnectedness of the endocrine and renal systems (Slee et al., 2012). Such interconnectedness underscores the importance of integrated management of endocrine disorders through collaboration among healthcare providers to offer integrative care. Lastly, the acceptance of the holistic definition of endocrinology helps clarify the broader importance of endocrine disorders in human health and encourages further research and clinical advancement in the field (Figure 5.2).

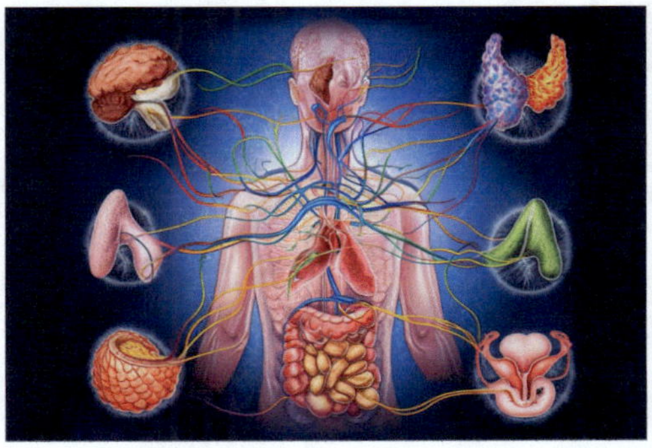

Figure 5.2. Endocrinology.

Source: https://vijaysuperspecialityhospital.in/wp-content/uploads/2024/08/a-captivating-and-educational-illustration-of-the-WRC8-LHTRKOHzEbV76x5Ug-a0JXnm_NT7ygxOblUMTjUA-1024x576.jpeg.

Importance of the Endocrine System

The endocrine system is responsible for the regulation of homeostasis in the human body by managing various physiological processes through hormone secretion. Hormones, released by glands such as the pituitary, thyroid, and adrenal glands, are chemical messengers that influence growth, metabolism, reproduction, and stress. The intricate relationship between the hypothalamus and pituitary gland, for instance, demonstrates the endocrine system's function as the regulatory center of the body for most of its functions. Interference with such regulatory pathways can lead to severe endocrine disease, thereby illustrating the important role a healthy endocrine system plays in general well-being. Studies have demonstrated that exposure to environmental chemicals interferes with key regulatory genes in the pituitary and hypothalamus, resulting in possible reproductive dysfunction, illustrating that both the environment and genetics play a role in endocrine well-being (Bellingham et al., 2016). A second major characteristic of the endocrine system is its relationship with the nervous system, which provides a framework for neuroendocrine signaling. This interaction regulates crucial processes, including the body's response to stress and mood control. The hypothalamic-pituitary-adrenal (HPA) axis is one of the most significant neuroendocrine systems and illustrates how stress may trigger hormonal responses that affect various systems in the body. Chronic endocrine axis dysregulation may be associated with disorders such as depression and anxiety, and it illustrates the interdependence of endocrine function and mental health. Disorders of sex development (DSD) underscore the complexities of the endocrine system even more, whereby hormonal dyshomeostasis may result in a variety of concomitant disorders. The international DSD Registry illustrates that a significant percentage of cases will be associated with other medical abnormalities, thus emphasizing the need for diligent clinical evaluation and integrated treatment (Ahmed et al., 2013). Given the endocrine system's crucial roles in health and disease, understanding its role in these contexts is essential for improving preventive and therapeutic interventions. The dysregulation of the system not only affects individual health outcomes but can also carry over into broader public health issues, especially in populations at risk of exposure to endocrine disruptors. The consideration of the effects of such exposures on major pathways, as evidenced by associations between maternal exposure to environmental chemicals, underscores the need for protective measures to mitigate health risks (Bellingham et al., 2016). Moreover, clinicians and researchers must give top priority to integral strategies considering the multidetermined causation of endocrinology disorders, given the fact that patients, many of whom will have co-morbidities, can complicate diagnosis and management. Emphasizing the importance of the endocrine system ultimately opens avenues for diagnosis, management, and public health interventions targeting endocrine dominance (Figure 5.3).

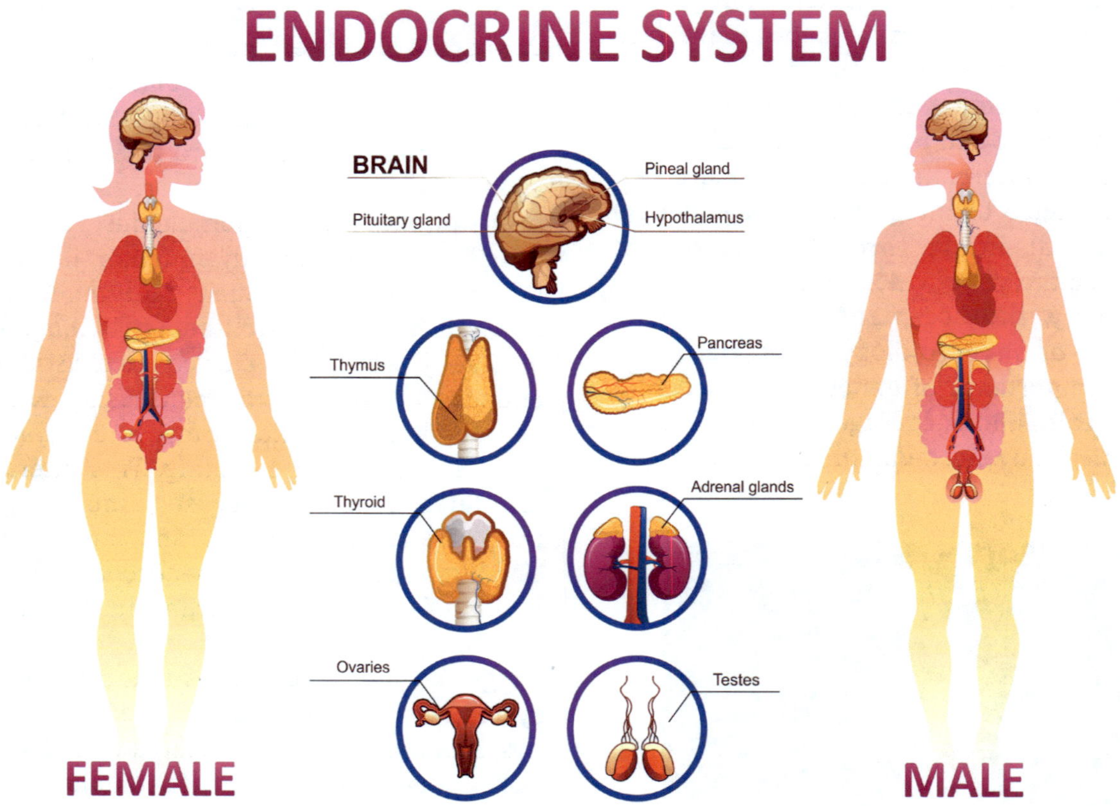

Figure 5.3. Endocrine system.

Source: https://mepss.vbatraining.org/file/29/endocrine-system.jpeg.

Overview of Common Endocrine Disorders

In endocrinology, most disorders result from deregulation of hormones secreted by endocrine glands. The most common endocrine disorders include adrenal insufficiency, thyroid disorders, and diabetes mellitus. Diabetes mellitus, which affects millions of individuals across the globe, is primarily divided into type 1, characterized by autoimmune destruction of beta cells of the pancreas, and type 2, a more common variant often coupled with obesity and genetic susceptibility. Both induce hyperglycemia and must be closely controlled to avoid the onset of complications such as cardiovascular disease, neuropathy, and retinopathy. Metabolic dysregulation from thyroid gland disorders, hypothyroidism, and hyperthyroidism, also inflicts great health impact with symptoms of fatigue, weight change, and mood disorders. Adrenal insufficiency, most commonly due to autoimmune destruction or prolonged corticosteroid therapy, disrupts the body's stress response and can leave a person compromised in performing daily activities.

Hypospadias is a classic example of a congenital illness associated with endocrine dysfunction. The condition where the urethral opening resides at the bottom of the penis typically occurs in conjunction with hormonal defects during fetal development. Notably, research has begun to uncover genetic factors that support this disorder, namely mutations in the steroidogenic factor 1 (SF-1, NR5A1) gene. Mutational evaluation of affected individuals has identified several heterozygous mutations associated with severe hypospadias, particularly with the presence of markers such as low testosterone and undescended testes.

These discoveries shed light on sex developmental disorders and the role of genetic analysis in severe cases of hypospadias. Lastly, linking structural defects such as hypospadias to hormonal and genetic causes enriches the discussion of endocrine disorders and widens the scope for clinical interventions (Achermann et al., 2009). Further, lifestyle choices play a significant role in determining the prevalence and severity of most endocrine disorders. For instance, lifestyle choices like the use of tobacco products, excessive alcohol consumption, and illicit drug use have been consistently linked with diminished reproductive functioning and infertility in both men and women. Cigarette smoking, while on the decline in some groups, remains prevalent and is associated with impaired sperm quality and hormonal disruption. Similarly, alcohol intake, while socially accepted, is increasingly known to affect gonadal and general reproductive function negatively. Drug addiction represents yet another significant danger, especially in young people, which introduces multi-dimensional endocrine dysfunctions to undermine fertility potential. Because of the multifactorial pathogenesis of such lifestyle disorders, prevention practices targeting lifestyle modification seem to be a viable option for promoting endocrine well-being (Angelis et al., 2018) (Figure 5.4).

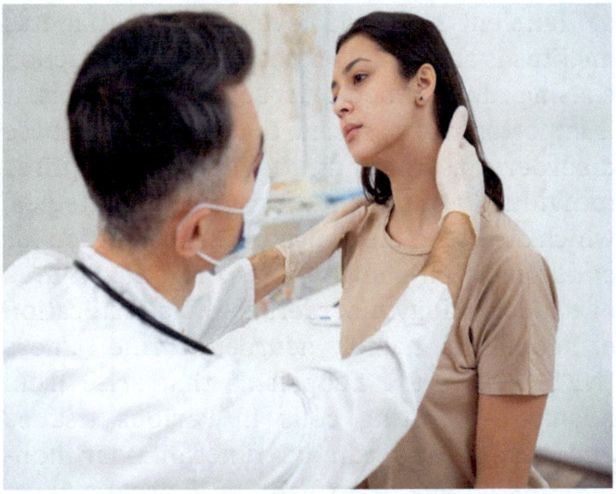

Figure 5.4. Common endocrine disorders.

Source: https://lh4.googleusercontent.com/zE_WB0HRr-WDAYdIGvmfnzu1DAAhU5C0EC-Ct6bKsQhtp0SfU-4XdmFGCYuWjO4bFxFfWWYJ8Vz7XW2xYJTU7yetVlQoAVbRVV6Tmt-ilOWFQGMjG3Cv6SdcVgISBfXeJ4fW1991oMXnXHUxnv_xLCc.

5.1. Types of Endocrinology Disorders

Learning Outcome

1. Describe diabetes mellitus
2. Know the thyroid disorders
3. Learn about adrenal disorders

Endocrinology encompasses a wide variety of conditions arising from abnormal hormone production, secretion, or action. One of the most visible types is hypersecretion diseases, which involve excessive hormones such as cortisol that may lead to severe health conditions. For instance, diseases such as Cushing's syndrome arise from excessive production of cortisol, which often occurs as a result of adrenal tumors or pituitary gland dysfunctions. This excess of cortisol can cause a range of symptoms such as hypertension, obesity, and muscle weakness. Conversely, hypo-secretion disorders consist of deficient hormone levels, where diabetes mellitus is an example of low insulin production causing raised blood glucose concentrations. It is important to appreciate the subtleties of these disorders, as their treatment often requires individually tailored therapeutic strategies, which attests to the delicate balance needed for endocrine well-being. Another significant area of endocrinology disorders is the classification of neoplasms, namely neuroendocrine tumors (NETs). NETs are neoplasms that arise from hormone-secreting cells in various tissues and organs and can be functional or non-functional. The treatment and prognosis of NETs significantly depend on multiple factors including tumor histology, primary site, and stage of disease. For instance, octreotide acetate has been used to manage symptoms of carcinoid syndrome associated with certain NETs, and medications such as sunitinib have demonstrated activity in advanced pNETs (Baldelli et al., 2018). As research continues, it is critical to establish the place of new treatment and biomarkers, such as chromogranin A, which may have the ability to make management of NETs less cumbersome and lead to improved patient outcomes. Finally, endocrine diseases are also caused by environmental factors, which increasingly become a public health matter. Exposure to toxic chemicals is able to disrupt endocrine functions, leading to developmental and disease states. Such endocrine disruption can lead to learning disabilities, behavioral disorders, and even reproductive health issues. Such environmental impacts necessitate policy reform to reduce exposure to harmful chemicals, underscoring the need to integrate public health strategies with endocrine research. Greater awareness of these associations can provide the foundation for preventive interventions and inform effective ones, as the interplay between environmental exposures and hormonal health becomes more grounded in the broader field of endocrinology (Hitchcock et al., 2011).

5.1.1. Diabetes Mellitus

Diabetes Mellitus is a collection of metabolic syndromes with defects in insulin secretion, insulin action, or both that are long-standing and lead to hyperglycemia. Type 1 and Type 2 diabetes are two principal types that are very different in etiology and pathogenesis. Type 1 diabetes is an autoimmune disease in which the immune system attacks pancreatic beta cells, leading to reduced or no insulin secretion. Conversely, Type 2 diabetes is driven by insulin resistance, accompanied by decreased insulin secretion. Varying clinical presentations and management approaches emphasize the importance of individualized treatment and follow-up in these patients. Also, it is crucial to appreciate these differences while considering complications related to them, like cardiovascular disease, neuropathy, and retinopathy, which are disproportionately affecting patients with diabetes, and this highlights the importance of continuous monitoring and integral care. Progress in immunotherapy has introduced unexpected complexities into the management of diabetes, particularly among patients with underlying or occult conditions. A case demonstrates this overlap, where a 56-year-old female patient was diagnosed with indigent diabetic ketoacidosis (DKA) following administration of nivolumab, an immune checkpoint agent for metastatic lung adenocarcinoma. The patient had no prior Diabetes Mellitus history, stressing the risk some treatments pose in causing endocrine states. Specifically, her rapid development of DKA with severe metabolic derangements underscores the critical need for careful monitoring of blood glucose levels in oncology patients receiving immunotherapy. The ever-growing connection between these therapies and the onset of new-onset autoimmune diabetes necessitates reviewing clinical guidelines for early intervention and optimal patient care in the face of such complications, further emphasizing the dynamic nature of endocrinology in modern medicine (Baker et al., 2018). In addition, research into the role of fibroblast growth factor 21 (FGF21) continues to advance knowledge of metabolic syndromes associated with Diabetes Mellitus. A study examining FGF21 levels in type 2 diabetic patients reported significantly elevated levels compared with those in normal controls, providing evidence of a potential biomarker for metabolic disturbance. The correlation of the levels of FGF21 with components of metabolic syndrome, such as body mass index (BMI) and HDL-cholesterol, indicates that it may be an important factor in glucose regulation and lipid metabolism. Such findings are important, in that they result in more research into the therapeutic application of FGF21 as a drug for type 2 diabetes patients presenting with comorbidities. Practitioners are made aware of these correlations so that they can tailor interventions while recognizing the interconnected nature of diabetes with other endocrine disorders, thereby emphasizing the importance of an integrated approach to endocrinology (Khoshnia et al., 2015) (Figure 5.5).

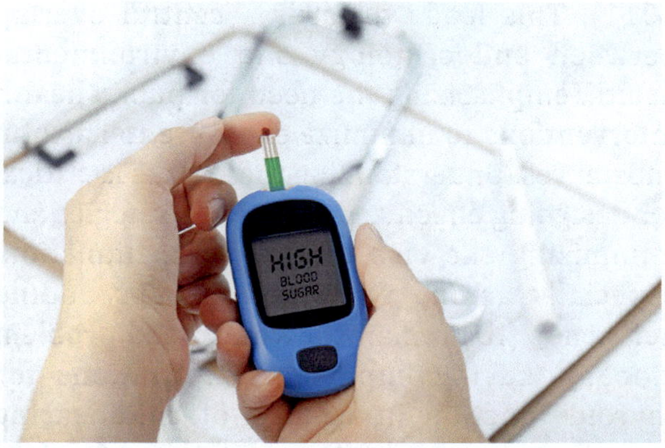

Figure 5.5. Diabetes mellitus.

Source: https://jsshospital.in/wp-content/uploads/2022/03/Blog.jpg.

5.1.2. Thyroid Disorders

Thyroid illnesses constitute a significant category of the endocrinopathies of man. The thyroid gland is located in the neck and regulates human metabolism, growth, and development by secreting the hormones thyroxine (T4) and triiodothyronine (T3). Hypothyroidism due to deficient hormone secretion and hyperthyroidism due to excessive hormone production can lead to various physiological and psychological symptoms. They may include weight changes, fatigue, and mood changes, ultimately disrupting quality of life. The multifactorial aspect of these disorders is that they require a thorough knowledge of their etiology, which typically consists of autoimmune associations, genetic predispositions, and environmental factors, thereby making them a point of emphasis in endocrine health research. Environmental factors also contribute to thyroid disease incidence. For instance, exposure to toxic chemicals has been known to be detrimental to thyroid function and, therefore, overall health and development. Exposure to toxic chemicals leads to neurodevelopmental complications like learning disabilities and behavioral disorders, largely among vulnerable groups like pregnant women and infants (Hitchcock et al.,

2011). This leads towards a central overlap between endocrinology and environmental health, emphasizing the need for public health interventions to minimize exposure to harmful substances. Understanding these links is critical for designing effective prevention strategies and minimizing the risk of thyroid malfunction, especially among vulnerable groups. Iodine deficiency (ID) remains a widespread problem globally, having important implications for thyroid function in women of childbearing age. ID can severely disrupt fetal and infant neurodevelopment, leading to irreversible cognitive impairment (Bouga et al., 2018). Yet, despite the global efforts, through salt iodization and food fortification programs, trends in some regions, the UK among them, still indicate low levels of iodine, with many pregnant women failing to meet the targeted intake. Such dietary deficiency, coupled with public ignorance about the source of iodine, remains a significant public health threat. Consequently, an increase in the consumption of foods containing iodine, such as dairy and seafood, is important for improving the iodine status of populations, particularly pregnant women, since this might reduce the harmful health impacts of iodine deficiency (Figure 5.6).

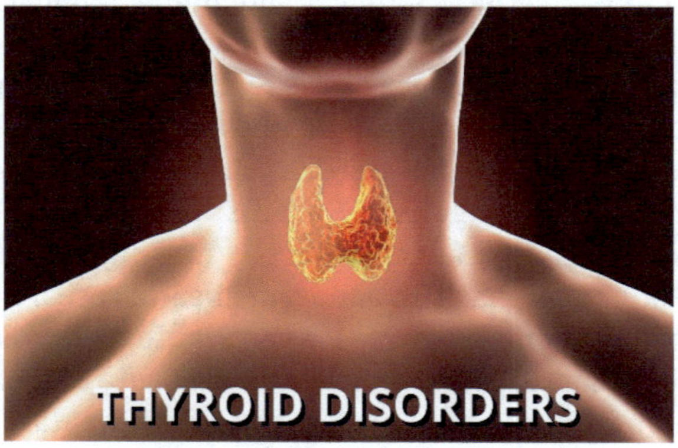

Figure 5.6. Thyroid disorders.

Source: https://i0.wp.com/districtendocrine.com/wp-content/uploads/2021/05/Thyroid-thumb.jpg?fit=2000%2C1428&ssl=1.

5.1.3. Adrenal Disorders

Adrenal disorders constitute a dominant category of endocrine disorders affecting the body's metabolism and stress response. The adrenal glands are located on top of each kidney and play a role in the secretion of the major hormones, including cortisol, aldosterone, and adrenaline. These hormones play significant roles in the body's metabolism, blood pressure, and stress response. Disturbances in these glands can result in a number of disorders, such as Cushing's syndrome, where excess cortisol is produced, and Addison's disease, where insufficient hormones are produced. The symptoms of adrenal disorders often overlap with those of other diseases, and this can complicate the diagnosis and treatment of the disorders. This complexity underscores the importance of understanding the intricate hormonal relationships governed by the hypothalamic-pituitary-adrenal (HPA) axis, whose dysfunction can trigger an array of physiological and psychological illnesses, including anxiety and depression (Chou et al., 2016). Cushing's syndrome is one of the more recognized adrenal disorders, caused by prolonged exposure to high doses of glucocorticoids, with cortisol being the primary one. It may be either endogenous, secondary to adrenal gland hyperactivity, or exogenous, typically secondary to chronic steroid treatment. Patients with Cushing's syndrome may show a typical clinical presentation of obesity, hypertension, and hyperglycemia, reflecting the widespread effect of the hormone on metabolic activity. Moreover, recent studies indicate the complexity of cortisol regulatory processes and determine that the' timing and duration of cortisol surges are key to deciding individuals' responses to stress and trauma recovery (Chou et al., 2016). Understanding such processes not only helps better establish adrenal disorders but also in creating more efficient therapeutic regimens to overcome their impact on patients' lives. However, Addison's disease, also called primary adrenal insufficiency, results from the failure of the adrenal glands to produce sufficient levels of cortisol and typically aldosterone. The condition can lead to disabling symptoms and signs like fatigue, weight loss, and hypotension, whose effects can be fatal if not dealt with early and diagnosed. Typically, as a result of autoimmune diseases, Addison's disease requires lifelong treatment, normally hormone replacement therapy to maintain cortisol levels. The association of Addison's disease with autoimmune mechanisms, and its potential identification with other endocrine disturbances, such as hypothyroidism, parallels Schmidt's syndrome in human beings. Recognition of the relationships among various endocrine dysfunctions is relevant to the development of integrated treatment strategies that not only address hormonal aberrations but also consider the far-reaching implications for patient morbidity and well-being (Figure 5.7).

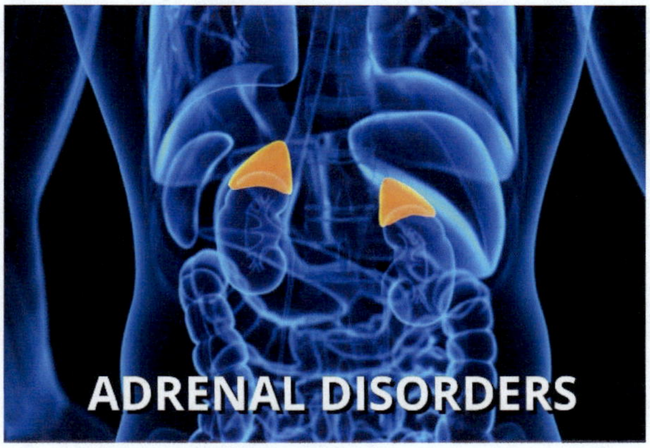

Figure 5.7. Adrenal disorders.

Source: https://i0.wp.com/districtendocrine.com/wp-content/uploads/2021/05/Adrenal-disorders-thumb.jpg?fit=2000%2C1428&ssl=1.

Test Your Knowledge

1. What does diabetes mellitus mean?
2. What are the most common thyroid disorders?

5.2. Causes of Endocrinology Disorders

Learning Outcome

1. Describe the genetic factors and endocrinology disorders
2. Know the impact of environmental factors on endocrinology disorders
3. Understand the role of lifestyle choices in the management and prevention of endocrinology disorders

The pathogenesis of endocrine diseases is polyetic and includes genetic, environmental, and physiological factors. Genetic mutations play a key role, particularly in endocrine disorders of hormone secretion and regulation. Genetic aberrations in the steroidogenic factor 1 gene (SF-1, NR5A1), for example, are associated with 46,XY disorders of sex development and thus hypospadias. Research has shown that heterozygous mutations in the NR5A1 gene are associated with severe forms of hypospadias, low testosterone levels, and other hormonal dysfunctions, highlighting the central role of genetics in such conditions. Genetic susceptibility is therefore a key factor in determining the severity and frequency of certain endocrinological conditions, and warrants comprehensive genetic screening among affected patients for diagnostic and therapeutic planning purposes (Achermann et al., 2009). Another vital feature of endocrinological disorders is hormonal disturbances that can arise as a result of multiple environmental and lifestyle influences. For instance, exposure to endocrine-disrupting chemicals, such as pesticides and plastics, can interfere with hormonal pathways, leading to disorders in both female and male reproductive systems. Besides, physiological states such as obesity and stress are also involved in hormone signaling defects, which could lead to disorders such as insulin resistance or thyroid disorders.

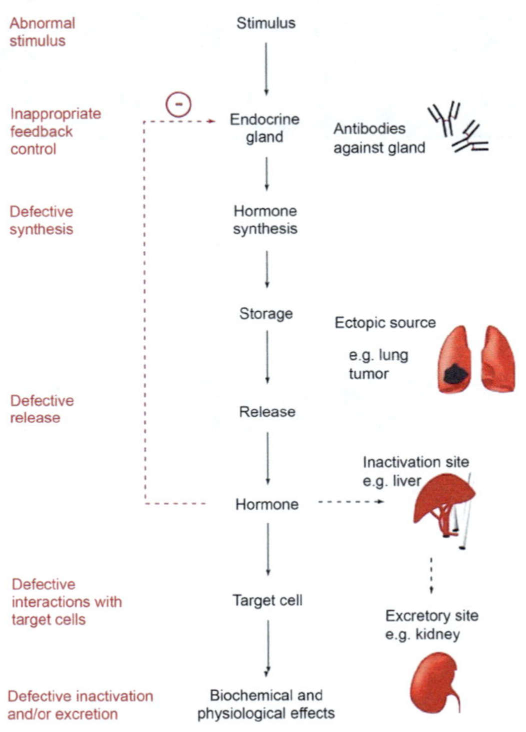

Figure 5.8. Overview of the causes of endocrine disorders.

Source: https://img.brainkart.com/imagebk17/LaIrzBr.jpg.

These states demonstrate the ripple effect of lifestyle choices on endocrine health, highlighting that, in addition to genetic factors, lifestyle and environmental factors need to be considered in diagnosing and treating endocrine disorders as well. This multifactorial awareness is central to prevention and management planning in the field (Machado et al., 2019). Lastly, one should appreciate the role of sex differences in the expression and severity of endocrinological disorders. Various studies have suggested that certain disorders, such as prolactinomas, occur more frequently and manifest differently in males and females. Estrogen levels and sex-specific genetic susceptibility are believed to affect the growth and evolution of these tumors, again showing that gender plays a central role in endocrinology. In particular, higher serum estradiol levels in women may lead to an earlier diagnosis of prolactinomas. By further exploring these sex differences, researchers gain clearer insight into the biological mechanisms underlying different disorders, which could result in more specific treatment strategies based on a person's sex and hormonal balance (Machado et al., 2019) (Figure 5.8).

5.2.1. Genetic Factors

The combination of , endocrine diseases, and genes typically explains issues of complicated development. One of the best examples is the association between SF-1 gene mutations (NR5A1) and cases of severe hypospadias, a condition of the male genitalia. In a study of patients with the condition in detail, heterozygous mutations in the NR5A1 gene were identified in three of 60 cases analyzed. These mutations were associated with penoscrotal hypospadias and hypotestosteronemia, suggesting a critical role for SF-1 in the regulation of male sexual differentiation. Specifically, the mutations disrupted transcriptional activation within hormone-sensitive mechanisms, further substantiating the suggestion that genetic defects can manifest as radical endocrinological dysregulation, ultimately influencing physical health and gender assignment outcomes in affected individuals (Achermann et al., 2009). In addition, genetic problems extend their effect deeper into more common issues of reproductive health, namely, infertility. For men's fertility, of utmost concern is the synergistic impact of lifestyle on genetic susceptibility. A review of literature shows how ubiquitous unhealthy lifestyle patterns, such as smoking and alcohol consumption, can negatively influence the reproductive capacity in men. Evidence indicates that while such behavior is environmentally determined, it could also be interacting with genetic risk factors for fertility disorders. The ubiquitous prevalence of tobacco smoking among reproductive-age individuals provokes an examination of the interplay between lifestyle and genetics, underlining once more the necessity of preventive measures. These are aspects that need to be addressed, since the implications of both genetic inclinations and self-destructive behaviors can cause amplified challenges for infertile couples (Angelis et al., 2018). Lastly, the relevance of genetic elements in endocrine disorders cannot be overemphasized, given that advances in genetic research continue to deepen insights into how various endocrine system dysfunctions arise. Genetic screening and bypass investigations can identify susceptible groups to disorders caused by specific mutations, permitting early interventions. For instance, understanding NR5A1 mutations in relation to hypospadias not only enables timely intervention by a medical professional but also guides reproductive planning within families. As genetic inheritance is complex and has implications for endocrine disorders, research must proceed. This can lead to more targeted therapeutic approaches and greater public awareness of the impact of genetic factors on reproductive well-being, enabling better outcomes for individuals with these conditions.

5.2.2. Environmental Influences

Environmental influences on endocrine disorders are identified as a key field of research within the general framework of human health. Various elements in our surroundings, including pollutants, lifestyle, and socioeconomic status, play a significant role in the function of endocrine systems. For instance, exposure to endocrine-disrupting chemicals (EDCs) in consumer products and agricultural pesticides has been linked to infertility and hormone imbalance. They can interfere with the body's hormonal communication, leading to conditions such as polycystic ovary syndrome and reduced fertility in men. Indeed, evidence suggests that, despite therapeutic regimes intended to control such conditions, primary prevention by minimizing environmental exposures remains important for maximizing aggregate reproductive health outcomes (Angelis et al., 2018). Besides, lifestyle factors such as tobacco use, alcohol consumption, and drug addiction also play a crucial role in endocrine function and fertility. Studies indicate that tobacco smoking is prevalent among individuals of reproductive age and is detrimental to male and female reproductive health. Nicotine and nicotine metabolites can interfere with hormonal mechanisms and exacerbate conditions such as low testosterone levels among men. In addition, socially acceptable drinking of alcohol has been shown to deteriorate gonadal function with the passage of time. The literature has consistently demonstrated detrimental effects on fertility in several studies, and this is regarded as a serious public health problem (Angelis et al., 2018). The findings necessitate re-evaluation of social norms for these drugs and recognition of their potential to cause instability in hormonal balance and result in endocrine disorders. Adding to the complexity of the interaction between endocrine disease and environmental factors is the role of steroid hormones, which are both highly influenced by hereditary predisposition and environmental factors. Steroid hormones such as estrogen and testosterone have been implicated in having a critical role in many neuroendocrine processes, affecting mental health, sexual orientation, and metabolic programming. In addition, environmental stressors are capable of shifting the activity and expression of such hormones, impacting individuals' possibilities of developing disorders like polycystic ovary syndrome. There is evidence to support that the protective roles of hormones, such as those of progesterone, can also be impacted by environmental factors, particularly in the prevention of neurodegenerative conditions. This intricate interaction highlights the necessity of integrative approaches to the understanding and control of endocrine diseases in the context of a person's environmental exposures (Figure 5.9).

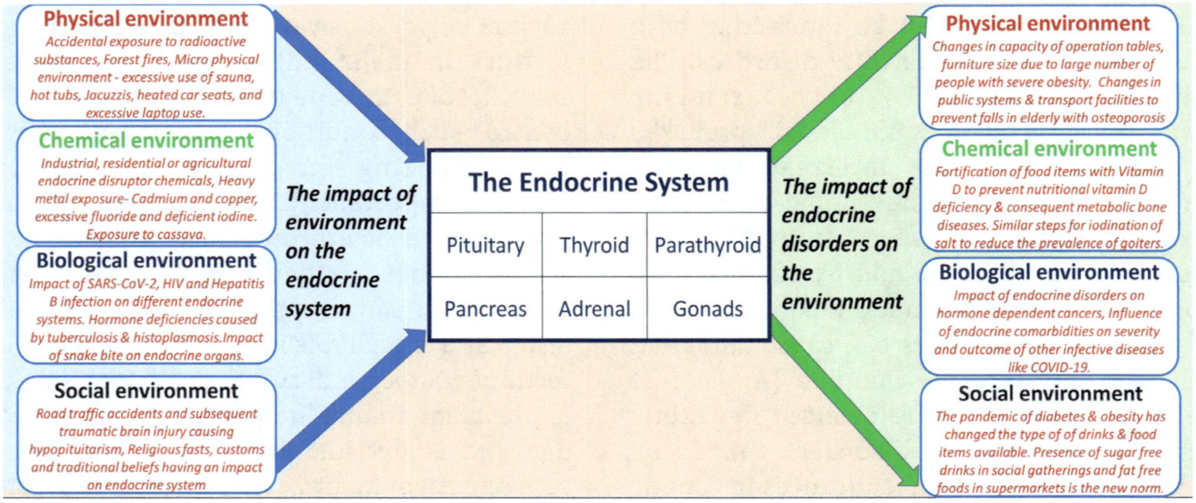

Figure 5.9. Relationship of the environment and endocrine system.

Source: https://www.ncbi.nlm.nih.gov/books/NBK568568/bin/trop_environmental-Image001.jpg.

5.2.3. Lifestyle Choices

Lifestyle choices are central to the management and prevention of endocrine conditions, particularly metabolic disorders. Diet, physical activity, and sleep all play important roles in maintaining hormonal balance within the body. Eating behaviors, including caloric intake and diet quality, have direct effects on insulin sensitivity and glucose metabolism in maintaining energy balance. Additionally, regular exercise is associated with improved hormone regulation, particularly in individuals aiming to avoid conditions like obesity or type 2 diabetes. Engaging in healthy activities such as these can help avoid risks associated with hormonal disorders. Thus, enhancing awareness of healthy lifestyle factors can be instrumental to overall endocrine well-being and disease avoidance. In addition, the specific food elements consumed directly impact the synthesis and control of hormones. For instance, iodine is an essential nutrient for thyroid hormone production, and insufficiency could lead to such conditions as hypothyroidism, which is gaining popularity in various populations. More so, in the UK, iodine deficiency in women of childbearing age is of concern due to possible implications for fetal brain development. Despite programs like iodization programs in most nations, most pregnant women remain iodine deficient. Estimates indicate that around 60% fail to meet levels stipulated under WHO guidelines (Bouga et al., 2018) This points to the need for public health interventions targeted at food consumption patterns so that women are exposed to sufficient quantities of foods rich in iodine to support their endocrine status and that of their potential offspring. In addition to food patterns, lifestyle options such as education and awareness of nutrients are vital in the prevention and management of endocrine disorders. Low levels of information about optimal nutrient sources, for instance, iodine from milk and seafood, limit people's ability to make informed food choices that promote health. As indicated in research papers in peer-reviewed journals, there is a perceived knowledge gap between healthcare workers and members of the public regarding the significance of iodine and other essential nutrients for health outcomes (Mercer et al., 2013). Closing such a knowledge gap is important in helping people make effective changes in what they eat, once more highlighting the link between education and lifestyle behavior. Promoting a multispectral strategy comprising awareness, accessibility, and dietary changes is of primary importance for the maintenance of long-term endocrine health and the avoidance of adverse effects from accompanying disorders.

Test Your Knowledge

1. What are the genetic disorders of the endocrine system?
2. What are the impact of environmental factors on endocrinology disorders?

5.3. Symptoms of Endocrinology Disorders

Learning Outcome

1. Describe the common symptoms across endocrinology disorders
2. Know the disease-specific symptoms
3. Know the impact of endocrinology disorders on quality of life

Endocrine disorders comprise a wonderfully varied array of symptoms that can vary significantly depending on the endocrine gland or organs involved and the nature of the dysfunction. Perhaps the best example is thyroid dysfunction, leading to hypothyroidism and hyperthyroidism. Hypothyroidism typically evolves with fatigue, weight gain, cold intolerance, and depression, whereas hyperthyroidism may be responsible for weight loss, increased appetite, sweating, and restlessness. Particularly notable, thyroid hormones also play critical roles in sexual and reproductive function. Abnormalities of thyroid function are associated with infertility in both men and women, illustrating the hormone's critical role in reproductive health (Carosa et al., 2018). Symptoms can often be mild, leading to subsequent misdiagnosis or delayed therapy, and careful evaluation of patients with unexplained changes in weight, mood, or reproductive health is thus required. Similarly, pituitary gland conditions such as prolactinomas show certain symptoms due to endocrine imbalance. Prolactinomas, characterized by elevated prolactin production, lead to infertility, galactorrhea, and menstrual abnormalities in women but decreased libido, impotency, and gynecomastia in men. The different presentations of these signs reflect the strong association between reproductive organs and hormonal control (Machado et al., 2019). Other determinants, such as gender, influence the size and activity of these tumors, which makes their clinical presentation more complex and highlights the significance of clinicians staying alert while identifying such symptoms, especially in women diagnosed sooner than men. Information regarding such symptoms is paramount for early and accurate diagnosis, which plays a significant role in determining the outcomes of patients. Also, symptoms of damaged adrenal glands, such as Cushing's syndrome and Addison's disease, demonstrate the diverse impact of endocrine disorders on overall health. Cushing's syndrome is characterized by excessive cortisol, leading to abdominal fat, skin changes, and muscular weakness. Addison's disease, on the other hand, is characterized by the underproduction of adrenal hormones, which results in weakness, hyperpigmentation, and hypotension. Such contradictory presentations necessitate a delicate balance in understanding the body's physiological functions of adrenal hormones and their regulating impact on body functions. Moreover, the psychological implications of these conditions, i.e., depression or mood swings due to hormonal imbalance, cannot be overlooked as they have a direct relationship with the quality of life and well-being of the patients, thus highlighting the importance of holistic treatment methods in managing the symptoms of endocrine disorders (Figure 5.10).

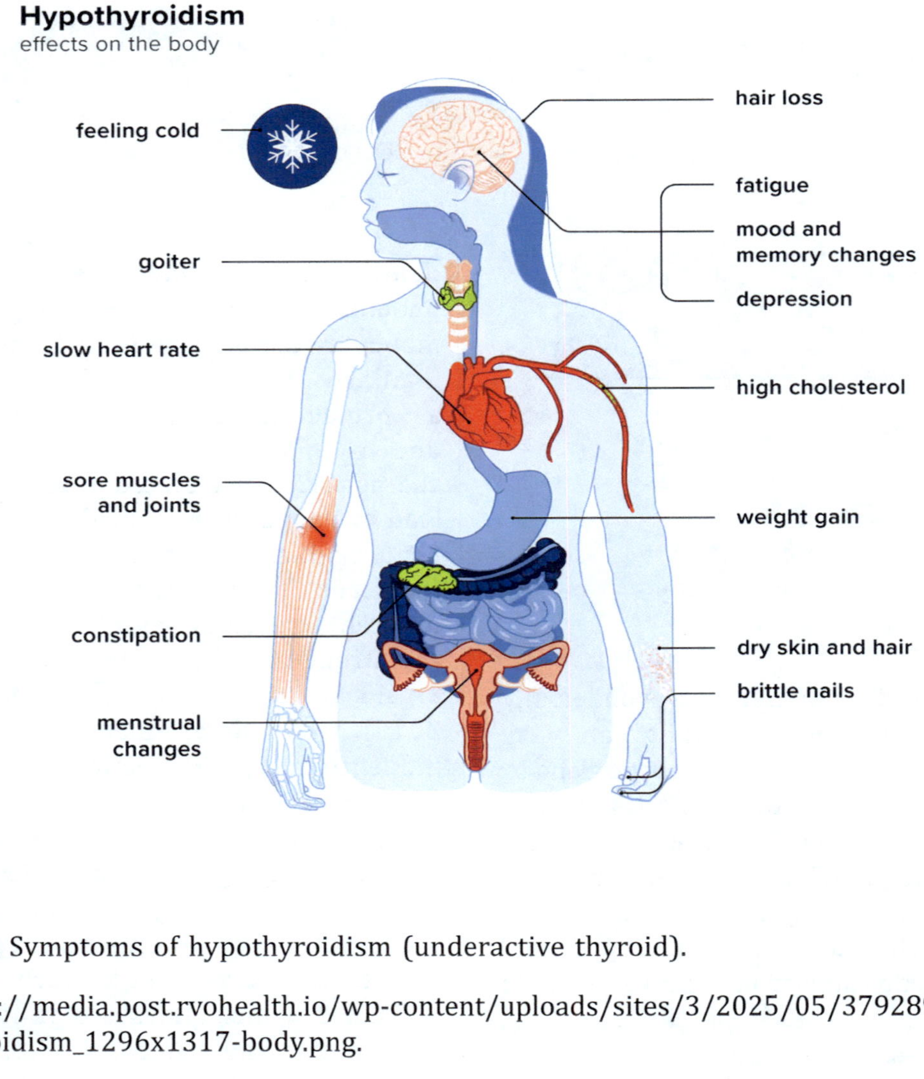

Figure 5.10. Symptoms of hypothyroidism (underactive thyroid).

Source: https://media.post.rvohealth.io/wp-content/uploads/sites/3/2025/05/3792894-symptoms-of-hypothyroidism_1296x1317-body.png.

5.3.1. Common Symptoms Across Disorders

Endocrinopathy disorders often present a variety of symptoms that, while heterogeneous in their etiology, share significant overlap between various conditions. Such generalized symptoms as fatigue, weight loss or gain, and mood change may occur in several disorders, including but not limited to thyroid disease, diabetes, and adrenal insufficiency. For instance, hypothyroid patients tend to have chronic fatigue and gain weight, just like with adrenal gland disease. Such symptom overlaps complicate diagnosis in endocrinology, since the doctor needs to untangle which disorder, if any, is the primary cause. The shared symptomatic presentation highlights the importance of strict screening for intrinsic physiological mechanisms and ensuring treatment measures are in place (Overy et al., 2014). An interesting observation in endocrinology is the psychological impact of hormonal imbalances. Cushing's syndrome, for example, through hypersecretion of cortisol, tends to cause significant mood disorders, including depression and anxiety. Similarly, individuals with diabetes may exhibit mood swings as a consequence of the immediate effects of blood sugar changes. The psychological of such disorders illustrate the interaction between body and mind because hormonal changes affect not only physiological condition but also behavior and mood.

This exchange illustrates how common symptoms, such as mood lability and fatigue, also cut across diagnostic lines, thereby complicating diagnosis and treatment of endocrine diseases (Hitchcock et al., 2011). This overlapping symptomatology across various endocrine conditions also underscores the need for an integrated approach to patient care. Symptom-oriented treatments are usually of use in several conditions; for instance, lifestyle modifications such as exercise and diet help symptoms of mood dysfunction and fatigue in both metabolic syndrome and thyroid disease. This holistic consideration of patient health makes clinicians appreciate learning about patient health in more comprehensive ways, leading them to be less attuned to single diagnoses. By recognizing similar signs, healthcare professionals can better tailor interventions to both the physical and psychological problems that individuals with endocrinology disorders suffer, and this leads to improved patient outcomes and quality of life (Overy et al., 2014).

5.3.2. Disease-Specific Symptoms

In endocrinology, symptoms of a specific disease are direct expressions of endocrine imbalances and reflect the dynamic interplay between hormone levels and body functions. As an illustration, prolactinomas, functioning pituitary adenomas with elevated serum prolactin, are associated with a variety of symptoms like galactorrhea, amenorrhea, and infertility in women and diminished libido and erectile dysfunction in men. Specifically, sex differences are integral to these presentations. Women are shown to be diagnosed earlier because the salience of reproductive symptoms, as being more conspicuous than men's subtle manifestations, makes them an easier target for attention and treatment. This disparity emphasizes the importance of recognizing gender-specific presentations in the diagnosis and treatment of endocrine disorders, as is highlighted by recent findings on the transforming growth factor beta 1 (TGFbeta1) system's involvement in prolactinoma pathogenesis (Machado et al., 2019). Thyroid disorders also demonstrate how disease-specific symptoms can significantly impact reproductive health. Thyroid hormones, triiodothyronine (T3), and thyroxine (T4), have a profound influence on sexual as well as reproductive functions. Altered levels of the hormones can lead to various symptoms, such as menstrual irregularities in women and altered sexual function in men, exemplified by documented relationships between thyroid disease and fertility in both men and women. Historically, our knowledge of this interrelationship evolved with the identification that thyroid hormone receptors (TRs) co-existed with the reproductive organs. This hormone dysregulation can have adverse effects on the sex steroid hormone axis, leading to adverse fertility outcomes; however, research still uncovers the complex impact of thyroid disease on sexuality, particularly in men, where conditions such as compromised libido and erectile dysfunction have been established (Carosa et al., 2018). The complexity of endocrinology illnesses signifies the interconnectedness of hormonal imbalances and symptomology of certain diseases, necessitating an integrated clinical approach in the healthcare environment. This interconnectedness matters most when determining treatment options, because regulating one endocrine disease will significantly alleviate symptoms of associated hormonal imbalances. Definition of the molecular mechanisms involved in these interactions not only enhances the therapeutic care of endocrine disease but also highlights the need for customized therapeutic intervention. By recognizing the unique symptomatic presentations in both genders and in various disorders, clinicians can tailor their treatment according to an understanding of the multifaceted problem posed by hormonal disease. Last but not least, constant research and clinical monitoring are necessary to clarify these complex systems further and ensure effective disease-specific symptom control across endocrinology (Carosa et al., 2018; Machado et al., 2019) (Figure 5.11).

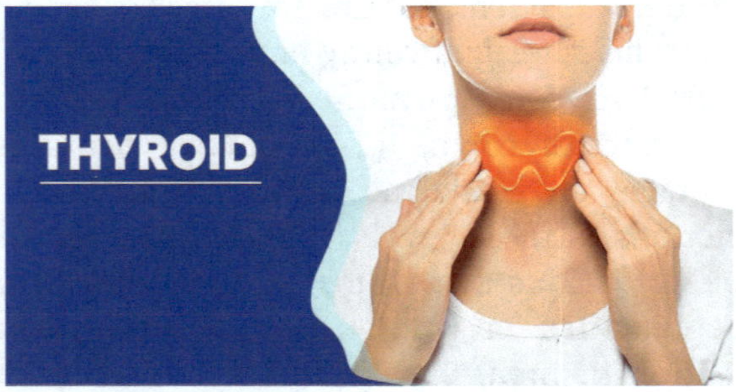

Figure 5.11. Thyroid symptoms.

Source: https://www.maxlab.co.in/categoryimage/1667462132.jpg.

5.3.3. Impact on Quality of Life

The impact of endocrine illnesses goes beyond the boundaries of physical health, reaching down to the quality of life of a person. Diabetes, thyroid illness, and fertility illness are not only clinical conditions; they encompass a variety of issues that influence mental health, social function, and daily activity. The chronicity of such illnesses typically leads to uninterrupted stress, anxiety, and depression, and therefore an emotional burden on the patients. Also, the necessity for ongoing medical check-ups and lifestyle modification may limit personal and professional activities, especially over the long term, finally undermining overall satisfaction. In a broader analysis of these disorders, one must consider how they can affect one's sense of self and meaning, as well as one's capacity to engage with their community and loved ones. Lifestyle choices are important factors in determining the quality of life for those suffering from endocrine disorders. Health-risk lifestyles such as tobacco use and alcohol misuse have always been linked with adverse effects on reproductive health, as well as the overall endocrine function. Cigarette smoking is still prevalent among the reproductive age group, posing a significant public health concern. The negative effects of smoking on fertility are severe, potentially aggravating the condition of already existing hormonal imbalances and reducing the likelihood of conception. Similarly, alcohol consumption, under regular circumstances, regardless of the social environment, can harm the gonadal activity, contributing to the health profiles of individuals with endocrine disorders. The significance of this is that managing such harmful conduct not only improves health outcomes but also aligns with interventions to enhance the quality of life for such individuals, inviting a holistic treatment and prevention model (Angelis et al., 2018). Environmental insults, including exposure to harmful chemicals, add burden to endocrinology disorder patients and occur in one of numerous deleterious forms, having a significant quality-of-life effect. Exposure has been linked to illnesses such as learning disability, behavioral disorder, asthma, and allergy, all of which collectively may disrupt normal development and function. Such disabilities can restrict educational and vocational pursuits, leading to frustration and diminished self-esteem. Additionally, the resulting psychological effects stemming from such medical comorbidities can discourage socialization, leading to further feelings of incompetence or isolation. Given the potential long-term implications of environmental toxins in this matter, policy reform addressing exposure risks needs to be implemented. Promoting safer surroundings not only helps prevent illness but also enhances the quality of life for infected persons, thereby improving their health and interactions with communities (Hitchcock et al., 2011; Streuning et al., 2011).

Test Your Knowledge

1. What are the symptoms of endocrine disorder?
2. What are the impact of endocrinology disorders on quality of life?

5.4. Diagnosis of Endocrinology Disorders

Learning Outcome

1. Understand the blood tests for hormone levels
2. Describe the imaging techniques for gland assessment
3. Learn about patient history and physical examination

Diagnosis of endocrine disorders involves a complete understanding of hormonal imbalances and their physiological manifestations. Practitioners, in most instances, use a collection of patient history, physical examination, and laboratory exams to determine specific disorders. Hormonal assays, as an example, play a significant role in deciding abnormal hormone levels like cortisol, insulin, and thyroid hormones. In hypothyroidism, measurement of thyroid-stimulating hormone (TSH) levels can indicate dysfunction and warrants further evaluation to determine the etiology. Imaging procedures such as ultrasound, MRI, and CT scans also aid in diagnosing structural endocrine organ disorders. A combination of these diagnostic tools provides an overall view of the patient's endocrine status and helps formulate effective treatment strategies. Endocrinological diseases, particularly sexual development diseases, disclose the complexity of diagnosis in the field. Diseases such as hypospadias require examination of genetic and hormonal factors to explain their causality. In an investigation on boys with various severities of hypospadias, scientists observed heterozygous mutations in the NR5A1 gene among those with severe forms, which refers to the genetic etiology of some disorders. The co-existence of low testosterone levels in these patients, along with other hormonal parameters, indicates the importance of a subtle diagnostic approach to discriminate between different types of congenital anomalies. The detection of such mutations emphasizes the importance of genetic counseling and personalized management in affected individuals, thereby improving health outcomes and understanding of 46,XY disorders of sex development (Achermann et al., 2009). Also, the endocrine tumor diagnosis of such tumors as prolactinomas presents distinctive challenges due to their heterogeneity of presentation and biological behavior. They are pituitary adenomas with prolactin production imbalance, which frequently results in infertility and other reproductive disorders. Epidemiological surveys have shown gender differences in prolactinoma incidence and diagnosis, but with a bias towards earlier diagnosis in females. This variation is not due to physiological parameters, such as serum estradiol levels and their influence on tumor growth. Additional research on the TGFbeta1 system has revealed its role in modulating lactotroph function, providing insight into the mechanisms of hormonal regulation that may dictate the development and progression of the tumors. Understanding these determinants is important for clinicians to optimize diagnostic strategy and management regimen in patients with manifestations of pituitary dysfunction (Machado et al., 2019) (Figure 5.12).

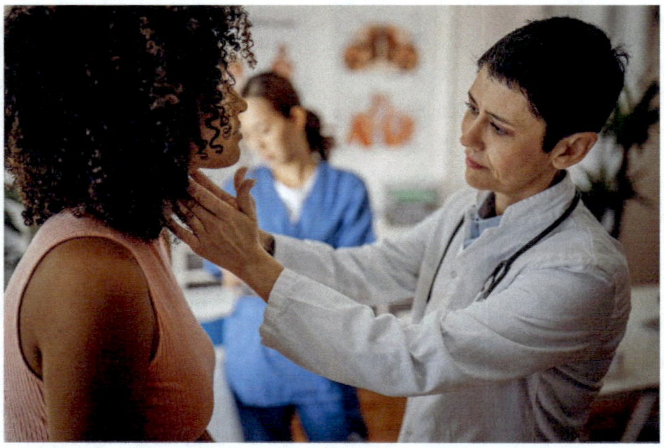

Figure 5.12. Diagnosis of endocrinology disorders.

Source: https://wp04-media.cdn.ihealthspot.com/wp-content/uploads/sites/464/2024/03/iStock-1345288567-1.jpeg.

5.4.1. Blood Tests and Hormone Levels

Blood work is a key diagnostic method in the field of endocrinology, particularly with regard to hormone levels. Blood work allows the body to provide critical information about the functioning of the thyroid, adrenal, and pituitary glands, which are all essential for maintaining homeostasis in the body. For example, thyroid hormone levels are measured using serum tests, which may indicate conditions such as hypothyroidism or hyperthyroidism that profoundly affect metabolism and energy status. By quantifying these hormone levels, clinicians can provide appropriate management, which is crucial for resetting endocrine balance and managing symptoms of endocrine disorders. The relationship between blood tests and accurate hormone level measurement underscores the importance of periodic health examinations to prevent such diseases. In addition to periodic testing of hormones, new evidence suggests that environmental pollutants can have an impact on endocrine function and hormone levels. Studies of dogs suggest exposure to polybrominated diphenyl ethers (PBDEs) and polychlorinated biphenyls (PCBs) may be linked with thyroid hormone imbalance. Although some logistic regression analyses indicated no statistically significant correlation of these pollutants and hypothyroxinemia in dogs, the mere presence of these chemicals in the environment raises questions about their impact on human endocrine health. Blood tests that measure not only hormones but also chemical toxicity might better establish how environmental pollutants contribute to endocrine disease. Understanding the interactions among these factors is important for developing preventive strategies to mitigate potential health risks posed by environmental pollutants (Kass et al., 2017). The impact of hormonal imbalance extends beyond mere body symptoms and reaches into cognitive development and overall well-being. Epidemiologic studies have found early exposure to endocrine-disrupting chemicals to be linked with adverse effects such as learning disability and behavioral disturbance, confirming evidence that toxic exposures can disrupt endocrine function (Hitchcock et al., 2011). These findings support the need for vigilance regarding internal hormonal testing and external influences that can disrupt endocrine health. By incorporating hormone and pollutant level tests in the environment, practitioners will be able to better evaluate patients' state of health and devise interventions that address endocrine disease as well as the disease cause. Such a multidimensional approach that incorporates blood testing for hormones, along with environmental assessment, would thus revolutionize our understanding of endocrine disorders and their treatment in humans (Figure 5.13).

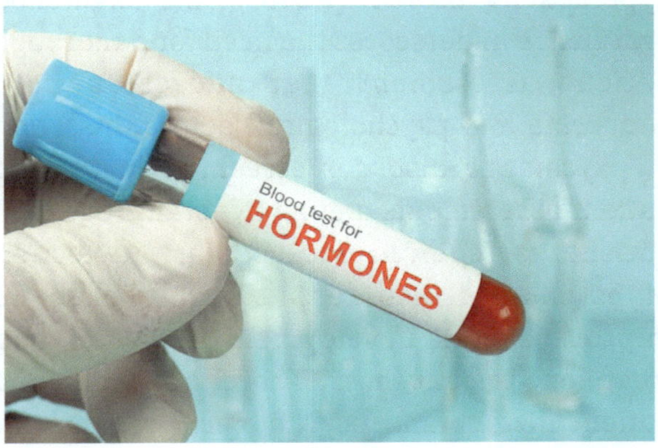

Figure 5.13. Blood tests for hormone levels.

Source: https://img.freepik.com/premium-photo/doctor-holding-blood-tube-analysis-hormones-biochemistry-lab-blood-sample-study-levels-hormone-tests_431724-9912.jpg.

5.4.2. Imaging Techniques

Imaging modalities are instrumental in the diagnosis and management of endocrine disorders in humans. Magnetic resonance imaging (MRI) and computed tomography (CT) have become strong modalities for imaging endocrine glands and related pathologies among the imaging modalities used. MRI, given its excellent soft-tissue contrast, is especially beneficial for evaluating pituitary gland tumors and the degree of local invasion in hypersecretion syndromes. In contrast, CT scans are valuable for identifying structural abnormalities of the adrenal glands and pancreas. The sensitivity of these imaging modalities in providing detailed anatomical and, at times, functional data significantly aids clinicians in developing appropriate interventions, thus maximizing patient outcomes in complicated endocrine disease. The use of ultrasound is impressive for evaluating thyroid pathology, especially given its availability and low cost. High-resolution ultrasound is able to assess thyroid nodules, determine size, composition, and vascularity, all of which are relevant in risk stratification. Ultrasound-guided fine-needle aspiration biopsy is also able to provide cytological samples from suspicious nodes and facilitate accelerated malignancy diagnosis. Imaging techniques such as positron emission tomography (PET) are invaluable in monitoring response to therapy when following the response to treatment. The combination of imaging modalities allows comprehensive evaluation of endocrine disorders, meeting the need for individualized and targeted therapy. Emerging imaging technologies, such as molecular imaging technologies, are changing the landscape of endocrine disorder diagnosis and treatment. Such technologies that involve hybrid imaging techniques, such as PET/MRI, allow simultaneous recording of anatomical and functional information, providing an integrated picture of the endocrine system. As revealed by research, there is room for these new approaches to increase our understanding of the pathophysiology of diseases such as hormonal imbalance and insulin resistance.

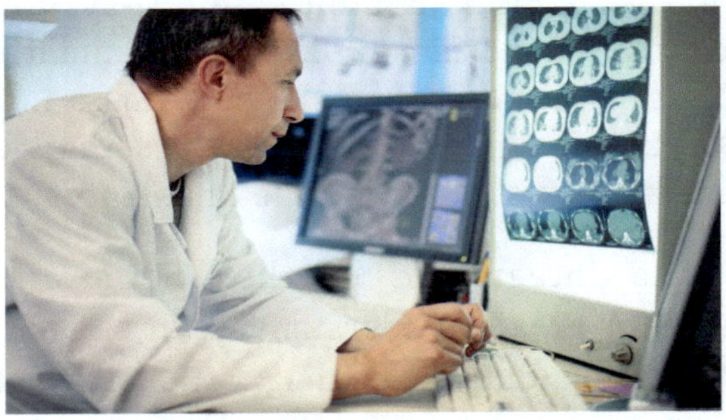

Figure 5.14. Diagnostic imaging techniques

Source: https://www.healthimages.com/content/uploads/sites/2/2019/10/radiologist.jpg.

Moreover, imaging how epicardial adipose tissue influences cardiac function can reveal new pathophysiological pathways for managing cardiovascular complications of endocrine disorders. Ongoing advancements in imaging modalities are not only revolutionizing paradigms in diagnosis but also improving research initiatives focused on demystifying the pathophysiologic intricacies of endocrine dysfunctions, as defined in existing literature on these conditions, that need to be further investigated and validated within clinical practice (Larauche et al., 2011; Agra et al., 2017) (Figure 5.14).

5.4.3. Patient History and Physical Examination

Thorough patient history and physical examination are key components in the assessment of endocrine disorders. These processes provide clinicians with valuable information regarding a patient's status, symptoms, and signs, and potential underlying pathologies. Taking a thorough patient history is not only the retrieval of the presenting complaints but also a systematic review of the patient's medical, family, and psychosocial histories. These differences are particularly evident in endocrinology, where numerous diseases exhibit complex, multi-systemic patterns. Furthermore, physical examination, using sensitive tests such as body mass index (BMI) and secondary sexual features, can yield immediate clues to endocrine imbalances.

The integration of these differences allows for greater understanding of endocrine disorders, guiding future diagnostic testing and management plans. Finally, effective patient history and physical examinations foster more individualized treatment of these disorders. The significance of mental health aspects in relation to endocrine disease cannot be exaggerated. There are certain diseases, such as congenital adrenal hyperplasia (CAH) and familial male precocious puberty (FMPP), that have been reported to have a high psychiatric morbidity. One such study that assessed children with the following conditions revealed that approximately 44.4% of patients with CAH and 55.6% of patients with FMPP met the criteria for at least one lifetime psychiatric diagnosis, such as anxiety disorders and attention-deficit hyperactivity disorder (ADHC). This heightened prevalence underscores the need for a thorough patient assessment that addresses both endocrine and psychological factors. Insertion of psychiatric disorder screening in routine patient assessments among hyperandrogenism patients is required because early detection of psychiatric disorders is highly likely to improve overall development outcomes and treatment effectiveness. Therefore, a detailed patient history and psychological assessment can help enhance care planning for patients with endocrine disorders such as CAH and FMPP. Moreover, the role of lifestyle factors in endocrine function underscores the importance of a thorough patient history and examination.

The modifiable risk of physical inactivity and obesity is intertwined with other hormonal disturbances like hypertension and insulin resistance. There is evidence that adding lifestyle interventions, such as exercise and weight management strategies, may substantially improve patient outcomes in endocrine disorders. These lifestyle risks are most significant in multicultural populations, whose health behaviors are culturally and socioeconomically mediated. For instance, a study on black South African adults' physical activity found that body weight and blood pressure control are strongly associated with each other, highlighting the necessity for personalized health interventions. Including such lifestyle considerations in patient assessment not only enhances understanding of endocrine status but also supports the development of holistic, patient-specific treatment plans conducive to long-term health.

Test Your Knowledge

1. What blood tests test hormone levels?
2. What are the two main types of diagnostic imaging techniques?

5.5. Treatment Options for Endocrinology Disorders

Learning Outcome

1. Learn about hormone replacement therapy
2. Describe the medications for endocrine disorders
3. Understand the role of lifestyle modifications in managing endocrine disorders

Treatment for endocrine diseases has also increased over the years with the progress of medical science, enabling patients to obtain personalized treatments to cure specific endocrine imbalances. For instance, hormone replacement therapy (HRT) is a common treatment for diseases such as hypothyroidism and adrenal insufficiency. In these cases, synthetic hormones are administered to restore appropriate hormone levels and counteract the symptoms of hormonal deficiencies. In addition, diet and exercise regimens, for instance, can be significant in the management of diseases like obesity and diabetes, which usually run in association with hormonal dysregulation. By emphasizing the use of customized treatment protocols that encompass pharmacologic and non-pharmacologic interventions, healthcare providers can enhance quality of life for individuals with endocrine disorders, offering them the care tailored to their unique healthcare needs. In the past few years, the role of Assisted Reproductive Technology (ART) has been the focal point of the specialty of endocrinology when treating endocrine-related infertility. ART is a term used to describe many treatments that attempt to conceive when other treatments are not successful, typically as a consequence of hormonal disorders such as polycystic ovary syndrome (PCOS) or thyroid disease. There are ethical implications of ART, particularly in the context of religious belief, in addition to the medical demand. Infertile couples have generated controversies regarding the balance between technological intervention and respect for moral values, particularly in embryo handling. Such ethical challenges need to be addressed to guarantee informed decision-making for couples receiving ART, as autonomy and dignity continue to be fundamental in healthcare services in reproductive endocrinology (Gresham et al., 2020).

Furthermore, conditions like obstructive sleep apnea (OSA) have turned into severe concerns in the management of endocrinology, particularly due to their association with metabolic diseases. Recent data indicate that OSA is a common condition impacting a high rate of the population and is highly correlated with obesity and diabetes (Arble et al., 2018). Treatment for OSA typically involves lifestyle changes, such as weight loss and education regarding sleep hygiene, as well as CPAP. As more is known about the bidirectional interaction between metabolic physiology and OSA, the endocrinologist must consider the role of hormones such as insulin and leptin in shaping overall treatment strategies. By addressing both comorbid illnesses and their root causes in endogenous hormonal states, healthcare practitioners can further optimize overall patient success and advance a more holistic approach to endocrine illness (Figure 5.15).

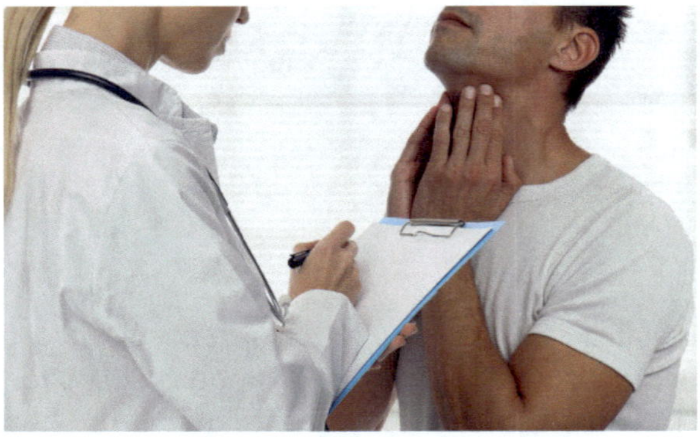

Figure 5.15. Treatment of endocrine disorders.

Source: https://ucfhealth.com/wp-content/uploads/2020/10/endoctrine-disorders.jpg.

5.5.1. Hormone Replacement Therapy

Hormone Replacement Therapy (HRT) has become an essential intervention for the treatment of several endocrinology disorders, the most significant examples of which are menopause and thyroid disturbances. HRT is a measure of alleviating the symptoms due to hormonal imbalance by supplementing exogenous hormones, i.e., estrogen and progesterone, in postmenopausal females. This therapy not only relieves common symptoms like hot flashes and mood swings but can also be especially vital in the prevention of osteoporosis. This condition is extremely common among postmenopausal populations. Research emphasizes the value of tailoring HRT regimens to patient profiles with an emphasis placed on the need for an in-depth understanding of the complexities of the endocrine system and of how hormones work together to promote overall health. The decision to pursue HRT needs to be made upon weighing potential benefits against risks, a process that continues to evolve within the medical community. The interaction between thyroid hormones and reproductive health also illustrates the necessity of HRT in the management of endocrine disease. Thyroid hormones (THs) of thyroxine (T4) and triiodothyronine (T3) are at the very center of sexual and reproductive function. Its effects are manifested in both genders, but the subtlety is less explored in female sexuality than in male models. Studies have substantiated that thyroid deficiency can adversely affect fertility, and THs are mediators of the hormonal axis governing reproductive physiology. Its dysregulation may lead to amenorrhea or other menstrual irregularities in females and also make it more difficult to regulate HRT. With more research being uncovered, the reality that understanding the intricate relationship between thyroid hormones, sex function, and replacement therapies can open up additional therapeutic paths for the management of endocrine disorders is well appreciated (Carosa et al., 2018). Additionally, HRT has purposes beyond reproductive medicine, providing a broader context for endocrine management in clinical practice.

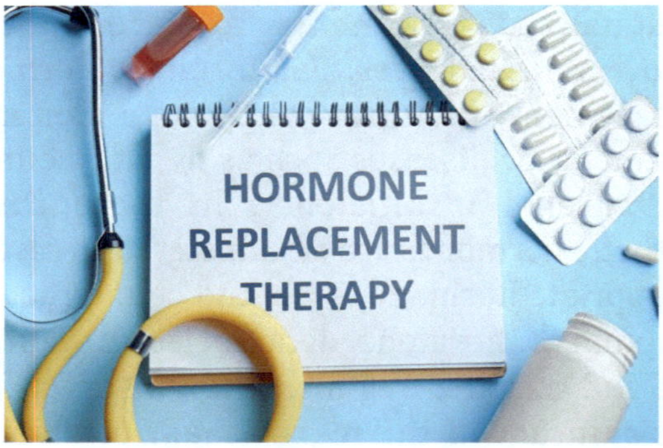

Figure 5.16. Hormone replacement therapy.

Source: https://sa1s3optim.patientpop.com/assets/images/provider/photos/2667109.jpg.

Hormonal therapies are becoming better understood to be used to treat a wide range of disorders outside traditional uses, such as weight management and metabolic syndrome. Physiological effects of these therapies should be carefully monitored and managed with multidisciplinary interventions, particularly given the varied responses people may have to HRT. As significant is the recognition of funding assistance for ongoing research and education in this area, underlining the collaborative effort needed to advance our understanding (Allen et al., 2015). Last but not least, the HRT in endocrine disorders discussion draws attention not only to the physiology involved but also to the ethical dimension to managing patients, necessitating careful deliberation based on changing evidence and treatment-specific appraisals (Figure 5.16).

5.5.2. Medications and Their Mechanisms

The pharmacological profile of drugs in the treatment of endocrine disorders has undergone a radical shift, necessitating a complex understanding of medications and their mechanisms of action. Targeted medications for hormonal deficiencies, such as thyroid hormone or insulin, act through complex mechanisms that significantly impact body functions. Levothyroxine, a man-made thyroxine hormone, acts by binding to nuclear receptors to control gene expression, thereby controlling metabolic processes. Correcting the normal thyroid activity alleviates hypothyroid symptoms, thus highlighting the importance of proper hormonal control. Insulin and insulin analogues also work by augmenting glucose uptake into peripheral tissues, particularly muscle and fat, therefore regulating blood glucose. Understanding such mechanisms reveals the intricate relationship between drugs and endocrine responses, which is relevant to the successful management of patients with endocrine diseases. The role of neurotransmitters in endocrine functions is another area where drugs have significant effects. New studies have highlighted the significance of serotonin in maternal behavior and reproductive functions, linking hormonal changes to neurological processes (Li et al., 2019). Certain drugs, particularly selective serotonin reuptake inhibitors (SSRIs), show this overlap by altering brain levels of serotonin and therefore impact mood and behavior during critical life events such as pregnancy and postpartum recovery. Such SSRIs can alleviate maternal mental disease symptoms but also overlap with the hormonal changes that characterize the maternal brain. Hence, the effects of these drugs on neuroendocrine responses call for an integrated approach to treating endocrine diseases and demonstrate how drugs can simultaneously influence physiological and psychological dimensions of health. It is also important to keep in mind that drugs debilitate endocrine functions. Although the majority of drugs are effective in curing hormonal disorders, they at times cause issues that can complicate the original disease.

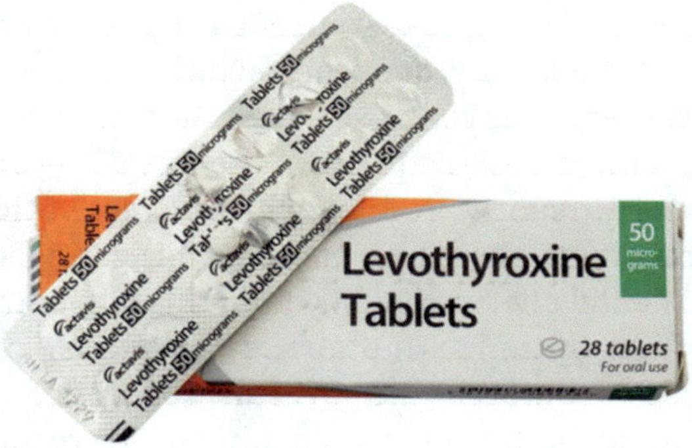

Figure 5.17. Levothyroxine is a thyroid hormone drug.

Source: https://countrymedicalpharmacy.com/wp-content/uploads/2023/06/levothyroxine-drug-watse-time-money-thyroid-treatment-942099.jpg.

For instance, glucocorticoids, which are extremely widely used in the treatment of many endocrine and autoimmune disorders, can disrupt the hypothalamic-pituitary-adrenal (HPA) axis, potentially leading to adrenal insufficiency and metabolic syndrome. Such drugs act by mimicking cortisol with anti-inflammatory effects, but long-term use can be harmful. Mechanism-based understanding of these drugs thus enters into action, because clinicians must weigh benefits against possible long-term endocrine deregulation. With ongoing pharmacologic advancements, research to enhance side effects and therapeutic efficacy will be central to the management of endocrine disorders (Billups et al., 2014) (Figure 5.17).

5.5.3. Lifestyle Modifications

Lifestyle modification is crucial for the management of endocrine diseases, especially for reducing the effect of chronic stress, which is increasingly being regarded as a factor for endocrine imbalance. Increased levels of stress can aggravate the body's physiological reactions controlled by the endocrine system, influence hormonal regulation, and leave a person vulnerable to diseases such as diabetes and thyroid illness. By adopting healthier lifestyle choices—such as continued exercise, a nutritious diet, and stress-reduction techniques—one can significantly reduce chronic activation of the stress response, thereby mitigating its detrimental effects. Not only does this preventive measure optimize metabolic functions, but it also promotes the overall resilience of hormonal pathways, which ultimately results in a healthier balance throughout the body's intricate mechanisms. The response to such changes is of primary concern, as it constitutes a protective measure against the development of endocrine disorders caused by stress and underscores the role of lifestyle in disease control. Furthermore, adequate sleep hygiene is an essential element of lifestyle change that can potentially influence endocrine function. Poor sleep patterns have been linked with dysregulation of hormones such as cortisol, insulin, and growth hormone, all of which are critical to maintaining overall well-being. Sleep deprivation can create a cascade of hormonal changes, leading to heightened stress reactions and increased inflammation. Studies have shown that improving the quality of sleep is not only able to normalize hormonal imbalances but also induce psychological resilience against stressors. With the integration of appropriate sleeping habits, such as a daily sleep schedule and sleeping conditions, the body becomes simpler to manage hormonally, and the risk of contracting long-term endocrine diseases is reduced. The link between improved sleep and balance of the hormones further illustrates how lifestyle adjustments can play an important role in managing endocrine disorders, as established in various studies on the subject. Further, food selection is central to facilitating major lifestyle modifications that cure endocrine disorders. Diet has a potent influence on hormonal health, and certain foods can exacerbate or alleviate symptoms associated with hormonal imbalance. For instance, eating highly processed sugar and trans fats can lead to insulin resistance and heightened inflammation—both tightly tied to diseases such as obesity and polycystic ovarian syndrome.

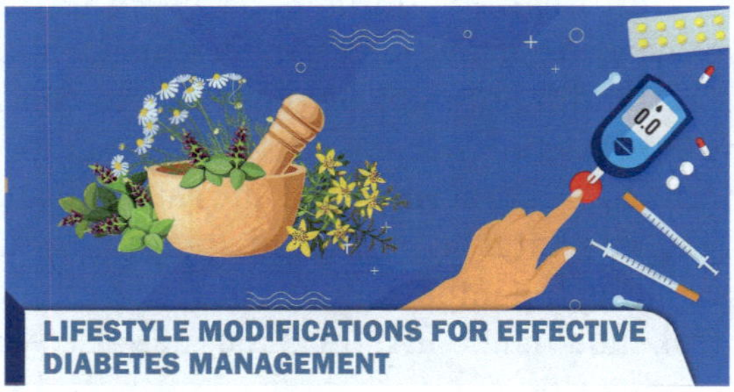

Figure 5.18. Lifestyle modifications for effective diabetes management.

Source: https://blogs.dpuerp.in/images/blog/61/580-lifestyle-modifications-for-effective-diabetes-management.jpg.

On the contrary, a diet rich in whole foods, with high concentrations of fruit, vegetables, lean protein, and healthy fat, has proven to sustain endocrine function and regulate blood sugar levels. By consciously choosing nutrient-rich foods, it is quite easy to support endocrine health and avoid exacerbating the disorder. The merging of these dietary shifts with other lifestyle adjustments enunciates the notion that holistic interventions play a pivotal role in the management of the nuances of endocrinology disorders and their treatment, particularly taking into consideration the intricate dynamics between diet, stress, and hormonal regulation (Baritaki et al., 2019; Cannizzaro et al., 2019) (Figure 5.18).

Test Your Knowledge

1. What is hormone replacement therapy (HRT)?
2. What is the significance of lifestyle modifications in managing endocrinology disorders?

5.6. Current Research and Advances in Endocrinology

Learning Outcome

1. Know the emerging therapies
2. Describe the genetic research and endocrinology
3. Understand the role of technology in diagnosis and treatment

Recent advancements in endocrinology have made more of the complex dynamics of hormonal imbalance and numerous conditions, such as infertility and metabolic disease, come to light. Science has revealed how chemicals in the environment, termed endocrine disruptors, communicate with the hormonal system and impact reproductive health and metabolic processes. For instance, it has been proven through research that endocrine-disrupting chemicals (EDCs) play a role in the etiology of disorders like polycystic ovary syndrome (PCOS) and obesity, where hormonal interference can exacerbate clinical symptoms and lead to chronic health complications. Knowledge of such interactions is thus important for developing specific interventions and therapeutic measures to treat endocrine disorders effectively. As researchers continue to examine the mechanisms of these endocrine interactions, they highlight the need for greater awareness and education about the implications of environmental exposures for endocrine function, as well as the necessity of policy changes to reduce exposure to toxic chemicals. A significant area of current research is the psychological and emotional meaning of endocrine disorders, particularly infertility. The problem of couples who are infertile is further compounded by the advancements in Assisted Reproductive Technology (ART), which creates ethical questions about the biological processes. Recent studies reveal three prevailing ethical frameworks among ART seekers: community health, ordered society, and human dignity. These strategies respond to the biological ambivalence inherent in ART, to an increasing desire to address the emotional and spiritual lives of treatment couples. The discussion further emphasizes the importance of constructing ethical foundations into the medical application of ART in a manner that is respectful not merely of the physical but also of the emotional dimensions of reproductive well-being. Hence, these discussions pave the way for future research that marries clinical findings with ethical considerations, thereby improving the treatment process for patients. Endocrinology research has also focused on the destructive effects of environmental toxic exposure on the endocrine system, particularly on how chemicals affect human development and growth. Recent studies have shown that exposure to toxicants can result in a vast array of health states, including learning impairments and behavioral disorders, which are likely to be induced by disrupted endocrine signaling. The implications of these discoveries are extensive, requiring policy changes to reduce exposure to harmful substances across the overall population and among special risk groups. Such evidence not only informs public health programs but also challenges the medical community to collaborate more closely with policymakers to address the root causes of endocrine disruption. Thus, ongoing research into the impacts of environmental toxicants on endocrine function is critical to safeguarding future generations and facilitating overall health gain in society. Lastly, in-depth examination of the factors can lead to visionary strategies that mitigate against the threats of endocrine disorders and improve population health outcomes (Figure 5.19).

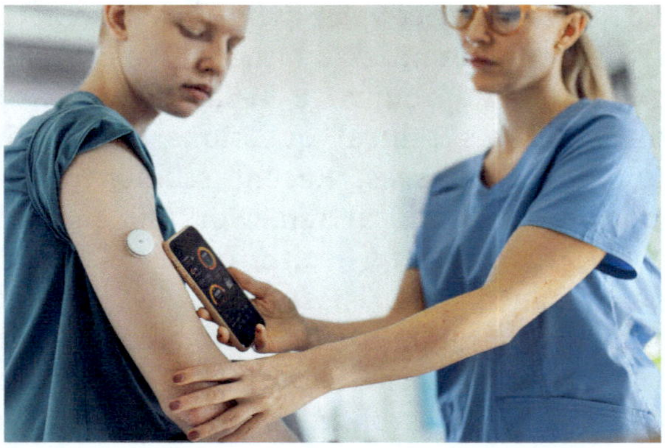

Figure 5.19. Advancements in Endocrinology: Emerging Trends and Research.

Source: https://wp04-media.cdn.ihealthspot.com/wp-content/uploads/sites/464/2024/03/iStock-1796960382-1.jpeg.

5.6.1. Emerging Therapies

Endocrinology is being subject to a range of new therapies that seek to battle the multidimensional nature of endocrine diseases. Traditional methods have been centered on suppression or replacement therapy with hormones; however, recent advances have opened new avenues for more precise modalities of treatment. For instance, treatments that are centered on targeting specific molecular pathways of the endocrine system, particularly in the case of glucocorticoid disorders, have taken center stage. This method not only enhances efficacy but also minimizes the side effects of broad-spectrum hormonal treatments. The expanding knowledge base of molecular mechanisms, combined with increasingly sophisticated genetic analysis, underscores the potential of individualized therapies. Newer biopharmaceutical developments, such as monoclonal antibodies and small-molecule inhibitors, have shown promising results in clinical trials and therefore represent a groundbreaking paradigm shift in endocrinology treatment. One particularly fascinating development is that of the 18-kDa translocator protein (TSPO). Already implicated in cholesterol trafficking and steroidogenesis, the protein is being explored for potential roles in a variety of endocrine disease states. With its ability to bind mitochondrial proteins and influence cellular processes such as apoptosis and autophagy, TSPO is an emerging prime target for future therapeutics. Recent studies have found that deciphering the high-resolution structure of TSPOs can catalyze the design of specific modulators that induce substantial metabolic changes. By revealing the extensive physiological mechanisms under TSPO control, scientists are unlocking drugs with the potential to have a profoundly modulating effect on endocrine signaling, thus providing new avenues for the treatment of diabetes, adrenal insufficiency, and other metabolic disorders, while at the same time improving patient outcomes and quality of life, as stated in (Aghazadeh et al., 2016). On a parallel front, the condition of congenital heart defects (CHDs), being primarily a cardiologic condition, has significant overlaps with endocrine therapy interventions. Current research reaffirms that the underlying genetic and environmental mechanisms for CHDs bear important implications for endocrine function and regulation in these subjects. By examining the intricate interaction between such defects and endocrine disturbances, it is conceivable that there can be an optimization of therapy, taking into consideration both cardiovascular and hormonal balance. Systematic approaches that combine next-generation sequencing with phenotypic analysis enable it to identify individual genetic variants associated with both conditions. Such a comprehensive understanding is crucial for the design of personalized therapy that not only repairs the structural abnormalities of CHDs but also optimizes endocrine function and metabolic health, as emphasized by Reemtsen et al. (2017). Consequently, this field serves to highlight the necessity of interdisciplinary collaboration in enhancing the care of patients with complex health issues.

5.6.2. Genetic Research and Endocrinology

The overlap between genetic research and endocrinology has revealed a number of intricacies of endocrine disease, namely the genetic etiology of hypospadias and other disorders. These have been highlighted by more recent research, which has highlighted the role of steroidogenic factor 1 (SF-1, NR5A1) in human sex development, revealing mutations that lead to 46, XY disorders of sex development. The identification of these mutations in individuals with severe hypospadias emphasizes genetic heterogeneity and the range of phenotypes for this disease. In fact, one cohort study demonstrated that heterozygous mutations of NR5A1 were identified in three cases, suggesting genetic mutations to be responsible for key clinical features such as low testosterone levels and cryptorchidism, which suggests a direct impact on endocrine function (Achermann et al., 2009). So, incorporating genetic screening into the clinical environment has the potential to enhance diagnostic accuracy and inform management in affected individuals. Furthermore, genetic inquiry has significant implications for more extensive endocrine diseases, like metabolic syndromes involving circadian biology. A workshop at the National Institute of Diabetes and Digestive and Kidney Diseases emphasized the need to determine how sleep and circadian rhythm affect metabolic function. As new research emerges, it is suggested that these biological cycles are altered in such a way that hormonal disturbances lead to hormonal imbalances, which further complicate conditions like diabetes. On this note, genomic and phenotypic assessments must be incorporated in a way that does not lead one to jump to conclusions about individual risk factors. Research must be directed not only towards measurements of insulin and glucose but also towards understanding the intricate dynamics among genetics, sleep, and metabolic health (Arble et al., 2015). Such a multidisciplinary approach may yield new ways to diminish the deleterious effects of disrupted circadian rhythms on endocrine function. Lastly, the future of endocrinology is, to a great extent, contingent upon the ongoing interplay between genetic research and clinical practice. Upon identifying the genetic components of endocrine disorders, this knowledge can guide the development of individualized treatment regimens and targeted interventions.

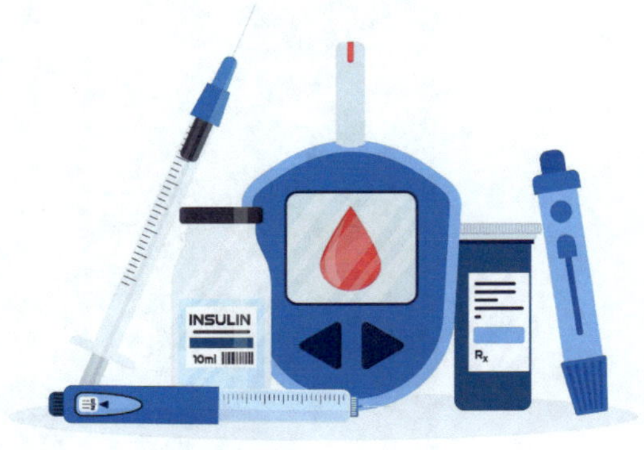

Figure 5.20. Genetic testing for diabetes.

Source: https://www.news-medical.net/images/Article_Images/ImageForArticle_23422_16717210961015802.jpg.

For instance, identifying specific genetic markers associated with heightened susceptibility to disorders such as adrenal insufficiency or thyroid disease will enable more rigorous management of health. Moreover, interdisciplinarity between endocrinologists and geneticists is a key component in translating basic genetic science into clinical contexts. Through such collaboration, new therapies may be explored, and ultimately, improved patient outcomes and insights into the intricate interface between endocrinology and genetics in human disease and health (Figure 5.20).

5.6.3. Role of Technology in Diagnosis and Treatment

Technology has revolutionized the diagnosis and treatment of endocrine disorders in endocrinology. Diagnostic methods, such as high-throughput genetic analysis and imaging modalities, have significantly enhanced the detection and characterization of endocrine abnormalities. For instance, the addition of next-generation sequencing enables scientists and clinicians to identify genetic mutations underlying disorders such as congenital adrenal hyperplasia or multiple endocrine neoplasia, thereby facilitating early intervention. Furthermore, imaging modalities like CT scans and MRI yield essential information about the structural disturbances of endocrine glands, enabling one to accurately localize tumors or hyperplastic tissue. Having the ability to utilize such superior technologies not only increases diagnostic accuracy but also lays the groundwork for tailor-made treatment regimens tailored to patients' genetic and phenotypic features in endocrine disease. Parallel to diagnostic innovation has also come the therapeutic history of endocrine disorders. Technology has revolutionized some of the newer therapies, such as targeted medication and newer hormonal replacement therapy.

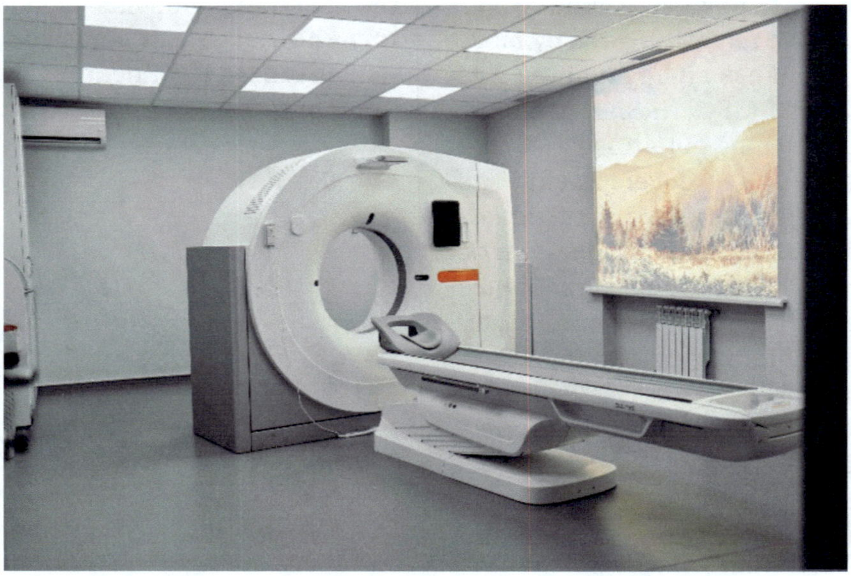

Figure 5.21. Magnetic resonance imaging (MRI).

Source: https://premierimaging.org/wp-content/uploads/2022/01/mri-magnetic-resonance-imaging-scan-device-mri-2021-09-02-07-55-40-utc-scaled.jpg.

For example, continuous glucose monitoring systems in diabetic patients provide real-time information, enabling instantaneous lifestyle adjustments and medication dose adjustments. Similarly, technological advances in telemedicine have increased patients' access to specialist consultations for thyroid dysfunction and other conditions, as remote monitoring systems enable healthcare providers to observe patients' responses and modify treatment protocols with ease. Not only do these kinds of technological interventions increase patient compliance and engagement, but they also improve clinical outcomes by implementing a proactive rather than reactive approach in healthcare. In addition, technology is also central to the application of data-driven information, significantly influencing endocrinology research and practice. The integration of electronic health records with artificial intelligence can automate the analysis of patient data, enabling predictive modeling and risk assessment across a wide range of endocrine diseases. This not only helps clinicians make informed decisions but also aligns with the concept of personalized medicine, in which therapy is tailored to the patient's individual profile. Big data in endocrinology can identify patterns and correlations across heterogeneous patient groups, translating into improved protocols and a greater understanding of disease mechanisms. Therefore, as technology continues to advance, their use in the diagnostic and therapeutic realms of endocrinology will certainly promote disease management and improve patients' quality of life (Overy et al., 2014; Allen et al., 2015) (Figure 5.21).

Test Your Knowledge

1. Do endocrinologists do genetic testing?
2. What is the role of technology in diagnosis and treatment?

SUMMARY

Finally, the interplay between endocrine diseases and other aspects of human function underscores the significance of these conditions in determining a person's quality of life. Hormone dynamics govern vital processes, from growth and metabolism to reproductive function. The case of the thyroid hormones is particularly revealing because it establishes an important nexus between thyroid and reproductive function, as it has an impact on fertility and sexual health in women and men. The findings presented in the chapter indicate that endocrine disturbances not only lead to physiological changes but also potentially create emotional and psychological problems, which is important to address with comprehensive treatment plans that address both the medical and mental health components (Carosa et al., 2018). Finally, the discussion of endocrinology disorders would be incomplete without discussing the socio-cultural aspects of these ailments. Infertility, say, is loaded with emotional toll, influencing the mental well-being of the individual, interpersonal relationships, and social functioning. Utilization of Assisted Reproductive Technology (ART) poses ethical questions of particular importance at this time. Where couples pursue solutions to infertility, the intersection of religion, ethics, and medical technology demands a delicate conversation among medical providers and community leaders. With this, the understanding of the endocrine system's role in reproductive disorders enables more compassionate and informed interventions for individuals in need (Gresham et al., 2020). Ultimately, the intervention for an endocrine disorder requires an interdisciplinary approach that involves medical, psychological, and ethical components. With the continued practice of endocrinology, research will be essential to the realization of early diagnosis, prevention, and intervention of endocrine disorders. By raising public consciousness of the principal health consequences of hormonal derangement and the need for an integrated understanding of health, society can contribute to better-assisted individuals who suffer from such disorders. Promoting integrative treatment models and free forum discussion of the consequences of endocrine action will optimize the quality of life of patients and drive towards an informed public debate (Carosa et al., 2018; Gresham et al., 2020).

Human endocrinology disorders comprise multiple conditions that affect hormone regulation and metabolism. Endocrine disorders can become a decisive determining factor of physical and mental health, causing a variety of complications that affect quality of life. For example, disruption of endocrine function may increase the risk of obesity, diabetes, and sterility. Both genetics and environmental factors play a role in the development of these illnesses. Recent evidence points to the hazard posed by exposure to toxic chemicals, which are harmful to health and development and predispose to early birth and learning disability, further underlining the need to address environmental risk in policy reform (Hitchcock et al., 2011). This mutual interplay between internal hormonal imbalance and external environmental insults underscores the complexity of endocrine disease. One of the most significant among such concerns is the incidence of male reproductive tract malformations, which has been linked to endocrine disruption in fetal development. The testicular dysgenesis syndrome (TDS) explains this condition in that pregnant women's exposure to estrogenic compounds is observed to increase the incidence of conditions such as hypospadias and cryptorchidism and potentially also result in testicular cancer later in life (Boobis et al., 2008). These findings highlight the urgent necessity to research further the extent to which prenatal exposure contributes to endocrine health, as the latest quantitative overviews on this subject have found a correlational relationship without delineating the mechanisms underlying it.

Systematic reviews are hence essential for developing efficacious preventive measures. In addition, the increasing prevalence of endocrine disorders necessitates an urgent requirement to enhance public health interventions focusing on both treatment and prevention. While scientists continue to identify associations between exposure to environmental pollutants and endocrine disorders, it is now essential to lobby for changes that will reduce causative exposures. Evidence-based policy can help prevent risks associated with endocrine disorders and, consequently, improve health outcomes. By establishing a greater understanding of the significant effects of environmental factors on hormonal well-being, overall strategies can be developed to combat these problems, thereby improving the quality of life for those involved.

KEY TERMS FROM THIS CHAPTER

- Adrenal glands
- Endocrine disruptors
- Growth hormone
- Hormonal regulation
- Hypothyroidism
- Reproductive health
- Thyroid dysfunction
- Cushing's syndrome
- Endocrinology
- Hormonal imbalances
- Hyperthyroidism
- Pituitary gland
- Steroid hormones
- Thyroxine

CRITICAL THINKING QUESTIONS

1. **Which hormone is deficient in Type 1 Diabetes Mellitus (T1DM)?**
   a. Glucagon
   b. Insulin
   c. Cortisol
   d. Thyroxine
2. **What is the most common cause of hyperthyroidism?**
   a. Hashimoto's thyroiditis
   b. Graves' disease
   c. Iodine deficiency
   d. Pituitary adenoma
3. **Which of the following is NOT a symptom of hypothyroidism?**
   a. Cold intolerance
   b. Weight gain
   c. Tachycardia
   d. Dry skin
4. **What is the primary laboratory finding in Cushing's syndrome?**
   a. Elevated serum cortisol levels
   b. Decreased serum glucose levels
   c. Increased thyroid hormone levels
   d. Reduced growth hormone levels
5. **Which diagnostic test is commonly used for diabetes mellitus?**
   a. Serum cortisol measurement
   b. Oral glucose tolerance test (OGTT)
   c. Thyroid function test
   d. Lipid profile

Short Answer Questions

1. Define the endocrinology.
2. What is the importance of the endocrine system?
3. List the types of endocrinology disorders.
4. What is the main cause of endocrine disorders?
5. What are the symptoms of endocrinology?

Answer to Critical Thinking Questions

1. (b); 2. (b); 3. (c); 4. (a); 5. (b).

REFERENCES

1. Köhler, B., Lin, L., Mazen, I., Cetindag, C., Biebermann, H., Akkurt, I., Rossi, R., Hiort, O., Grüters, A., & Achermann, J. C. (2009). The spectrum of phenotypes associated with mutations in steroidogenic factor 1 (SF-1, NR5A1, Ad4BP) includes severe penoscrotal hypospadias in 46,XY males without adrenal insufficiency. *European Journal of Endocrinology, 161*(2), 237–242. https://doi.org/10.1530/eje-09-0067Aghazadeh, A., Amitani, A., et al. (2016). TSPO: Kaleidoscopic 18-kDa amid biochemical pharmacology, control, and targeting of mitochondria. https://core.ac.uk/download/36779164.pdf (accessed on 12th July 2025).
2. Agra, A., Alexander, A., Alexopoulos, A., et al. (2017). Investigating interactions between epicardial adipose tissue and cardiac myocytes: What can we learn from different approaches? https://core.ac.uk/download/82983603.pdf (accessed on 12th July 2025).
3. Ahmed, A., Akre, A. B., et al. (2013). Novel associations in disorders of sex development: Findings from the I-DSD registry. https://core.ac.uk/download/16459200.pdf (accessed on 12th July 2025).
4. Allen, A., Badylak, S., Bancos, J., et al. (2015). New directions for the treatment of adrenal insufficiency. https://core.ac.uk/download/30697715.pdf (accessed on 12th July 2025).
5. Arble, D. M., & Framnes, S. N. (2018). The bidirectional relationship between obstructive sleep apnea and metabolic disease. https://core.ac.uk/download/213087655.pdf (accessed on 12th July 2025).
6. Arble, D. M., Bass, J., Behn, C. D., et al. (2015). Impact of sleep and circadian disruption on energy balance and diabetes: A summary of workshop discussions. https://core.ac.uk/download/213087763.pdf (accessed on 12th July 2025).
7. Baker, E., Corbett, R. W., Doulgeraki, T., et al. (2018). Nivolumab-induced fulminant diabetic ketoacidosis followed by thyroiditis. https://core.ac.uk/download/156738919.pdf (accessed on 12th July 2025).
8. Baldelli, R., Campana, D., Di Giacinto, P., et al. (2018). Chromogranin A: From laboratory to clinical aspects of patients with neuroendocrine tumors. https://core.ac.uk/download/188822602.pdf (accessed on 12th July 2025).
9. Baritaki, S., Chatzaki, E., de Bree, E., et al. (2019). Chronic stress, inflammation, and colon cancer: A CRH system-driven molecular crosstalk. https://core.ac.uk/download/323076588.pdf (accessed on 12th July 2025).
10. Bellingham, M., Cotinot, C., Evans, N. P., et al. (2016). Timing of maternal exposure and fetal sex determine the effects of low-level chemical mixture exposure on the fetal neuroendocrine system in sheep. https://core.ac.uk/download/74230048.pdf (accessed on 12th July 2025).
11. Billups, B., Burdakov, D., Burke, L. K., et al. (2014). 5-HT obesity medication efficacy via POMC activation is maintained during aging. https://core.ac.uk/download/29151000.pdf (accessed on 12th July 2025).
12. Binst, D., Daminet, S., Martlé, V., et al. (2016). Combined atypical primary hypoadrenocorticism and primary hypothyroidism in a dog. https://core.ac.uk/download/84045655.pdf (accessed on 12th July 2025).
13. Boobis, A. R., Lester, J. N., Martin, O. V., et al. (2008). Defective spermatogenesis: Martin et al. respond. https://core.ac.uk/download/337379.pdf (accessed on 12th July 2025).

14. Bouga, M., Combet, E., & Lean, M. E. J. (2018). Contemporary challenges to iodine status and nutrition: The role of foods, dietary recommendations, fortification, and supplementation. https://core.ac.uk/download/151395796.pdf (accessed on 12th July 2025).
15. Cannizzaro, E., Plescia, F., Cirrincione, L., & Ramaci, T. (2019). Work-related stress, physio-pathological mechanisms, and the influence of environmental genetic factors. https://core.ac.uk/download/287859255.pdf (accessed on 12th July 2025).
16. Carosa, E., Jannini, E. A., & Lenzi, A. (2018). Thyroid hormone receptors and ligand, tissue distribution, and sexual behavior. https://core.ac.uk/download/160052696.pdf (accessed on 12th July 2025).
17. Chou, T., D'Orsogna, M. R., & Kim, L. U. (2016). Onset, timing, and exposure therapy of stress disorders: Mechanistic insight from a mathematical model of oscillating neuroendocrine dynamics. https://core.ac.uk/download/323078037.pdf (accessed on 12th July 2025).
18. Collard, J., Gafane, L., Nell, T., et al. (2014). Physical activity and hypertension in South African adults. https://core.ac.uk/download/29852228.pdf (accessed on 12th July 2025).
19. De Angelis, C. C., Di Dato, C., Gianfrilli, D., et al. (2018). Smoke, alcohol, and drug addiction and male fertility. https://core.ac.uk/download/153370850.pdf (accessed on 12th July 2025).
20. Ernst, M., Green-Golan, L., Leschek, E., et al. (2010). Psychiatric characterization of children with genetic causes of hyperandrogenism. https://core.ac.uk/download/55802070.pdf (accessed on 12th July 2025).
21. Gonzalez Deniselle, M. C., Lara, H. E., Recabarren, S. E., et al. (2016). Developmental and functional effects of steroid hormones on the neuroendocrine axis and spinal cord. https://core.ac.uk/download/159294623.pdf (accessed on 12th July 2025).
22. Gresham, M. E. (2020). Inconceivable: An analysis of assisted reproductive technology for the church. https://core.ac.uk/download/322850911.pdf (accessed on 12th July 2025).
23. Hitchcock, E., & Madsen, T. (2011). Growing up toxic: Chemical exposures and increases in developmental disease. https://core.ac.uk/download/71358334.pdf (accessed on 12th July 2025).
24. Kass, P., Lau, G., Puschner, B., et al. (2017). Comparison of polybrominated diphenyl ethers (PBDEs) and polychlorinated biphenyls (PCBs) in the serum of hypothyroxinemia and euthyroid dogs. https://core.ac.uk/download/323070337.pdf (accessed on 12th July 2025).
25. Khoshnia, M., Marjani, A., & Shafaei, A. (2015). Serum level of fibroblast growth factor 21 in type 2 diabetic patients with and without metabolic syndrome. https://core.ac.uk/download/52205725.pdf (accessed on 12th July 2025).
26. Larauche, M., Mulak, A., & Taché, Y. (2011). Stress-related alterations of visceral sensation: Animal models for irritable bowel syndrome study. https://core.ac.uk/download/323080393.pdf (accessed on 12th July 2025).
27. Li, M., Lonstein, J. S., & Pawluski, J. L. (2019). Serotonin and motherhood: From molecules to mood. https://core.ac.uk/download/286364516.pdf (accessed on 12th July 2025).
28. Machado, A. I., Camilletti, M. A., Diaz, G. S., et al. (2019). Sex differences in the pituitary TGFβ1 system: The role of TGFβ1 in prolactinoma development. https://core.ac.uk/download/159292815.pdf (accessed on 12th July 2025).

29. Mercer, J. G., & Murphy, M. (2013). Diet-regulated anxiety. https://core.ac.uk/download/19506489.pdf (accessed on 12th July 2025).

30. Overy, C., & Tansey, E. M. (2014). The recent history of seasonal affective disorder (SAD). https://core.ac.uk/download/30696938.pdf (accessed on 12th July 2025).

31. Reemtsen, B., Finn, J. P., Alejos, J., Touma, M., Halnon, N., Nelson, S. F., et al. (2017). A path to implement precision child health cardiovascular medicine. https://core.ac.uk/download/323077346.pdf (accessed on 12th July 2025).

GASTROINTESTINAL DISORDERS

6

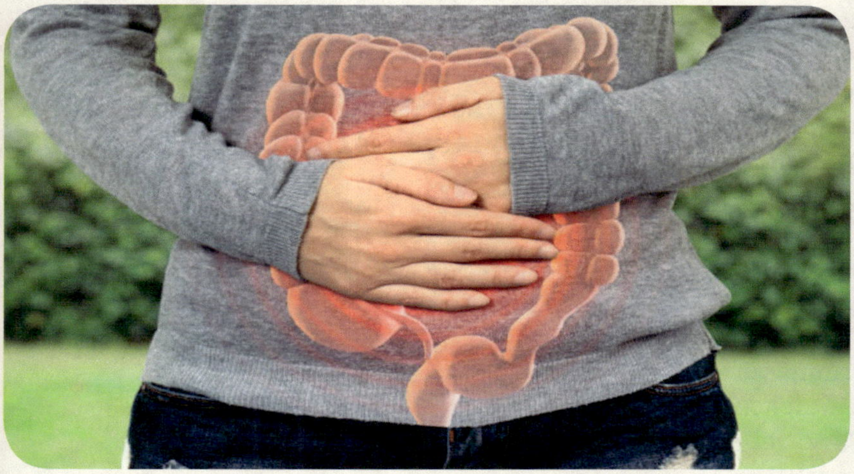

LEARNING OBJECTIVES

After studying this chapter, you will be able to:

1. Describe the anatomy of the gastrointestinal tract
2. Describe the common gastrointestinal disorders
3. Learn about causes and risk factors associated with gastrointestinal disorders
4. Describe the symptoms and diagnosis of gastrointestinal disorders
5. Know the treatment options of gastrointestinal disorders

Introduction

The GI system plays a key role in maintaining overall health and functioning, reflecting the intricate interaction among various physiological processes. Gastrointestinal disorders, comprising a broad array of digestive tract disorders, may significantly affect quality of life and compromise performance during daily functioning. These conditions, from the comparatively frequent ones such as irritable bowel syndrome (IBS) through more severe ones such as inflammatory bowel disease (IBD) and gastrointestinal cancers, are typically the outcome of multifactorial etiology. Emerging evidence favors the potential for a role of gut microbiota in the pathogenesis of these conditions, with emphasis placed on the complex relationship between microbial communities, the immune system, and the gut-brain axis. For instance, gut microbial abnormalities—dysbiosis—have been found to influence gastrointestinal motility and inflammatory reactions, raising the question of whether therapeutic intervention aimed at modifying these microbial profiles (Cicala et al., 2016). The more studies that have come out in contemporary times, the more it has become known that environmental, psychological, and physiological stressors contribute to exacerbating gastrointestinal disorders. Indeed, conditions like IBS have been shown to have a strong correlation with psychological parameters such as anxiety and stress, thereby highlighting the significance of the brain-gut axis. Stressful life events might trigger or worsen symptoms, leading to enhanced visceral hypersensitivity and pain sensitivity. Experimental stress models have been developed, and researchers are now able to explore the patterns of stress across life periods and its relevance for accounting for vulnerability in the persons at risk for GI dysfunction. The biological processes mediating stress-induced changes in GI sensitivity are typically multifaceted and encompass peripheral and central sensitization, underscoring the imperative for integrated treatment regimens that address both psychological and physical determinants (Larauche et al., 2011). The increased prevalence of gastrointestinal conditions in today's society necessitates the urgency of effective prevention and treatment. With ongoing progress in the field of gastrointestinal health, current research into the function of the gut microbiota and the intricate interactions within the gut-brain axis is promising for therapeutic advances. In particular, probiotics and lifestyle interventions aimed at restoring microbial balance could play central roles in managing these disorders, thereby improving patient outcomes. Moreover, a holistic approach encompassing dietary, psychological, and pharmacological interventions will be vital to addressing the complexities of these conditions. A comprehension of the root factors resulting in gastrointestinal disorders will eventually lead the way towards new approaches that improve the quality of life for patients suffering from these frequently debilitating diseases, a remarkable achievement in gastrointestinal medicine and research (Cicala et al., 2016) (Figure 6.1).

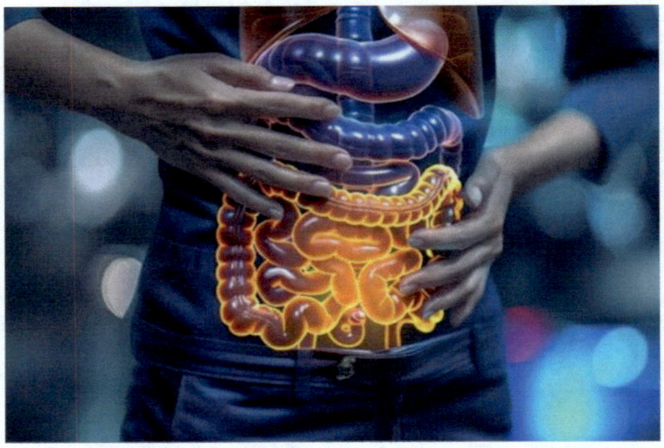

Figure 6.1. Gastrointestinal disorders.

Source: https://neumedclinics.com/wp-content/uploads/sites/143/2024/12/Gastrointestinal-Disorders.1.webp.

Definition of Gastrointestinal Disorders

Gastrointestinal illness is a broad range of illnesses that affect the gastrointestinal (GI) tract, which is comprised of organs from the mouth to the anus, responsible for digestion and elimination. Gastrointestinal illness may present with a range of symptoms, including abdominal cramps, bloating, diarrhea, constipation, and systemic illnesses such as malnutrition or dehydration. The complexity of the GI tract offers space for a vast array of disorders, from functional disorders like irritable bowel syndrome (IBS) to the more severe pathological conditions like inflammatory bowel diseases (IBD), such as Crohn's disease and ulcerative colitis. Understanding these disorders requires an interdisciplinary approach that integrates anatomy, physiology, and pathology, with a focus on the complex interdependence among these components and their impact on overall health. Innovations in gastroenterology technology during recent years have facilitated increased understanding of the etiology and pathophysiology of GI diseases. For example, the development of fiberoptic endoscopy has revolutionized diagnosis and therapy by allowing direct visualization and intervention in the GI tract. It is one of the major reasons for increased understanding of diseases that could not be diagnosed easily with traditional techniques. The implications of such practices extend beyond mere detection; they have significant therapeutic management and, by association, patient outcome implications. Notably, the development of more advanced pharmacological treatments has had a profound influence on the management of most gastrointestinal disorders, thereby improving quality of life in patients (Camilleri et al., 1999). Additionally, emerging research also highlights the role of the gut microbiome in gastrointestinal health and disease. Changes in gut microbiota composition have been associated with many gastrointestinal diseases, highlighting a potential mechanism for novel therapeutic interventions. For instance, studies have shown that patients and children with autistic spectrum disorders (ASD) have a distinctive difference in the composition of gut microbiota compared to their neurotypical counterparts, leading to hypotheses on the potential interaction of microbiome status and gastrointestinal symptoms. Through advanced experimental strategies, researchers attempt to clarify causal relationships within this complex system, highlighting the multifactorial nature of gastrointestinal diseases. By integrating evidence from citizen-science projects and controlled studies, a general understanding of the microbiome's role in gastrointestinal health may be established, further informing our treatment and management strategies in this field (Debelius et al., 2015).

Importance of Studying Gastrointestinal Health

It is of most relevance to know about gastrointestinal health because of its effects on overall well-being and quality of life. The gastrointestinal (GI) tract is responsible for nutrition, metabolism, and immune function, providing the body with essential nutrients and serving as a protective barrier against pathogens. Studies have demonstrated that changes in gastrointestinal health have been linked to a variety of systemic diseases, including malnutrition, autoimmune disease, and even mental illness. For instance, the gut-brain axis illustrates the profound relationship between GI health and neurologic health, where a healthy, balanced gut microbiota is essential. In light of these relations, detailed research into gastrointestinal health can enable quicker identification and improved treatment of often-recurring disorders, thereby highlighting its place in the broader picture of human health. In addition, the growing prevalence of GI illnesses, such as irritable bowel syndrome, inflammatory bowel disease, and celiac disease, underscores the necessity of investing in research on gastrointestinal health. Such disorders tend to generate debilitating symptoms and compromised quality of life for millions of individuals. Defining the mechanisms and causative factors of such illnesses can provide a potential avenue for developing new treatments and prophylactic measures. Also, because diet, exercise, and stress have been shown to play important functions in gastrointestinal function, taking an interdisciplinary approach to gastrointestinal health can prove beneficial. Research can help identify risk factors for GI disorders, thereby facilitating therapeutic interventions and increasing public awareness of the importance of a healthy gastrointestinal tract. Lastly, the influence of external factors such as environmental poisons should also be taken into account in the search for gastrointestinal health. New evidence indicates that the twentieth century's industrial activities have led to widespread exposure to heavy metals, which are harmful to GI health as well as to other body systems (M-Mood et al., 2021). Chronic exposure to such toxins can disrupt normal cellular function, which may result in gastrointestinal disease. Aside from that, learning how these toxic substances influence the gut microbiota is also important since emerging evidence suggests that derangement of the microbial balance can also lead to further deterioration in health status. Interdisciplinary research that integrates environmental science, toxicology, and gastroenterology can provide insights into how these factors interact and influence gastrointestinal health, informing strategies to reduce the incidence of related diseases (Alaggio et al., 2022) (Figure 6.2).

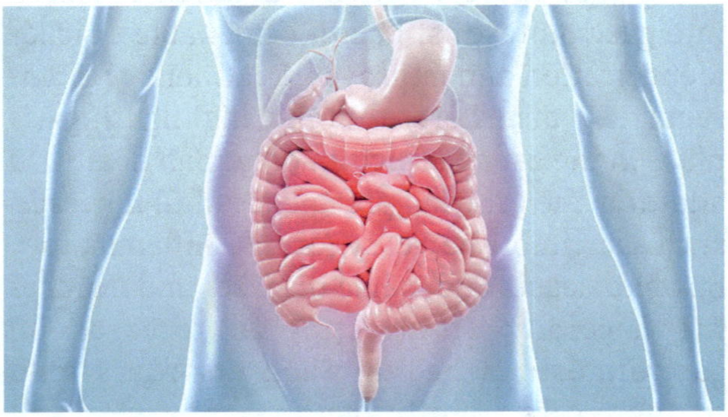

Figure 6.2. Importance of gastrointestinal health.

Source: https://theaeonclinic.com/wp-content/uploads/2024/09/what-is-gut-health.webp.

6.1. Anatomy of the Gastrointestinal Tract

Learning Outcome

1. Describe the structure and function of the digestive system
2. Understand the role of the gastrointestinal tract in nutrient absorption
3. Know the interaction between the gastrointestinal tract and other body systems

The gastrointestinal system is a complex system that plays a role in breaking down and absorbing nutrients, as well as the process of eliminating waste. Comprising the esophagus, stomach, small intestine, large intestine, and accessory organs such as the liver and pancreas, the GI system functions as a coordinated system to perform these activities. All organs perform some function, e.g., that of the stomach, not only chemically breaking down food with gastric juice but also mechanically with muscle contraction. Derangement of this intricate anatomy can lead to severe gastrointestinal illness, affecting nutrient uptake and overall well-being. It is necessary to know this anatomy, as it determines the diagnosis and treatment of many conditions that occur along the path of the digestive tract; for example, here the interdependence of functions and organs is evident. Pancreatic exocrine insufficiency (PEI) is a good example of anatomical alteration post-surgery, e.g., bariatric surgery, as a source of complications. The restructuring of the GI tract, although designed to enhance metabolic health and weight control, can inadvertently cause suboptimal pancreatic enzyme secretion, resulting in overlapping symptoms of maldigestion and malabsorption. Indeed, steatorrhea, weight loss, and malnutrition result from these alterations, rendering diagnosis and treatment complicated. The relevance of fecal elastase-1 (FE1) testing is evident here, as it can assist in diagnosing PEI in patients with chronic gastrointestinal symptoms following surgery. Thus, the multifaceted understanding of the anatomical changes that occur during surgery is paramount for effective clinical management of postoperative complications, emphasizing the need for continuous monitoring and therapeutic intervention in affected persons (Arnelo et al., 2017). It cannot be stressed too strongly how the relationship between diet, metabolism, and GI health is essential. Food interacts with GI anatomy in a manner that plays a major role in homeostasis and the prevention of disorders. For instance, dietary fiber content regulates bowel movements, effectively preventing constipation and increasing gut microbial diversity. Additionally, the biochemical function underlying the digestion of macronutrients requires an efficient GI tract to facilitate the absorption of vital vitamins and minerals.

Interruptions in this system may result in metabolic dysfunctions that have a lasting effect on the individual's overall well-being. Understanding these interactions informs the nutritional interventions and advice that aim to prevent gastrointestinal disease, with the suggestion of an integrative approach that engages biochemistry, human physiology, and dietary strategy (Sarmidi et al., 2012) (Figure 6.3).

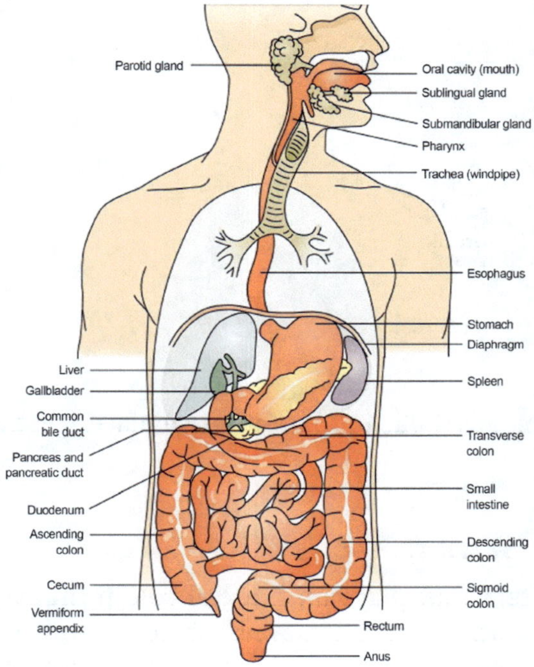

Figure 6.3. Anatomy of the gastrointestinal tract.

Source: https://img.brainkart.com/article/article-Anatomy-of-the-Gastr-eWX.jpg.

6.1.1. Structure and Function of the Digestive System

The digestive system is an intricate group of organs that are designed to break down food, absorb nutrients, and eliminate waste. It begins in the oral cavity, where the enzymatic process begins carbohydrate digestion, followed by the esophagus that transports consumed food into the stomach. Food is also broken down further in the stomach by gastric acids and enzymes into a liquid-like substance known as chyme. This is crucial to the following step of nutrient absorption, which occurs primarily in the small intestine. The small intestine is lined with villi and microvilli, significantly increasing the surface area available for absorption. This complexity illustrates the system's ingenious design, as it can effectively cope with a variety of foods and maintain homeostasis by regulating the nutrient content in the blood. The role of the digestive system is closely linked to its structural components, which work in harmony to enable processing and absorption. There are specialized cells and structures in each organ that play specific roles; for example, the liver produces bile, which is vital in fat emulsification, while the pancreas secretes enzymes to facilitate carbohydrate, protein, and fat digestion. Coordination between the organs is important to prevent malabsorption and gastrointestinal disease. Studies have also noted that changes in regulatory mechanisms, such as those involving sodium-proton exchanger 3 (NHE3) mediation, can result in fluid absorption dysfunctions and pH imbalances that can cause renal and digestive system diseases, indicating the interdependence of functions within the body (Dong et al., 2022). Secondly, the mechanisms of the gastrointestinal system place top priority not only on nutrient absorption but also on the potential effects of antimicrobial resistance (AMR), which play a pivotal role in gut health. AMR can contribute to treatment failure in gastrointestinal infections caused by various pathogens and further exacerbate existing gastrointestinal disorders (Murray et al., 2022). For instance, common pathogens of gastrointestinal disease, such as Escherichia coli and Staphylococcus aureus, can become resistant to treatment, leading to increased morbidity. Such understanding of the dynamics highlights the importance of keeping a healthy digestive system, while also the ongoing need for research into the subject to better determine the correct interventions and prevention against gastrointestinal diseases, which will, in the long run, improve outcomes and quality of life (Figure 6.4).

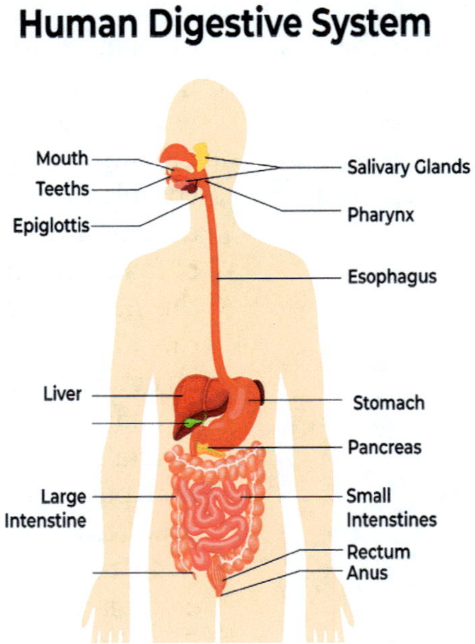

Figure 6.4. Human digestive system.

Source: https://media.geeksforgeeks.org/wp-content/uploads/20231113145954/Human-Digestive-System.png.

6.1.2. Role of the Gastrointestinal Tract in Nutrient Absorption

The gastrointestinal (GI) tract is a complex organ system that plays an integral role in nutrient absorption, helping maintain homeostasis and overall health. It involves several structures, such as the esophagus, stomach, small intestine, and large intestine, which are all designed to degrade and absorb food into usable units. The duodenum is where most nutrient absorption occurring with bile and enzymes contributing to the chemical digestion of macronutrients. With lumen content passage in the portions, nutrients such as carbohydrates, proteins, and fats are broken down into their simpler molecules, which can be efficiently absorbed into the blood system, a demonstration of the GI tract's critical role in energy and nutrition balance. Aging also has a strong impact on GI tract function, affecting nutrient absorption and overall health. Changes in the mechanical and motility functions of the GI tract and in chemical digestion processes all contribute to impaired ability to absorb vital nutrients such as vitamins and minerals. For instance, alterations in the functional state of the intestinal mucosa are responsible for malabsorption syndromes, such as in older subjects who tend to have difficulty with nutrient intake and bioavailability. Given these conditions, understanding the intricate relationship among aging, gut integrity, and nutrient uptake becomes essential, particularly when malnutrition heightens risk factors for a variety of pathologies, such as cardiovascular and immune system diseases, demonstrating the far-reaching implications of suboptimal GI health among elderly individuals (Bordoni et al., 2015). Moreover, nutrient absorption is not limited to macronutrients, with micronutrients also playing a key role in maintaining body functions. Gastrointestinal diseases can complicate absorption kinetics and induce severe health effects. Celiac disease, Crohn's disease, and irritable bowel syndrome are just some diseases that can significantly impair nutrient absorption, leading to deficiencies that may not always be easily revealed. For example, vitamin B12 deficiency is frequent in Crohn's disease patients due to impaired ileal absorption, while patients with celiac disease may exhibit fat-soluble vitamin deficiencies due to malabsorption. These issues need to be resolved with a holistic view of the mechanisms that regulate nutrient absorption in the GI tract and an evaluation of dietary options that foster maximum health in patients (Baal et al., 2011) (Figure 6.5).

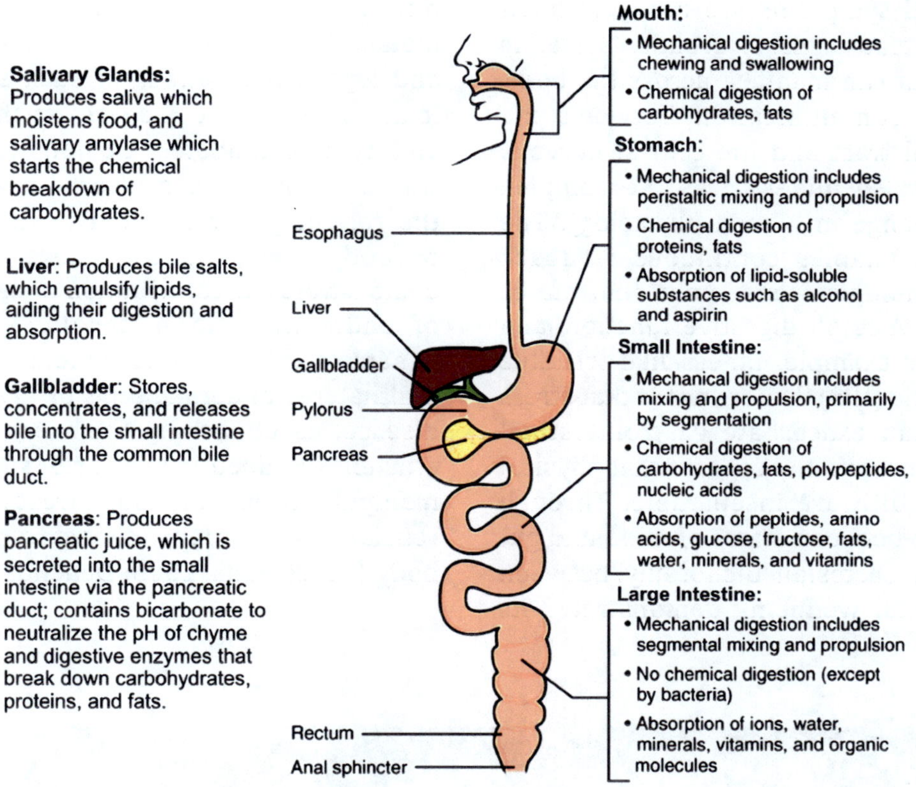

Figure 6.5. Summary of digestion and absorption. Digestion begins in the mouth and continues as food travels through the small intestine. Most absorption occurs in the small intestine.

Source: https://openoregon.pressbooks.pub/app/uploads/sites/98/2020/03/digestive-tract-summary.png.

6.1.3. Interaction Between the Gastrointestinal Tract and Other Body Systems

The GI tract is a key hub that controls and communicates with various body systems and, consequently, plays a basic role in health. One of its chief functions is communication with the immune system, as the gut-associated lymphoid tissue (GALT) regulates immune responses and provides a line of defense against pathogen invasion. Due to such close interaction, disturbances in gut microbiome have been associated with a variety of autoimmune and inflammatory diseases. For instance, dysbiosis—a gut bacterial imbalance—can cause systemic inflammation that, in addition to impacting digestive health, also contributes to diseases such as arthritis and inflammatory bowel disease. Probing such associations underscores the value of understanding that gastrointestinal symptoms are rarely isolated events but instead signs of broader systemic disruptions that can manifest across the body. The two-way communication between the gastrointestinal tract and the central nervous system (CNS) also underscores the complex nature of exchange in human physiology. The gut-brain axis enables continuous feedback wherein psychological and emotional states can exert influence on digestive function, and conversely. For example, illness like Irritable Bowel Syndrome (IBS) demonstrates that stress and anxiety can exacerbate gastrointestinal symptoms in line with the concept that physical and mental health are inseparable. Through the correlation between states of mind and gut operation, the Cartesian dichotomy between body and mental wellbeing demonstrates its limitations in explaining health events in totality. Understanding these interactions makes it possible to identify integrative approaches, with multimodal treatment strategies that consider both the psychological and physiological to enhance patient outcomes. Furthermore, the role of the gastrointestinal tract in metabolic regulation and endocrine function also complicates its connection with other body systems. Not only is the gut a digestive system, but it also actively participates in energy metabolism, regulating hormones like insulin and leptin. Disruptions of such signaling can lead to metabolic disease, such as obesity and type 2 diabetes, demonstrating the GI tract's contribution to overall health. Further, the role of gut microbiota in the modulation of body weight and glucose homeostasis demonstrates its contribution to the modulation of endocrine and metabolic systems. The dynamics of these interactions necessitate a multilateral understanding of gastrointestinal disease, as unpacking them can guide more efficient therapeutic measures, such as dietary manipulation and microbial treatment aimed at rebalancing interdependent systems within the body (Felice et al., 2003; Debelius et al., 2015).

Test Your Knowledge

1. What are the structures and functions of the digestive system?
2. What is the role of the gastrointestinal tract in nutrient absorption?

6.2. Common Gastrointestinal Disorders

Learning Outcome

1. Describe the irritable bowel syndrome (IBS)
2. Understand the inflammatory bowel diseases (IBD)
3. Understand the gastroesophageal reflux disease (GERD)

One of the most prevalent gastrointestinal disorders affecting millions worldwide is irritable bowel syndrome (IBS), a disease characterized by abdominal pain and altered bowel function, diarrhea or constipation. The pathophysiology of IBS is complex and multifactorial, typically involving interactions among gut microbial communities, the gut-brain axis, and psychosocial factors. Patients may present with complaints of worsening quality of life due to the chronic nature of the symptomatology. In addition, recent studies have highlighted the role of the gut microbiota in IBS, suggesting that dysbiosis, or microbial imbalance, may increase symptom severity and symptomatology. As researchers examine the use of dietary therapy and probiotics, it is clear that IBS may require treatment that accounts for unique gut microbiota patterns and food intake to allow for a more comprehensive understanding of this disorder's intricate presentation and therapy (Debelius et al., 2015). Another significant gastrointestinal disorder is the occurrence of *Helicobacter pylori* (*H. pylori*) infection, one of the primary causes of various gastric pathologies, including peptic ulcers and gastric carcinoma. The organisms are implicated in the breakdown of the gastric mucosal barrier, leading to inflammation and predisposing to more serious diseases if left untreated. Early diagnosis and effective eradication therapy are of fundamental importance in the prevention of *H. pylori* associated complications, with guidelines suggesting repeated screening in patients with high prevalence rates. However, failure of therapy in the treatment of H. pylori infection, observed in approximately 20% of cases, reflects the challenges in treating this infection. With clinicians encountering antibiotic resistance and heterogeneity in treatment response, the importance of patient support and education comes into focus for ensuring improved treatment and adherence to long-term treatment regimens in the context of H. pylori infection (Ciorbagiu et al., 2016). In addition to IBS and H. pylori, inflammatory bowel diseases (IBD), consisting of Crohn's disease and ulcerative colitis, represent significant challenges in the field of gastrointestinal health. Such relapsing illnesses are characterized by episodes of inflammation within the gastrointestinal tract and can potentially induce debilitating symptoms such as severe abdominal pain, diarrhea, and malnutrition.

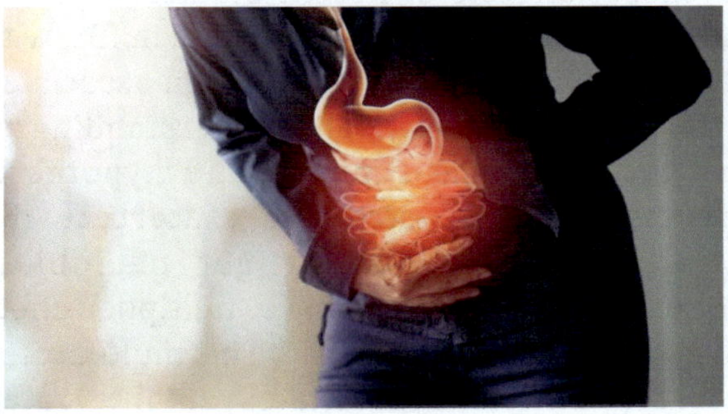

Figure 6.6. Common gastrointestinal disorders.

Source: https://www.drbhushan.in/wp-content/uploads/2024/10/Common-Gastrointestinal-Disorders-and-How-to-Manage-Them.jpg.

The etiology of IBD is thought to be the result of a combination of genetic predisposition, environmental influences, and immune response dysregulation. Recent advances in biologic therapy have opened new therapeutic possibilities for management, with success in alleviating inflammation and achieving remission. However, long-term management of IBD still requires a multidisciplinary team with patient follow-up at frequent intervals and psychological therapy for the patients to achieve an integrated understanding of the disorder's impact on their quality of life. With advancing research, a deeper understanding of the underlying pathogenic mechanisms of IBD may uncover new therapies that improve patient outcomes and quality of life (Figure 6.6).

6.2.1. Irritable Bowel Syndrome (IBS)

Irritable Bowel Syndrome (IBS) is a prevalent gastrointestinal disorder characterized by a group of symptoms such as abdominal discomfort, bloating, and disturbance of bowel habits manifested as diarrhea, constipation, or their alternating combination. The pathophysiology of IBS remains multifactorial and complex, including gut motility, visceral sensitivity, and psychosocial factors. Recent studies highlight the pivotal role of the gut microbiota in IBS, with variations in microbial composition associated with disease severity. The understanding of the gut-brain axis supports the hypothesis that psychological stressors exacerbate IBS symptoms by modulating gut microbiota composition, thereby having a multiplier effect on mental and gut well-being. This multifaceted interdependence necessitates an integrated management strategy that addresses both gastrointestinal and psychological aspects of the condition. Recent studies have highlighted the significance of diet in managing IBS symptoms, showing that particular diet patterns can influence the gut microbiota. Studies find that high-fiber diets, with greater proportions of fermentable oligosaccharides, disaccharides, monosaccharides, and polyols (FODMAPs), could avert IBS symptoms and maintain gut health by promoting a healthy microbiota. The production of short-chain fatty acids through dietary fiber fermentation helps reduce inflammation and preserve gut integrity, thereby establishing a direct link between the diet consumed and the microbiota-gut-brain axis. These findings are consistent with the observation that individuals with IBS may notice symptom improvement when provided with personalized dietary care, thereby addressing both physiological and psychological facets of the disease. With GIT's involvement in health management, nutritional methods form a critical component of overall treatment programs. Growing evidence suggests a relationship between IBS and various chronic disorders, including psychiatric disorders such as depression and anxiety. Indeed, the gut-brain axis comes into play here, where the composition of gut microbiota might influence neurochemical mechanisms and, as a consequence, mood and cognition. The findings of these studies extend beyond clinical practice into research, as subsequent studies have sought to clarify the mechanisms underlying such associations. As health care professionals deal with the increasing prevalence of IBS and associated disorders, the union of microbiome research and therapeutic methods opens new frontiers for intervention. The exploration of microbial-based therapies and dietary treatments can pave the way for novel treatment approaches, emphasizing the role of integrative medicine in IBS management and underscoring the appeal of further exploring its pathophysiology (Figure 6.7).

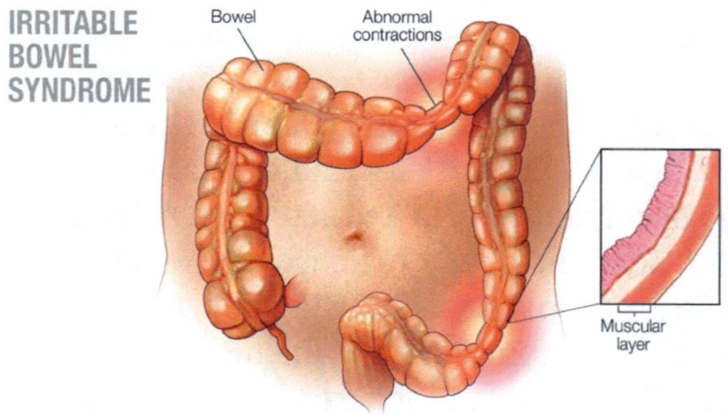

Figure 6.7. Irritable bowel syndrome.

Source: https://drrohitgoyalgastro.com/wp-content/uploads/2024/06/Untitled-design.png.

6.2.2. Inflammatory Bowel Disease (IBD)

The fulminans of Inflammatory Bowel Disease (IBD) are not only in its pathological manifestation, but also the variability of symptoms expressed by the patients. IBD is predominantly characterized by Crohn's disease and ulcerative colitis, both of which are characterized by chronic inflammation of the gastrointestinal tract. The variable nature of symptoms such as abdominal pain, diarrhea, and weight loss suggests that there are biochemical determinants of symptom expression. Research has established that hormonal factors, i.e., interactions among intestinal hormones such as progesterone, may play a significant role in such oscillatory patterns of symptoms. By examining the hormonal mechanisms implicated, new therapeutic modalities would be made available and hope provided to those patients who currently experience no benefit from the disabling symptoms of IBD with present treatments (Linson et al., 2013). Environmental factors, and in particular dietary factors, are increasingly recognized as critical agents of the etiology and perpetuation of IBD. Recent data have shown that dietary exposure may interact with the gut microbiota to induce inflammatory responses in genetically predisposed individuals. The D-ECCO working party emphasizes the necessity of understanding diets' double role: its possible role as an environmental precipitant for IBD and as part of nutritional management. With aspects such as fiber intake, native and acquired immunity-governed fatty acids, and food additives as targets, researchers look to shed more light on the potential means by which specific dietary interventions may not only be employed for prevention but also for the treatment of IBD. In this manner, aside from highlighting the position of nutrition in IBD etiology, the gaps in knowledge in existing research requiring further study are highlighted (Allan et al., 2017). Based on current studies, the treatment of IBD must be an integrated approach using medical and diet interventions. Most importantly, the nutritional condition of the patients with IBD should be treated, as malnutrition is detrimental to the disease's impact and could be a hindrance to healing. Supportive nutrition therapy combined with drug interventions can minimize complications and improve the quality of life of patients suffering from IBD. Furthermore, creating awareness about the beneficial effects of certain eating habits can help patients become more engaged actors in their care. By stimulating a broad understanding of how eating habits and hormones interact, clinicians are able to create more effective, patient-centric treatment plans that take into account both the physiological and lifestyle aspects of living with IBD (Figure 6.8).

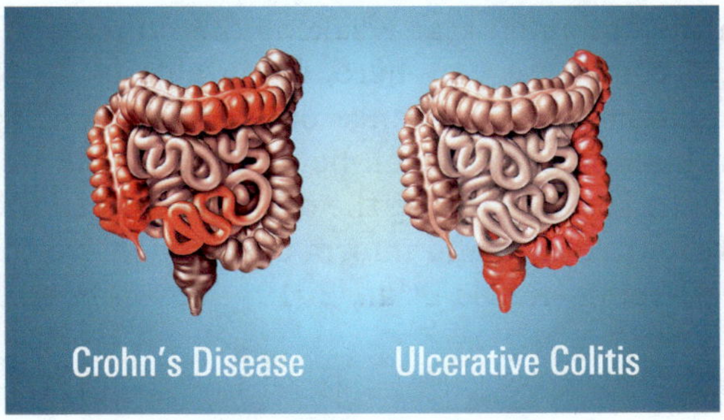

Figure 6.8. Inflammatory bowel diseases (IBD): Crohn's disease and ulcerative colitis.

Source: https://marley-storage.imgix.net/4b0d9083-03ba-4cea-a6d2-9b1268230ca9/IBD-crohnsvscolitis.png.

6.2.3. Gastroesophageal Reflux Disease (GERD)

Gastroesophageal Reflux Disease (GERD) is a chronic condition in which stomach contents are regurgitated into the esophagus, which causes a variety of unpleasant symptoms and potential complications. GERD's pathophysiology is largely based on a defect in the lower esophageal sphincter (LES), which plays a crucial role in preventing reflux. Such a weakened barrier not only allows acidic stomach contents to flow into the esophagus but also creates inflammation, esophagitis, and other complications, such as Barrett's esophagus, which predisposes one to esophageal cancer. Knowing these mechanisms is crucial, since GERD is prevalent in the general population, where its symptoms occur in an estimated 10–20% of adults on a routine basis. The consequences of GERD are greater than mere discomfort, since it can considerably reduce the quality of life and cause more complex gastrointestinal disease if left untreated. Therapy for GERD typically employs a multi-faceted approach, incorporating lifestyle modifications, pharmacologic management, and surgery when necessary. Lifestyle modifications, such as dietary alteration, weight loss, and avoidance of irritants like tobacco and alcohol, can abate symptoms in most patients. Pharmacologic therapy also primarily consists of proton pump inhibitors (PPIs), which effectively inhibit gastric acid secretion and promote healing of the esophageal mucosa. PPIs have proven to be very effective, while an issue with long-term therapy is the side effects that can impose more danger for some infections and malnutrition. Continued evaluation of GERD therapy-related risks and benefits is essential for clinicians to enable the most beneficial and safest treatment appropriate to each patient's condition. More research into the epidemiology and risk factors for GERD is ongoing, and evidence points towards lifestyle, genetic predisposition, and comorbidities having a significant input into the prevalence and severity of GERD. Studies have shown that there exists a strong correlation between obesity and increased GERD symptoms, most likely due to higher pressure in the abdomen that weakens the function of the LES. Demographic factors, age and gender, may also come into play here, for in elderly groups, GERD seems to be more prevalent. New studies highlight the significance of considering GERD not just as a separate disorder but in the totality of gastrointestinal well-being because its impact may overlap with many other gastrointestinal conditions. Identifying the overlap between GERD and other gastrointestinal conditions can enhance preventive care and inform comprehensive treatment plans, thus improving patient outcomes and well-being (Rawla et al., 2019; Beeson et al., 2020) (Figure 6.9).

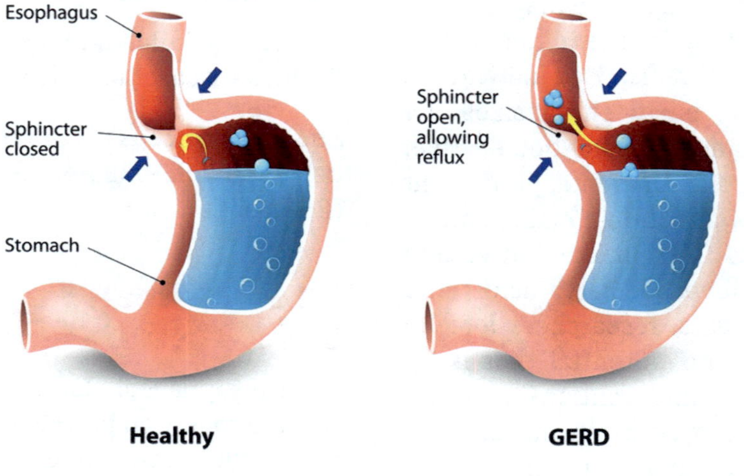

Figure 6.9. Gastroesophageal reflux disease (GERD).

Source: https://gastrohealth.com/-/media/news/patient-care-photos/gastroesophageal-reflux-disease-1024x676.ashx.

Test Your Knowledge

1. What are the inflammatory bowel diseases (IBD)?
2. What is gastroesophageal reflux disease (GERD)?

6.3. Causes and Risk Factors

Learning Outcome

1. Know the genetic predisposition to gastrointestinal disorders
2. Understand the environmental factors and lifestyle choices of study concerning gastrointestinal disorders
3. Describe the impact of diet on gastrointestinal health

A multifactorial pattern is prevalent in identifying the various causes and risk factors underlying gastrointestinal illness. One key factor is the incidence of infections, particularly from pathogens such as Helicobacter pylori. This bacterium leads to chronic gastritis and, consequently, severe types of peptic ulcers and even gastric cancer. The integrity of mucosal barriers is lost in *H. pylori* infections, which could lead to life-threatening complications in the event of no treatment. Failure of conventional therapies, which has been shown to occur in approximately 20% of the cases, underscores the importance of ongoing monitoring and adaptive therapies. Successful management is not only aimed at tackling the infection but also necessitates the clinician in providing moral encouragement and informing the patient about the possible complications of *H. pylori* infection, which emphasizes the effectiveness of integrative treatment approaches (Ciorbagiu et al., 2016). Psychological stress is yet another essential element influencing gastrointestinal disorders and is a determining factor in conditions such as irritable bowel syndrome (IBS). It has been established that various categories of stressors—psychological, physical, or immune—play an essential role in IBS pathophysiology, influencing symptoms and treatment effectiveness. Experimental models have been successful in demonstrating the manner in which stress amplifies visceral sensitivity, explaining the intricate interrelationship between the central nervous system and gut physiology. To develop effective treatments, an understanding of the mechanisms by which stress affects pain processing, such as peripheral and central sensitization, is necessary. Consequently, treating the psychological dimension of gastrointestinal disorders is as important as treating their physiological manifestations, and this is a consideration that holds water within holistic health care (Larauche et al., 2011).

The interplay between genetic predispositions and environmental exposures further complicates this scenario. An individual with a family history of gastrointestinal diseases is at greater risk of contracting the same, indicating a genetic reason. Diet, lifestyle habits, and socio-economic conditions are also responsible for susceptibility to causative factors in individuals for diseases such as Crohn's disease and ulcerative colitis. Low fiber consumption of processed foods, coupled with a lack of physical activity, has proven to exacerbate gastrointestinal ailments. The environment, through exposure to toxins or irritating chemicals, can also trigger inflammatory signals that lead to chronic gastrointestinal diseases. An appreciation of such multifactorial causes and risk factors is necessary to establish effective preventive interventions and tailored treatment plans in clinical practice (Figure 6.10).

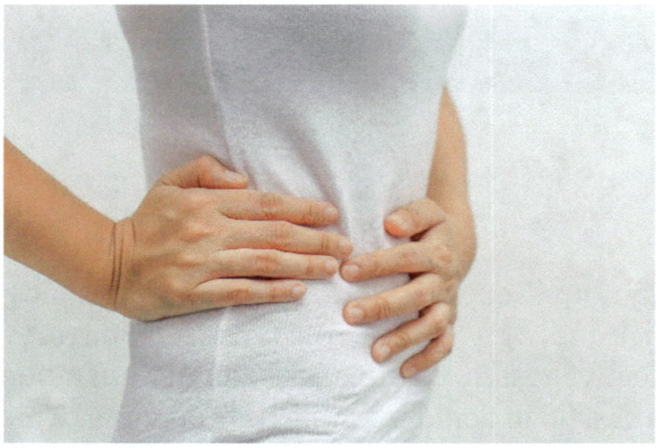

Figure 6.10. Common causes of gastrointestinal conditions.

Source: https://bgapc.com/wp-content/uploads/2021/02/image2.jpg.

6.3.1. Genetic Predisposition to Gastrointestinal Disorders

The genetic predisposition to gastrointestinal disorders highlights the intricate interplay between heredity and environment in their pathogenesis. A case in point is celiac disease (CeD), which occurs in genetically predisposed individuals upon exposure to gluten. Celiac disease is not only a localized condition within the gastrointestinal tract but also a systemic illness with multifactorial genetic factors. Specifically, individuals with a history of autoimmune diseases, such as Type 1 Diabetes (T1D), are predisposed to CeD because both diseases have a genetic component and immune system dysregulation. It is crucial to understand these connections for timely diagnosis and treatment, especially in high-risk patients, as misdiagnosis can lead to additional complications due to delayed treatment (Tharunika et al., 2025). The second significant aspect of genetic susceptibility is illustrated by colonic diverticulosis, a common condition in old individuals with pouches in the colon wall. Genetic and transcriptomic studies have identified specific genes involved in this condition, demonstrating a direct physiological correlation. The formation of diverticula was determined by scientists to be pivotal in the differential manifestation of various genes in diverticulosis. Specifically, genes such as ENTPD7 have been linked to the disease, suggesting potential causal relationships between genetic variants and diverticulosis severity. The genetic architecture not only enables understanding of the etiology of diverticulosis but also highlights the importance of genetic testing in assessing individual risk profiles for gastrointestinal conditions (Seo et al., 2024). The implications of genetic predispositions are not only important for diagnostic considerations but also for treatment and management approaches to gastrointestinal disease. Identifying individuals at higher genetic risk can be of great help for prevention and intervention. For example, patients with a genetic predisposition to conditions such as CeD should consider early dietary changes to avoid gluten, thereby preventing disease onset. Similarly, identification of genetic risk factors for diverticulosis can facilitate intensified colon health monitoring, thereby avoiding complications such as diverticulitis. Moreover, as the genetic mechanisms underlying these diseases are gradually elucidated by scientific inquiry, the way lies ahead with personalized medicine, in which therapy is tailored to individual genetic constitution. These advances offer the prospect of enhancing healthcare outcomes for patients with gastrointestinal diseases through more rational and targeted interventions.

6.3.2. Environmental Factors and Lifestyle Choices

The combination of environmental and lifestyle conditions also became a large field of research for human gastrointestinal diseases. Chronic stress, which is instigated by an individual's environment, has been increasingly recognized by researchers to significantly affect the body's physiological responses, including gastrointestinal conditions. Socioeconomic, work, and family stressors may initiate dysregulation of gut function and result in disorders such as irritable bowel syndrome (IBS) and inflammatory bowel disease (IBD). This correlation underscores the need for healthcare practitioners to adopt a holistic perspective that balances mind-body knowledge, recognizing that chronic stress has far-reaching effects on gut function and nutrition (Estrine et al., 2006). Thus, this integrated method is paramount to developing holistic treatment plans and prevention programs for high-risk groups. Besides, environmental influences, including diet and nutrient status, play a significant role in defining gastrointestinal health, particularly in the elderly. As people age, the aging GI tract undergoes several alterations that adversely affect digestion and nutrient uptake. These physiological alterations may increase the prevalence of malnutrition, significantly increasing the predisposition to GI diseases. Pay attention to the environmental factors, including accessibility of foods in the right quantity and socioeconomic status, becomes crucial while organizing the diet based on the requirements of older individuals (Bordoni et al., 2015).

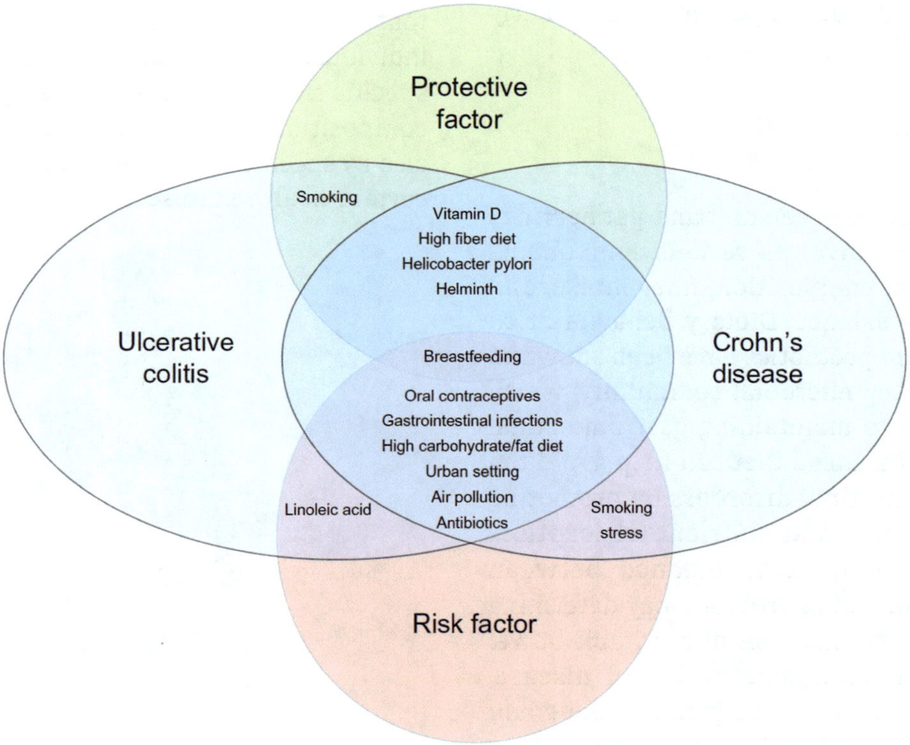

Figure 6.11. The relationship between environmental factors and the development of Crohn's disease and ulcerative colitis.

Source: https://www.researchgate.net/publication/255695171/figure/fig1/AS:203349019369472@1425493592031/The-relationship-between-environmental-factors-and-development-of-Crohns-disease-and.png.

By focusing interventions on the decline in functional ability of the gastrointestinal system among the elderly, health professionals can organize specific interventions that target not only disorders but also malnutrition and its outcomes. In conclusion, the interrelation between lifestyle, environmental issues, and gastrointestinal disorders is complex and multifaceted. Individuals' living environments and lifestyle choices dictate their overall well-being and the development of gastrointestinal ailments. Emphasis on education on stress management, dietary consumption, and access to healthcare plays a key role in reducing the prevalence of such conditions. Further, while addressing lifestyle factors such as exercise and diet, scientists and doctors can establish preventive practices that reduce the risk of gastrointestinal illness. This multifaceted model should incorporate interdisciplinary methods that consider psychological, social, and biological factors to optimize gastrointestinal health and promote more desirable lifestyle patterns across various populations, particularly among the susceptible (Figure 6.11).

6.3.3. Impact of Diet on Gastrointestinal Health

The relationship between diet and gut health is multifaceted and involves various components such as nutrient composition, fiber intake, and gut microbiota balance. Dietary behaviors rich in prebiotics and probiotics have been shown to support a healthy microbial community, which is fundamental to maintaining gastrointestinal health. A well-balanced diet can help avoid the risk of gastrointestinal disorders by promoting optimal digestion and nutrient absorption. Particularly, the delicate balance between dietary fiber and gut microbiota may determine the development of diseases like irritable bowel syndrome and inflammatory bowel disease, suggesting that intervention through diet could be a therapy. In addition, understanding how diet influences gut health is increasingly being suggested as a pertinent area of research, given the rising prevalence of gastrointestinal disorders and allied complications in modern society. Dietary fiber intake is one of the factors that plays a major role in ensuring gastrointestinal health by modulating gut microbiome and motility. Fiber, particularly prebiotic fibers, enhances the growth of beneficial microbes, and thereby improves the integrity of the intestinal barrier as well as keeps inflammation at a minimum. For people with disease states such as acute pancreatitis, fiber-rich diets have been reported to play a protective role, including reduced infection rates and improved recovery. Evidence exists that prebiotic-supplemented diet patients experience fewer gastrointestinal complications, which suggests the role of fiber in the dietary care of gastrointestinal illness. The association between fiber intake and pancreatic health is complicated, in that high levels can have adverse consequences, including impaired nutrient absorption. This is in support of the need for personalized dietary recommendations that control fiber intake while responding to individual health conditions, in line with patient-specific treatment. Furthermore, gut microbiota composition is influenced not only by diet, but also by specific dietary regimens associated with certain health statuses.

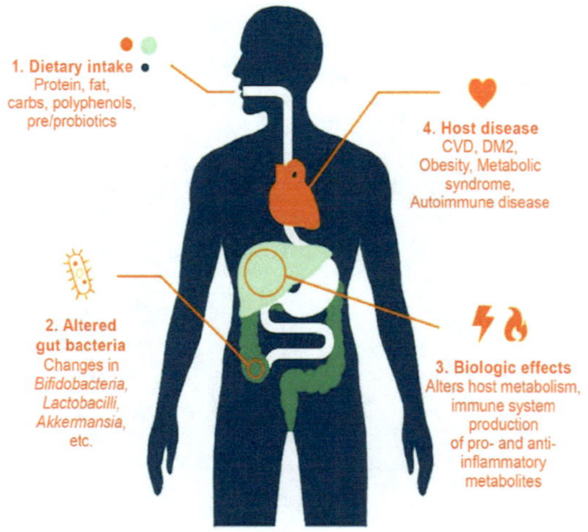

Figure 6.12. Impact of diet on the gut microbiome and human health.

Source: https://www.researchgate.net/publication/315978151/figure/fig1/AS:963516475383820@1606731637652/Impact-of-diet-on-the-gut-microbiome-and-human-health.gif.

Research has indicated that patients with specific gastrointestinal illnesses, such as autism spectrum disorders, possess characteristic differences in their gut microbiota compared to neurotypical individuals. This raises the question of how far diet can be harnessed to control the microbiome and, consequently, the associated clinical symptoms. Causality between dietary interventions and changes in the microbiome must be established by future studies, including large-scale longitudinal cohorts and citizen-science endeavors like the American Gut Project, if evidence-based dietary advice is to be made. This intricate interplay among diet, gut microbiota, and gastrointestinal disease suggests that dietary interventions may hold tremendous promise for the prevention and treatment of gastrointestinal disease, and further research to understand the role of each dietary constituent in shaping gut health is warranted (Figure 6.12).

Test Your Knowledge

1. What is celiac disease?
2. What is the impact of diet on gastrointestinal health?

6.4. Symptoms and Diagnosis

Learning Outcome

1. Describe the common symptoms associated with gastrointestinal disorders
2. Learn about diagnostic procedures and tests
3. Understand the importance of early diagnosis for treatment outcomes

Symptoms of gastrointestinal illness are diverse and can significantly affect a patient's quality of life. Abdominal pain, bloating, diarrhea, constipation, and changes in appetite are some of the common manifestations. They can result from a wide array of underlying pathologies varying from simple functional disorders like IBS to more severe pathologies like IBD or gastrointestinal cancers. Identification of the intangible character of these symptoms is critical to effective diagnosis. Indeed, the randomness of symptom presentation can make it challenging to identify the specific disorder affecting the patient. Thus, a comprehensive understanding of the symptomatology of various gastrointestinal illnesses is essential for clinicians seeking to provide precise and timely diagnoses, thereby improving patient outcomes. Diagnosis of gastrointestinal illness most commonly involves a combination of clinical examination, endoscopic examination, imaging, and laboratory tests. Traditional techniques, such as endoscopy, revolutionized the science by offering direct visualization of the gastrointestinal tract and enabling biopsies for diagnosis. As mentioned, recent decades have seen vast improvements in gastroenterology, especially through fiberoptic endoscopic methods, which have increased diagnostic yields for conditions such as colorectal cancer and chronic inflammation (Camilleri et al., 1999). These techniques, although crucial in the information they yield, are not without their faults. Availability of specialized centers where such procedures can be carried out has often proven to be the bottleneck in diagnosis, making it possible for many patients to have their symptoms remaining unsolved for extended periods. Given the complexity of gastrointestinal disease, advanced diagnostic technology is playing an increasingly important role. Technologies such as the electrogastrogram (EGG) offer promising noninvasive techniques for surveillance of electrical activity of the gastrointestinal tract, a key component to symptomatology. While promising, widespread application of EGG is limited by technical inconsistency and interpretive challenges. New technologies, such as multi-channel wearable devices that improve data collection and analysis, hold the promise of a future in which these noninvasive techniques could be applied to enhance diagnosis across a larger patient population. If these new techniques are integrated, clinicians can better diagnose abdominal symptoms, ultimately leading to timely and accurate diagnoses that result in tailored treatment programs for gastrointestinal disease (Coleman et al., 2018) (Figure 6.13).

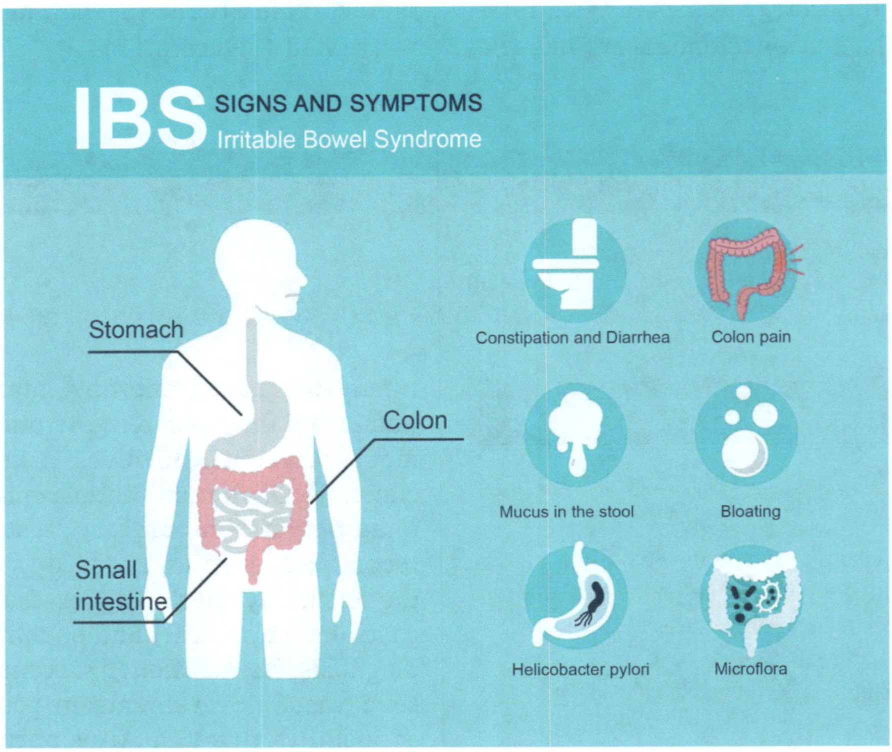

Figure 6.13. Sign and symptoms of irritable bowel syndrome.

Source: https://novagastro.org/wp-content/uploads/2023/02/iStock-965546890.jpg.

6.4.1. Common Symptoms Associated with Gastrointestinal Disorders

Gastrointestinal disease encompasses a wide range of conditions that affect the gastrointestinal system and cause a variety of unpleasant symptoms. Abdominal pain is complained of by most patients, and the frequency and severity of this pain vary from patient to patient. This pain is typically associated with irritable bowel syndrome (IBS), inflammatory bowel disease (IBD), and functional dyspepsia. Secondly, bloating is Please replace with CCBY 4also a common symptom, with a sense of fullness and abdominal distension. These symptoms are capable of having a significant impact on the quality of life of individuals, leading to both physical discomfort and psychological distress. The complexity of these gastrointestinal symptoms needs to be well understood to diagnose and treat them successfully, to the point that there is a need for further evolution in gastroenterological research and clinical practice (Camilleri et al., 1999). Another prevalent symptom of gastrointestinal disorders is disrupted bowel habits, which may manifest in the form of constipation, diarrhea, or alternating patterns between the two. Such changes in bowel movements may be indicative of several underlying disorders, like celiac disease, lactose intolerance, or more serious disorders like colorectal cancer. The necessity to pass one's bowels typically accompanies these changes, which only serve to exacerbate the issue that those who suffer from such disorders are facing. The social and individual implications of such symptoms can give a background of embarrassment and anxiety and add to the patient's condition. Thus, health practitioners have not only the responsibility of identifying the precise gastrointestinal disorder but also of addressing the concurrent psychosocial factors that complicate management and treatment (Debelius et al., 2015).

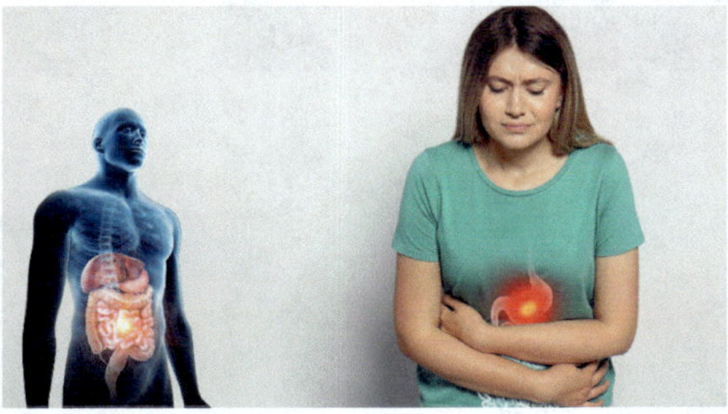

Figure 6.14. Symptoms of gastrointestinal disorders.

Source: https://ayurhridayam.com/wp-content/uploads/2024/11/Gastrointestinal-Diseases-Symptoms.png.

In addition to physical symptoms, gastrointestinal illnesses frequently cause systemic manifestations such as weight loss and fatigue. Fatigue could be due to nutrient malabsorption or chronic pain and discomfort, and could impact the quality of one's daily life and overall well-being. Weight loss, whether conscious or unconscious, could be a sign of some deeper pathology, and therefore vigorous medical evaluation is necessary. The co-occurrence of such symptoms underscores the need for a synthesis of evaluations that encompass the physiological and emotional health of patients with gastrointestinal diseases. By understanding the multicomponent nature of such ailments, medical professionals can tailor interventions that not only manage gastrointestinal symptoms but also enhance patients' overall quality of life (Camilleri et al., 1999) (Figure 6.14).

6.4.2. Diagnostic Procedures and Tests

Effective diagnosis of gastrointestinal illness depends largely on existing diagnostic techniques and tests that can help identify the proximate causes of symptoms in patients. Traditional methods, such as endoscopy and colonoscopy, allow for direct visualization of the GI tract and facilitate the collection of biopsy samples. These procedures have been instrumental in the identification of diseases such as inflammatory bowel disease and colorectal cancer. Notwithstanding this, the array of diagnostics is expanding, and new technologies are being introduced into the clinic to bypass some of the limitations of more established methods. For example, noninvasive techniques such as the electrogastrogram (EGG) are being evaluated for their potential to monitor gastric electrical activity, which might be useful for the analysis of functional disorders (Coleman et al., 2018). Thus, the evolution of diagnostic methods not only enhances precision but also expands access to appropriate treatment for patients with gastrointestinal illness. In parasitic disease, the diagnostic setting has specific challenges and possibilities. Soil-transmitted helminths, such as Ascaris lumbricoides, impose significant health burdens worldwide and require precise and effective diagnostic methods. Traditional methods such as the Kato-Katz thick smear are prevalent despite being less sensitive, primarily because of their simplicity and low cost. Improvements in microscopy technology, such as FLOTAC®, have increased sensitivity, hence the need for continued improvement in diagnostic techniques (Jourdan et al., 2015).

Furthermore, molecular diagnostics can also increase the sensitivity and specificity of detection but are often accompanied by higher operating expenses that limit their application to specific environments. As such, improving diagnostic procedures for STHs contributes not only to the individual case of a patient but also to the development of more comprehensive public health programs to control and eliminate infections. With regard to advances in diagnostic testing, the demand for noninvasive approaches cannot be overstated. Innovations such as wearable, multi-channel gastric activity monitoring systems using EGG have been developed to address the limitations of conventional diagnostic practices (Coleman et al., 2018). These new systems can continuously monitor gastrointestinal functions without invading the body, which improves patient comfort and compliance with monitoring protocols. By establishing a clearer conception of myoelectric dynamics and their correlation with meal response and circadian rhythms, such technologies would enhance diagnostic accuracy for functional gastrointestinal disorders. More sensitive diagnostic procedures in this context not only enable enhanced patient management but also contribute to a more comprehensive approach to appreciating the multifactorial character of gastrointestinal disorders in humans (Figure 6.15).

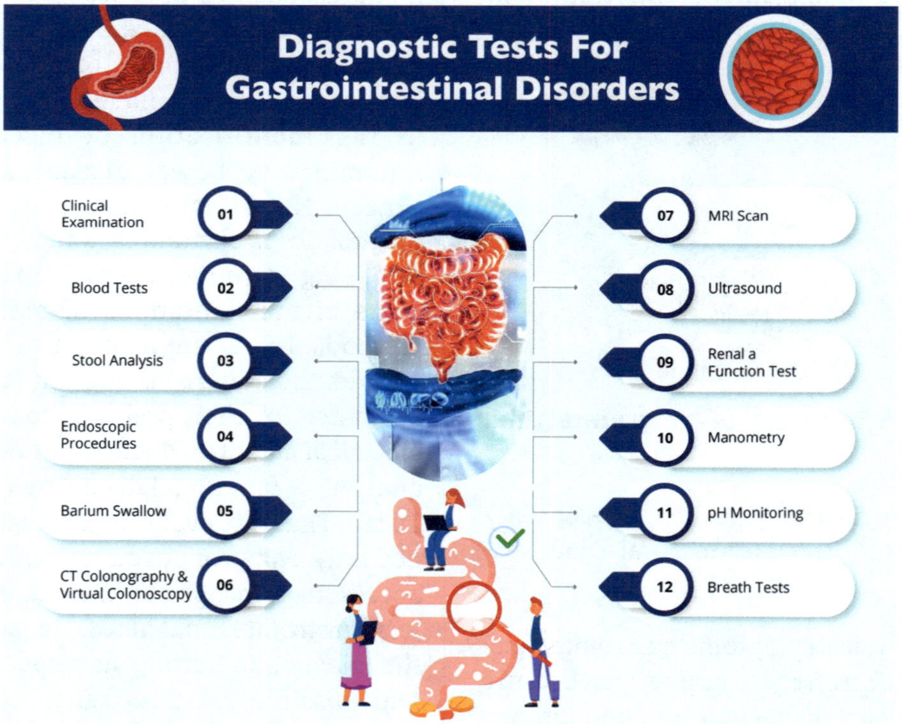

Figure 6.15. Diagnostic tests for gastrointestinal disorders.

Source: https://images.ctfassets.net/eexbcii1ci83/7ve6grc8ek4EYSrLoTDRJ/ddfb6e24f2332bbd1643b3417f549361/Diagnostic_Tests_For_Gastrointestinal_Disorders.jpg.

6.4.3. Importance of Early Diagnosis for Treatment Outcomes

Early detection of gastrointestinal disorders is important to maximize treatment outcomes, since the success of intervention usually decreases with increasing delay in diagnosis. Most gastrointestinal disorders, such as those caused by genetic defects such as 22q11.2 deletion syndrome, present with a wide range of signs and symptoms that may be misinterpreted or missed. The disorders can result in serious health consequences, which require treatment to involve multiple strategies involving medical, surgical, and psychological methods. In addition, identifying these disorders early allows for prompt management of comorbid conditions and thus for an enhanced prognosis. The ability to initiate specific treatment strategies soon after diagnosis can substantially contribute to improving the quality of life among patients afflicted with such varied gastrointestinal conditions, highlighting the paramount importance of early intervention in ensuring better health outcomes. Technical advances in diagnostic techniques also highlight the importance of early diagnosis of gastrointestinal illnesses. For instance, an imaging technique such as the electrogastrogram (EGG) has shown promise in monitoring gastric electrical activity to provide information about gastrointestinal tract muscle coordination. Use of new technology, like multi-channel wearable devices, also indicates the need for improved diagnostic devices to enable screening for GI disorders in larger populations. These advancements not only improve diagnostic accuracy but also enable more personalized treatment plans tailored to patients' individual needs. Bridging the gap between technology and clinical practice allows healthcare professionals to maximize early detection, ultimately resulting in improved therapeutic outcomes and a reduction of the burden of gastrointestinal disorders on patients and healthcare systems. Besides that, early detection is also crucial in reducing the economic costs associated with gastrointestinal illnesses. Delayed detection and treatment can result in longer healthcare expenses since patients may receive more invasive treatments, multiple hospitalizations, or even surgery due to complications from untreated illnesses. For example, patient management of patients with syndromes such as 22q11.2 deletion syndrome requires a team-based effort by various healthcare professionals due to the syndrome's widespread effects, including gastrointestinal issues. This complexity not only increases the sophistication in the treatment process but also contributes to increased healthcare spending. Accordingly, the implementation of universal screening and early intervention strategies not only positively affects patient health outcomes but also serves to reduce the costs of the overall healthcare system, and therefore, there are compelling reasons for putting high emphasis on early diagnosis in managing gastrointestinal diseases.

Test Your Knowledge

1. What are the most common symptoms of gastrointestinal disorders?
2. What is the importance of early diagnosis for treatment outcomes?

6.5. Treatment Options

Learning Outcome

1. Understand the role of dietary modifications and nutritional therapy in managing gastrointestinal disorders
2. Describe the pharmacological treatments and medications for gastrointestinal disorders
3. Know the surgical interventions for gastrointestinal disorders

Therapy for diseases of the gastrointestinal tract should be multifaceted, tailored to the condition and the patient's needs. Dietary adjustments are a significant area of therapy for diseases such as eosinophilic gastrointestinal diseases. These diseases are very responsive to the removal of food allergens, which can reduce symptoms and inflammation. However, excessive reliance on elimination diets has potentially adverse implications on quality of life, especially in the pediatric group, such that healthcare professionals are forced to seek alternative therapies. The absence of randomized prospective studies in the area underscores the need for more rigorous research to validate dietary interventions and examine possible alternatives that minimize the long-term risk posed by such therapies as corticosteroids, which are commonly used but have questions about their side effects (Gupta et al., 2018). In certain gastrointestinal diseases, particularly those associated with Helicobacter pylori infection, antibiotic use plays a leading role.

Effective treatment regimens usually include antibiotics and proton pump inhibitors to clear bacteria and facilitate mucosal healing. The hindrance posed by antibiotic resistance, however, prevents treatments from being effective, with approximately 20% of the cases not responding to treatment. Continuous follow-up of the patients, along with a good understanding of resistance patterns, is critical to obtain maximum therapeutic gains. Furthermore, therapists must provide moral support and make patients aware of the complication risk through uncontrolled Helicobacter pylori infection, such as peptic ulcers and gastric cancer, emphasizing the need for active patient participation in treatment success (Ciorbagiu et al., 2016). Apart from dietary changes and antibiotic treatment, a range of interventions are in the pipeline for the management of gastrointestinal diseases. New biologic therapies, particularly those targeting the specific inflammatory pathways, have promise in controlling chronic illnesses such as inflammatory bowel disease. Such therapies, however, need to be watched closely due to their complex mechanism and potential side effects. Further advances in pharmacological treatments, such as drugs that modulate the gut microbiota and enhance gut barrier function, pave the way for more personalized therapeutic strategies. At last, an integrated strategy that includes dietary management, drug therapy, and patient education is needed to manage gastrointestinal disorders effectively, improve patient outcomes, and maximize quality of life (Figure 6.16).

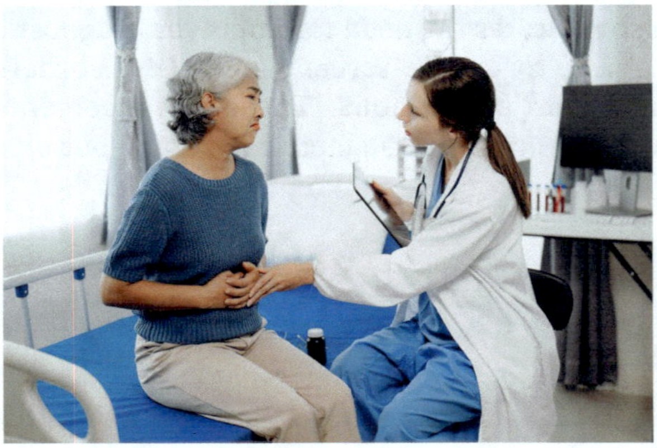

Figure 6.16. Most common GI disorders and their treatment.

Source: https://images.squarespace-cdn.com/content/v1/5acf6a542971141b99b9195a/2e6b937d-8741-4daa-9770-8885631ffd22/gi+doctors+in+okc.

6.5.1. Dietary Modifications and Nutritional Therapy

Dietary change is especially relevant to the management of gastrointestinal disease, particularly in terms of addressing the specific nutritional needs of a person with such a disease. In disorders such as irritable bowel syndrome (IBS), celiac disease, or inflammatory bowel disease (IBD), specific dietary changes can enhance symptoms as well as maximize overall gut function. Application of a low-FODMAP diet among patients with IBS, for example, has resulted in dramatic symptom control through the lowering of fermentable carbohydrates that irritate the intestines. Gluten-free diets are also important in celiac disease to prevent immune responses to gluten, thereby highlighting direct dietary interference with gastrointestinal health. By incrementally adding or removing food groups, patients can identify offending foods and tailor their nutrition to improve gastrointestinal function. Nutritional therapy is also gaining mainstream acceptance as a key component of the multidisciplinary approach to gastrointestinal disease. It is more than dietary advice; it is a holistic approach that addresses the biochemical and physiological aspects of gastrointestinal health. For example, the introduction of tailored nutritional regimens can provide the lacking nutrients in patients with malabsorption syndromes to ensure that deficiencies would not aggravate their condition. Moreover, nutritional therapy emphasizes dietary choices that support the health-enhancing gut microbiota, which are essential for maintaining microbial homeostasis and avoiding dysbiosis. The interaction of diet and microbiome suggests that some dietary changes will have a modulatory influence upon immune responses and inflammatory processes, which could offer new therapeutic management of immune-mediated gastrointestinal disease (Zheng et al., 2020). Alongside conventional dietary changes, examination of the gut-brain axis underscores the complexities of nutritional therapy in the treatment of gastrointestinal disease. Scientific studies have illuminated two-way communication between the gut microbiota and the central nervous system, proving that diet effects can extend far beyond digestive well-being to neurological function and mental health. The evolving linkage between the microbiota profile and psychological conditions highlights the importance of an equilibrated, diverse diet in promoting not only gastrointestinal health but also mental resilience and cognitive function (Cryan et al., 2019). Through the identification of such interactions, clinicians can design more holistic dietary regimens that incorporate physiological and psychological factors. This interdisciplinary model is significant because it acknowledges the intricate interplay among diet, microbiome, and overall health and sets the stage for the future direction of nutritional therapy in gastrointestinal care (Figure 6.17).

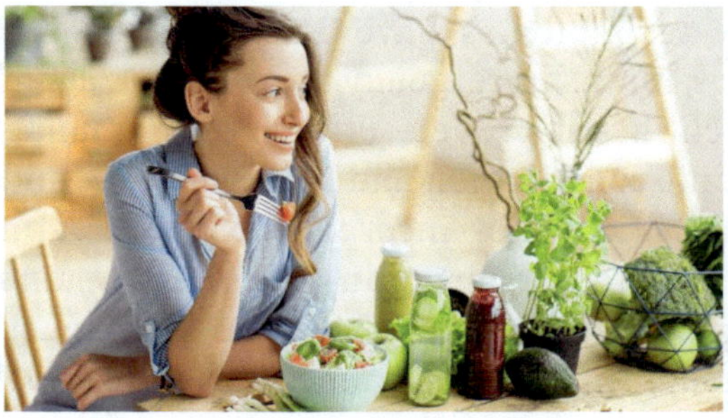

Figure 6.17. Diet changes to ease gastrointestinal issues.

Source: https://www.gastroconsa.com/wp-content/uploads/2021/04/Healthy-Diet-Changes-870x488.jpg.

6.5.2. Pharmacological Treatments and Medications

Pharmacotherapies for gastrointestinal illnesses are highly crucial for controlling diverse symptoms and etiopathologies. Proton pump inhibitors (PPIs) and H2 receptor antagonists are two of the most commonly used medications to prevent conditions such as gastroesophageal reflux disease (GERD) and peptic ulcers, both of which are characterized by hypersecretion of gastric acid. PPIs, for instance, have been shown to effectively suppress acid production, provide symptomatic relief, and enable healing of the esophageal mucosa. Additionally, antacids can produce relief from acidity discomfort instantly but only as a temporary measure. The complexity of gastrointestinal illness often necessitates the use of multi-drug pharmacological strategies to achieve optimal patient outcomes, ensure symptom control, and minimize the risk of adverse effects from long-term drug treatment (Declercq et al., 2018). Pharmacological therapy of acid-independent disorders, excluding acid-related disorders, is also being increasingly applied for functional gastrointestinal disorders such as irritable bowel syndrome (IBS). Drugs like loperamide are used to manage diarrhea, and antispasmodics can help in relieving abdominal cramping that comes with them. New technologies have also introduced new drugs, for instance, guanylate cyclase-C agonists, which have proved effective in managing chronic constipation and IBS with predominant constipation. Their incorporation into treatment regimes is a testament to a greater understanding of gastrointestinal motility and its impact on patients' quality of life. Moreover, psychological facets of gastrointestinal disorders must be given attention, as studies underpin the interface of psychological status and gastrointestinal well-being (Declercq et al., 2018). The influence of placebo effects in pharmaceutical treatment is increasingly becoming a significant research area, particularly in gastrointestinal disorders. Placebo responses can influence patient outcomes by enhancing the efficacy of active pharmacologic agents or even providing relief without the presence of drugs. The phenomenon is complex to drug approval processes, as it questions the efficacy of drugs per se against predicted effects. Understanding mechanisms behind placebo responses can facilitate the modulation of treatment approaches so that patients experience maximum benefits from their medications. Thus, by integrating research on placebo effects in the treatment of gastrointestinal disorders, potentially more effective treatment regimens and increased patient compliance may be made possible, with a resultant improvement in health outcomes. Future research must investigate how to maximize these effects and measure their impact on drug intake and patient perception (Figure 6.18).

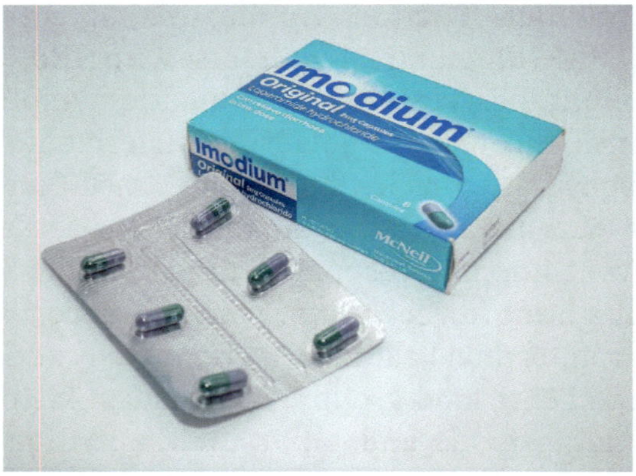

Figure 6.18. Loperamide, marketed as Imodium, is an antidiarrheal drug that works by slowing intestinal motility and thereby reducing the frequency of diarrhea.

Source: https://cdn.britannica.com/43/183143-050-42D3506D/Loperamide-Imodium-motility-frequency-diarrhea.jpg.

6.5.3. Surgical Interventions for Severe Cases

Surgical interventions are indicated for the management of gastrointestinal disease in extreme cases when non-surgical interventions are found to be unsatisfactory or inadequate to improve the condition. Complications such as severe inflammatory bowel disease (IBD), colorectal cancer, and complicated diverticulitis are generally managed using surgery to prevent further complications or manage disabling symptoms. For patients with acute pancreatitis, for example, treatment may include drainage or pancreatectomy if necrotizing complications arise. These are procedures that aim to restore the normal functioning of the gastrointestinal tract or remove affected tissues, significantly improving the patient's quality of life. For such a purpose, a multi-disciplinary approach that unites surgical expertise and gastroenterological management is extremely important for tailoring procedures to individual patient conditions and needs. In addition, the choice of proceeding with surgical interventions has to be complemented with a reasonable assessment of the severity of gastrointestinal diseases as well as the overall condition of health of the patients. Preoperative imaging examinations, such as MRI or CT scans, can provide useful information on the anatomy and pathology of the gastrointestinal tract. Besides, information about patients, such as age, comorbidities, and a history of surgery, must be evaluated to exclude potential postoperative complications. Surgical teams must balance all aspects of a patient's condition so as to ensure that the benefits of surgery outweigh the risks of the operation. This careful evaluation helps inform decisions consistent with best clinical practices to achieve maximum patient outcomes. After surgery, patients must be closely monitored and cared for in the long term to address any complications that can develop and support the healing process. Surgical interventions are apt to impact the management of gastrointestinal function in patients significantly and, as such, management of dietary lifestyles and nutritional supplementation. With resection surgery, such as for cancer of the colon and rectum, the risk of short bowel syndrome has to be managed to prevent malnutrition and ensure adequate absorption of nutrients. Moreover, the psychological implications of surgeries—especially in conditions such as surgical intervention for congenital disorders, including those that occur among patients suffering from 22q11.2 deletion syndrome that can present with gastrointestinal malformations—should not be ignored. As such, an integrated process with psychological rehabilitation services and support is imperative in the continuum of care following surgery to provide a smooth framework for recovery and promote long-term health outcomes (Figure 6.19).

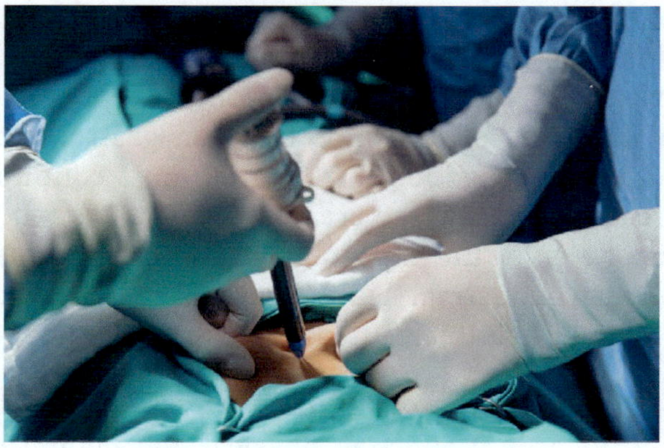

Figure 6.19. Best gastrointestinal (GI) surgery and treatment.

Source: https://regalhospital.com/wp-content/uploads/2022/03/Gastrointestinal-surgery.jpg.

Test Your Knowledge

1. What is the role of dietary modifications in managing gastrointestinal disorders?
2. What are the pharmacological treatments for gastrointestinal disorders?

SUMMARY

The quest for etiologies of gastrointestinal diseases in humans reflects a mix of factors, including genetic predisposition, environmental determinants, and lifestyle choices. These disorders are not individual pathologies but affect an individual's quality of life and serve as etiological factors in the development of other complications. For instance, the increasing prevalence of venous thromboembolism (VTE) in cystic fibrosis patients illustrates how some gastrointestinal presentations may be indicators of life-threatening outcomes. As such, complete clinical management is essential. Gastrointestinal health care is essential, especially given the rising incidence of such disorders in various populations, which necessitates preventive interventions and early treatment to avoid their effect (Trocchia et al., 2025). Moreover, the relationship between psychosocial factors and gastrointestinal disorders is increasingly being accepted in clinical research. The sequelae of postoperative Kinesio phobia, for example, may significantly augment gastrointestinal symptoms following lower limb surgery to produce augmented discomfort and complications. This relationship underscores the need to adopt an integrated treatment approach that addresses both the physiological and psychological aspects of gastrointestinal integrity (Gunes et al., 2025). Patient care practitioners can thereby augment patient recovery by accelerating the restoration of physiological integrity while reducing the incidence of secondary complications. In general, the treatment of gastrointestinal diseases requires a multidisciplinary approach that combines medical treatment, lifestyle modifications, and psychological support. As more evidence becomes available of the interrelationships between gastrointestinal function and general systemic consequences, future investigation in this area must continue to delineate these relationships if more effective treatments are to be created. Knowledge and education regarding gastrointestinal diseases are of most significant importance to both clinicians and patients. Ultimately, an overall understanding of gastrointestinal health can lead to better prevention measures and management strategies and facilitate healthier outcomes across various populations with these conditions.

There is a growing body of research indicating the intricate relationship between GI health and disorders affecting physical and mental health. The focus of this dialogue is the role of the gut microbiota in influencing brain function through mechanisms such as the gut-brain axis. Most notably, alterations in gut microbiota composition have been linked to cognitive impairment and psychiatric disease, suggesting the crucial involvement of these microorganisms in modulating neurotransmitter systems and neurotrophic factors, most notably Brain-Derived Neurotrophic Factor (BDNF). Abnormal signaling by BDNF, most often attributable to dysfunction in N-methyl-d-aspartate receptor (NMDAR), renders synaptic plasticity challenging and is implicated in the pathophysiology of schizophrenia. Clarifying these interactions can have the potential of new therapeutic strategies to treat not only gastrointestinal disease but also neuropsychiatric disease, identifying intestinal health as being dependent on cognitive functions as essential elements in the holistic vision of health care programs (Maqsood et al., 2016). Apart from neuropsychiatric factors, diet also plays a significant role in modulating inflammatory mechanisms in gastrointestinal disease. Dietary intake of dairy, for instance, has been formally studied in several clinical trials examining inflammatory markers in relation to dairy intake. Surprisingly, data suggest a discernible anti-inflammatory effect with dairy intake, particularly among individuals with metabolic disorders. These findings expand on what has previously been seen regarding nutrition's contribution to inflammatory status in the body. However, data stratification shows that, while low-fat and high-fat dairy products, especially fermented ones, exhibit protective effects, this is not a universal principle, as milk-allergic subjects may experience adverse effects. The complexity of dietary interactions calls for more serious investigation into the bioavailability of bioactive nutrients required to regulate GI tract inflammation (Bordoni et al., 2015). Lastly, the interplay between systemic inflammation and gastrointestinal health underscores the vital role of strategic dietary regimens in the treatment of gastrointestinal diseases. The research suggests that probiotics, prebiotics, and possibly certain aspects of diet may be therapeutic in alleviating behavioral deficits associated with gastrointestinal disorders. By ensuring a healthy gut microbiome, one can augment the production and activity of important neuroactive molecules, such as short-chain fatty acids (SCFAs), which are crucial for CNS homeostasis. This also promotes the use of an interdisciplinary approach integrating food and nutritional science with clinical modalities to formulate comprehensive treatment regimens. These integrative strategies have the potential to revolutionize not only the management of GI disease but also its systemic implications, paving the way for improved patient outcomes and public health (Bordoni et al., 2015; Maqsood et al., 2016).

KEY TERMS FROM THIS CHAPTER

- Carbohydrates
- Digestive tract
- Gastric acids
- Gastrointestinal disorders
- Inflammatory bowel diseases
- Metabolic health
- Oral cavity
- Crohn's disease
- Enzymes
- Gastroenterology
- Gastrointestinal system
- Irritable bowel syndrome
- Nutrient absorption
- Short-chain fatty acids

CRITICAL THINKING QUESTIONS

1. **Which of the following is the most common cause of peptic ulcer disease (PUD)?**
    a. Helicobacter pylori infection
    b. High-fiber diet
    c. Viral hepatitis
    d. Excessive water intake
2. **Which of the following is NOT a symptom of gastroesophageal reflux disease (GERD)?**
    a. Heartburn
    b. Regurgitation
    c. Difficulty swallowing (dysphagia)
    d. Chronic diarrhea
3. **What is the most common cause of acute pancreatitis?**
    a. Viral infection
    b. Gallstones and alcohol abuse
    c. Peptic ulcer disease
    d. Irritable bowel syndrome
4. **Which test is most commonly used to confirm the diagnosis of celiac disease?**
    a. Colonoscopy
    b. Small bowel biopsy
    c. Barium swallow test
    d. Abdominal ultrasound
5. **In Crohn's disease, which part of the gastrointestinal tract is most commonly affected?**
    a. Esophagus
    b. Stomach
    c. Terminal ileum and colon
    d. Rectum only

Short Answer Questions

1. What is a gastrointestinal disorder?
2. Why is gastrointestinal health important?
3. List the organs of the GI tract.
4. Name the three types of gastrointestinal disorders.
5. What is the treatment of gastrointestinal disorders?

Answer to Critical Thinking Questions

1. (a); 2. (d); 3. (b); 4. (b); 5. (c).

REFERENCES

1. Alaggio, R., Amador, C., Anagnostopoulos, I., Attygalle, A. D., Araújo, I., Berti, E., Bhagat, G., et al. (2022). The 5th edition of the World Health Organization classification of hematolymphoid tumors: Lymphoid neoplasms. *Leukemia*, *36*, 1720–1748. https://doi.org/10.1038/s41375-022-01620-2 (accessed on 12th July 2025).
2. Sigall-Boneh, R., Levine, A., Lomer, M., Wierdsma, N., Allan, P., Fiorino, G., Gatti, S., Jonkers, D., Kierkuś, J., Katsanos, K. H., Melgar, S., Yuksel, E. S., Whelan, K., Wine, E., & Gerasimidis, K. (2017). Research Gaps in diet and nutrition in inflammatory bowel disease. A topical review by D-ECCO Working Group [Dietitians of ECCO]. *Journal of Crohn S and Colitis*, *11*(12), 1407–1419. https://doi.org/10.1093/ecco-jcc/jjx109Arnelo, U., Haas, S. L., Löhr, J. M., et al. (2017). Pancreatic exocrine insufficiency after bariatric surgery. https://core.ac.uk/download/188827229.pdf (accessed on 12th July 2025).
3. Aytur, S., Bucci, J., & Wake, C. P. (2014). An assessment of the impact of climate change on human health in New Hampshire. https://core.ac.uk/download/84123597.pdf (accessed on 12th July 2025).
4. Baal, J. van, Dijcker, J. C., Hendriks, W. H., et al. (2011). Influence of nutrition on feline calcium oxalate urolithiasis with emphasis on endogenous oxalate synthesis. https://core.ac.uk/download/pdf/29235447.pdf (accessed on 12th July 2025).
5. Badiali, D., Bruno, G., Ribichini, E., et al. (2019). Role of fibre in nutritional management of pancreatic diseases. https://core.ac.uk/download/231748461.pdf (accessed on 12th July 2025).
6. Baker, J. S., & Grant, M. C. (2016). An overview of the effect of probiotics and exercise on mood and associated health conditions. https://core.ac.uk/download/141567244.pdf (accessed on 12th July 2025).
7. Balali-Mood, M., Naseri, K., Tahergorabi, Z., Khazdair, M. R., & Sadeghi, M. (2021). Toxic mechanisms of five heavy metals: Mercury, lead, chromium, cadmium, and arsenic. *Frontiers in Pharmacology*, *12*. https://doi.org/10.3389/fphar.2021.643972 (accessed on 12th July 2025).
8. Bassett, A. S., Emanuel, B. S., Marino, B., et al. (2015). 22q11.2 deletion syndrome. https://core.ac.uk/download/188828218.pdf (accessed on 12th July 2025).
9. Beeson, M. S., Ankel, F., Bhat, R., Broder, J., Paradise, S., Gorgas, D. L., Jones, J. S., et al. (2020). The 2019 model of the clinical practice of emergency medicine. *Journal of Emergency Medicine*, *59*, 96–120. https://doi.org/10.1016/j.jemermed.2020.03.018 (accessed on 12th July 2025).
10. Bordoni, A., Dansesi, F., Dardevet, D., et al. (2015). Dairy products and inflammation: A review of the clinical evidence. https://core.ac.uk/download/161844950.pdf (accessed on 12th July 2025).
11. Bordoni, A., Dupont, D., Gille, D., et al. (2015). Understanding the gastrointestinal tract of the elderly to develop dietary solutions that prevent malnutrition. https://core.ac.uk/download/286575279.pdf (accessed on 12th July 2025).
12. Calabrese, E., Dietrich, C. F., Dirks, K., et al. (2016). EFSUMB recommendations and guidelines for gastrointestinal ultrasound–Part 1: Examination techniques and normal findings (long version). https://core.ac.uk/download/74321241.pdf (accessed on 12th July 2025).

13. Camilleri, M. (1999). Functional bowel disease: A challenging frontier in gastroenterology. https://core.ac.uk/download/46601769.pdf (accessed on 12th July 2025).
14. Cicala, M., Guarino, M. P., Putignani, L., et al. (2016). Gastrointestinal neuromuscular apparatus: An underestimated target of gut microbiota. https://core.ac.uk/download/98336463.pdf (accessed on 12th July 2025).
15. Ciorbagiu, M. C., Mirea, C. S., Moraru, E., et al. (2016). *Helicobacter pylori*: Types of diseases, diagnosis, treatment, and causes of therapeutic failure. https://core.ac.uk/download/144552985.pdf (accessed on 12th July 2025).
16. Coleman, T. P., Gharibans, A. A., Kriegsfeld, L. J., et al. (2018). Artifact rejection methodology enables continuous, noninvasive measurement of gastric myoelectric activity in ambulatory subjects. https://core.ac.uk/download/323082131.pdf (accessed on 12th July 2025).
17. Cryan, J. F., O'Riordan, K. J., Cowan, C. S. M., Sandhu, K. V., Bastiaanssen, T. F. S., Boehme, M., Codagnone, M. G., et al. (2019). The microbiota-gut-brain axis. *Physiological Reviews*, *99*, 1877–2013. https://doi.org/10.1152/physrev.00018.2018 (accessed on 12th July 2025).
18. Debelius, J., Gilbert, J. A., Hornig, M., et al. (2015). Towards large-cohort comparative studies to define the factors influencing the gut microbial community structure of ASD patients. https://core.ac.uk/download/323065966.pdf (accessed on 12th July 2025).
19. Declercq, T., Lemey, L., Petrovic, M., et al. (2018). Late-life depression: Issues for the general practitioner. https://core.ac.uk/download/154408401.pdf (accessed on 12th July 2025).
20. Dong, Y., Li, H., Ilie, A., Gao, Y., Boucher, A., Zhang, X. C., Orlowski, J., et al. (2022). Structural basis of autoinhibition of the human NHE3-CHP1 complex. *Science Advances*, *8*. https://doi.org/10.1126/sciadv.abn3925 (accessed on 12th July 2025).
21. Estrine, J., & DeLisle, L. (2006). Stress: Putting the brain back into medicine. https://core.ac.uk/download/71356692.pdf (accessed on 12th July 2025).
22. Farkas, D. K., Galea, S., Gradus, J. L., et al. (2020). Associations between adjustment disorder and hospital-based infections in the Danish population. https://core.ac.uk/download/288432803.pdf (accessed on 12th July 2025).
23. Felice, A. G. (2003). Of mind over...matter. https://core.ac.uk/download/46601844.pdf (accessed on 12th July 2025).
24. Grabska-Kobyłecka, I., Szpakowski, P., Król, A., Książek-Winiarek, D., Kobyłecki, A., Głąbiński, A., & Nowak, D. (2023). Polyphenols and their impact on the prevention of neurodegenerative diseases and development. *Nutrients*, *15*, 3454. https://doi.org/10.3390/nu15153454 (accessed on 12th July 2025).
25. Gunes, H., Bulbuloglu, S., Sarıtaş, S., & Ozdemir, A. (2025). The effect of kinesiophobia on gastrointestinal disorders in patients with lower extremity orthopedic surgery. *Frontiers in Surgery*, *12*. https://www.semanticscholar.org/paper/fc921d1c816e0fd6310f4a8799aa461530991bbc (accessed on 12th July 2025).
26. Gupta, A. K., & Maity, C. (2021). Efficacy and safety of *Bacillus coagulans* LBSC in irritable bowel syndrome. *Medicine*, *100*, e23641. https://doi.org/10.1097/md.0000000000023641 (accessed on 12th July 2025).
27. Gupta, S. K., & Naramore, S. (2018). Nonesophageal eosinophilic gastrointestinal disorders: Clinical care and future directions. https://core.ac.uk/download/228066333.pdf (accessed on 12th July 2025).

28. Hills, R. D., Pontefract, B., Mishcon, H. R., Black, C. A., Sutton, S. C., & Theberge, C. R. (2019). Gut microbiome: Profound implications for diet and disease. *Nutrients*, *11*, 1613. https://doi.org/10.3390/nu11071613 (accessed on 12th July 2025).

29. Jourdan, P. M., & Lamberton, P. H. L. (2015). Human ascariasis: Diagnostics update. https://core.ac.uk/download/46559165.pdf (accessed on 12th July 2025).

30. Larauche, M., Mulak, A., & Taché, Y. (2011). Stress-related alterations of visceral sensation: Animal models for irritable bowel syndrome study. https://core.ac.uk/download/323080393.pdf (accessed on 12th July 2025).

31. Linson, E. A. (2013). The interplay between hormones and irritable bowel disease. https://open.bu.edu/bitstream/2144/12149/6/Linson_Elyse_2013_nosig_nocv.pdf (accessed on 12th July 2025).

32. Lopez, M. T., & Verstegen, M. W. A. (2011). A novel model to explain dietary factors affecting hypocalcemia in dairy cattle. https://core.ac.uk/download/pdf/29230002.pdf (accessed on 12th July 2025).

33. Malani, A. (2008). Regulation with placebo effects. https://core.ac.uk/download/62548544.pdf (accessed on 12th July 2025).

34. Maqsood, R., & Stone, T. W. (2016). The gut-brain axis, BDNF, NMDA, and CNS disorders. https://core.ac.uk/download/46558496.pdf (accessed on 12th July 2025).

35. Mueller, S., & Riedmueller, R. (2017). Ethical implications of the mild encephalitis hypothesis of schizophrenia. https://core.ac.uk/download/199422708.pdf (accessed on 12th July 2025).

36. Murray, C. J. L., Ikuta, K. S., Sharara, F., Swetschinski, L. R., Robles Aguilar, G., Gray, A. P., Han, C., et al. (2022). Global burden of bacterial antimicrobial resistance in 2019: A systematic analysis. *The Lancet*, *399*, 629–655. https://doi.org/10.1016/s0140-6736(21)02724-0 (accessed on 12th July 2025).

37. Rawla, P., & Barsouk, A. (2019). Epidemiology of gastric cancer: Global trends, risk factors, and prevention. *Gastroenterology Review*, *14*, 26–38. https://doi.org/10.5114/pg.2018.80001 (accessed on 12th July 2025).

38. Sarmidi, M. R. (2012). Food is our medicine. https://core.ac.uk/download/11801185.pdf (accessed on 12th July 2025).

39. Seo, J., Liu, H., Young, K. L., Zhang, X., Keku, T., Jones, C. D., North, K. E., et al. (2024). Genetic and transcriptomic landscape of colonic diverticulosis. *Gut*, *73*, 932–940. https://www.semanticscholar.org/paper/dd81342f2a768afe5bdb6b2ba3c857f09a87ab57 (accessed on 12th July 2025).

40. Tharunika, S., Mohan, V., Anjana, R., & Amutha, A. (2025). A narrative review of celiac disease in India with a focus on its link with type 1 diabetes. *Journal of Diabetology*. https://www.semanticscholar.org/paper/8d6a725b0c4d37b5d6d8f6c5f9c6adb7799e9e6c (accessed on 12th July 2025).

41. Trocchia, C., Ashour, D., Mosha, M., Hamner, B., Betensky, M., Goldenberg, N. A., & Khalaf, R. (2025). Venous thromboembolism occurrence and association with gastrointestinal disorders in children with cystic fibrosis: An analysis from the TriNetX Research Network global multicenter real-world dataset. *Seminars in Thrombosis and Hemostasis*. https://www.semanticscholar.org/paper/be79bdce39ad13b9bb8e1410d8856cf025ec1dd7 (accessed on 12th July 2025).

MUSCULOSKELETAL DISORDERS

7

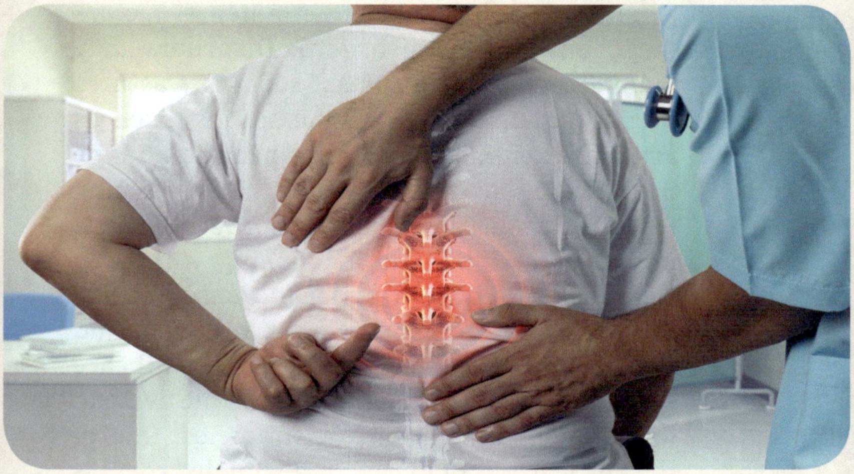

LEARNING OBJECTIVES

After studying this chapter, you will be able to:

1. Describe the types of musculoskeletal disorders
2. Learn about causes and risk factors associated with musculoskeletal disorders
3. Learn about symptoms and diagnosis of musculoskeletal disorders
4. Describe the treatment options of musculoskeletal disorders
5. Understand the impact of musculoskeletal disorders on quality of life
6. Know the prevention strategies for musculoskeletal disorders

Introduction

Musculoskeletal disorders (MSDs) constitute a broad spectrum of conditions affecting muscles, bones, tendons, and ligaments, with a considerable impact on individuals' health and well-being, as well as on the quality of their lives. They characteristically entail pain, inflammation, and functional impairment, resulting in interference with a person's normal functioning and potential to integrate into the labor force. Incidence of MSDs has been on the rise, driven by factors such as demographic dynamics, rising occupational hazards, and sedentary lifestyles. In this case, there is a need to understand several etiological factors responsible for the causation of MSDs, including their impact from ergonomics practices and work environment variation among individuals. For instance, typical manufacturing work practices often neglect human variability in favor of repeated musculoskeletal stress, which can lead to long-term injuries (Case et al., 2013). The effects of MSDs extend beyond the individual, as they pose serious economic challenges to healthcare systems and employers (Case et al., 2013). Treatment, rehabilitation, and lost productivity expenses are high, which calls for successful measures to minimize risks associated with MSDs. Ergonomic assessments and programs play a critical role in addressing such problems by enabling safer working practices and minimizing the inherent risks of specific tasks. For example, methods such as the Occupational Health Assessment Scale (OWAS) and Rapid Entire Body Assessment (REBA) have been used to identify and reduce ergonomic risks related to manual handling. By integrating such methods into work planning, organizations can establish healthier and more productive environments, thereby limiting the occurrence of musculoskeletal disorders (Case et al., 2013).

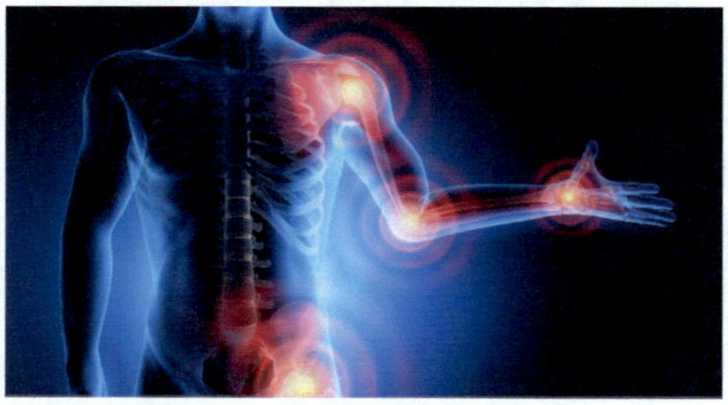

Figure 7.1. Musculoskeletal disorders.

Source: https://www.uhsussex.nhs.uk/wp-content/uploads/2023/08/musculoskeletal-disorders.jpg.

New MSD treatments are also in development, with significant interest in regenerative medicine and tissue engineering. Existing treatments pose some logistical and cost-related challenges, especially those derived from autologous cell culture. Recent advances in endogenous tissue engineering are, however, aimed at leveraging the body's own natural healing processes, which hold the key to transforming musculoskeletal disorder treatment. This paradigm is aimed at the need to develop methodologies that enable the regeneration of damaged tissue without the complexity inherent in *ex vivo* cell culture. As progress in this field continues, greater insight into prevention and treatment modalities will be essential to tackle the mounting burden of MSDs, creating a better society and enhancing quality of life overall (Figure 7.1).

Definition of Musculoskeletal Disorders

Musculoskeletal disorders represent a broad range of diseases affecting the musculoskeletal system's bones, muscles, ligaments, tendons, and nerves. A variety of factors, including age, genetics, lifestyle, and environmental factors may cause these disorders. Disorders may manifest as acute traumas, such as fractures or strains, or as chronic conditions, such as arthritis, tendinitis, and back pain. Italic type is not applied in this answer. The defining feature of musculoskeletal disorders is their impact on mobility and functioning, which can significantly reduce a patient's quality of life. Moreover, they are prevalent worldwide and become a significant burden for healthcare systems in terms of expenditure and the demand for long-term management strategies. One of the key features of musculoskeletal disorders is the complex interplay between structural and physiological factors that underlie dysfunction and pain. The majority of disorders are depicted by underlying pathophysiological processes that can lead to chronic pain disorders. For instance, conditions like chronic idiopathic neck pain are challenging to diagnose and treat due to the indeterminate relationship between structural problems and patient complaints. While imaging studies often reveal changes of aging within the musculoskeletal system, these findings are not always corroborative of the patient's sense of disability or pain, raising the possibility that other contributing elements, such as central sensitization, may be at play. Central sensitization, the augmentation of nervous system signaling in the central nervous system, can complicate the clinical presentation, making the definitions of these conditions not only complexcomplex but also highly related to subjective and objective findings (Bramer et al., 2015). New treatment and management techniques for musculoskeletal disorders are being pursued regularly, and tissue engineering techniques are at the forefront. These methods use a patient's own cells and aim to harness their regenerative potential, thereby circumventing limitations built into traditional ex vivo approaches to cell culture and transplantation. Although musculoskeletal conditions remain difficult to treat due to their complexity and heterogeneity in patient response, endogenous tissue engineering methods aim to promote natural regeneration without complications arising from the introduction of foreign tissue. This paradigm emphasizes the need to develop more targeted strategies to address the diverse manifestations of musculoskeletal disorders, which continue to pose significant challenges in both clinical and public health (Adam et al., 2012).

7.1. Types of Musculoskeletal Disorders

Learning Outcome

1. Define the osteoarthritis
2. Describe the rheumatoid arthritis
3. Understand the tendinitis

The classification of musculoskeletal disorders encompasses a broad range of conditions affecting bones, joints, and soft tissues and plays an important role in patients' quality of life. Among them, osteoarthritis is one of the most prevalent forms. Osteoarthritis, a degenerative joint disease, is characterized by cartilage degeneration, leading to pain, stiffness, and loss of mobility. While age is the primary predisposing factor, obesity and repetitive stress injuries also play significant roles in the development and evolution of such conditions. In contrast, inflammatory diseases, such as rheumatoid arthritis, are characterized by their autoimmune etiology, in which the body's immune response mistakenly targets the joint tissues for destruction, resulting in inflammation, pain, and ultimately deformities. Understanding these various types of musculoskeletal disorders is critical because it directs treatment methods that can best avoid pain and improve patient outcomes (Antal et al., 2008).

Soft tissue injuries are another significant type of musculoskeletal disorder, such as tendinitis, bursitis, and myofascial pain syndrome. Tendinitis occurs when tendons that connect muscles to bones swell, typically due to overuse or repetitive activity. This condition is commonly found in the shoulder, elbow, and knee, and severely limits physical function and activities of daily living. Bursitis, or inflammation of the bursae—the fluid-filled sacs that pad joints—can also create significant pain, particularly in areas surrounding the shoulder and hips. Myofascial pain syndrome results from trigger points in muscles that generate localized pain, which frequently presents as persistent, nagging pain and reduced movement.

Physiotherapy and ergonomic management can be particularly beneficial in treating these soft tissue injuries because they target the underlying pathology, enabling recovery and minimizing recurrence (Dul et al., 2025). Fractures constitute another prevalent type of musculoskeletal disorder, ranging from an extensive range of bone injury, from complete fractures to stress fractures. Fractures are caused by trauma, such as falls or accidents, but may also result from underlying conditions like osteoporosis, in which bones weaken and become more susceptible to fracture. Healing of fractures is usually achieved with immobilization in casts or braces, with surgical intervention at times. Rehabilitation following fractures is also crucial for functional recovery and the prevention of further injury. Effective fracture management requires a comprehensive understanding of bone health, including lifestyle factors such as diet and exercise, to maximize healing and skeletal integrity throughout an individual's lifetime (Antal et al., 2008) (Figure 7.2).

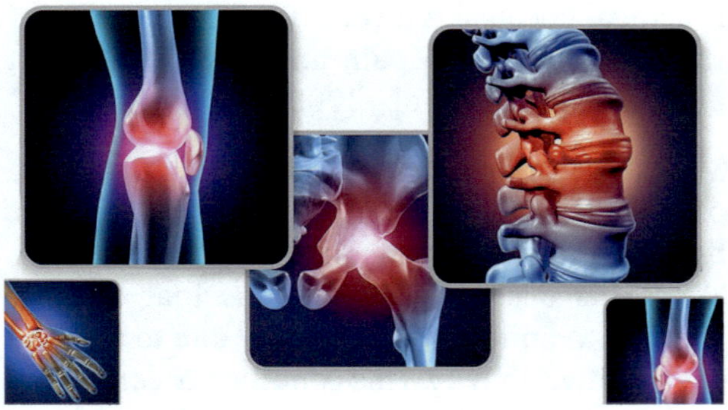

Figure 7.2. Types of musculoskeletal disorders.

Source: https://www.wearwell.com/media/magefan_blog/m/s/msd-header-image.jpg.

7.1.1. Osteoarthritis

Osteoarthritis (OA) is one of the most prevalent musculoskeletal conditions that affects adults, and the degeneration of the cartilage and the underlying bone is the main characteristic. As joints begin to deteriorate, OA results in cartilage degeneration, leading to pain, stiffness, and loss of mobility, ultimately compromising quality of life. It characteristically occurs in weight-bearing joints such as the hips, knees, and hands, where joint wear is greatest. The development of OA is determined by age, obesity, heredity, and previous joint trauma. Osteoarthritis is important not only for pain control and recovery of function but also for preventing additional joint breakdown, thereby reducing the disability and costs associated with it. Emerging work has explored novel therapeutic strategies intended to reverse the structural changes of osteoarthritis, with particular focus on intra-articular approaches. In this regard, studies on recombinant human BMP-7 (bone morphogenetic protein-7) have emerged as a promising area. Preclinical data indicate that BMP-7 exerts reparative effects on cartilage, which may result in symptom improvement of knee OA. A Phase 1 trial evaluated the tolerability and safety of intra-articular BMP-7 administration in symptomatic patients with knee OA. The outcome was mild side effects, with the most frequent being pain at the injection site, but no dose-limiting toxicity was observed, further urging further studies on the application of BMP-7 as a therapy.

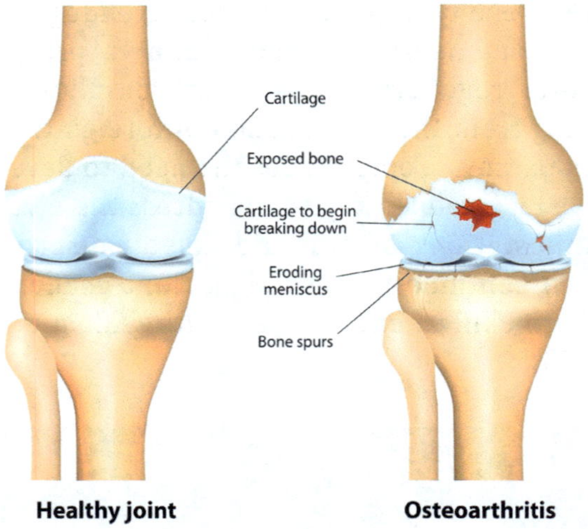

Figure 7.3. Osteoarthritis.

Source: https://novusspinecenter.com/wp-content/uploads/2019/02/osteoarthritis_1500x1386.jpg.

This emphasizes the need for ongoing research into disease-modifying treatments that target the underlying pathophysiology of OA, rather than merely symptomatic relief (Hunter et al., 2010). In addition to new treatments, understanding of the demographic and clinical profiles of at-risk groups to osteoarthritis is essential to successful intervention and management. For instance, some dog breeds, such as the German Shepherd Dog, have been studied to assess hereditary and breed-related susceptibility to musculoskeletal disease, including OA. Clinical data analysis through initiatives like the VetCompassTM Program enables exploration of clinical data gathered within practice, creating breed health information and informing breeding practice. This perspective is critical because it highlights the importance of the roles of both genetic predisposition and environmental influences on osteoarthritis pathology and emphasizes the multifaceted nature of the disease. Such studies can provide valuable information not only to veterinary medicine but also to the development of knowledge of OA in humans, as there are analogies in musculoskeletal anatomy and pathological processes that offer insights in both directions (Agresti et al., 2017) (Figure 7.3).

7.1.2. Rheumatoid Arthritis

Rheumatoid arthritis (RA) is a chronic systemic autoimmune disease characterized by inflammation targeting the joints and producing progressive disability and decreased quality of life in affected individuals. RA pathophysiology is an inappropriate immune response against synovial joints, causing synovitis and subsequent cartilage and bone loss. Destruction is usually accompanied by extra-articular manifestations, including fatigue, malaise, and even cardiovascular disease. The typical clinical picture in RA is symmetric polyarthritis, with morning stiffness and joint inflammation common presenting features. At more advanced phases of the disease, chronic inflammation compromises activity of daily living and functional autonomy, thereby necessitating ongoing rheumatological care and management. The impact of RA also extends beyond the physical condition, profoundly affecting mental health and overall quality of life. It has been found that RA patients report increased levels of depression and anxiety, which could be due to the disease's chronic pain and functional damage. Moreover, the complexity of RA management leads to greater evidence of a pain-disability cycle leading to undermined self-efficacy and, therefore, to worsening psychological distress. Evidence has shown that patients reporting lower self-efficacy present with more severe pain, describing an evident correlation between perceived control of the condition and pain severity. As a consequence, healthcare providers are increasingly being called upon to integrate an integrated method of patient care regarding RA, such as psychological support in addition to pain control in the therapeutic framework, in order to maximize health results as well as enhance quality of life in RA patients (Bandura et al., 2009). Foot complications are incredibly prevalent in RA patients, although these issues frequently go undersized in actual clinical practice. Research places in the spotlight that problems of the foot significantly contribute to disability in RA patients, and the necessity is greater for increased awareness and management of such issues in rheumatology care. While such problems are very common, specialist podiatry services remain inaccessible, especially in nations like New Zealand. Enhanced coordination between podiatric treatment and rheumatology services would yield a more integrated management regimen, addressing RA's multi-faceted problems. While healthcare systems attempt to improve the accessibility of services for chronic musculoskeletal diseases, it is imperative that the specific needs of RA patients, for example, foot care, be met to minimize pain and optimize functional capacity (Chapman et al., 2010) (Figure 7.4).

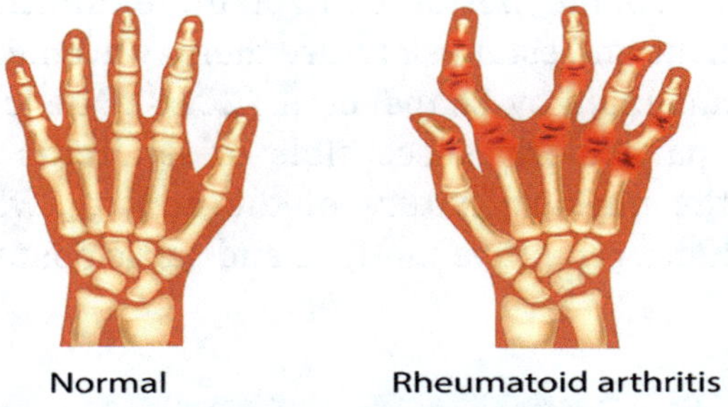

Figure 7.4. Rheumatoid arthritis (RA).

Source: https://www.birlahospital.com/wp-content/uploads/2024/03/Rheumatoid-Arthritis.webp.

7.1.3. Tendinitis

Tendinitis, or tenderness of a tendon, is an overuse musculoskeletal disorder seen in many groups, especially athletes and participants in repetitive activities. It most often happens through overuse, illustrating the mechanics of sports and daily activities. Tendons, which connect muscles to bones, are important for movement and stability. The etiology of tendinitis is characterized by pain, swelling, and stiffness in a specific location, which can significantly compromise one's quality of life and range of motion. It is crucial to be aware of the causative factors of this condition, such as poor technique and inadequate warm-ups, to prevent and treat it early. Ongoing studies have witnessed growing enthusiasm for the application of mesenchymal stromal cells (MSC) in treating tendinitis, particularly in veterinary medicine, which would find potential human therapeutic applications. MSCs injected into lesions have been shown to transiently increase inflammation but could also trigger long-term healing. Complexities explored in equine models provide valuable information on strategic approaches to translation for use in humans. Even though the initial inflammatory response is problematic, it also suggests that MSCs may influence tendon healing in a new way compared with traditional treatments. As we keep on exploring MSCs' influence, it may lead to revolutionary treatment approaches that provide better control of tendinitis in humans and establish future therapy avenues as documented by Chapel et al. (2018). Musicians are particularly susceptible to tendinitis due to the physical nature of the activity, which includes repetitive motions and static postures. The intricate movements involved in playing various instruments tend to put specific muscle groups under strain, leading to pain and discomfort primarily focused in the shoulders, wrists, and back. A study of music students and teachers found that a large percentage reported experiencing pain during or after play, reflecting the prevalence of tendinitis in this population. It highlights the importance of preventive interventions and good physical conditioning to mitigate such risks. As indicated by Bažon et al. (2016), preventive interventions and therapeutic treatments are key to maintaining the health and longevity of musicians, highlighting the importance of awareness and proactive management in minimizing the occurrence of tendinitis and overall performance (Figure 7.5).

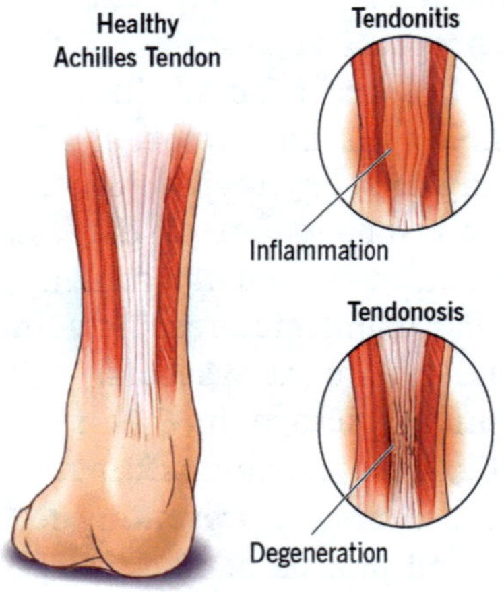

Figure 7.5. Tendinopathy is a painful condition that causes pain and swelling.

Source: https://my.clevelandclinic.org/-/scassets/Images/org/health/articles/22289-tendinopathy.

Test Your Knowledge

1. What is osteoarthritis?
2. What is rheumatoid arthritis?

7.2. Causes and Risk Factors

Learning Outcome

1. Understand the genetic predisposition
2. Describe the lifestyle factors
3. Know the occupational hazards

Musculoskeletal disorders (MSDs) result from a multifactorial interplay of several causes and risk factors with significant effects on individual health as well as workplace efficiency. An overarching factor leading to MSDs is repetitive motion, which is prevalent in sedentary employment, manufacturing, and assembly work. Overemphasis on productivity and work speed often leads to adverse ergonomic practices that can cause injury. For instance, while conventional manufacturing norms may not allow for variation, different workers react differently to repetitive work based on age, gender, and skill levels. Variability has the potential to enhance musculoskeletal loading, underscoring the need for ergonomic assessments that account for such variations (Agresti et al., 2017). These issues can be mitigated by redesigning the work environment and conducting individual assessments to minimize the risk of MSDs, thereby enhancing the overall well-being of workers. Environmental factors also play a central role in the causation of musculoskeletal diseases. Inadequate light, inadequate space, and improper workstations lead to improper posture and increased physical strain when performing tasks. Where working conditions fail to accommodate such ergonomic issues, workers are generally compelled to undertake abnormal postures, which over time lead to chronic pain and injury. Furthermore, organizational health and safety culture may influence the incidence of MSDs. Organizations that prioritize employee well-being through education and the availability of ergonomic gear will experience fewer musculoskeletal injuries. The data collected in projects like the VetCompassTM Program underscore the importance of accounting for demographic features and work environment, factors that can play a significant role in generating disorders in specific groups, such as the populations covered in the study on breeds like the German Shepherd Dog (Agresti et al., 2017). Psychological conditions, including stress and mental illness, are also among the risk factors for musculoskeletal disorders. Worth noting: stress can cause muscle tension and exacerbate underlying physical health, creating a cycle that leads to chronic pain. Furthermore, physical performance is also directly linked to mental health; workers with elevated levels of depression or anxiety are less likely to implement preventive health practices, such as good stretching or ergonomic adjustments.

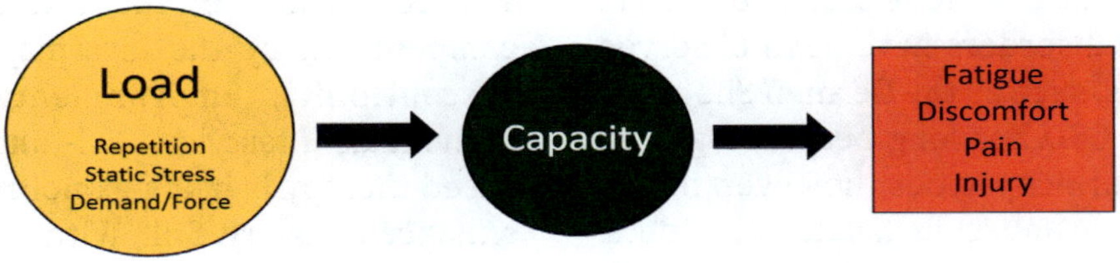

Figure 7.6. Causes of musculoskeletal disorders.

Source: https://rmi.colostate.edu/wp-content/uploads/sites/9/2021/07/ERGO_MSD-Causes-1536x471.png.

To solve this issue, organizations must adopt holistic approaches to their workers' health that encompass physical and psychological well-being. It not only helps prevent MSDs but also helps create a more robust workforce. Lastly, understanding these multifaceted causes and risk factors enables effective prevention strategies and interventions to reduce the prevalence of musculoskeletal disorders across diverse working populations (Case et al., 2013) (Figure 7.6).

7.2.1. Genetic Predisposition

Understanding genetic predisposition is crucial in the study of musculoskeletal disorders because certain genetic factors contribute significantly to determining how susceptible an individual is to such disorders. Genetic predisposition refers to the inherited tendency to develop particular illnesses, including most musculoskeletal diseases, such as osteoarthritis, rheumatoid arthritis, and hereditary connective tissue diseases. These genetic factors not only contribute to the structural integrity of musculoskeletal tissue but also to its repair. Research has shown that specific genes involved in cartilage metabolism and inflammation may alter a person's susceptibility to degenerative joint diseases. With the discovery of genetic markers for musculoskeletal disorders, clinicians can tailor prevention strategies to a patient's unique genetic profile, potentially reducing disease burden and improving musculoskeletal health overall. Implications of genetic predisposition in musculoskeletal disorders have been observed in animal models, such as the German Shepherd Dog (GSD). The GSD has long been recognized for its varied work capacities; however, health issues, specifically musculoskeletal disorders, have recently come into question. According to research within the VetCompassTM Program, demographic and clinical data for GSDs indicate an excess prevalence of musculoskeletal disease for this breed and point towards the influence of genetics upon their causation. Specifically, inherited traits such as joint configuration and cartilage resilience can especially impact the likelihood of diseases such as hip dysplasia or degenerative joint disease. These findings reinforce the necessity of knowledge-based breeding programs that incorporate genetic susceptibility to improve the overall health and longevity of at-risk breeds for musculoskeletal disorders (Agresti et al., 2017).

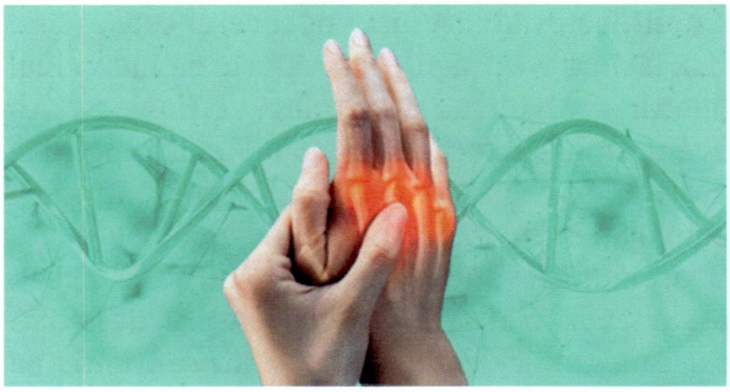

Figure 7.7. Understanding the role of genetics in rheumatoid arthritis.

Source: https://www.indushealthplus.com/front/media/article_img/rheumatoid-arthritis.jpg.

Furthermore, genetic susceptibility involves multiple risk factors, which presents challenges for the management and treatment of musculoskeletal disorders in sport and active populations. Tendinous and ligamentous injuries, often linked with intrinsic genetic etiology, result in extreme disability both in sports and in daily functional activities. The complexity of these injuries is further compounded by the interplay among genetic susceptibility, environmental factors, and individuals' lifestyles. Cell- and growth factor-based therapy is being explored as a therapy to enhance recovery. Still, with a risk for abuse in high-performance settings, and it creates ethical concerns regarding genetic enhancement for athletics. As has been demonstrated through surveillance by the International Olympic Committee, genetic insights into such injuries are essential for designing equitable standards in sporting performance while safeguarding the welfare and health of the persons involved in these sporting contexts (Bachl et al., 2008) (Figure 7.7).

7.2.2. Lifestyle Factors (e.g., Diet, Exercise)

The pathogenesis of lifestyle-related factors and musculoskeletal disorders is complex and multifactorial, and includes diet and exercise in prevention and management. A well-balanced diet, complemented with vital nutrients such as vitamin D and calcium, is important for maintaining bone mineral density and overall musculoskeletal health. In certain research studies, inadequate nutritional intake has been reported to impair bone mineralization, increasing susceptibility to fractures and other musculoskeletal issues. Thus, the individual who adheres to regular, health-related dietary patterns is at lower risk of disorders such as osteoporosis. With the integration of dietary and nutritional adjustments and specific exercise routines, individuals can maintain musculoskeletal health, immune to debilitating illnesses resulting from sedentary lifestyles and poor nutrition. In addition, exercise is also necessary to enhance musculoskeletal strength and flexibility. Daily aerobic and resistance training physical activity has been shown to increase muscular endurance, joint stability, and functional ability. When individuals make time for regular physical activity, they not only build up their musculoskeletal systems but also lower the risk of obesity-related disorders, which are linked to musculoskeletal disorders. To the elderly, this association holds even greater importance; while body weight declines with adopting an active lifestyle, so does the likelihood of acquiring musculoskeletal injuries related to weight-bearing. Surprisingly, research indicates that even among older persons, e.g., women aged 65-74 years, significant health benefits result from lifestyle modifications that include weight loss and exercise, supporting the relevance of movement in avoiding musculoskeletal challenges (Daniels et al., 2013). Lastly, lifestyle determinants of psychology also play a role in musculoskeletal health. Exercise has also been found to have its positive mental health impacts, such as lower anxiety and depression levels, which indirectly impact the experience and perception of pain due to musculoskeletal disease. Interestingly enough, it is relatively uniformly misconceived that musculoskeletal pain is caused only by physical injury; yet, acquaintance with the biopsychosocial model highlights the importance of psychological well-being in mitigating these conditions. If individuals perceive the body as weak or damaged, based on profound assumptions dictated by clinical diagnosis, they may form inappropriate habits, such as activity avoidance, which exacerbate their condition (Lewis et al., 2018). Therefore, creating a habit of consuming well-proportioned food and physical exercise with handling mental health disorders is imperative for effective prevention and treatment of musculoskeletal disorders (Figure 7.8).

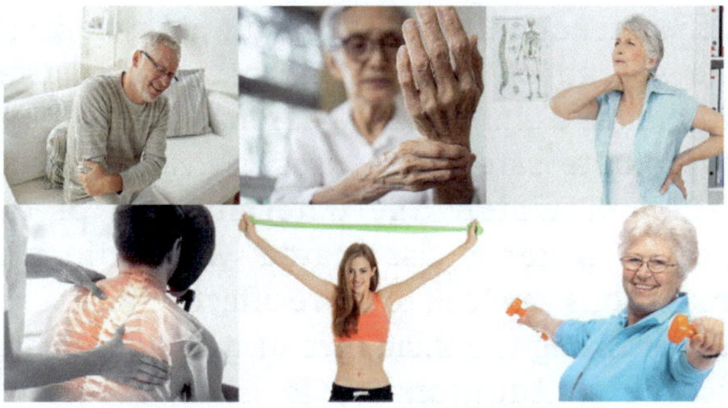

Figure 7.8. Exercise for musculoskeletal health.

Source: https://www.howdenmedicalcentre.nhs.uk/assets/img/Musculoskeletal%20portal%201200x650px.jpg?h=f77122ffa755e831e2e8da37cf28721c.

7.2.3. Occupational Hazards

When it comes to musculoskeletal disorders (MSDs), occupational risks play a significant part in becoming mindful of the connection between the work environment and health. Various professions expose workers to a range of risks, including repetitive strain injuries, awkward postures, and heavy lifting. Research indicates that these factors significantly contribute to the prevalence of MSDs, with impacts on individual workers and organizational effectiveness. Moreover, long-term occupational exposure to these agents has been linked with chronic pain and compromised quality of life, suggesting that prevention is critical. Improving these risks through workplace ergonomic practices and design interventions has the potential to minimize them, further supporting the need for an occupational health paradigm to safeguard worker welfare and enhance productivity (Kriebel et al., 2011). Occupational risk terrain is also compounded by the variety of workplace environments that carry inherent risks. For instance, healthcare professionals are often plagued with issues of patient handling, which lead to spinal injury and musculoskeletal pain. Similarly, manufacturing workers are exposed to prolonged repetitive activity that overworks joints and muscles, resulting in common MSDs such as tendonitis and carpal tunnel syndrome. The spread of these conditions necessitates individual training and awareness workshops to promote safe procedures (Srivastav et al., 2011). Ultimately, the determination of the specific hazards associated with different professions can lead to more effective measures in preventing the incidence of musculoskeletal disorders. Additionally, it is necessary to campaign for general policies addressing occupational health and safety measures. Both employers and regulators must collaborate to provide guidelines on ergonomic testing and safety measures. Experience indicates that even with sensitization, many industries fail to enforce proper preventive measures against occupational hazards. As studies emphasize, restricting exposure to risk factors not only reduces the prevalence of MSDs but also enhances the overall morale and productivity of the workforce. Ergonomic interventions, i.e., modified workstations and employee training in safe lifting techniques, can be highly effective in reducing the frequency of musculoskeletal disorders, underscoring the imperative need for an integrated approach to occupational health (Kriebel et al., 2011) (Figure 7.9).

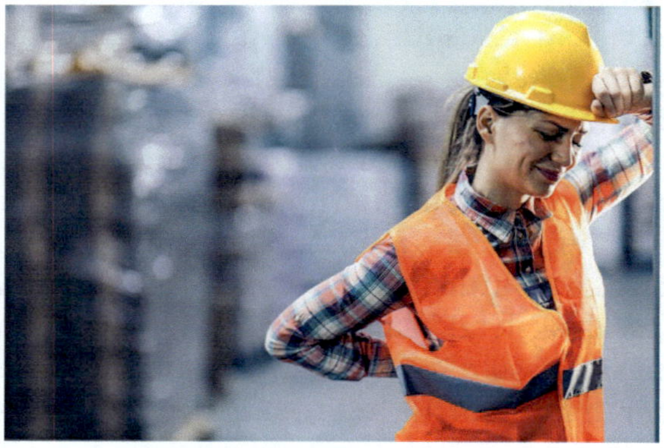

Figure 7.9. Work-related musculoskeletal disorders.

Source: https://humanfocus.co.uk/wp-content/uploads/how-to-prevent-musculoskeletal-disorders-in-the-workplace.jpg.

Test Your Knowledge

1. What disease is caused by genetic predisposition?
2. What are occupational hazards?

7.3. Symptoms and Diagnosis

Learning Outcome

1. Learn about common symptoms of musculoskeletal disorders
2. Know the diagnostic methods of musculoskeletal disorders
3. Understand the importance of early diagnosis in musculoskeletal disorders

Manifestation of the disease in musculoskeletal disorders varies, and it poses significant challenges to accurate diagnosis and treatment. Most frequently reported symptoms include persistent pain, stiffness, swelling, and functional impairment in involved locations. These kinds of symptoms may be precipitated by a range of underlying pathologies, such as osteoarthritis, rheumatoid arthritis, or fibromyalgia, each presenting unique features which medical professionals must scrupulously distinguish. Doctors typically rely on a broad-based assessment, for example, the patient's medical history, physical examination, and imaging studies, to illuminate the specific type of the disorder. Though technology in diagnosis has advanced, the inherent subjective nature of pain and distress can result in variability in diagnosis because what is incapacitating to one patient would be gauged differently by another, complicating clinical management. Diagnostic evaluation of musculoskeletal disorders generally involves a systematic approach, with initial assessments augmented by more sophisticated imaging technologies. X-rays, MRIs, and CT scans are invaluable in imaging the integrity of joints, bones, as well as the nearby soft tissue, allowing pathologies such as fractures or degeneration to be identified. Moreover, laboratory tests might play an important role in detecting inflammatory markers or specific pathogens that may be responsible for diseases such as rheumatoid arthritis or infections. Their interpretation, however, must always be made within the clinical presentation of the patient. Efficacy is often compromised by heterogeneity in musculoskeletal symptoms, highlighting the necessity for individualized evaluation strategies to account for differences in symptomology and disease courses, as outlined in previous studies on chronic pain disorders (Antal et al., 2008). Psychological factors may also contribute to the diagnostic complexity of musculoskeletal disorders beyond symptoms. Patients may also have associated emotional upset, depression, or anxiety, which themselves exacerbate the physical symptoms. The chronicity of pain in such illnesses as chronic low back pain is also linked with alterations in brain function and perception of pain that imply central psychological and neurologic involvement in understanding and managing pain. For instance, evidence has shown that chronic pain is linked to cortical reorganization that affects the efficacy of traditional therapeutic interventions, and accordingly, treatment models need to be remodeled (Barbanti et al., 2015). Therefore, an interdisciplinary treatment that combines psychological support and mainstream medical treatment could enhance prognosis in such complex conditions and eventually lead to improved patient satisfaction and quality of life.

7.3.1. Common Symptoms (e.g., Pain, Stiffness)

Musculoskeletal disorders (MSDs) are prevalent conditions that are primarily characterized by typical symptoms such as pain and stiffness. Musculoskeletal pain has numerous causes, including injury, inflammation, and degenerative joint and bone disease. For instance, osteoarthritis generally results in musculoskeletal pain that can significantly impair an individual's quality of life. The character of such pain can vary, ranging from dull ache to searing discomfort, depending upon the condition. Further, stiffness of these disorders can be particularly prominent on arising or after periods of rest, adding difficulty to activities of daily living. Because the degree of stiffness generally corresponds to the presence and severity of pain, familiarity with these symptomatology is significant for diagnosis and management of musculoskeletal disorders. A probe of post-major medical event pain incidence, e.g., post-stroke, demonstrates a more nuanced appreciation of symptom experience across populations.

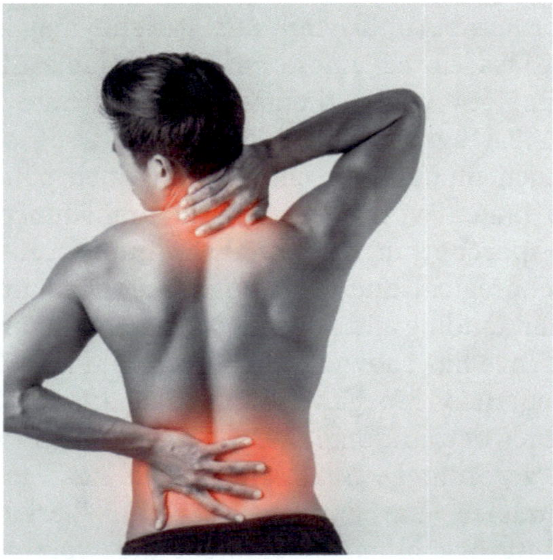

Figure 7.10. Musculoskeletal pain.

Source: https://www.southgatephysio.co.uk/wp-content/uploads/bfi_thumb/close-up-man-rubbing-his-painful-back-isolated-white-background-scaled-3itbohf8txyn27hmhgwdfu.jpg.

Research indicates that various types of post-stroke pain, e.g., musculoskeletal pain, express themselves differently at different stages of recovery. Specifically, studies have shown that the prevalence of pain is most significant at the subacute and chronic stages after a stroke, when patients mostly indicate excessive but uncontrolled levels of musculoskeletal and shoulder pain (Barbanti et al., 2015). This highlights the necessity for personalized approaches to pain management for pain-affected stroke survivors who might not respond to standard interventions. The potential for musculoskeletal pain to increase over time necessitates continued research into effective treatment modalities. In addition to stroke pain, osteoarthritis also illustrates the significant interplay of pain and stiffness as common manifestations of musculoskeletal disorders. Clinical trials on the effects of intra-articular BMP-7 are among those that have sought to treat these symptoms by way of potential therapy ((Hunter et al., 2010)). The observed increase in pain and perceived stiffness points to difficulty in symptom control in conditions affecting mobility and function. Notably, the progressive course of osteoarthritis, in which pain and stiffness increase with disease severity, requires ongoing searching for novel treatment approaches. The management of these common symptoms not only aims to provide relief but also to enhance the overall functional capacity and quality of life of patients with musculoskeletal disorders (Figure 7.10).

7.3.2. Diagnostic Methods (e.g., Imaging, Physical Exams)

Diagnosis of musculoskeletal disorders is multifaceted and highly reliant on physical examinations and advanced imaging modalities. Physical examination is usually the initial component of evaluating the status of a patient, allowing health practitioners to assess the range of motion, tenderness, and inflammation in regions of distress. Physical examinations can provide rich information about the nature of the disorder, distinguishing between inflammatory, degenerative, or traumatic origins. Furthermore, they allow for the identification of potential concomitant disorders. Although physical exams are necessarythey are not always guaranteed, particularly in the case of complex musculoskeletal disorders. Imaging methods, such as X-rays, MRI, and ultrasound, are then frequently employed to corroborate initial findings and provide a clearer image of internal anatomical structures. Imaging modalities are important for precise diagnosis of musculoskeletal diseases, as they enable clinicians to see inside organs without invading them. For example, X-rays are the initial imaging modality used to diagnose fractures, joint disease, and changes seen in arthritis. Magnetic resonance imaging (MRI), on the other hand, is better than the rest in viewing soft tissues such as tendons, ligaments, and cartilage and is therefore a godsend for diagnosing ligament strain and tendonitis.

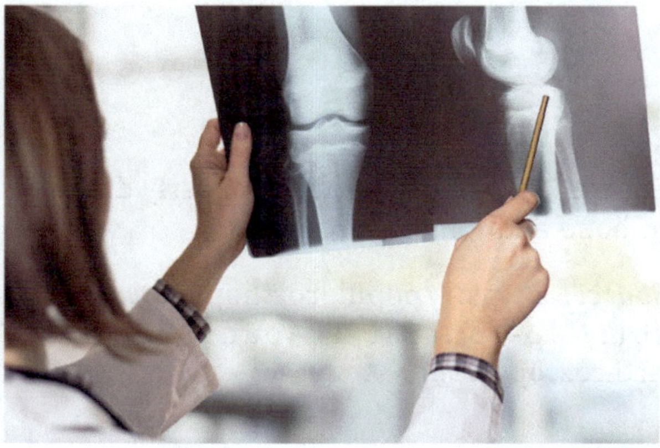

Figure 7.11. Imaging tests for musculoskeletal disorders and muscle damage.

Source: https://www.envrad.com/content/uploads/2021/04/muscologo.jpg.

However, excessive reliance on imaging at times leads to diagnostic errors due to the complexity of interpretation. Studies reveal that diagnostic accuracy varies from 85% in musculoskeletal conditions that are essentially diagnosed based on imaging alone, highlighting the need to incorporate clinical judgment and imaging diagnostics (Junior et al., 2009). In addition, the integration of imaging data with clinical observations significantly enhances diagnosis accuracy and treatment outcomes of musculoskeletal disorders. While advanced imaging provides critical information, doctors must remain alert to the potential for misdiagnosis arising from nonspecific findings or overinterpretation. For example, ultrasonography, while useful for assessing soft tissue injury, can yield false positives, leading to unnecessary procedures (Junior et al., 2009). Moreover, the clinician's ability to integrate imaging findings with physical examination data is paramount; adequate training and experience directly influence diagnostic precision. The acknowledgment that misdiagnosis can lead to ineffective treatment is a testament to the importance of ongoing training and standardized guidelines in musculoskeletal diagnostics. This multi-parameter diagnosis method ultimately aims to reduce error and improve the treatment of individuals suffering from musculoskeletal disease (Figure 7.11).

7.3.3. Importance of Early Diagnosis

The significance of early diagnosis in musculoskeletal disorders cannot be overstated, as it is a key predictor of long-term patient outcomes. Early identification of disorders, ranging from arthritis to injuries of the bone and soft tissues, enables early intervention. Early intervention not only lessens pain but also ensures functional mobility, which is necessary for maintaining the quality of life. Collectively, these factors underscore the importance of comprehensive screening protocols to identify musculoskeletal disorders at their onset. By utilizing early diagnosis as a priority, medical systems are able to largely reduce the burdens of chronic disease while ultimately improving patient prognosis as a whole, while saving healthcare expenses in the long run. Early diagnosis is consistently shown in research to be linked to better management of musculoskeletal disorders, thereby leading to more effective treatment. For instance, the VetCompass™ Programme has been used to identify common musculoskeletal conditions in specific dog breeds, providing valuable data for veterinary practices that can also be applied to human conditions. An understanding of the demographic and clinical presentation enables healthcare professionals to individualize treatment plans efficiently, providing patients with the most appropriate treatment for their diagnosis. This collaboration in the diagnosis and management of disorders meets the critical need for high-level educational efforts that alert practitioners and patients to the signs and symptoms of musculoskeletal disease, promoting an active response to health. Far more significant, however, are the long-term effects of delayed diagnosis, calling for early intervention strategies not only in veterinary medicine but also in human health. When musculoskeletal disorders are misdiagnosed or not diagnosed, patients tend to experience more severe worsening of their condition and disability or chronic pain-type outcomes. As explored in various healthcare settings, effective diagnosis pathways ensure rapid referrals and access to specialty care when required, which is especially imperative for managing conditions that may otherwise rapidly progress. By adopting an active approach to early diagnosis, medical professionals can engage with not only clinical efficacy but also patient education and self-management, ultimately leading to improved outcomes for patients with musculoskeletal disorders (Figure 7.12).

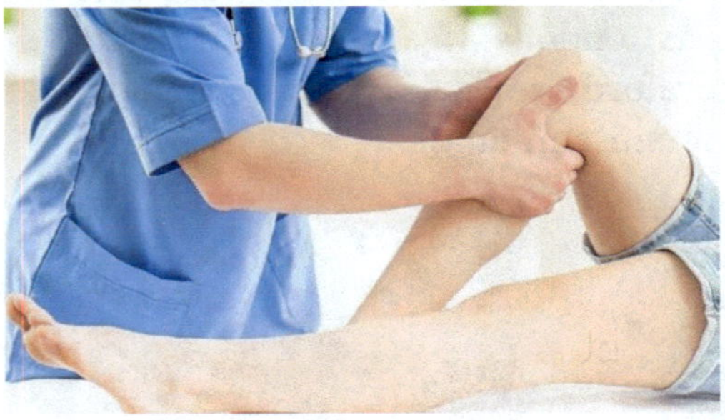

Figure 7.12. The importance of early diagnosis in bone and joint disorders.

Source: https://popularorthopaedichospital.com/wp-content/uploads/2024/12/Arthroscopy.webp.

Test Your Knowledge

1. What are the common symptoms of musculoskeletal disorders?
2. What are the diagnostic methods of musculoskeletal disorders?

7.4. Treatment Options

Learning Outcome

1. Understand the role of pharmacological treatments in managing musculoskeletal disorders
2. Describe the physical therapy and rehabilitation in the management of musculoskeletal disorders
3. Understand the role of surgical interventions in the management of musculoskeletal disorders

In musculoskeletal disorder treatment, choices vary widely depending on the disorder, its severity, and the patient's general health. Non-surgical treatments are most typically the first line of treatment, such as physical therapy, medications, and lifestyle modification. Physiotherapy is one method used to improve mobility, reduce pain, and regain function through specific exercise and modalities such as ultrasound or electrical stimulation. For instance, rotator cuff syndrome and bursitis can be successfully treated conservatively. : The efficacy of such a treatment was demonstrated in clinical trials comparing various interventions, e.g., injections of Traumeel and corticosteroids. The study indicates a paradigm shift toward combining less-invasive methods with existing treatment regimens, thereby expanding the range of options for patients in need of musculoskeletal pain relief (Bossche et al., 2015). When conservative management fails, more advanced interventions must be explored. In the case of those with acute pain from musculoskeletal conditions, medication therapies take center stage. NSAIDs, acetaminophen, and corticosteroids are commonly used to reduce pain and inflammation. If there is chronic pain or symptoms, injections such as corticosteroid injections into affected joints are effective in managing conditions like rotator cuff syndrome. Research emphasizes the necessity of counterbalancing such drug treatments with rehabilitative therapies in order to ensure complete treatment. Additionally, an understanding of the prevalence of pain types among specific populations, such as stroke patients, suggests the importance of individualized management strategies that consider new patient experiences and optimize functional outcomes (Barbanti et al., 2015). Surgical intervention is considered when conservative and pharmacologic options are unsuccessful in the relief of symptoms or when there is a structural compromise amenable to repair. Arthroscopy, joint replacement, and tendon reconstruction are now commonplace for severe musculoskeletal disease, giving patients a chance at true recovery and improved quality of life. However, opting to undergo surgical correction involves considering potential risks, benefits, and the general health condition of the patient. Medical practitioners must engage patients in discussions about their treatment course, educating them on the details of their situation and options available. Through an educated therapeutic relationship, patients are enabled to make informed treatment decisions that align with their health hopes and recovery expectations within the general framework of musculoskeletal disorder management (Bossche et al., 2015).

7.4.1. Pharmacological Treatments (e.g., Pain Relievers, Anti-Inflammatories)

Pharmacological treatment is critical for musculoskeletal disorders, particularly for pain relief and anti-inflammatory effects. Acetaminophen and NSAIDs are usually the first line of drugs when treating patients with musculoskeletal pain because they offer symptomatic relief with fewer side effects compared to aggressive medications. However, although these drugs are widely used, they may not always be effective enough in giving patients with chronic non-cancer pain adequate pain relief. As emphasized by studies, a majority of the patients end up using drug combinations to achieve an optimum amount of analgesia, which demonstrates a higher degree of complexity in managing pain for musculoskeletal conditions. Heterogeneity in patient response requires a personalized approach, with both pharmacological and non-pharmacological treatments in treatment plans (Carey et al., 2018). In the context of the complexities in drug therapy, opioids are an unpleasant option for severe musculoskeletal pain. Initially termed non-addictive, the sudden rise in opioid prescription since 1999 has caused a veritable epidemic of addiction and overdose in the United States. The misuse of these potent analgesics not only contributed to increased patient mortality but also put prescribing ethics in doubt. Since opioids are associated with disastrous consequences, doctors now have no alternative but to reexamine their pain drug prescribing methods, with more emphasis on assessing risks and educating patients on addiction risk. Finally, a supervised opioid regimen might be justified, but with caution and under the protection of other therapeutic interventions to counteract risk (Carey et al., 2018). Moreover, addiction to multi-modal pharmacotherapy for treatment necessitates the role of combined care in treating musculoskeletal disorders. As research shows, co-prescription of two or more drugs, like NSAIDs, antidepressants, and opioids, tends to exacerbate drug-related problems (MRPs). Patients often complain of a wide range of adverse effects, making it hard for them to perform optimally during daily activities. Further, even after receiving a mixture of different pharmacologic interventions, most patients remain with ongoing pain and functional disabilities. This raises questions about the suitability of existing therapeutic protocols and underscores the importance of health professionals increasing their capacity to manage MRPs and to create more efficient pain management programs. The ultimate effect is the streamlining of treatment procedures, so that not only do they eliminate pain but also contribute to overall well-being among individuals suffering from musculoskeletal disorders (Hoban et al., 2018) (Figure 7.13).

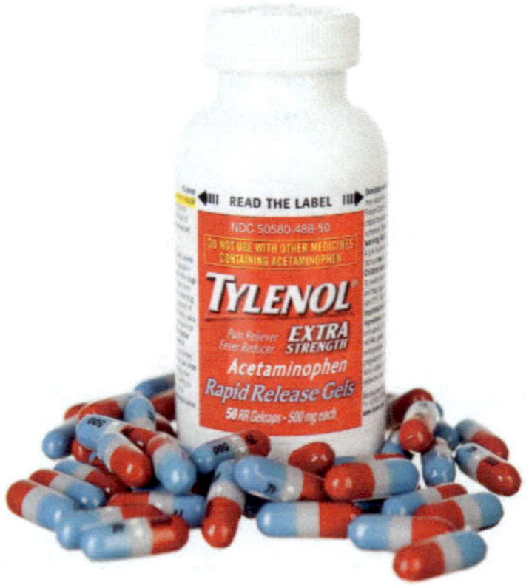

Figure 7.13. Acetaminophen.

Source: https://cdn.britannica.com/23/130223-050-99065995/acetaminophen-suppositories.jpg.

7.4.2. Physical Therapy and Rehabilitation

Physical rehabilitation and physical therapy are integral components of the management of musculoskeletal disorders, offering patients a way to regain function and reduce pain. The variety of therapeutic techniques—ranging from manual therapy, exercise prescription, and heat therapy—constitutes significant factors in providing recovery and protection from future damage. Furthermore, customized rehabilitation programs tailored to specific patient needs may prove to be of considerable help. Evidence also shows that such programs should not only provide for the physical restorative requirements but also the psychological requirements, since mental health can influence healing processes significantly. This approach enables healthcare professionals to devise comprehensive treatment plans that cover both the physical and emotional aspects of rehabilitation. The efficacy of physical therapy is also supported by recent expert consensus statements in the field, which highlight the value of multiple therapeutic modalities for treating musculoskeletal conditions. A case in point is the spa therapy, which has been the subject of much recent attention as a complementary therapy modality, with experts citing its capacity to treat multiple musculoskeletal pathologies (Bernetti et al., 2017).

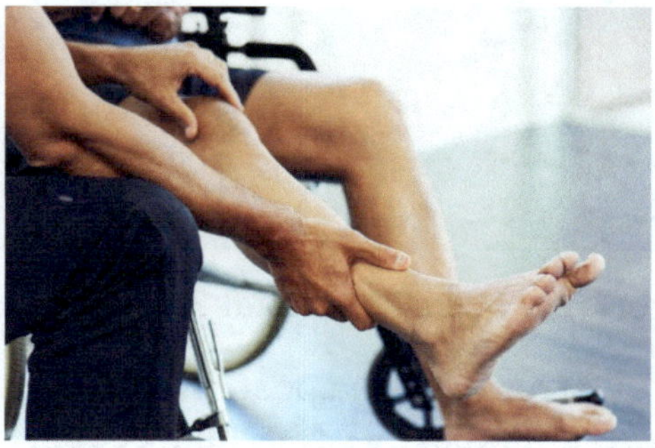

Figure 7.14. Musculoskeletal physiotherapy.

Source: https://aimst.edu.my/wp-content/uploads/2021/01/male-physiotherapist-assisting-a-senior-patient-in-recovery.jpg.

The positive outcomes of this kind of therapy demonstrate that integrating conventional and innovative methods can enhance the quality of patient care. Furthermore, consensus among clinicians regarding treatment indications and effectiveness can serve as a valuable guide for medical practitioners aiming to maximize rehabilitation options based on customized patient profiles. Adherence to prescribed exercise regimens is yet another decisive factor in the success of patients with musculoskeletal disorders in physical rehabilitation and physical therapy. Physical activity is necessary regularly to maintain mobility and prevent further musculoskeletal deterioration, but acquiring and sustaining compliance is difficult. Evidence from recent research has emphasized the need to develop measures to assess exercise adherence, ultimately guiding clinicians in developing patient compliance plans (Williams et al., 2014). Healthcare practitioners can achieve better rehabilitation outcomes by identifying appropriate measures and creating a supportive environment. Successful interventions are those that not only elicit patients to engage in the first place but also maintain commitment over the long term, thereby maximizing the impact of physical therapy on the treatment of musculoskeletal disorders (Figure 7.14).

7.4.3. Surgical Interventions

A major characteristic of the management of musculoskeletal disorders is surgical intervention, particularly when non-surgical methods are not improving symptoms or restoring function. Some commonly performed surgical procedures include arthroscopy, joint replacement, and osteotomy, each intended to address specific pathologies such as osteoarthritis, fractures, or tendon damage. The pressing need for effective surgical techniques is underscored by the significant burden upper limb disorders impose, contributing to excess work loss and impaired quality of life in affected individuals. As recognized in the latest studies, neither biomedical treatment nor ergonomic treatment alone optimizes results for these conditions, but instead a multimodal treatment plan incorporating surgical treatment as an adjunct to rehabilitation effort promises great hope for the best attainment of occupational status and enabling timeliness of return to work (Burton et al., 2008). Among the most important surgical interventions is hip hemiarthroplasty for patients with intracapsular femoral neck fractures. With mortality as high as 10-40% in the first year following surgery, it is important to address complications arising from the surgery. Surprisingly, surgical site infection (SSI) is one of the biggest causes of such a high rate of mortality, happening to roughly 4.68% of all those undergoing the surgery. Taking these figures into account, new treatment concepts, such as the use of high-dose antibiotic-impregnated cement, are being explored in clinical settings. This novel therapy should reduce the incidence of SSI and improve long-term outcomes, representing an important advancement in the operative treatment of hip fractures (Sprowson et al., 2013). Integration of surgical interventions into a comprehensive treatment program requires careful consideration of several variables, including patients' overall health, the severity of the condition, and psychosocial factors. A biopsychosocial approach, considering biological, psychological, and social variables, will be required to develop effective management systems, as research indicates. Successful interventions will need to engage all concerned parties—like healthcare workers, patients, and employers—who are significant to the recovery process. As indicated by the necessity of synchronized actions in surgical and non-surgical fields of management, a movement towards an integrated approach can substantially improve rehabilitation and occupational recovery for patients with musculoskeletal disorders (Burton et al., 2008) (Figure 7.15).

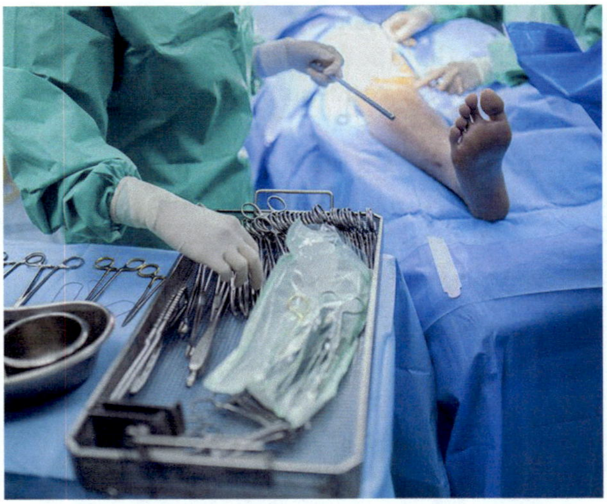

Figure 7.15. Musculoskeletal Surgeries.

Source: https://media.post.rvohealth.io/wp-content/uploads/2023/09/unrecognizable-doctors-surgeon-surgical-equipment-operating-operation-room-732x549-thumbnail-732x549.jpg.

Test Your Knowledge

1. What medication is used for musculoskeletal disorders?
2. Why is physical therapy and rehabilitation necessary?

7.5. Impact on Quality of Life

Learning Outcome

1. Understand the physical limitations and disability
2. Describe the psychological effects of musculoskeletal disorders
3. Address the economic burden of musculoskeletal disorders on individuals and healthcare systems

Musculoskeletal disorders (MSDs) significantly affect an individual's quality of life, influencing multiple aspects of functioning and psychological well-being. Physical limitations resulting from conditions such as arthritis, osteoporosis, and back pain can hinder mobility, reducing the ability to perform activities of daily living and attend social gatherings. Consequently, an individual may become withdrawn as the inability to function correctly in their environment may contribute to lowered social contact. Furthermore, chronic pain from these disorders tends to induce sleep disruptions and fatigue, further contributing to the undesired effect on emotional well-being. Reduced physical activity is also associated with a high probability of weight gain and associated health effects, further building on the initial musculoskeletal pathology. It is therefore imperative to appreciate the multidimensional impact of MSDs in order to implement effective interventions that seek to address both physical and psychological factors affecting quality of life. The connection between musculoskeletal disorders and overall quality of life extends beyond physical challenges. Psychological impact remains a significant concern, as chronic conditions can cause such problems as depression and anxiety. Individuals suffering from MSDs may struggle with coming to terms with their sense of self and purpose, particularly if their conditions limit previously enjoyed activities. Managing the chronic pain and functional disability to engender a chain of negative feelings, which deters the victims from seeking social support or evaluating treatment options. This loneliness leads to deterioration of their mental state, ultimately impacting their resilience and ability to deal with their conditions. Therefore, mental health support is required for managing musculoskeletal disorders and to allow individuals to regain control over their lives as well as improve their quality of life by implementing coping strategies for managing physical as well as emotional problems. The impact of musculoskeletal disorders can extend to other areas of quality of life, including sexual function and gastrointestinal function. Research indicates that as a person ages, there can be an increase in sexual dysfunction and incontinence, two issues that are associated with changes in musculoskeletal well-being. The resulting decline in sex can be detrimental to sex lives, causing the development of feelings of inadequacy and reduced self-esteem. In addition, gastrointestinal problems such as chronic constipation and fecal impaction are also prevalent among older individuals, which further adds to the health scenario in individuals with musculoskeletal disorders (Black et al., 2013; Colyer et al., 2013). These issues together reflect the need for a holistic approach to the treatment and care of individuals with musculoskeletal disorders, which not only addresses the physical symptoms of musculoskeletal disorders but also the emotional, social, and gastrointestinal well-being of the individual. By considering these many steps, medical practitioners can improve the quality of life for MSD patients (Figure 7.16).

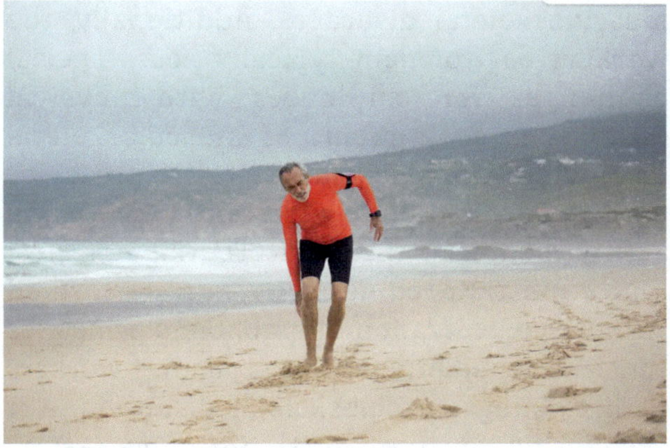

Figure 7.16. Impact of musculoskeletal pain on quality of life.

Source: https://cdn.prod.website-files.com/66bd9da1417f66a31d1d0a79/66dd6587930b82790d1c606e_pexels-kampus-production-8638045.webp.

7.5.1. Physical Limitations and Disability

Physical impairments that result from musculoskeletal disorders take a remarkable toll on individuals' functioning, social lives, and overall health. Chronic low back pain is a perfect example of how physical impairment can truncate mobility and functioning and develop in a cycle of inactivity and deteriorating physical health. The majority of patients with such disorders are also unable to adhere to conventional rehabilitation therapies, possibly due to a lack of understanding or a lack of motivation. Empirical findings show that improved communication between patients and healthcare practitioners can increase treatment adherence, leading to better outcomes. Physiotherapist autonomy-supportive communication has been shown to heighten patients' intrinsic motivation, thereby resulting in long-term adherence to prescribed exercise and physical activity, as concluded in a recent study (Black et al., 2012). This highlights the central role of not just medical treatment, but also good interpersonal communication in adapting to the physical limitations of musculoskeletal disorders. Additionally, the working environment typically poses special challenges for employees with physical disabilities as a result of musculoskeletal disorders. Traditional manufacturing processes barely accommodate diversity in human ability, hence further exacerbating physical limitations. Repeated activities performed without consideration of ergonomic principles can lead to additional injury among workers with existing musculoskeletal disorders. Not accounting for individual differences—e.g., gender, age, and anthropometry—can seriously hinder work performance and increase the risk of injury (Case et al., 2013). Therefore, it is critical to address these ergonomic problems by examining work processes to promote an inclusive, safer work environment for people with physical disabilities. By adopting risk assessment methods sensitive to human variation, organizations can establish work designs that lower exposure to risk and decrease musculoskeletal disorder incidence. Finally, the overlap of physical limitation and disability brings to focus more universal societal implications of musculoskeletal disorders. Not only do they affect the individual, but also healthcare systems and the labor market, with high costs. Individuals with long-term musculoskeletal conditions can be limited in their work and economically and socially disadvantaged. This process needs a collaborative approach among healthcare professionals, employers, and policymakers to create accommodative facilities for individuals with disabilities. Granting access to appropriate rehabilitation services and adaptive workspaces can reduce the impact of physical impairments. In total, constructing an inclusive society through rehabilitation can enable people with musculoskeletal disorders to be more active and empowered, thereby enhancing the quality of their lives and enabling participation in various aspects of work and community life.

7.5.2. Psychological Effects (e.g., Depression, Anxiety)

The interface between musculoskeletal disorders (MSDs) and psychological symptoms such as depression and anxiety is a complex landscape that needs to be thoroughly examined. MSDs, which encompass many different conditions affecting the muscles, joints, and bones, often lead to chronic pain that can significantly affect a person's quality of life. Individuals with conditions like chronic low back pain also usually experience co-occurring psychological distress, the result being a cycle in which physical pain acts to amplify emotional pain. Current research indicates that this co-relationship is not coincidental but that the chronic pain associated with MSDs can result in neurobiological changes that render individuals susceptible to mood disorders. Thus, it is crucial to understand this dynamic to properly design comprehensive treatment plans that address both the physical and mental components of these disorders. Furthermore, the role exercise plays in alleviating the psychological effects of MSDs cannot be overlooked. Frequent exercise is extensively proven to have a positive impact on the condition of mental health, serving as a potential antidote to depression and anxiety related to chronic pain. Physical training has been shown to enhance mood and may even reverse neurobiological changes observed in chronic MSDs. This underscores the necessity of physical rehabilitation as an integral part of treatment protocols for patients with these diseases. Research assesses the impact of exercise on health not only for improving body function but also for its therapeutic benefits for mood disorders, and it is suggested that the addition of physical activity to treatment regimens will enhance psychological function and address the physical disability of patients (Baker et al., 2016). Additionally, the efficacy of current treatments for MSDs has been challenged, in particular, their effectiveness psychologically. Even though chronic non-specific low back pain is common and numerous therapeutic approaches have been developed, patients gain minimal relief with continuing feelings of hopelessness and frustration. The sub-grouping paradigm widely used in clinical settings may constrain effective treatment protocols because it fails to account for common psychological aspects of such disorders. Thus, both clinicians and researchers share an immediate need to re-evaluate treatment strategies, taking into account the psychological implications of chronic physical conditions. Understanding the cognitive and affective barriers created by chronic pain can lead to more effective interventions into both the somatic and psychological domains of MSDs (Antal et al., 2008) (Figure 7.17).

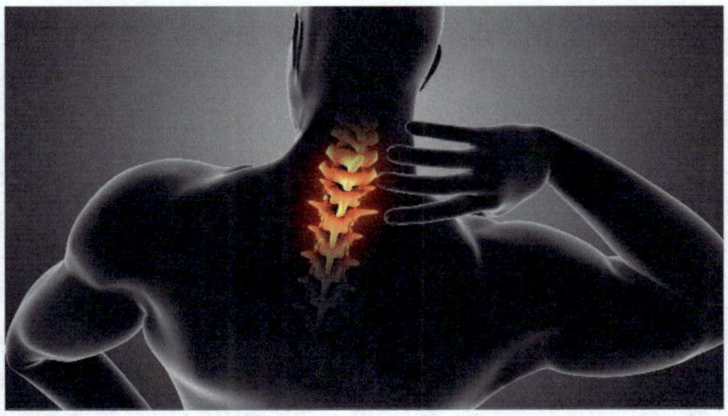

Figure 7.17. The psychological impact of chronic pain.

Source: https://nkjinstitute.com/wp-content/uploads/2024/09/psychological-effects-of-chronic-pain.jpg.

7.5.3. Economic Burden on Individuals and Healthcare Systems

The economic burden of disabilities and chronic pain due to MSDs is staggering and creates a cycle of economic strain to both patients and society. Disability and chronic pain due to MSDs result in lower productivity, higher healthcare costs, and more usage of social services. In fact, individuals suffering from these conditions tend to accrue lost income and diminished quality of life that can exacerbate underlying financial vulnerabilities. This becomes worse by a healthcare system that could potentially neglect the provision of special needs treatment to MSD patients, resulting in limited options for treatment and escalating medical costs in the long run. While these conditions become increasingly prevalent, their financial impacts on patients and the health care system become more pronounced, yet again validating the need for enhanced policy responses and better resource planning at healthcare centers. In addition to financial impacts at the personal level, the health care system in general has a considerable economic impact based on the prevalence of musculoskeletal disorders. The costs of diagnosis, treatments, and rehabilitation for MSDs can strain health budgets, diverting resources from other vital services. Hospitals and clinics face greater operational strain as they struggle to cope with the increased number of patients requiring assistance for these conditions. In addition, the burden is passed on to insurance companies, which could face higher claims for musculoskeletal treatment. This process can lead to higher premiums for employers and patients alike, and to a cycle of economic loss affecting numerous stakeholders. Efforts aimed at maximizing healthcare provision, such as the utilization of evidence-based practice and the application of full-care protocols, are key to eluding these economic consequences and ensuring sustainable healthcare provision (Burton et al., 2016). Lastly, addressing the economic burden of musculoskeletal disorders should be done through a multi-disciplinary approach that recognizes the intertwined complexities among patient experience, healthcare practice, and policy. Evidence suggests that integrating prevention approaches, such as workplace interventions and early access to care, can result in significant long-term cost reductions for MSDs. Further, specific programs aimed at diminishing disparities in access to and treatment outcomes by gender can assist in alleviating some of the economic load that women endure, as they have dissimilar obstructions to coexisting with males compared to women. By prioritizing research into the differences and promoting gender-sensitive health policy, it is not only possible to enhance individual health outcomes but also to reduce the overall economic burden on individuals and on health systems. With investment and a commitment to integrated care, society can facilitate a more equitable and effective response to the challenge of managing musculoskeletal disorders and their cost (Burton et al., 2016).

Test Your Knowledge

1. What are the physical limitations?
2. What are the psychological effects of musculoskeletal disorders?

7.6. Prevention Strategies

Learning Outcome

1. Understand the importance of regular exercise
2. Understand the importance of nutrition in maintaining musculoskeletal health
3. Describe the ergonomic practices in daily activities

Prevention of musculoskeletal disorders (MSDs) is crucial for reducing injury and enhancing workplace safety. Due to the etiologic complexity of the disorders, multiple actions can be taken to minimize exposure to risk factors. Ergonomic interventions are a fundamental part of these measures because they involve modifying the work environment to suit workers' capabilities. This approach includes task redesign, workstation fitting, and posture care in work. For instance, the use of adaptable equipment and tools that minimize strain can significantly reduce the prevalence of MSDs across various workplaces. As evidenced by recent findings, anticipatory actions promote workers' health and productivity and consequently foster a more sustainable workplace centered on the preservation of worker well-being (Kriebel et al., 2011). The benefits of a successful ergonomically designed intervention go beyond injury prevention to enable an organizational safety culture. Physical well-being and wellness programs also play a key role in MSD prevention. Wellness programs are likely to include activities to promote physical fitness, strengthening, and flexibility training relevant to reducing the risk of musculoskeletal trauma. Such intervention is especially justified in high-risk populations, especially those with reduced muscle mass or other disease-related conditions. For instance, as outlined in recent research, exercise interventions have been shown to reduce treatment-related side effects in patients with cancer, underscoring the importance of maintaining physical strength and functioning (Fairman et al., 2018). Promoting regular exercise and education on good body mechanics can help individuals be more self-motivated toward their well-being, ultimately resulting in a decreased incidence of MSD. These preventive steps emphasize the need for an integrative paradigm in health care encompassing exercise, education, and environmental change. Also, employer-driven initiatives can ensure an all-around approach towards preventing musculoskeletal disorders. They must be trained in safe lifting techniques and the importance of taking frequent breaks to avoid sustained strain. Such training courses can encourage greater sensitivity among workers to their own physical capability and foster an active health emphasis. Moreover, frequent ergonomic evaluations in the workplace can help detect potential hazards and resolve them before they become a problem. As noted in the convergence of findings from recent studies, such preventive practices not only help reduce the economic burden of MSDs on organizations but also enhance overall employee satisfaction and job retention (Kriebel et al., 2011). By prioritizing such preventive measures, employers and workers can collaborate to achieve better health outcomes and maintain a healthy, unimpaired work environment (Figure 7.18).

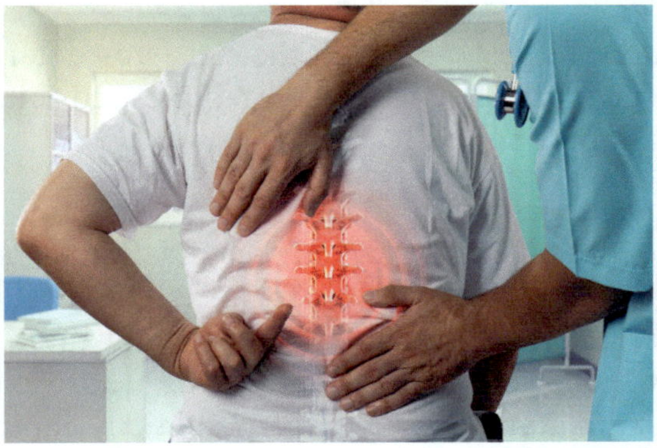

Figure 7.18. Prevention of musculoskeletal disorders.

Source: https://carrierchronicles.com/wp-content/uploads/2023/04/GettyImages-1050434764.jpg.

7.6.1. Importance of Regular Exercise

The significance of regular physical activity cannot be overstated, particularly in the context of musculoskeletal disorders, which place a significant burden on public and individual health. Regular physical activity is an essential determinant of muscle strength, flexibility, and joint stability, all of which are significant factors in preventing musculoskeletal injury and disorder. Furthermore, exercise is a vital mechanism for improving total physical function and quality of life. Studies have shown that adherence to a routine exercise program can alleviate pain and stiffness in conditions such as arthritis, thereby enhancing mobility and activities of daily living. Regular exercise integrated into daily activity can prevent the onset of chronic musculoskeletal disorders, ultimately contributing to a healthier, more active lifestyle. In addition to physical benefits, regular exercise is a prime element of mental well-being, which indirectly could influence musculoskeletal well-being. The physical exercise correlates with improved mood and reduced levels of depression and anxiety. The mental well-being element is crucial in patients who have chronic pain or musculoskeletal conditions because emotional stress could exacerbate pain perception and limit the extent of physical activity. There is a self-perpetuating cycle generally; increased psychological health promotes mental functioning in exercise, adding to psychological health. Therefore, the development of a culture that encourages regular exercise not only enhances physical health but also addresses mental illnesses, thus resulting in a cyclical process of managing musculoskeletal disorders. Recommendations for pain management in patients with musculoskeletal disorders also enhance the application of exercise as an adjuvant non-pharmacological treatment. For instance, the CDC provides detailed recommendations on using exercises to effectively treat various types of pain and encourages their use alongside traditional medical treatments (Dowell et al., 2022). Similarly, during the COVID-19 pandemic, rehabilitation practices emphasized the need to stay active, detailing its role in ensuring lung function, muscle mass, and overall physical health while in quarantine (Zhao et al., 2020). Thus, the inclusion of regular exercise as a part of an overall treatment regimen can not merely dislodge acute presentations of musculoskeletal disorders but enhance long-term health, promoting an active rather than passive approach to health (Figure 7.19).

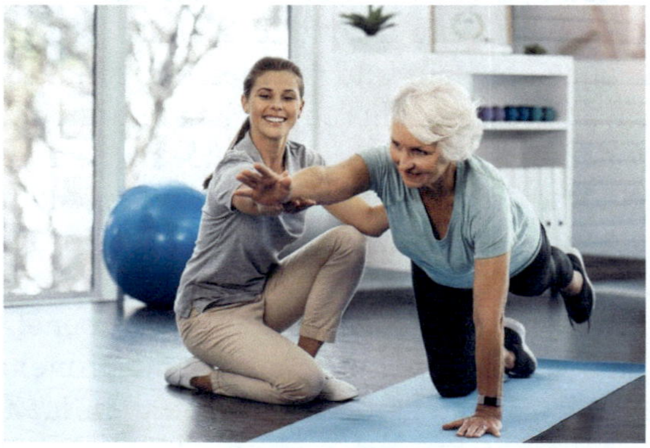

Figure 7.19. Importance of physical therapy for patients with musculoskeletal conditions.

Source: https://custom-images.strikinglycdn.com/res/hrscywv4p/image/upload/c_limit,fl_lossy,h_9000,w_1200,f_auto,q_auto/3450126/372972_572549.jpeg.

7.6.2. Nutritional Considerations for Musculoskeletal Health

The function of nutrition in maintaining musculoskeletal health cannot be overstated, as the right food factors play an important role in disease prevention and recovery. Nutrients such as proteins, vitamins, and minerals contribute considerably to the development of strong bones and healthier muscles. Amino acids are particularly important for muscle protein synthesis, and per studies, leucine enhances the activity by triggering specific signaling pathways (Abuja et al., 2018). In addition, vitamins C and D play roles in collagen formation and bone mineralization, thus exemplifying the interdependence of these nutrients in the preservation of musculoskeletal structures. The addition of an equilibrious diet that contains these nutrients is required, especially in individuals who engage in vigorous physical exercise or competitive sports, where the risk for musculoskeletal injury is high. Recent research has already begun to establish the specific roles of various dietary supplements in musculoskeletal wellness. For instance, vitamin C possesses antioxidant properties that indirectly aid in tendon repair, while vitamin E exhibits an antiproliferative effect on collagen deposition during healing (Abuja et al., 2018).

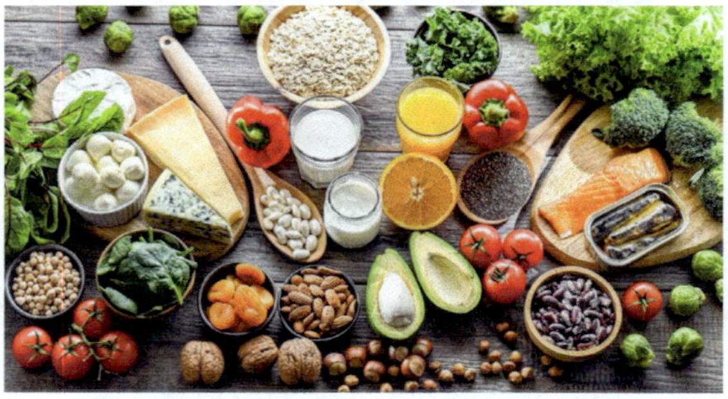

Figure 7.20. Nutrition for bone & joint health.

Source: https://premierortho.com/wp-content/uploads/2025/04/foods-for-bone-and-joint-health.webp.

This suggests that including such vitamins in one's diet will not only aid recovery from injury but also strengthen musculoskeletal tissues overall. On top of that, there is growing interest in the effects of omega-3 fatty acids, whose anti-inflammatory activity may potentially inhibit pain in various musculoskeletal disorders. The clinical application of such results remains cautious because of the differential levels of evidence of their effectiveness in human populations. It is also significant to consider the potential impacts of sport specialization on children and its influence on nutritional needs. As physical training is becoming increasingly specialized for elite performance, the nutritional needs of child athletes are rising, necessitating a balance between skill acquisition and general health. While sport expertise can enable rapid skill mastery, it may also pose risks, e.g., overuse injuries, which are further exacerbated by improper nutrition. Keeping a balanced diet that not only supports physical functioning but also mental comfort and social ease is paramount as the young athletes work through their respective competitive fields. Therefore, integrally meeting these nutritional factors can lead to maximal growth, development, and longevity in both sports and daily life (Figure 7.20).

7.6.3. Ergonomic Practices in Daily Activities

Ergonomic behaviors play a vital part in avoiding the risk of musculoskeletal disorders (MSDs) in everyday work. By designing work and environments to match human body capacities and limitations, ergonomic concepts are able to minimize strain and prevent injury to a large extent. For instance, proper workstation setup, such as an ideal chair position and monitor height, can improve posture and reduce discomfort while working at a computer for longer hours. Also, encouraging regular breaks and adding flexibility exercises into work routines can aid in physical well-being. Incorporation of such practices is vital in offices and manufacturing units, where repetitive movements and strained postures are prevalent. Not only do such ergonomic practices encourage staff wellness but also productivity, as more comfortable workers can work more efficiently (Kriebel et al., 2011). Moreover, the ergonomics strategy at work aims to highlight knowledge of organizational culture to improve musculoskeletal well-being. Effective prevention initiatives should align with the organization's overall policies. Research has proven that ergonomic intervention should not be a one-off exercise but should engage workers actively and promote ownership of health programs. For instance, a successful Musculoskeletal Disorders Prevention Program may include worker-environment evaluations and feedback procedures that promote cooperation across all staff levels. Tailoring ergonomic solutions to specific workplace issues is most significant, as it ensures interventions are relevant and effective in addressing the diverse needs of workers (Cruz et al., 2012). This collective practice enables one to develop a culture whereby ergonomic practices become the normal mode of doing things, and as such, enjoy long-term benefits to health. Beyond workplace settings, ergonomic practices can be applied to various daily activities that do not involve formal work. Simple adjustments in day-to-day activities—how one picks up items, uses assistive devices for heavy loads, and maintains proper posture while performing domestic work—can help prevent the onset of MSDs. For instance, gardening or household activities can be complemented by applying body mechanics that distribute weight evenly and reduce tension on joints and the spine. Moreover, greater awareness of ergonomics in leisure activities, such as exercise or sports, would boost overall wellness. Ultimately, the inclusion of ergonomic principles in daily life not only applies to work environments but also to musculoskeletal health, the interconnectedness of routine, and the avoidance of harm being the predominant factors (Cruz et al., 2012).

Test Your Knowledge

1. What is the importance of regular exercise?
2. What is the importance of nutrition in maintaining musculoskeletal health?

SUMMARY

In discussing musculoskeletal disorders, it is evident that they have a significant impact on both personal lives and overall public health. Chronic musculoskeletal pain, such as low back pain, has garnered important interest and study; nonetheless, the clinical effectiveness of numerous treatment interventions remains contentious. Studies indicate that most widely used treatments are of minimal benefit, and this has been underscored by recent evidence against traditional treatment models. Clinicians often find a disconnection between clinical practice and trial results, necessitating reexamining ongoing interventions and a call to tailor treatment approaches. The supposition that chronic pain may be a function of more widespread neural changes necessitates a move toward the explication of pain mechanisms rather than sole symptom targeting, as in recent controversies within the discipline (Antal et al., 2008). Moreover, the variability in patients' responses to interventions underscores the imperative of individualized care. Population heterogeneity in musculoskeletal disorders renders a single treatment modality difficult. For instance, the effectiveness of interventions is diluted in addressing changing patient needs in chronic low back pain when structural and psychological facets become hopelessly intermixed. Researchers are increasingly recognizing the value of subgrouping patients not just by body symptoms but also by psychosocial factors that may contribute to outcomes. Such depth of understanding can facilitate a more effective management approach, correlating treatment with the unique characteristics of each patient (Antal et al., 2008). Ultimately, a reconceptualization of musculoskeletal disorders through multifactorial models may lead to pioneering advances in treatment effectiveness. Last but not least, the evolution of surgical procedures, such as hip arthroplasties, reflects the dynamic environment of managing musculoskeletal disorders. Research comparing various implant designs and their respective mechanical performance has enabled the design of more effective surgical procedures, demonstrating that a personalized approach can yield improved patient outcomes. For instance, findings from research studies have determined that cemented short-stem prostheses are capable of offering better stability to certain population groups. In contrast, porous designs imply effects to others, with emphasis placed on the development of customized treatment protocols based on individual patient conditions. Such new approaches underscore the need for interdisciplinarity in treating musculoskeletal disorders by integrating biomechanical principles with clinical methods. As the understanding of these complex conditions deepens, so too can the ability to implement comprehensive, patient-centered care that ultimately improves the quality of life for those affected.

Musculoskeletal conditions are a serious health problem as they encompass a wide range of disease categories involving bones, muscles, cartilage, and connective tissues. Key information on these conditions indicates their occurrence, compounded by risk factors including age, obesity, and work hazards. Specifically, workplace settings are prone to health risks because certain ergonomic factors contribute to musculoskeletal problems among workers. The findings from case studies provide evidence that implementing control measures and reviewing design choices can significantly mitigate these risks and enhance occupational health and safety outcomes. The evidence synthesis emphasizes the importance of both preventive interventions and effective intervention strategies in addressing musculoskeletal disorders across diverse populations and workplaces. In keeping these dynamics in mind, it is evident that the management of these conditions in human beings depends heavily on integrated concepts (Kriebel et al., 2011). Furthermore, chronic pain disorders such as neck pain particularly point towards the complexity of musculoskeletal disorders. Chronic idiopathic neck pain has been observed to remain a widespread condition where patients can have moderate disability that has a substantial impact on their quality of life. This type of pain does not usually present with significant structural pathology, rendering diagnosis and treatment problematic. Recent literature has described central sensitization (CS) as an advocated mechanism for pain hypersensitivity, yet its primary role in the idiopathic condition is disputed. The findings report that the contribution of CS differentiates between patient groups with traumatic neck pain and chronic non-traumatic neck pain, criticizing the implementation of individualized treatment protocols. These findings not only highlight the specific concerns faced by patients but also underscore the need for further research to identify effective interventions for specific subgroups within the musculoskeletal disorder population (Bramer et al., 2015). In reviewing the key points on musculoskeletal disorders, including the implications of these findings within a broader context of health care provision, is necessary. Integration of multidimensional pain management programs, ergonomic assessments, and prevention education into clinical practices offers a viable path to reducing the prevalence and severity of these disorders among affected individuals. Additionally, recognition of the multicausality of musculoskeletal disorders allows practitioners to create a whole-person treatment, addressing not only physical status but also psychosocial status that can lead to pain experience. This interdisciplinary process calls for the coordination of healthcare professionals from various disciplines to provide a platform for improved clinical outcomes for patients. Lastly, accepting complexity and interrelating features of musculoskeletal disorders is crucial for further advancing the field and improving patient care (Kriebel et al., 2011; Bramer et al., 2015).

KEY TERMS FROM THIS CHAPTER

- Back pain
- Chronic ailments
- Genetics
- Inflammatory disorders
- Mesenchymal stromal cells
- Musculoskeletal system
- Rheumatoid arthritis
- Bones
- Fractures
- Healthcare systems
- Ligaments
- Muscles
- Occupational hazards
- Strains

CRITICAL THINKING QUESTIONS

1. **Which of the following is the most common cause of osteoarthritis?**
   a. Autoimmune disease
   b. Aging and joint wear-and-tear
   c. Bacterial infection
   d. Vitamin D deficiency
2. **What is the hallmark symptom of rheumatoid arthritis (RA)?**
   a. Joint pain and stiffness that improves with activity
   b. Acute, localized joint swelling after trauma
   c. Joint pain that worsens with movement and improves with rest
   d. Fever without joint involvement
3. **Which of the following is the most common site of a herniated disc?**
   a. Thoracic spine
   b. Cervical spine
   c. Lumbar spine
   d. Sacral spine
4. **In osteoporosis, which cells are primarily responsible for bone resorption?**
   a. Osteoblasts
   b. Osteocytes
   c. Chondrocytes
   d. Osteoclasts
5. **Which of the following laboratory markers is elevated in polymyositis?**
   a. Creatine kinase (CK)
   b. Alkaline phosphatase (ALP)
   c. Hemoglobin
   d. Serum bilirubin

Short Answer Questions

1. What is a musculoskeletal disorder?
2. List the types of musculoskeletal disorders.
3. What is tendinitis?
4. What are the risk factors of musculoskeletal disorders?
5. What is the importance of early diagnosis in musculoskeletal disorders?

Answer to Critical Thinking Questions

1. (b); 2. (a); 3. (c); 4. (d); 5. (a).

REFERENCES

1. Tack, C., Shorthouse, F., & Kass, L. (2017). The Physiological Mechanisms of Effect of vitamins and amino acids on tendon and muscle healing: a systematic review. *International Journal of Sport Nutrition and Exercise Metabolism, 28*(3), 294–311. https://doi.org/10.1123/ijsnem.2017-0267Agresti, A., Egenvall, A., Gough, A., Kathrani, A., Kyriazis, A., Peiravan, A., German, A. J., et al. (2017). Demography and disorders of German Shepherd Dogs under primary veterinary care in the UK. https://core.ac.uk/download/84659839.pdf (accessed on 12th July 2025).
2. Antal, A., Antal, A., Delitto, A., Keller, A., Moore, A., Pascual-Leone, A., Radebold, A., et al. (2008). Chronic non-specific low back pain–sub-groups or a single mechanism? https://core.ac.uk/download/335445.pdf (accessed on 12th July 2025).
3. Bachl, N., Collins, M., Cook, J., Derman, W., et al. (2008). International Olympic Committee consensus statement: Molecular basis of connective tissue and muscle injuries in sport. https://core.ac.uk/download/2776587.pdf (accessed on 12th July 2025).
4. Bai, B., Chen, H. Y., Hu, Y., et al. (2017). Finite element analysis of porously punched prosthetic short stem virtually designed for simulative uncemented hip arthroplasty. https://core.ac.uk/download/84591439.pdf (accessed on 12th July 2025).
5. Baker, J. S., & Grant, M. C. (2016). An overview of the effect of probiotics and exercise on mood and associated health conditions. https://core.ac.uk/download/141567244.pdf (accessed on 12th July 2025).
6. Bandura, A., Harrison, A. L., Berry, D., Kalso, E., Viller, F., Wolfe, F., Keefe, F. J., et al. (2009). Patterns of analgesic use, pain, and self-efficacy: A cross-sectional study of patients attending a hospital rheumatology clinic. https://core.ac.uk/download/pdf/19185.pdf (accessed on 12th July 2025).
7. Barbanti, P., Bovi, P., Candeloro, E., et al. (2015). Prevalence and time course of post-stroke pain: A multicenter prospective hospital-based study. https://core.ac.uk/download/54530964.pdf (accessed on 12th July 2025).
8. Bažon, I., Pišot, R., & Plevnik, M. (2016). Playing-related health risks among students and teachers of the music department at the Koper Art School. https://core.ac.uk/download/52491120.pdf (accessed on 12th July 2025).
9. Bernetti, A., Brignoli, O., Coclite, D., et al. (2017). Appropriateness and efficacy of spa therapy for musculoskeletal disorders: A Delphi method consensus initiative among experts in Italy. https://core.ac.uk/download/84928671.pdf (accessed on 12th July 2025).
10. Black, A. E., Halvari, A. E. M., Murray, A., Hall, A. M., Walker, B. F., Craig, C., Leonhardt, C., et al. (2012). Communication style and exercise compliance in physiotherapy (CONNECT): A cluster randomized controlled trial to test a theory-based intervention to increase chronic low back pain patients' adherence to physiotherapists' recommendations: Study rationale, design, and methods. https://core.ac.uk/download/pdf/9837538.pdf (accessed on 12th July 2025).
11. Black, G., Ranson, R. N., Saffrey, M. J., et al. (2013). Age-related changes to lumbosacral spinal cord motoneurons that modulate bladder and bowel functions in male C57BL/6 mice. https://core.ac.uk/download/82978019.pdf (accessed on 12th July 2025).
12. Bramer, W., Cagnie, B., Danneels, L., et al. (2015). Lack of evidence for central sensitization in idiopathic, non-traumatic neck pain: A systematic review. https://core.ac.uk/

download/55807729.pdf (accessed on 12th July 2025).

13. Burton, A. K., Abasolo, L., Alizadehkhaiyat, B. G., Pearce, B. G., Baldwin, M., Beaton, D., & Bonde, J. (2008). Management of work-relevant upper limb disorders: A review. https://core.ac.uk/download/1649687.pdf (accessed on 12th July 2025).
14. Burton, A. K., Daniels, K., Health & Safety Laboratory, Kendall, N. A. S., et al. (2016). Developing an intervention toolbox for the common health problems in the workplace. https://core.ac.uk/download/30734335.pdf (accessed on 12th July 2025).
15. Carey, M. R. (2018). An evaluation of the treatment modality and management of acute and chronic low back pain individuals in rural southeast Kansas. https://core.ac.uk/download/217281799.pdf (accessed on 12th July 2025).
16. Case, K., Hussain, A., Marshall, R., et al. (2013). Achieving workplace inclusiveness by using ergonomics risk assessment. https://core.ac.uk/download/42143922.pdf (accessed on 12th July 2025).
17. Chapel, A., De Becker, A., Hillmann, A. B., Ahrberg, A., Hillmann, A. J., Nixon, A. J., & Carvalho, A. M. (2018). Effects of mesenchymal stromal cells versus serum on tendon healing in a controlled experimental trial in an equine model. https://core.ac.uk/download/160499874.pdf (accessed on 12th July 2025).
18. Chapman, J., Dalbeth, N., Gow, P., et al. (2010). Podiatry services for patients with arthritis: An unmet need. https://core.ac.uk/download/1662153.pdf (accessed on 12th July 2025).
19. Clayton, A. (2012). Endogenous musculoskeletal tissue engineering – A focused perspective. https://core.ac.uk/download/10908942.pdf (accessed on 12th July 2025).
20. Colyer, F., Davies, H., Gamage, P., et al. (2013). Ultrastructural analysis of changes in neurons of the mouse internal anal sphincter during ageing. https://core.ac.uk/download/82978021.pdf (accessed on 12th July 2025).
21. Cruz, R. M., Merino, E. A. D., Silveira, A. L. D., et al. (2012). Critical analysis of a musculoskeletal disorder's prevention program. https://core.ac.uk/download/30354079.pdf (accessed on 12th July 2025).
22. Daniels, M. J., Middleton, K. R., Milsom, V. A., et al. (2013). Benefits and risks of weight-loss treatment for older, obese women. https://core.ac.uk/download/211342010.pdf (accessed on 12th July 2025).
23. Dowell, D., Ragan, K., Jones, C. M., Baldwin, G., & Chou, R. (2022). CDC clinical practice guideline for prescribing opioids for pain—United States, 2022. *MMWR Recommendations and Reports*, *71*, 1–95. https://doi.org/10.15585/mmwr.rr7103a1 (accessed on 12th July 2025).
24. Dul, J., & Neumann, W. P. (2025). Ergonomics contributions to company strategies. https://core.ac.uk/download/pdf/6904965.pdf (accessed on 12th July 2025).
25. Fairman, C. M., Galvao, D. A., Hart, N. H., et al. (2018). The potential therapeutic effects of creatine supplementation on body composition and muscle function in cancer. https://core.ac.uk/download/213607833.pdf (accessed on 12th July 2025).
26. Garshnek, V., Hooke, L. R., Radtke, M., et al. (2025). USSR Space Life Sciences Digest, issue 3. https://core.ac.uk/download/pdf/42842161.pdf (accessed on 12th July 2025).
27. Hecimovich, M. (2004). Sport specialization in youth: A literature review. https://core.ac.uk/download/11234954.pdf (accessed on 12th July 2025).

28. Helfenstein Junior, M., & Siena, C. (2009). Diagnostic mistakes involving tendonitis: Medical, social, legal, and economic impact. https://core.ac.uk/download/37708783.pdf (accessed on 12th July 2025).

29. Hoban, B. (2018). Associations between multiple medication use and medication-related problems among people with chronic non-cancer pain who are prescribed opioids. https://unsworks.unsw.edu.au/bitstreams/b15b24d0-8891-4696-b51a-2fbe1a10574d/download (accessed on 12th July 2025).

30. Hooke, L. R., & Teeter, R. (2025). USSR Space Life Sciences Digest. Index to issues 1–4. https://core.ac.uk/download/pdf/42841024.pdf (accessed on 12th July 2025).

31. Hunter, D. J., Jonas, B. L., Kissin, E., et al. (2010). Phase 1 safety and tolerability study of BMP-7 in symptomatic knee osteoarthritis. https://core.ac.uk/download/142040210.pdf (accessed on 12th July 2025).

32. Kriebel, D., Tickner, J., Jacobs, M., & Markkanen, P. (2011). Lessons learned: Solutions for workplace safety and health. https://core.ac.uk/download/71352756.pdf (accessed on 12th July 2025).

33. Lewis, J., & O'Sullivan, P. (2018). Is it time to reframe how we care for people with non-traumatic musculoskeletal pain? https://core.ac.uk/download/287581134.pdf (accessed on 12th July 2025).

34. Sprowson, A., Stewart, A., Sprowson, A. P., Murty, A. N., Nivbrant, B., Todd, C. J., & Jensen, C. D. (2013). The effect of high dose antibiotic impregnated cement on rate of surgical site infection after hip hemiarthroplasty for fractured neck of femur: A protocol for a double-blind quasi-randomized controlled trial. https://core.ac.uk/download/19210671.pdf (accessed on 12th July 2025).

35. Vanden Bossche, L., & Vanderstraeten, G. (2015). A multi-center, double-blind, randomized, placebo-controlled trial protocol to assess Traumeel injection vs dexamethasone injection in rotator cuff syndrome: The TRAumeel in ROtator cuff syndrome (TRARO) study protocol. https://core.ac.uk/download/55799136.pdf (accessed on 12th July 2025).

36. Williams, A., Beswick, A. D., Woolf, A. D., Martin, C., Terwee, C. B., Terwee, C. B., & Abrams, D. (2014). Recommendations for exercise adherence measures in musculoskeletal settings: A systematic review and consensus meeting (protocol). https://core.ac.uk/download/19553903.pdf (accessed on 12th July 2025).

37. Zhao, L., Xie, Y. X., & Wang, C. (2020). Recommendations for respiratory rehabilitation in adults with coronavirus disease 2019. *Chinese Medical Journal*, *133*, 1595–1602. https://doi.org/10.1097/cm9.0000000000000848 (accessed on 12th July 2025).

DERMATOLOGY IN FAMILY MEDICINE

8

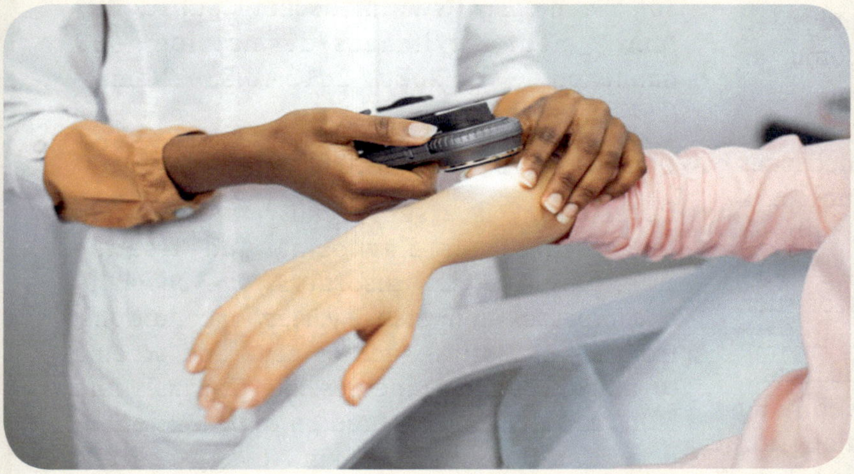

LEARNING OBJECTIVES

After studying this chapter, you will be able to:

1. Describe the common dermatological conditions
2. Understand the role of family physicians in dermatology
3. Know the diagnostic techniques in dermatology
4. Describe the treatment modalities and preventive dermatology

Introduction

Over the past decade, the incorporation of dermatology into family medicine has been increasingly recognized, as family physicians are playing a growing role in treating skin-related diseases. This is part of a general trend in healthcare in which sweeping, rather than narrow, approaches are preferred, especially in primary care. Given that family medicine doctors encounter a broad range of dermatological issues, from benign tumors to complex autoimmune conditions, their education and exposure to dermatological knowledge play a pivotal role. This ongoing change demands an understanding of diverse dermatological concerns through an increased emphasis on cultural competence and consideration of various patient backgrounds. (Bray et al., 2020) indicates the contribution of diversity to enhancing patient care by making dermatological practice more diverse, thereby reflecting the multicultural patient society. Enhancement of these elements within family medicine would result in a significantly higher diagnostic yield and efficacy of treatment. Furthermore, the contribution of dermatology to family medicine is indicated through its impact on public health outcomes. Skin diseases, although not typically accorded the same level of urgency as other illnesses, can result in considerable morbidity and a significant impact on the physical status and also the mental health of the patients. Primary care physicians are well-positioned to identify and manage these diseases as they engage in continuous relationships with patients and establish a culture of trust and comprehensive care. Notably, studies indicate that an integrated approach can yield better health outcomes as family providers are typically the first point of contact for patients with dermatologic complaints. As noted earlier, the heightened focus on diversity in dermatology literature suggests a broadening recognition of the need for tailored approaches that resonate with various groups. (Bray et al., 2020) presents evidence of such programs, a consideration that is significant to enable health equity in dermatological care. Lastly, the way recertification and continuing education mandates have developed alongside medical boards, particularly in dermatology, plays a crucial role in shaping competencies in family medicine. As defined in contemporary controversy surrounding board recertification procedures and their efficacy, this increasing demand for more streamlined and efficient pathways that further diminish the skillsets of family physicians in dermatology comes about puts particular importance on the possible benefits of the reforms that are able to eliminate some of the issues raised by doctors about the inadequacy of traditional methods of recertification. Proper training in dermatology, on the other hand, enables family medicine specialists to manage the complexity of skin diseases better, hence enhancing patient satisfaction and outcome. Introducing new recertification programs offers an opportunity to bridge knowledge gaps and make family doctors more effective in addressing dermatological issues amid a rapidly evolving health environment (Figure 8.1).

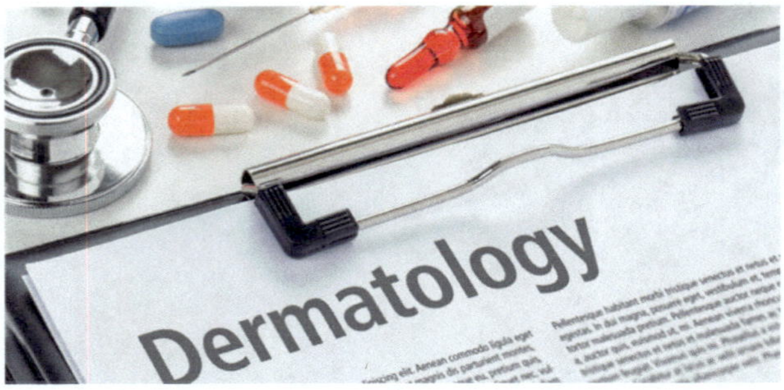

Figure 8.1. Dermatology in family medicine.

Source: https://www.medschool.lsuhsc.edu/family_medicine/images/dermatology%20banner.png?3/16/2020%2012:40:53%20pm.

Definition of Dermatology

Dermatology is a subspecialty medical field that focuses on diagnosing and treating skin, hair, and nail disorders. The specialty encompasses an immense variety of conditions, from simple issues such as acne and eczema to more disabling illnesses like psoriasis and skin cancer. Family medicine practitioners often encounter dermatology-related concerns among their patient base; therefore, familiarity with dermatology is required to provide comprehensive care. The inclusion of dermatology in family medicine not only adds treatment options but also provides holistic management of patients' health, as skin diseases can be expressions of systemic disease and make direct contributions to patients' quality of life and their families'. Therefore, understanding the definition and extent of dermatology becomes crucial to appreciating its significance in the broader arena of healthcare in family medicine. The significance of dermatology extends beyond the patient to influence family relationships and health-related quality of life. Chronic skin diseases have been found to affect the emotional well-being of patients and their families significantly. In one study comparing family quality of life across various medical specialties, 92% of participants reported emotional impact, underscoring the far-reaching consequences of skin conditions for families (Basra et al., 2013). The findings of the study show that issues arising from skin disorders most frequently disrupt daily routines and cause tension in family relationships. As family physicians treat these complex dermatologic diseases, they are also key players in establishing support structures that can better-balanced and more supportive household life. Apart from this, the economic aspects of dermatology in family practice cannot be overlooked. Current research indicates that subspecialist physicians, including dermatologists, earn much more money than their primary care counterparts. This has created patterns whereby medical students are prepared to pay for dermatology residency positions over generalist ones because of the economically beneficial prospects in dermatology clinics (Nicholson S). This economic reality, therefore, influences the availability and accessibility of dermatology services in family clinics. As family medicine continues to evolve, doctors must be cognizant of budgetary concerns and able to appropriately represent their patients while facilitating the integration of dermatology into overall family health planning (Figure 8.2).

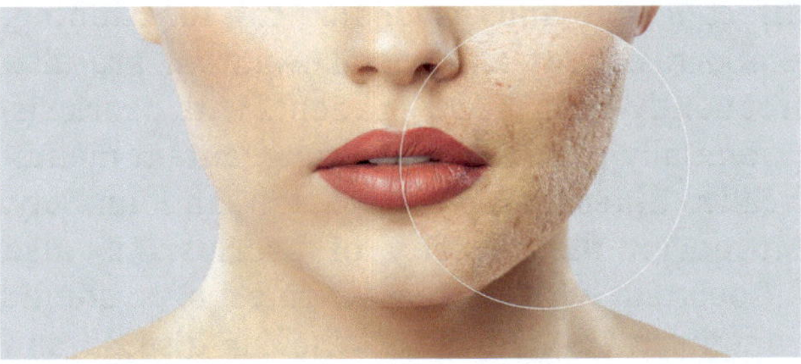

Figure 8.2. Dermatology.

Source: https://media.fmp-data.bliss.build/original_images/Dermatology.jpg.

Importance of Dermatology in Family Medicine

The role of dermatology in family medicine is significant due to the prevalence of skin ailments across all age groups of patients. Family physicians are the first line of contact for diagnosing and treating most skin conditions, ranging from benign eruptions to severe skin ailments. This initial function delivers early intervention, which is essential for good treatment and improved patient care. Moreover, family physicians can detect dermatological conditions, which can be pointers to systemic diseases. Early diagnosis of diseases such as diabetes, autoimmune diseases, and even cancer is made possible by detecting skin symptoms, underscoring the importance of dermatology in an integrated model of patient care. Family physicians must thus be properly trained in dermatological aspects to provide an integrated model which reflects enhanced health status among patients. In recent years, advances in dermatology have also identified the necessity for continuing education and training among family medicine physicians. With new treatment modalities being introduced at a rapid pace and growing insights into the pathophysiology of the skin, family physicians must be familiar with the most recent evidence in dermatological practice. This ongoing education is needed not only to manage common skin diseases effectively but also to manage complex cases that may require referral to specialists. Recent evidence indicates that many primary care physicians lack knowledge of dermatologic genetic services, thereby hindering their ability to provide comprehensive care (Jenevein et al., 2015). Therefore, enhancing the knowledge base of family medicine practitioners in dermatology can significantly improve patient care, ensuring that skin diseases are recognized and treated promptly. Moreover, the integration of dermatology into family medicine enhances the overall quality of patient interactions and care provision. By addressing skin issues in the setting of a family practice, doctors can gain a more holistic view of their patients' overall health and build closer relationships with them. Having this close connection allows better communication of treatment options and lifestyle modifications that can influence the skin.

Additionally, ongoing research in dermatology has led to new treatment advances that are increasingly used in family medicine, such as biologic therapy for conditions such as eczema and psoriasis (Boffa et al., 2004). The above indicates the necessity for family practitioners to incorporate dermatology into their practices, in order to offer modern, efficient care that meets patients' diverse needs.

8.1. Common Dermatological Conditions

Learning Outcome

1. Describe the acne and its impact on patients
2. Understand the eczema and its management in family practice
3. Know the psoriasis and treatment options

The most frequent dermatoses encountered in family practice are acne vulgaris, which is seen in millions of individuals of all ages, but mostly adolescents. Acne is defined as a chronic inflammatory cutaneous pilosebaceous disease. Acne arises from the interaction of an overproduction of sebum, faulty keratinization, inflammation, and bacterial colonization. Research has indicated that dietary factors, especially dairy intake, can affect the development of acne through hormonal changes that increase the severity of the condition. Although there is evidence of an association between dairy consumption—particularly skim milk—and high acne incidence, conclusive randomized controlled trials are still needed to establish these connections. Knowledge of these correlations not only aids in treatment planning but also helps practitioners provide comprehensive care by attending to the many lifestyle factors that may be contributing to patients' acne problems (Patton et al., 2016). Another skin condition commonly seen in family practice is eczema, or more specifically, atopic dermatitis, involving chronic inflammation and a compromised skin barrier. Dry, pruritic skin occurs frequently in patients and has a highly detrimental effect on quality of life. Chronic eczema is a challenge, as exacerbations may follow environmental triggers, such as irritants and allergens. The psychological impact of eczema is essential; many patients complain about anxiety, frustration, and even depression from coping with evident eruptions on the skin and discomfort.

Family doctors must adopt a holistic strategy for managing eczema that involves not only pharmacological strategies to reduce inflammation but also health education on lifestyle change and avoidance of triggers. Effective management can ultimately contribute significantly to improving patients' well-being, hence the necessity of long-term support and follow-up (Abeni et al., 2016). Psoriasis, another frequent dermatological presentation, is an autoimmune, chronic illness characterized by increased skin cell proliferation that forms scaly plaques. Psoriasis affects the population at a frequency of roughly 2-3% and tends to co-occur with physical symptoms that significantly affect social and psychological functioning. Embarrassment and social isolation are also frequently described by patients with psoriasis, potentially contributing to concomitant mental health illnesses of depression and anxiety. Moreover, the severity of psoriasis is also associated with increased rates of systemic complications like cardiovascular disease and metabolic syndrome. Thus, family medicine doctors must adopt an integrative treatment strategy that addresses both the physical and psychological impacts of psoriasis. This includes engaging in dialogue about the patient's psychosocial health and referring to therapeutic counseling as needed, promoting an integrated care plan that addresses the complex issues of psoriasis (Abeni et al., 2016) (Figure 8.3).

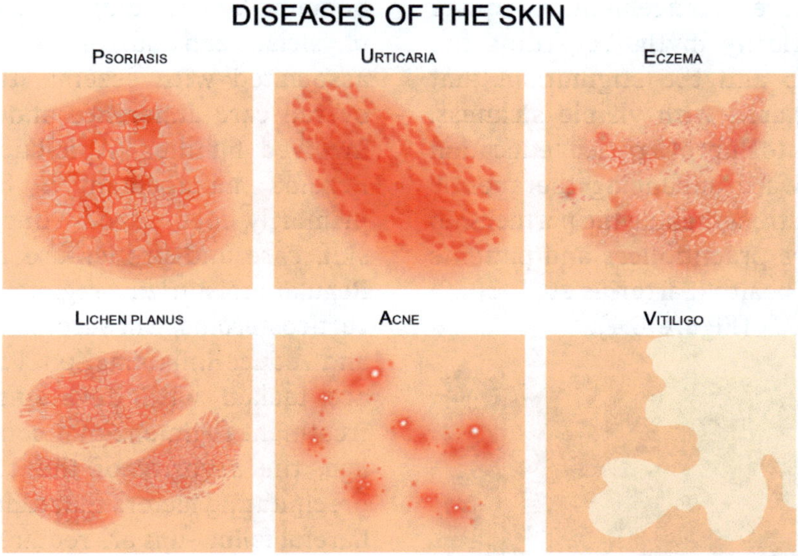

Figure 8.3. Diseases of the skin.

Source: https://www.fionawaring.com/wp-content/uploads/2019/07/shutterstock_1154905705-2-1.jpg.

8.1.1. Acne and Its Impact on Patients

Acne, a common dermatologic condition, significantly influences patients' physical and psychological well-being. For the majority of individuals, particularly adolescents and young adults, acne may trigger great emotional distress, negatively affecting self-image and social functioning. The constant visibility of acne eruptions tends to increase concern over interpersonal relationships, leading to some patients' reclusion from society or avoiding social contacts. As acne strikes mostly during formative years, its psychological impact is drastic, and the outcome can be diseases such as depression and social phobia. This is the reason that it is crucial to deal not only with the physical symptoms of acne in family practice but also with the psychological impacts that might ensue from the disease with treatment and care that targets the entire person. In addition, the socio-economic component of acne cannot be eluded. Patients with severe or moderate acne have generally commented on increased medical costs and absenteeism from work, impacting their overall quality of life. Therapy regimens can be prolonged and expensive, spanning topical treatments, oral antibiotics, and in extreme instances, even surgical intervention. The cost of acne care falls particularly heavily on individuals with inadequate health coverage or limited economic resources, leading to disparities in treatment access and outcomes. Financial aspects of such concerns for acne and its treatment point to the very significant role that family physicians play in guiding patients through cost-efficient treatment while promoting systemic assistance to mitigate the cost burden of such chronic skin diseases as acne. Patient education then becomes an integral component of acne care, with emphasis on individualized treatment and informed decision-making. Dermatology clinicians and nurses play crucial roles in educating patients about their conditions to ensure treatment adherence. By providing clear information on the character of acne, its causes, and how to properly manage it, healthcare professionals can enable individuals to be proactive in skincare management. Adequate information can clarify myths regarding the treatment of acne and the stigmatism that is generally associated with visible sickness. Additionally, efforts to improve patient education go a long way toward enhancing therapeutic outcomes, thereby strengthening the partnership between healthcare practitioners and patients on the path to skin health (Sartorius et al., 2010; Chukwu et al., 2018) (Figure 8.4).

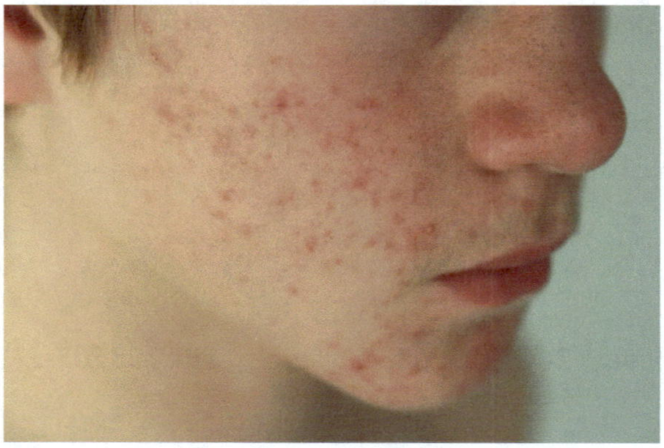

Figure 8.4. Acne.

Source: https://www.health.com/thmb/27qfo5VzSeLF0b9FndNIHbL0HvU=/1500x0/filters:no_upscale():max_bytes(150000):strip_icc():format(webp)/GettyImages-157144963-2000-64093d43108e4bfcaf4b377ac87f5f6a.jpg.

8.1.2. Eczema and Its Management in Family Practice

Eczema, particularly atopic dermatitis, is a challenging condition in family practice due to its chronic nature and increasing prevalence among children. With a multifactorial etiology, the condition affects patients' and their families' quality of life. Recent studies emphasize the key role of skin barrier dysfunction in the etiology of eczema, thereby requiring integrated management that considers preventive as well as therapeutic strategies. Family doctors play an important role in educating families about the condition and its potential impacts, ensuring that proper and timely treatment is provided to patients. By providing a common environment, physicians can address the psychosocial factors associated with eczema, thereby improving overall care adherence and quality of life for involved families (Apfelbacher et al., 2014). Eczema management in family practice is primarily focused on educating patients on skin care and proper use of topical therapy. Regular moisturizing regimens, as well as topical corticosteroids, will successfully suppress flares and reduce inflammation. Family practitioners are tasked with developing individualized treatment regimens that consider the patient's age, the severity of the condition, and the precipitating factors that exacerbate symptoms. Careful follow-ups are required not just to assess skin status but also to assess family dynamics and the psychological impact that ensues from the condition.

Proactive management entails educating families to recognize flare causes and implement lifestyle changes, which can significantly enhance control of the condition and overall patients' well-being (BEEP study team et al., 2020).

The recent advances in eczema prevention suggest that early intervention may reduce the incidence of atopic dermatitis in high-risk individuals. Clinical trials have demonstrated that early use of emollients can be a preventive intervention, albeit with highly heterogeneous results. While some research suggests a notable reduction in eczema incidence with emollient use during infancy, others have reported no significant preventative benefit, and further work is required. Family doctors must stay current with evolving evidence to provide patients and their families with well-informed advice. Lastly, an individualized, evidence-based family practice plan for the care of eczema is essential to improve disease outcomes, enhance family quality of life, and create an environment of support (Apfelbacher et al., 2014) (Figure 8.5).

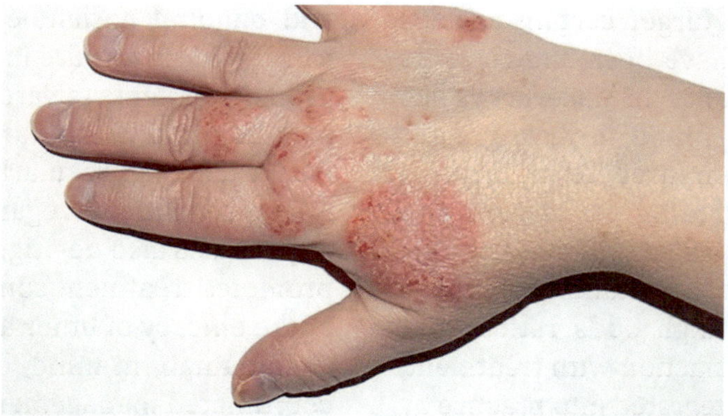

Figure 8.5. Eczema.

Source: https://images.apollo247.in/pd-cms/cms/2024-05/eczema_0.jpg?tr=q-80,f-webp,w-400,dpr-2.5,c-at_max%201000w.

8.1.3. Psoriasis and Treatment Options

Psoriasis, a chronic inflammatory skin condition, impacts patients' quality of life due to its visible signs and associated comorbidities. It is characterized by thick, scaly plaques on the skin due to the rapid growth of keratinocytes. Since its etiology is multifactorial, with genetic, immunologic, and environmental contributions, management plans are as well. Family doctors play a crucial role in the diagnostic process for psoriasis and in selecting treatment options that can range from topical therapy to systemic medication.

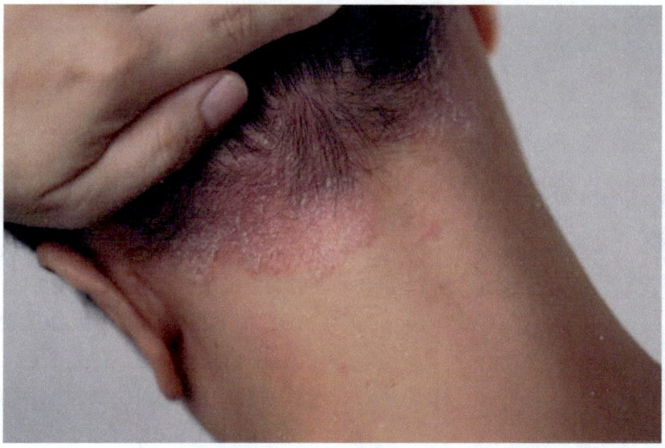

Figure 8.6. Psoriasis.

Source: https://www.health.com/thmb/aEJdBYX_7D88134f1aaKx1yWIB8=/750x0/filters:no_upscale():max_bytes(150000):strip_icc():format(webp)/Health-GettyImages-1604751312-be3c174df1b04084877ff6717123c13f.jpg.

Disease severity, skin involvement, and patient preference are significant determinants of treatment, underlining the value of an individualized care plan. Recent years have witnessed new advances in dermatology, opening the door to new treatments for psoriasis. New biologic agents that specifically target certain aspects of the immune system have been shown to be effective in clinical trials. For instance, drugs like adalimumab have been found to have greater drug survival rates compared to traditional treatment options, including etanercept and infliximab. Adalimumab, as per studies, not only offers a greater chance of maintaining response rates—documented by high odds ratios—but also general patient satisfaction with treatment. As these therapies are integrated into practice by family physicians, it is important to stay abreast of the latest information on the treatment of psoriasis to optimize patient management and provide effective treatment options (Boffa et al., 2004). Psoriasis treatment extends beyond pharmacotherapy; lifestyle changes and ongoing patient education are involved. Family physicians are in an excellent position to promote patients toward healthier lifestyles that may help moderate flare-ups, including eating well, exercising regularly, and managing stress. Educating patients regarding the chronic nature of psoriasis also de-stigmatizes the disease and promotes treatment compliance. With evidence of the efficacy of other anti-TNF agents, notably adalimumab, in mind, clinicians must develop coordinated management plans to monitor side effects and tailor treatment based on response (Berardesca et al., 2018). Such coordinated care not only ensures effective management of psoriasis but also improves the overall health and well-being of the patients (Figure 8.6).

Test Your Knowledge

1. What is acne?
2. What is eczema?

8.2. Role of Family Physicians in Dermatology

Learning Outcome

1. Understand the initial assessment and diagnosis in dermatology
2. Describe the treatment protocols and referrals for dermatological conditions
3. Understand the role of patient education in fostering self-care strategies for skin health

In family medicine dermatology, family physicians are integral healthcare providers, offering comprehensive assessment and initial treatment options for a range of dermatological conditions. These physicians are ordinarily the initial referral source for patients presenting with dermatologic issues, from benign eruptions to more complex presentations such as dermatitis and skin cancers. Depending on their training, they can perform important procedures, such as skin biopsies and cryotherapy, thus enabling early intervention that can be crucial in influencing outcomes. Integrating dermatology into family practice not only enhances patient access to specialist services but also enables continuity of care since family physicians understand their patients' general medical histories and underlying conditions. Although essential to their work, many family practitioners find dermatology wanting in terms of knowledge gaps and scarce availability of expert resources. Evidence indicates that despite the fact that most family physicians comprehend the extent to which genetics contributes to dermatologic conditions, there remains a lack of application of this understanding in practice (Jenevein et al., 2015). Apart from that, implementation issues in genetic testing and counseling within routine care can delay control of hereditary skin conditions, suggesting a need for specific education programs. Given the growing number of skin diseases against the backdrop of a changing population age structure, family doctors should be newly trained in dermatology to provide high-quality patient care.

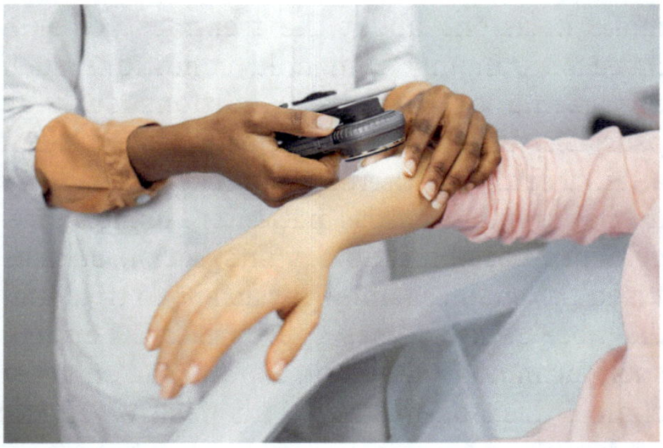

Figure 8.7. Role of a dermatologist.

Source: https://medical.rossu.edu/sites/g/files/krcnkv261/files/styles/atge_3_2_crop_md/public/2022-04/Dermatology.jpg?h=f9d06ff2&itok=ktvUIeL9.

Moreover, the evolving climate of dermatologic practice also overlaps with the influence of industry payments, which can shape physicians' experience and engagement with novel practices. Results indicate that payment incentives have the potential to skew patient care prioritization across specialties, even dermatology (Blumenthal et al., 2019). Family physicians must therefore navigate such factors and make ethical considerations within practice. Since they are looking to develop their dermatology skills, ongoing professional development is required. It could involve working alongside dermatology specialists, attending workshops, and staying up to date with the latest developments in dermatological procedures. Through ongoing learning, family doctors can enhance their practices, ultimately leading to improved dermatologic care and patient satisfaction (Figure 8.7).

8.2.1. Initial Assessment and Diagnosis

An accurate initial assessment in dermatology is necessary to attain precise diagnosis and subsequent management of many skin disorders. During the first patient consultation, the doctors must perform a comprehensive assessment that includes a thorough medical history, including the history of disease onset, disease duration, previous treatment, and associated symptoms. Particular importance should be given to identifying precipitating factors, such as environmental precipitates or recent dietary changes. With insight into the patient's background and symptomatology, healthcare professionals can create a differential diagnosis list and prioritize conditions appropriate to the patient's demographics and clinical presentation. This is a methodical approach that is particularly important, especially with heterogeneous conditions such as atopic eczema, in which initial evaluation informs management strategies and follow-up treatment as indicated by the consensus of the TREatment of ATopic eczema (TREAT) Registry Taskforce. This foundation enables clinicians to employ standardized treatment effectiveness measures (Apfelbacher et al., 2019). Physical examination's contribution to the diagnostic evaluation cannot be overstated since it provides crucial details about the diagnosis. The clinician must witness a thorough examination of the affected area, observing characteristics such as lesion morphology, distribution, and associated inflammatory features. In the case of acne vulgaris, clinicians are to evaluate the severity according to the presence of papules, pustules, or cysts, as well as evaluating potential psychosocial impact (Patton et al., 2016). The process is very applicable because the multifactorial etiology of acne extends beyond the skin with the possibility of compromising patients' quality of life. The results of the assessment are to be thoroughly documented to enable future comparison and guide treatment planning. Besides, certain diagnostic tools such as dermoscopy can be used in complex cases, enhancing the clinician's ability to assess condition severity and treatment response.

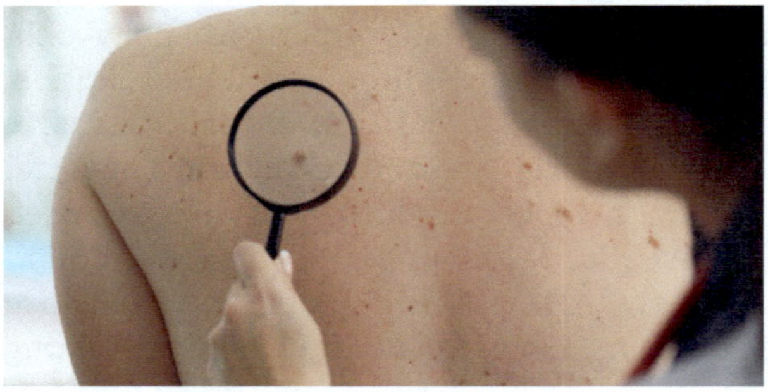

Figure 8.8. Diagnosing skin conditions.

Source: https://www.dermatologist.org.uk/wp-content/uploads/2022/02/Diagnosing-skin-conditions.jpg.

Following the initial assessment, the establishment of an accurate diagnosis determines the strategy of management. The diagnostic process can involve additional studies such as skin scrapings, cultures, or even a biopsy in doubtful cases, particularly if dermatoses overlap. For conditions like atopic eczema, inclusion of standardized information facilitates comprehensive observation of treatment and assessment of long-term consequences, including the fact that a consensus-oriented approach makes a more systematic follow-up schedule (Apfelbacher et al., 2019). At the same time, controversy surrounding the potential contribution of diet to dermatological illness, exemplified by anecdotal evidence in acne vulgaris, underscores the complexity of diagnoses that goes beyond "dermatological symptom" (Patton et al., 2016). Family physicians must remain vigilant in valuing all aspects of dermatologic health, not only medical management but also patient education and lifestyle modification, thereby enhancing patient-centered care in dermatology in family medicine (Figure 8.8).

8.2.2. Treatment Protocols and Referrals

In family medicine, developing evidence-based treatment protocols for skin diseases is essential to optimizing patient outcomes. Evidence-based guidelines allow family physicians to make decisions about the treatment of skin diseases, ranging from mild conditions such as eczema to complex conditions such as psoriasis. Adherence to treatment protocols can align treatment, thereby reducing variability in management across patients. Furthermore, evidence-based technology integration, such as VisualDx, enables family physicians to treat and diagnose skin diseases appropriately. Through such technology adoption, experts can enhance clinical decision-making, with positive effects on health outcomes and patient satisfaction. However, as identified in contemporary studies, such use does not have a significant impact on problem-solving speed or follow-up consultations, and research indicates the need for further research into the determinants influencing the effectiveness of the treatment (Burke et al., 2018). Referral to dermatologists often plays a critical role in the management of multifaceted skin diseases beyond the domain of primary care. Family doctors must be adept at determining when, or whether, patients need a referral, particularly for patients with suspected cutaneous malignancies or severe dermatologic diseases. Prompt and appropriate referrals can facilitate access to specialist services, and this can facilitate the provision of targeted treatment in a timely fashion. Moreover, establishing strong interprofessional collaboration with dermatologists facilitates working together to manage patients and enables open communication about what patients require. Referrals should also consider patients' socio-economic status and health literacy, as these factors significantly affect their ability to navigate the healthcare system. Facilitating discussions with patients regarding referral will aid their understanding and adherence to the management plan and enhance long-term outcomes.

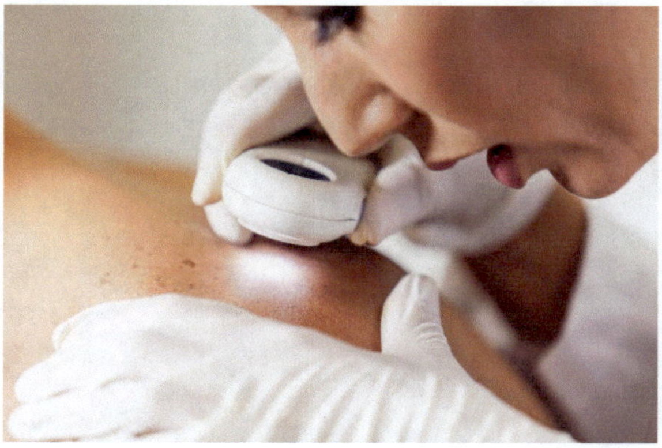

Figure 8.9. Rational referrals: dermatology.

Source: https://www.pulsetoday.co.uk/wp-content/uploads/2022/10/dermatology-referral-advice-and-guidance.jpg.

The integration of empowering technologies into primary care settings is one potential way to enhance treatment protocols and referral patterns in dermatology. By using tools that facilitate more productive patient-provider communication, family physicians are better able to treat chronic diseases and engage patients as more active partners in their own medical care. For example, technology can be leveraged to monitor patient outcomes and treatment adherence, thereby offering practitioners rich feedback to adjust their protocols. Furthermore, adopting these technologies in family practice enables comprehensive management that focuses on patient education and self-management strategies. Although the advantages are highlighted, there remain difficulties in adopting such technologies into everyday practice, including workflow disruptions and the need for ongoing training and support for primary care physicians (Nesbitt et al., 2017). Such difficulties have to be eliminated in the process of optimizing treatment protocol and referral possibilities in dermatology, and consequently optimizing patient-centered care (Figure 8.9).

8.2.3. Patient Education and Self-Care Strategies

In family medicine dermatology, patient education is important for promoting self-care measures to maintain healthy skin. Educating the patient on prevalent dermatological issues empowers them and helps them take the necessary measures to reduce mismanagement and complications. For example, awareness of the importance of sun protection and proper moisturization can greatly reduce the risk of skin cancer and eczema. In addition, it instills a sense of empowerment in patients, prompting them to take on active roles in their treatment plans, rather than being passive recipients. These educational sessions are supplemented by interactive visual aids or hands-on demonstrations, which have been found to enhance retention and understanding and, in turn, lead to better patient outcomes. Last but not least, self-care strategies, as one of the foundations of patient education, are important in dermatology. Patients must be instructed in how to perform regular skin checks, recognize the warning signs of possible issues, and the importance of following prescribed regimens. To illustrate, incorporating customized skincare regimens will greatly improve the management of chronic diseases such as acne and psoriasis. Moreover, education needs to extend into the realm of product selection—patients need to be taught about what various ingredients in skincare products mean and how to decide which are useful and which are not. Engaging patients in dialogue about their unique health goals not only maximizes adherence to treatment regimens but also allows healthcare providers to tailor their advice to changing lifestyles and mindsets. Coordination among community resources and healthcare professionals is an important strategy to enhance patient education and self-management in dermatologic clinics. Local agency-aligned programs can be utilized to plan workshops and presentations, market skin health awareness, and make resources available. Knowing these benefits, family medicine clinicians can significantly improve their outreach ability. As claimed, placing importance on the advantages of inter-organizational collaboration serves to maximize efforts in patient education (Bluestein et al., 2020). Furthermore, the rapid advancements in genetic testing and its utilization in dermatologic care underscore the importance of continually updating patient information. Physicians should be able to bridge the knowledge gap regarding the genetic component of skin conditions and refer patients to specialists when needed, thereby fostering an integrative approach to skin health (Jenevein et al., 2015).

Test Your Knowledge

1. What is a procedure for the treatment of a skin condition?
2. What is the role of patient education in fostering self-care strategies for skin health?

8.3. Diagnostic Techniques in Dermatology

Learning Outcome

1. Describe the visual examination and history taking
2. Know the dermatoscopy and its applications
3. Understand the biopsy procedures and interpretation

Dermatological diagnostic techniques have evolved significantly, and family medicine practitioners are now more capable of detecting and treating skin conditions. One of the most notable advancements is the use of clinical evidence technologies (CETs), such as VisualDx, to enhance diagnostic accuracy. Despite their potential, relatively user-friendly, but helpful in dealing with skin problems only occasionally. Findings revealed several barriers to the optimal use of CETs, including interface difficulties and a bias toward traditional sources of information. Nevertheless, despite this, these technologies remain valuable additions to diagnostic and treatment communication, supporting the need for ongoing improvement to maximize their advantage in everyday practice (Burke et al., 2020). In the last few years, data mining techniques have proven to be revolutionary tools in dermatology, with large medical datasets examined to show patterns associated with cutaneous diseases. These techniques encompass classification, association mining, and clustering, with wide-ranging applications in diagnosis. Classification, for instance, has proven particularly beneficial for diagnosing erythematous-squamous diseases, employing algorithms such as Neural Networks and Genetic Algorithms to improve accuracy. Clustering, conversely, aids in establishing commonalities of medical image data, enabling more structured exploration of dermatology conditions. With these data mining methods, dermatology has the capacity to leverage results from enormous volumes of data towards clinical decision-making and improved patient outcomes (Adibi et al., 2011). Also, the application of advanced diagnostic tools not only benefits family physicians' practices but also advances patient care in the community. The application of CETs and data mining facilitates multidisciplinary care, allowing PCPs to handle skin disorders more comprehensively. However, effective deployment of these technologies requires ongoing training and education to address challenges such as clinicians' comfort and confidence in dermatological practices. Emphasizing these elements of education can foster a culture of continuous improvement, thereby advancing the role of family medicine in dermatology. Ultimately, the integration of sound diagnostic techniques is necessary to enhance further family medicine's ability to offer quality skin care so that the patient may receive informed and effective care appropriate to their own dermatological needs (Adibi et al., 2011; Burke et al., 2020) (Figure 8.10).

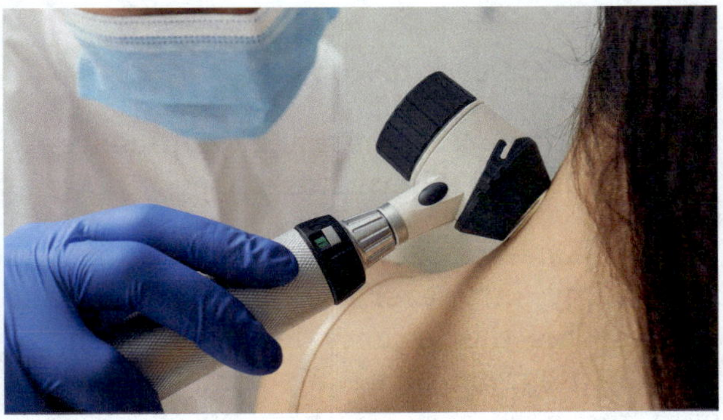

Figure 8.10. Diagnostic methods used by dermatologists.

Source: https://assets.medpagetoday.net/media/images/112xxx/112906.jpg?width=0.8.

8.3.1. Visual Examination and History Taking

In family medicine dermatology, visual examination and taking history are fundamental aspects of the diagnostic evaluation. Visual examination allows the clinician to record skin morphology, color, and lesion distribution, which provide significant information about a patient's dermatological status. By assessing these visual findings, clinicians can begin making differential diagnoses. In addition, detailed history-taking precedes this inspection to obtain relevant patient information, including prior skin problems, genetic predisposition, and lifestyle. Visual assessments, coupled with history-taking, enable doctors to develop an accurate understanding of patients' dermatological conditions, ultimately leading to improved patient outcomes. Communication plays a significant role in the history of dermatology. The provider's skill in taking complete patient histories, such as the onset and character of skin lesions, associated symptoms, and precipitants, is essential in diagnosing well. Questions about family history might uncover genetic associations that will influence the patient's presentation. Providers can establish a rapport and engage patients to offer sensitive information that is potentially diagnostic. In addition, awareness of the socio-cultural setup of the home environment where the patients reside will shed light on aggravating factors for skin diseases and contribute further to clinical decisions. Interdependence between good communication and empathetic examination thus elevates the quality of care provided in family medicine. The application of newer diagnostic tools, such as autofluorescence imaging, to the visual examination process can significantly support traditional methods. Recent developments embrace the use of autofluorescence properties as significant indicators of cellular and tissue well-being, particularly in dermatology. Visualization of endogenous fluorophores, for instance, aids in monitoring pathological changes without resort to invasive therapies. The technique, while still very much in its relative infancy for dermatological use, demonstrates a clear trajectory toward future clinical use that can be achieved with fewer resources and less time. With advances in science, further research is needed to make these technologies more sophisticated and establish standard operating procedures. Therefore, the addition of such advanced methodologies will not only enhance visual examinations but also allow family physicians to offer informed and accurate dermatological care (Aigner et al., 2020; Cole et al., 2020) (Figure 8.11).

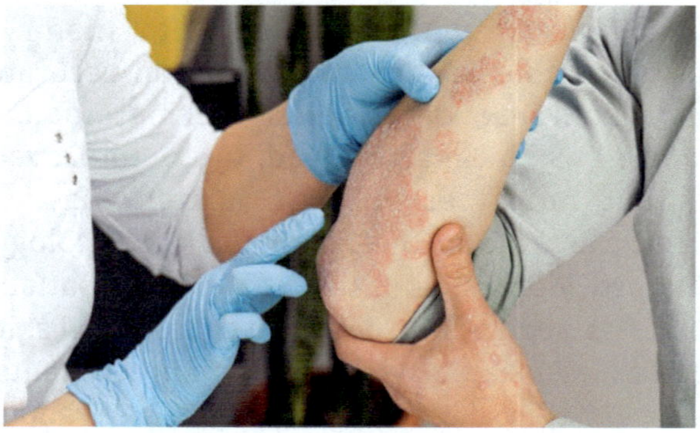

Figure 8.11. Dermatological assessment: history-taking and examination.

Source: https://www.practicenursing.com/media/mqkn5fnt/adobestock_393573411.jpeg?width=1002&height=564&bgcolor=White&v=1db887b55986fd0.

8.3.2. Dermatoscopy and Its Applications

The application of dermatoscopy is one significant advancement in dermatology, especially in family medicine practice. Dermatoscopy is an invasive-free procedure that allows primary care physicians to introduce greater accuracy into their diagnosis of skin lesions, discerning benign conditions from potential malignancies such as melanoma. This ability to visualize skin structures below the superficial layer enables clinicians to make more accurate judgments about when excisions or referrals are warranted. It is discovered by research that family doctors can do better in their diagnosis, to reduce unnecessary procedures and alleviate patient anxiety regarding indeterminate skin lesions, when well-trained (Burrows et al., 2019). As a result, incorporating dermatoscopy into routine examinations can allow primary care physicians to be more proactive in early detection and prevention of skin cancer. In addition, using dermatoscopy in primary care is not without challenges, including the need for proper training and equipment. A systematic review has highlighted that while dermoscopy enhances diagnostic accuracy, the failure to provide training to unoccupied clinicians may not yield greater accuracy than traditional visual inspection (Burrows et al., 2019).

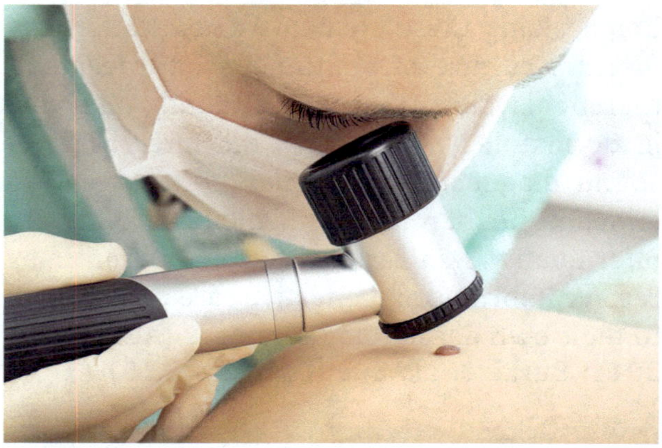

Figure 8.12. Dermatoscopy.

Source: https://kalmed.co.uk/wp-content/uploads/2023/01/Dermatoskop.jpg.

The brilliance of successfully integrating this technology into everyday practice further underscores the urgency for comprehensive training programs that equip family physicians with the necessary competency to practice dermatoscopy with confidence. Furthermore, practice settings must consider the time and expense required to apply this technology. Therefore, removal of these barriers is essential to optimize the clinical benefits of dermatoscopy in family medicine practice. Within the scope of patient care, the role of dermatology nurses alongside dermatoscopy cannot be overestimated. These specialists play a significant role in educating patients and providing important information about skin diseases and treatments. Research shows that more informed patients are more likely to adhere to medical regimens, thereby achieving better health outcomes. Dermatology nurses facilitate this process of education by developing trusting relationships with the patients, enhancing their cooperation and adherence to the medical regimen. These collaborations between primary care physicians and dermatology nurses promote a holistic approach to skin diseases, thereby enhancing the uniform application of dermatoscopy. Through this partnership, medical practitioners can provide quality diagnosis and treatment of skin conditions, further reinforcing the core role of dermatology in family medicine (Figure 8.12).

8.3.3. Biopsy Procedures and Interpretation

Biopsy procedures are a valuable diagnostic tool in dermatology, particularly in family practice, where accurate interpretations have a significant impact on patient management. Biopsy procedures involve the removal of a small amount of skin tissue for microscopy to aid in the diagnosis of several dermatological diseases. Excisional, incisional, shave, and punch biopsies are the most commonly used types, each applied based on the nature of the lesion and clinical suspicion. The choice of technique has not only implications for the diagnostic yield but also for therapeutic potential. For instance, excisional biopsies may be selected in cases of suspected malignancy to enable full excision, while punch biopsies may be used for small lesions or when histological understanding of the disease is required without being invasive. Once a biopsy has been performed, interpretation of the tissue specimen is based on histopathological examination by a specialist pathologist. Histopathological examination involves evaluation of the architectural and cytological features of the tissue, which may reveal underlying conditions such as autoimmune diseases, infections, and neoplasms. Of particular interest is the role of newer techniques, such as immunohistochemistry and molecular pathology, in enhancing diagnostic accuracy. For instance, in conditions such as dystrophic epidermolysis bullosa, genetic mutations in genes such as COL7A1, as deciphered from biopsy findings, can inform clinicians about the pathogenesis of the disease and guide family counseling on inheritance patterns (Abiri et al., 2017).

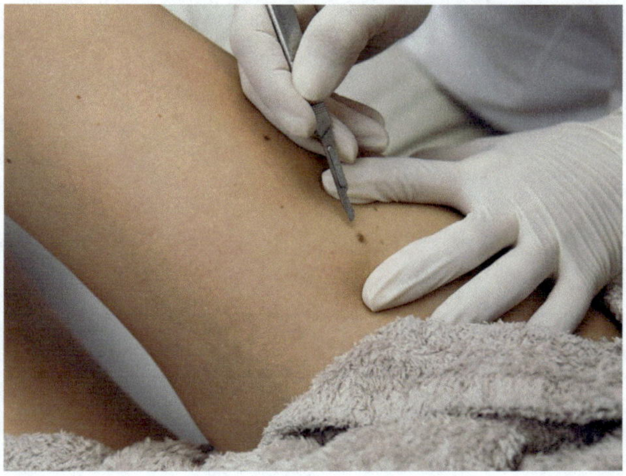

Figure 8.13. Skin biopsies and diagnosing dermatological conditions.

Source: https://epidermatology.com.sg/wp-content/uploads/2024/02/skin-biopsy-featured-image-1024x682.jpg.

Thus, correlating biopsy findings with clinical observation can inform holistic management regimens to concerned families, and pathology is an indispensable intervention in dermatology. Furthermore, the interpretation of biopsy results is not merely about a diagnosis; it often determines treatment regimens and prognostic calculations. For example, when it comes to suspected skin cancers, not only must one determine the type of cancer from the biopsy, but staging and treatment planning must also be based on histological grade and the margins achieved. This is particularly significant in family medicine, as dermatological health overlaps with patterns of hereditary disease. Deductive examination of biopsy results is imperative, especially in hereditary skin conditions, and underscores that family members need to be aware of the implications of diagnoses resulting from genetic mutations ascertained from biopsies. Advances in dermatopathology may make genetic information from routine biopsies an additional pathway for familial risk estimation and therapeutic management, thereby becoming another way to improve patient care in family medicine (Adaskevich et al., 2014) (Figure 8.13).

Test Your Knowledge

1. What is the use of dermatoscopy?
2. What are the procedures for a biopsy?

8.4. Treatment Modalities

Learning Outcome

1. Understand the topical therapies and their effectiveness
2. Describe the systemic treatments for severe conditions
3. Know the emerging therapies and innovations

In dermatology and family medicine, a close understanding of treatment modalities is required for the management of patients. The list of treatments that can be offered ranges from topical therapy and systemic medications to phototherapy and innovative surgery. Topical drugs such as corticosteroids and retinoids are first-line treatments for conditions such as eczema and psoriasis and provide benefit through localized action and a decreased risk of systemic side effects. Systemic agents, such as biologics, are now used to treat more severe dermatological conditions, with specific mechanisms of action that improve overall patient outcomes. Furthermore, phototherapy uses ultraviolet light to treat cutaneous diseases, penetrating deeper into the skin and effectively reducing inflammation and pathological cutaneous lesions. Such a diverse treatment paradigm suggests that family physicians need to stay current with the latest dermatologic treatment strategies. Education and prevention are the primary factors in dermatologic treatment modalities, the most significant of which are diseases prevalent in specific populations, e.g., skin cancer in Vermont. As the state has the highest melanoma incidence in the nation, awareness of sun protection is crucial. A study was conducted to establish that regular use of sunscreen, particularly in children, could greatly reduce the incidence of squamous and basal cell carcinomas (Sullivan et al., 2017). Family medicine providers can be proactive by teaching during well-child encounters, thereby ensuring families have the necessary information to protect themselves from the sun. By integrating preventive services and risk education into standard care, providers can avert subsequent dermatological conditions. The development of complex educational materials can further enhance patient knowledge and compliance, with an emphasis on teamwork between prevention and dermatology within the family medicine paradigm. Moreover, advances in dermatological treatments call for ongoing physician education. Incorporation of new technologies and treatment modalities, such as teledermatology, has improved access to care and enabled family physicians to collaborate effectively with dermatology specialists. The European Innovation Partnership on Active and Healthy Ageing calls for implementing innovative solutions to enhance the delivery of health care, with an emphasis on accessibility and patient-oriented care (Agache et al., 2016). By embracing these new methodologies in practice, family medicine can enhance patient outcomes and make the care process more efficient for dermatological diseases. Ongoing professional education, combined with working with specialists, will help medical professionals maintain proficiency in the use of the most effective treatment modalities. This global and modern perspective on dermatological healthcare enhances family medicine practice, ultimately improving patients' health and well-being (Figure 8.14).

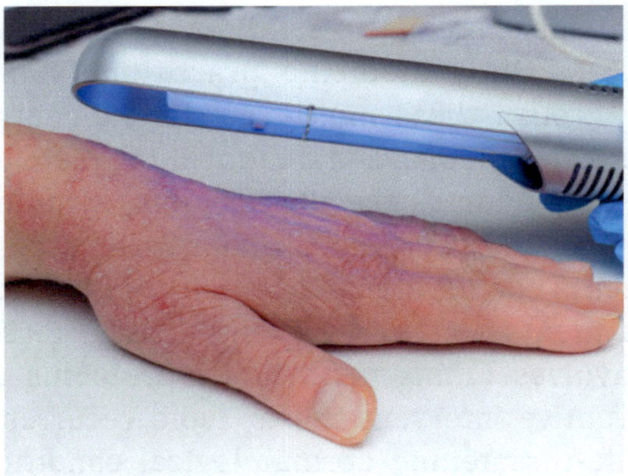

Figure 8.14. Phototherapy.

Source: https://skinhealthinstitute.org.au/wp-content/uploads/2023/03/Phototherapy.png.

8.4.1. Topical Therapies and Their Effectiveness

Topical therapy is foundational to the management of all dermatological conditions, particularly in family medicine, where patient care needs to be holistic. The therapies encompass a diverse group of drugs such as corticosteroids, calcineurin inhibitors, and retinoids, each being formulated to manage specific skin disorders. Whether they work depends heavily on the type of disorder and how diligently patients adhere to prescribed regimens. However, there is a long-standing intricacy because most individuals experience challenges in maintaining compliance owing to the chronic nature of skin illnesses. For instance, psoriasis patients typically present emotional suffering concerning their disorders, which in turn can hinder their drug regimen compliance. It is essential for medical professionals to understand these psychological and emotional factors to achieve better treatment outcomes and maximize the efficacy of topical treatments (Baker et al., 2016). Topical treatments also depend on the method of application and the drug's composition. Creams and ointments, for instance, may have variable rates of absorption, which will affect the drug's strength and overall action on the disease in question. Choice of a particular formulation must also consider the patient's own dermatological issue, lifestyle, and comfort factors. Moreover, advances in dermatology research emphasize the importance of an individualized approach to treatment, which can radically enhance compliance and efficiency. In the case of atopic eczema, good management, for example, requires careful documentation and follow-up on treatment response using standardized protocols (Apfelbacher et al., 2019). By addressing it with a tailored approach, family medicine doctors can deliver optimal results, thereby improving patients' quality of care across varying skin diseases. While there has been an increase in topical treatments, achieving optimal adherence among patients remains challenging. Research has shown that most patients find their medication regimens cumbersome, particularly those with diseases such as psoriasis. Psychological and emotional barriers have been found to cause nonadherence as the patient will find it hard to manage symptoms of the disease on the skin and the associated psychological stress. Interventions that target such barriers have been effective at improving adherence and thus clinical outcomes. In addition, patient engagement in co-decision-making for treatment plans has the potential to give patients a sense of ownership of their healthcare process and to further optimize treatment adherence. Therefore, addressing multi-dimensionality of adherence is central to enhancing the viability of topical treatments in family medicine practice (Baker et al., 2016) (Figure 8.15).

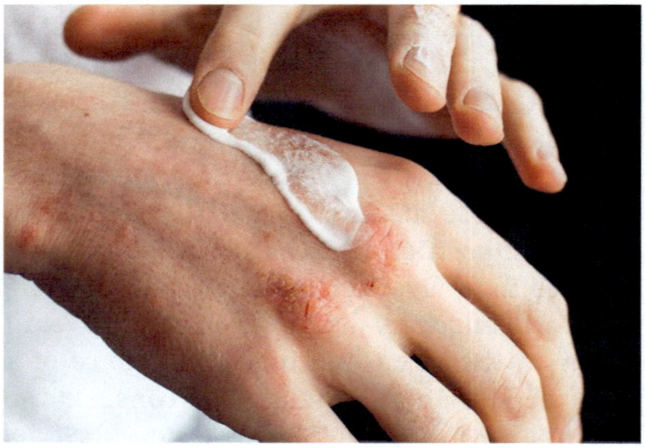

Figure 8.15. Topical treatments for skin problems.

Source: https://apollodermclinic.com/wp-content/uploads/2023/03/Topical-Steroids-Treatment-for-Various-Skin-Conditions-Apollo-Dermatology-Troy-MI.jpg.

8.4.2. Systemic Treatments for Severe Conditions

In dermatology, systemic treatments play an important role in managing severe skin illnesses with a highly dramatic effect on patients' quality of life. In diseases such as atopic dermatitis, characterized by intense itching and inflammation, systemic treatment often becomes necessary when topical treatment is not effective. A typical case in point is the instance of a young child who presents with an unhappy rash accompanied by persistent discomfort. In such a condition, systemic corticosteroids or immunomodulators are ordered to alleviate symptoms and control flares. Treatment of complicated atopic eczema not only includes effective medication but also requires an overall approach that considers possible psychosocial aspects and the need for ongoing patient education, thereby underscoring the key role of family physicians in integrated patient care (Formosa et al., 2007). Acne vulgaris is another skin condition that often requires systemic treatment, particularly in moderate to severe forms refractory to primary treatments such as topical retinoids or antibiotics. The multifactorial pathogenesis of acne, involving hormonal fluctuations, sebum hypersecretion, and inflammation, can further affect a patient's mental health and self-esteem. Recent studies have suggested potential dietary influences on acne severity, and thus, there is greater interest in knowing how systemic treatment, like oral isotretinoin, can optimally address the fundamental causes of this dermatological condition (Patton et al., 2016). Family medicine practitioners must sift through these multi-factorial elements to formulate personalized treatment regimens that not only address the physiological symptoms but also the psychological dimensions of the patient. Furthermore, discussion of systemic treatments extends beyond drug therapy; it involves taking up lifestyle problems and preventive interventions to avoid recurrences of life-threatening dermatological conditions. Systemic therapies hold promise for dramatic symptom and functioning improvement but also carry risks, such as side effects that require careful monitoring. As family medicine clinicians guide their patients through system-based care alternatives, they must provide extensive teaching on taking medications as prescribed, potential risks, and the necessity of follow-up appointments. By integrating these system-based care alternatives with continuous patient dialogue, clinicians enable the successful treatment of severe skin disease while establishing long-term patient relationships that lead to improved health outcomes and quality of life (Patton et al., 2016) (Figure 8.16).

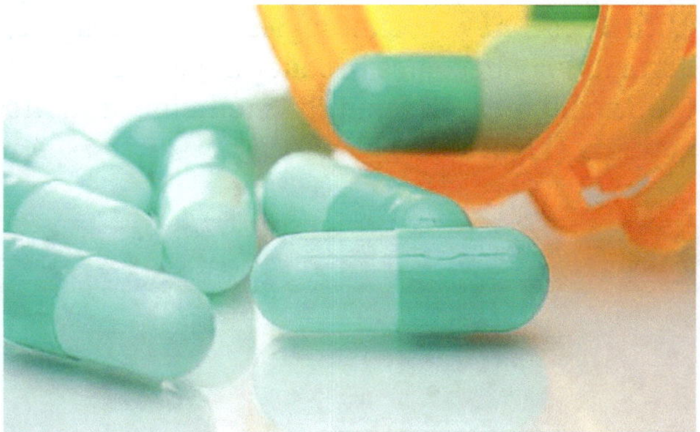

Figure 8.16. Systemic treatments for psoriasis.

Source: https://img.lb.wbmdstatic.com/vim/live/webmd/consumer_assets/site_images/article_thumbnails/reference_guide/systemic_treatments_for_psoriasis_ref_guide/650x350_systemic_treatments_for_psoriasis_ref_guide.jpg.

8.4.3. Emerging Therapies and Innovations

The last few years have witnessed significant progress in new therapies and technologies that enhance patient care in family medicine. A key area of interest is hyperhidrosis, an affliction affecting millions. In the past, therapy was confined to topical measures such as aluminum-based antiperspirants, which remain a first-line therapy option due to their immediate availability and cost-effectiveness (Jarrett et al., 2017). Nevertheless, current treatment approaches include newer modalities such as botulinum toxin injection and iontophoresis to offer options for individuals who are refractory to standard therapy. These new methods, in addition to improving patients' quality of life, also expand the array of therapeutic options available to family medicine providers so they can tailor therapies on a case-by-case basis. Another significant skin care innovation is the use of teledermatology and digital health technologies, which are best applied in family medicine practices. Teledermatology enables consultation from afar, more optimally allowing access for patients who may otherwise have difficulty accessing specialist visits. Using high-quality imaging and secure communication platforms, primary care providers can effectively triage dermatologic disorders and refer appropriately.

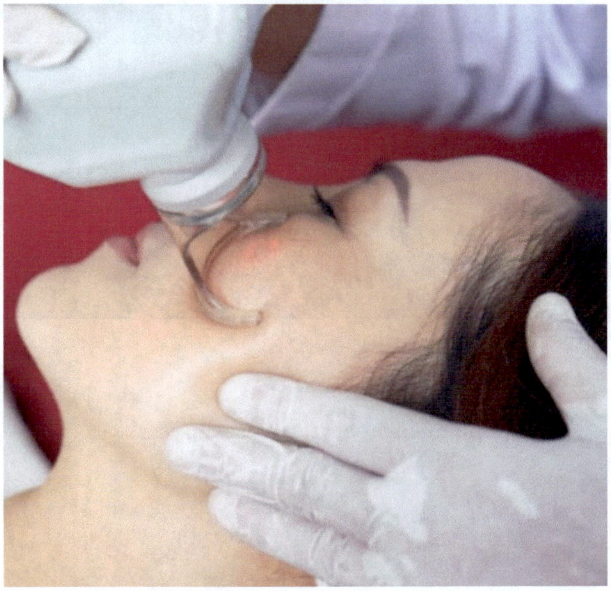

Figure 8.17. Innovations in dermatology: emerging technologies and trends.

Source: https://themedermatology.com/wp-content/uploads/2024/04/2.png.

This system not only reduces healthcare inefficiency costs but also enhances patient participation and compliance by facilitating timely follow-up. As these technologies advance, family medicine practitioners can treat a wide range of dermatologic disorders, from day-to-day skin complaints to complex diseases, thereby providing an all-around solution to patient care. Moreover, the introduction of biologic therapy is a revolutionary wave in dermatology. Biologics, aimed at specific mechanisms in the immune system, have been extremely useful in the treatment of chronic cutaneous conditions such as psoriasis and atopic dermatitis. These therapies mark a new plateau in therapy, especially for severely ill patients who are refractory to traditional therapy. The addition of biologics to family practice dermatology not only reflects progress in understanding the pathogenic processes of skin disorders but also signals a transition toward personalized medicine in family practice. This transition is marked by accumulating evidence of the safety and efficacy of biologics, honing family physicians' ability to deliver state-of-the-art, patient-tailored care (Baldo et al., 2015). With these new technologies and therapies, dermatology becomes broader in nature, which eventually benefits family medicine and its patients (Figure 8.17).

Test Your Knowledge

1. What are topical treatments?
2. What is a systemic treatment for skin disease?

8.5. Preventive Dermatology

Learning Outcome

1. Describe the skin cancer screening and awareness
2. Know the sun protection strategies
3. Understand the lifestyle modifications for skin health

Combining preventive dermatology with family medicine is crucial to ensure skin health and prevent dermatological disease. Preventive dermatology emphasizes early diagnosis and intervention procedures to manage probable skin disorders effectively. Incorporating routine skin checks into a regular family checkup enables the healthcare team to identify early warning signs of dermatological disorders, such as melanoma or eczema, and begin appropriate treatment in the proper time. Such preventive measures can markedly decrease the healthcare burden of chronic skin diseases on patients and the healthcare system overall. Moreover, patient education is important in reducing disease prevalence and improving quality of life, with regard to sun protection, skin cleansing, and lifestyle adjustments. The proactive approach of preventive dermatology is ideally suited to the goals of family medicine, where comprehensive patient care is the focus and encouraging a more comprehensive healthcare experience that addresses medical and preventive concerns. The integration of dermatology nurses into preventive dermatology adds another valuable dimension to patient care through family medicine. Dermatological nurses are central to patient education on skin health, risk factors, and the prevention of most dermatological conditions. Dermatological nurses are also central to motivating compliance through education, ensuring patients are adequately informed about their dermatological condition and the necessity of pre-emptive treatment. The communication offers a degree of trust with the patient, and hence, patients are encouraged and compliant with preventive measures and honest communication regarding their concerns. Besides that, dermatology nurses also tend to work closely with dermatologists and family physicians, which supports a multidisciplinary practice pattern that enhances patient outcomes. Appropriate collaboration among healthcare providers optimizes the likelihood of identifying risk factors across various populations and thus the efficacy of preventive dermatology in family practice (Chukwu et al., 2018). In addition, support for preventive dermatology is reinforced by findings indicating an increasing prevalence of skin disease in certain populations. Increasing urbanization and environmental changes have significantly contributed to the rise in cases of diseases such as canine atopic dermatitis—a comparison highlighting the need for integrative preventive measures. Such similarities in veterinary dermatology can teach family medicine practitioners about potential environmental factors affecting patients' skin health (Nødtvedt et al., 2007). Recognizing the community's epidemiological trends, family medicine doctors can adjust prevention methods to make them more applicable and impactful. Hence, preventive dermatology not only coexists comfortably with family medicine principles but also provides an opportunity for clinicians to apply knowledge derived from more universal dermatological science to enhance patient outcomes and, ultimately, healthier populations (Figure 8.18).

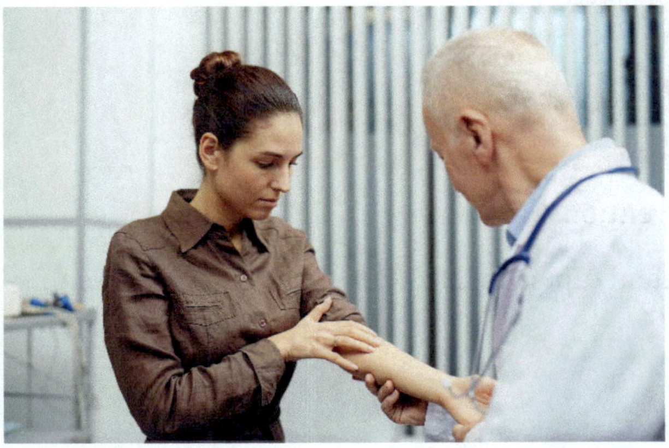

Figure 8.18. Prevention and management of skin disorders.

Source: https://www.health.com/thmb/j05U--EQnUu5uIGjpWJKqYT311Q=/2121x0/filters:no_upscale():max_bytes(150000):strip_icc()/Health-GettyImages-886098366-5a2b34568cc04e26ac9e1e72ce19c589.jpg.

8.5.1. Skin Cancer Screening and Awareness

Effective skin cancer examination and education are central components of family medicine dermatology as they play an immediate role in early diagnosis and patient prognosis. Patients tend to care about the skin, but most are not adequately educated about when to seek a specialist. As an illustration, a study conducted in Vermont found that patients are concerned about their nevi but lack specific knowledge of the features that warrant a referral to a specialist. To close this knowledge gap, educational resources, such as information pamphlets, have been developed to assist healthcare professionals in counseling their patients. The pamphlets describe the characteristics of melanocytic nevi and encourage individuals to be proactive with their healthcare providers when encountering suspicious results. This forward-thinking approach fosters an awareness and alertness culture, ultimately leading to higher rates of early detection and reducing the mortality rate of skin cancers such as melanoma (Logan et al., 2019). The work of health professionals goes beyond screening; education is at the core of providing patients with knowledge about skin cancer. Dermatological nurses, in particular, play a prominent role in this multifaceted approach by facilitating patient understanding and participation. Such experts are best suited to create patient-physician relationships of trust that will significantly enhance screening compliance and treatment adherence rates. Dermatology nurses teach patients through patient education programs to empower them with the skills and knowledge to recognize potential skin issues at an early stage. Education is very important because informed patients are likely to get medical assistance early, thus enhancing the overall efficiency of dermatological treatment. As such, expanding the role of nursing in ways that increase awareness of skin cancer benefits patients themselves as well as the broader agenda of family medicine in promoting preventive care (Chukwu et al., 2018). Furthermore, the challenges associated with screening for skin cancer can have significant impacts on patient compliance and awareness. Socioeconomic status, cultural issues, and limited knowledge of skin ailments can be impediments to patients' access to necessary healthcare services. Patients sometimes have misconceptions about the need for frequent skin check-ups or feel embarrassed when discussing their problems. Hence, education and accessibility must become priorities for family medicine doctors in clinics. Integrating skin cancer education programs within routine care can address such issues, thereby making a more participatory concept of health. By directly engaging patients through modified education campaigns and information, family medicine can develop a system in which skin cancer screening is an integral component of healthcare, ultimately improving early detection rates and outcomes for patients at risk (Chukwu et al., 2018; Logan et al., 2019) (Figure 8.19).

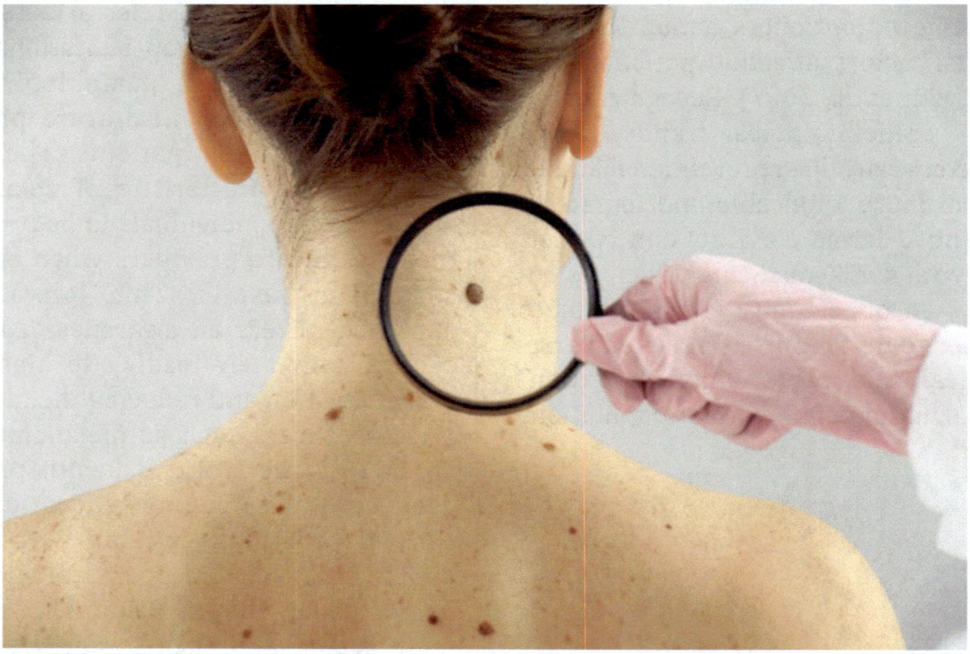

Figure 8.19. Skin cancer awareness: prioritize prevention.

Source: https://www.newportbeachdps.com/wp-content/uploads/2024/06/Skin-Cancer-Screening-scaled-1.jpg

8.5.2. Sun Protection Strategies

Sun protection strategies are part of dermatological practice in family medicine, primarily aimed at preventing skin cancer and photoaging. Education campaigns have been a significant part of informing the population about the risks of sun exposure. In Malta, a rise in the incidence of skin cancer, for instance, prompted targeted campaigns that were significantly responsible for raising awareness and changing behavior for this purpose. A review of survey results reveals that, while knowledge of sunscreen application was stable, there were disconcerting trends, including a decline in hat use and greater participation in outdoor leisure activities during peak sun periods, indicating that education must be revolutionary to address shifting attitudes and actions (Amato-Gauci et al., 2008).

Dermatologists are able to capitalize on such data along with family practitioners to revamp community health programs that promote awareness and adherence to sun protection. Furthermore, a well-executed sun protection regimen encompasses several practical aspects, including the use of broad-spectrum sunscreen, protective clothing, and behavioral changes.

The dermatological community promotes the utilization of sunscreen with at least SPF 30, which protects against UVA and UVB radiation. In addition to sunscreen, hats and long-sleeved shirts can also provide valuable protection from harmful sun exposure during outdoor activities. These strategies, combined with family lifestyles, can promote a lifetime of sun-protection practices, significantly reducing the risk of melanoma and other skin cancers. The responsibility does not only lie with the healthcare practitioners to encourage these practices but also falls on the families to adopt sun-safe habits themselves so that their children would pick it up by imitation, and sun protection becomes a habit for them (Birlea et al., 2018).

Finally, the inclusion of recent advances in melanocyte biology and skin cancer pathogenesis gives better insight into effective sun protection. Current advances illustrate how a knowledge of the molecular pathways of the skin's response to ultraviolet radiation informs dermatologists practice in prescribing preventive measures. Discussion of immunotherapy and genetic predisposition further underscores the need for individualized sun protection measures, particularly for those at higher risk of skin cancer. These focused strategies, ideally, would include learning about sun exposure limits, as well as dermatological assessments tailored to an individual's skin type and history. Thus, translating these findings into family practice enables a greater impact on public health, as families become aware of their own risk factors and of protection against the sun (Amato-Gauci et al., 2008; Birlea et al., 2018).

8.5.3. Lifestyle Modifications for Skin Health

Lifestyle modifications are key to maximizing skin health in family medicine dermatology. The skin is a barrier that expresses overall health and well-being. Family physicians are best suited to encourage lifestyle changes to preserve skin integrity, such as dietary modifications, hydration, and sun protection.

Dietary lifestyles that emphasize high intake of antioxidants, vitamins, and essential fats can also affect the appearance and functioning of the skin. Foods high in omega-3 fatty acids, vitamins E and C, and polyphenols have been found to alleviate inflammatory skin disorders and promote overall dermatological well-being. With the integration of these dietary alterations into patient care, family physicians can encourage an active approach to dermatological issues, thereby enhancing patients' quality of life (Alhuthayli et al., 2023). Even proper hydration is a lifestyle change that requires attention in both prevention and treatment of skin disorders.

The water content of the skin directly affects its resilience and elasticity, and therefore its appearance and function. It is imperative that family physicians emphasize adequate fluid intake as an easy yet effective way to maintain hydrated skin. Additionally, it is important to encourage patients to avoid excessive alcohol and caffeine use, which causes dehydration. Education on the benefits of moisturizing agents, particularly for people who live in dry environments or have dry skin, may be integral to overall skin health management. General practitioners can empower patients through these discussions to make good decisions that enhance skin wellness (Alhuthayli et al., 2023). Sun protection is among the lifestyle modifications for skin health that cannot be excluded in family medicine practice. Ultraviolet (UV) radiation overexposure is a major risk factor for premature aging of the skin and skin cancers, and sun protection thus falls under patient education. Family physicians should encourage the use of daily broad-spectrum sunscreen application, protective clothing, and shade, particularly during peak sun exposure times. Additionally, emphasizing the importance of periodic skin examinations for diagnosing potential malignancies can empower patients with the tools to effectively protect their skin. By establishing a setting that optimizes sun protection and includes periodic skin examinations, family practitioners can significantly reduce the long-term sequelae of UV exposure, thereby ensuring overall dermatological health and patient well-being (Figure 8.20).

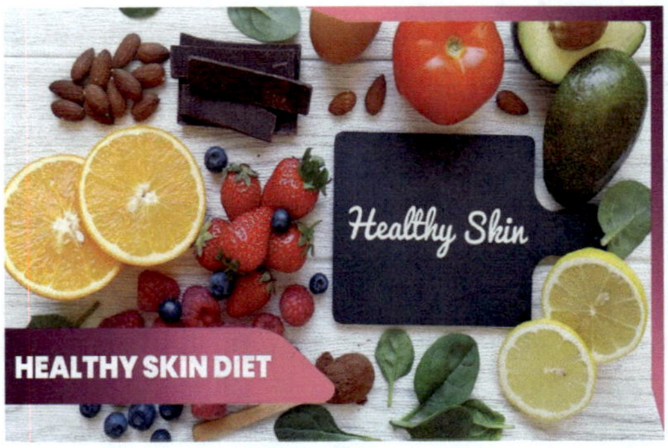

Figure 8.20. Healthy skin diet.

Source: https://fitnesswithnidhi.com/wp-content/uploads/2024/06/Healthy-Skin-Diet-scaled.jpg.

Test Your Knowledge

1. What is a skin cancer screening?
2. What are the sun protection strategies?

SUMMARY

In documenting the emergence of dermatology in family medicine, it is important to recognize that dermatologic conditions are central to patient health and well-being across diverse populations. Family medicine is a core healthcare model in which practitioners are often the first point of entry for patients with dermatological concerns. As such, they must be equipped with the knowledge needed to diagnose and manage these prevalent skin conditions. The increasing number of diseases such as atopic dermatitis, as observed among both dogs and human beings, is an indication of the necessity for a better understanding of skin diseases against the background of family medicine. Through a focus on dermatoses training and education, family physicians can create more potential to provide complete care that addresses physical and psychological aspects of skin health and ultimately treat a multicultural patient population (Nødtvedt et al., 2007). Furthermore, the impact of industry affiliations and payment models on dermatology practices cannot be overlooked. The association between physician profiles and industry payment value reveals significant disparities in the delivery and access to dermatologic services. With high industry payments to a select number of physicians, based on years of experience and specialty, family medicine may be at a disadvantage in delivering equal dermatology care. These forces are essential to recognize, particularly since management of skin conditions typically requires referral to dermatologists and continuing professional development in skin-related matters (Blumenthal et al., 2019). Knowledge of these forces shaping the industry can inform family medicine practitioners' prescribing practices and communication with pharmaceutical representatives, so that patient care remains at the forefront of their practice. Finally, the future of dermatology in family medicine requires joint initiatives in research and innovation that can influence patient care. As the field continues to evolve and new technologies and treatments are introduced, family physicians need to be well-versed and quick to respond. Emphasis on preventive treatment and early intervention will be critical in the treatment of chronic skin conditions whose effects can extend far into patients' lives. Furthermore, closing gaps in interdisciplinarity between dermatologists and family physicians can lead to more comprehensive approaches and better health outcomes for patients. As the urban-rural relationship, with its increased incidence of certain dermatological disorders, illustrates, more research is indicated to address the environmental determinants of skin health. Lastly, the integration of dermatological science into family medicine fosters improved patient care and health promotion among multicultural populations (Nødtvedt et al., 2007; Blumenthal et al., 2019).

In family medicine practices, several key considerations arise that lead to the inclusion of dermatologic services within primary health care centers. Increased participation by primary care doctors is necessary for dermatologic care to become more accessible. By educating and training family doctors in the identification and treatment of common skin disorders, the healthcare system can relieve pressure on specialists. This shift not only makes patient treatment easier but also encourages a healthier approach to health, allowing early diagnosis and treatment of dermatologic diseases in an established health care system. This integration also aligns with broader healthcare programs aimed at improving service delivery, such as managed care and team-based care, and, overall, leads to better health outcomes for patients across diverse populations. Moreover, family medicine doctors' contributions to the management of dermatological problems reflect a greater understanding of the interplay between skin health and patients' overall well-being. With an increased number of family doctors adept at diagnosing and treating dermatologic problems, there is potential to better manage chronic diseases such as psoriasis and eczema, which have a profound effect on patients' quality of life. Enhanced access to dermatology evaluation and treatment via primary care reduces healthcare spending on avoidable referrals as well as improves patient satisfaction and outcomes. Programs such as those supporting team practice and integrated service provision enable this trend by embracing interprofessional practice among health professionals to address comprehensive patient needs, both physical and psychological. Last but not least, alternative treatments and holistic healing have become prominent. Such conferences emphasize the need for family medicine physicians to be knowledgeable about all treatment modalities, including lifestyle modification and wellness interventions. Identifying these alternative therapies can enable family medicine practitioners to offer patients whole-person care options, thereby fostering treatment adherence and enhancing health literacy. Addressing skin health from multiple angles enables healthcare professionals to treat dermatological conditions with greater attention to patients' psychosocial circumstances. This expansive approach finally fits into larger patterns in family medicine to offer patient-centered care that acknowledges the multi-dimensional nature of health and healing in the community.

KEY TERMS FROM THIS CHAPTER

- Acne
- Autoimmune disorders
- Cryotherapy
- Diabetes
- Healthcare
- Nail disorders
- Psoriasis
- Anxiety
- Cardiovascular disease
- Dermatology
- Eczema
- Metabolic syndrome
- Patient satisfaction
- Skin biopsies

CRITICAL THINKING QUESTIONS

1. **Which of the following is the most common skin condition seen in primary care?**
   a. Psoriasis
   b. Acne vulgaris
   c. Melanoma
   d. Lichen planus
2. **What is the most common cause of contact dermatitis?**
   a. Allergic reaction to a substance
   b. Genetic predisposition
   c. Viral infection
   d. Bacterial overgrowth
3. **Which skin lesion is most characteristic of psoriasis?**
   a. Pearly, umbilicated papules
   b. Silvery scaly plaques on extensor surfaces
   c. Irregular pigmented patches with raised edges
   d. Honey-colored crusts on an erythematous base
4. **Which condition is commonly associated with the "herald patch"?**
   a. Pityriasis rosea
   b. Psoriasis
   c. Eczema
   d. Tinea corporis
5. **What is the first-line treatment for mild to moderate acne vulgaris?**
   a. Systemic corticosteroids
   b. Topical retinoids and benzoyl peroxide
   c. Oral isotretinoin
   d. Antifungal creams

Short Answer Questions

1. What is dermatology?
2. What is the importance of dermatology in family medicine?
3. What are the most common dermatological conditions?
4. Describe the role of family physicians in dermatology.
5. What are the treatment modalities of?

Answer to Critical Thinking Questions

1. (b); 2. (a); 3. (b); 4. (a); 5. (b).

REFERENCES

1. Sampogna, F., Abeni, D., Gieler, U., Tomas-Aragones, L., Lien, L., Titeca, G., Jemec, G. B. E., Misery, L., Szabó, C., Linder, M. D., Evers, A. W. M., Halvorsen, J. A., Balieva, F., Szepietowski, J. C., Romanov, D. V., Marron, S. E., Altunay, I. K., Finlay, A. Y., Salek, S. S., . . . Dalgard, F. (2016). Impairment of sexual life in 3,485 dermatological outpatients from a multicentre study in 13 European countries. *Acta Dermato Venereologica*, *97*(4), 478–482. https://doi.org/10.2340/00015555-2561Abiri, M., Barzegar, M., Ertel, A., et al. (2017). Dystrophic epidermolysis bullosa: COL7A1 mutation landscape in a multi-ethnic cohort of 152 extended families with high degree of customary consanguineous marriages. https://core.ac.uk/download/98337377.pdf (accessed on 12th July 2025).
2. Adaskevich, V. P., Katsina, M. A., & Tsikhanouskaya, I. V. (2014). Basic dermatology. https://core.ac.uk/download/80151520.pdf (accessed on 12th July 2025).
3. Adibi, N., Ahmadzadeh, M. R., Barati, E., et al. (2011). A survey on utilization of data mining approaches for dermatological (skin) diseases prediction. https://core.ac.uk/download/1667194.pdf (accessed on 12th July 2025).
4. Agache, I., Bachert, C., Bedbrook, A., et al. (2016). ARIA 2016: Care pathways implementing emerging technologies for predictive medicine in rhinitis and asthma across the life cycle. https://core.ac.uk/download/77614616.pdf (accessed on 12th July 2025).
5. Aigner, F., Pratschke, J., Schumann, T., et al. (2020). Recent advances and the potential for clinical use of autofluorescence detection of extra-ophthalmic tissues. https://core.ac.uk/download/323257980.pdf (accessed on 12th July 2025).
6. Alhuthayli, A. K. A., Almalki, A. S. O., Alharbi, A. S. A., Alneami, A. M., Fadl, A. A., Alsahli, H. M., Alshammari, H. S. A., et al. (2023). Pediatric dermatology in family medicine: Common conditions and management strategies. https://core.ac.uk/download/603897541.pdf (accessed on 12th July 2025).
7. Amato-Gauci, A. J., Aquilina, S., Calleja, N., et al. (2008). Trends in sun exposure awareness and protection practices in Malta: 1999–2004. https://core.ac.uk/download/46602201.pdf (accessed on 12th July 2025).
8. Apfelbacher, B., Blume-Peytavi, U., Boguniewicz, M., et al. (2014). Emollient enhancement of the skin barrier from birth offers effective atopic dermatitis prevention. https://core.ac.uk/download/30662564.pdf (accessed on 12th July 2025).
9. Apfelbacher, C. J., Arents, B. W. M., Barbarot, S., et al. (2019). TREatment of ATopic eczema (TREAT) Registry Taskforce: Consensus on how and when to measure the core dataset for atopic eczema treatment research registries. https://core.ac.uk/download/323310740.pdf (accessed on 12th July 2025).
10. Baker, T., Baumeister, D., Carver, C., Cohen, S., Detweiler-Bedell, J., DiMatteo, M., et al. (2016). Nonadherence to psoriasis medication as an outcome of limited coping resources and conflicting goals: Findings from a qualitative interview study with people with psoriasis. https://core.ac.uk/download/286713998.pdf (accessed on 12th July 2025).
11. Baldo, V., Buja, A., Carraro, D., et al. (2015). Out-of-hours primary care services: Demands and patient referral patterns in a Veneto region (Italy) Local Health Authority. https://core.ac.uk/download/53516100.pdf (accessed on 12th July 2025).

12. Basra, M. K. A., Finlay, A. Y., Golics, C. J., et al. (2013). The impact of patients' chronic disease on family quality of life: An experience from 26 specialties. https://core.ac.uk/download/287581121.pdf (accessed on 12th July 2025).

13. Beck, K., Bhutani, T., Chang, A. Y., et al. (2020). Implementation of an ultraviolet phototherapy service at a national referral hospital in Western Kenya: Reflections on challenges and lessons learned. https://core.ac.uk/download/323072276.pdf (accessed on 12th July 2025).

14. BEEP study team, Boyle, R. J., Bradshaw, L. E., Brown, S. J., et al. (2020). Daily emollient during infancy for prevention of eczema: The BEEP randomised controlled trial. https://core.ac.uk/download/287649733.pdf (accessed on 12th July 2025).

15. Berardesca, E., Bernardini, N., Bianchi, L., et al. (2018). Use of biological drugs in patients with psoriasis and psoriatic arthritis in Italy: Results from the PSONG survey. https://core.ac.uk/download/154948747.pdf (accessed on 12th July 2025).

16. Birlea, S., Bosenberg, M. W., Box, N. F., et al. (2018). Frontiers in pigment cell and melanoma research. http://arxiv.org/abs/1808.01869 (accessed on 12th July 2025).

17. Bluestein, D., Gnilka, B., & Lazernick, B. (2020). The Health Empowerment Program: A primary care – area agency on aging partnership. https://core.ac.uk/download/287016545.pdf (accessed on 12th July 2025).

18. Blumenthal, D. M., Elashoff, D., Inoue, K., et al. (2019). Association between physician characteristics and payments from industry in 2015–2017: Observational study. https://core.ac.uk/download/323076301.pdf (accessed on 12th July 2025).

19. Boffa, M. J. (2004). Dermatology. https://core.ac.uk/download/46601884.pdf (accessed on 12th July 2025).

20. Bray, J. K., Feldman, S. R., Huang, W. W., et al. (2020). Publication rates on the topic of racial and ethnic diversity in dermatology versus other specialties. https://core.ac.uk/download/322493872.pdf (accessed on 12th July 2025).

21. Burke, M. (2018). Effect of a clinical evidence technology on patient skin disease outcomes in primary care: A cluster-randomized controlled trial. https://core.ac.uk/download/215154033.pdf (accessed on 12th July 2025).

22. Burke, M. D., Littenberg, B., et al. (2020). Barriers and facilitators to use of a clinical evidence technology in the management of skin problems in primary care: Insights from mixed methods. https://core.ac.uk/download/289036096.pdf (accessed on 12th July 2025).

23. Burrows, N. P., Emery, J., Hall, P. N., et al. (2019). Dermoscopy for melanoma detection and triage in primary care: A systematic review. https://core.ac.uk/download/222832482.pdf (accessed on 12th July 2025).

24. Carlson, C., Sholk, J., Nanni, J., Peterson, K., Smith, L. A., & Bhavaraju, N. (2016). Breaking the barriers to specialty care: Practical ideas to improve health equity and reduce cost–Increasing specialty care availability. https://core.ac.uk/download/75785770.pdf (accessed on 12th July 2025).

25. Chukwu, R., & Mankila, J. (2018). Dermatology nurses' job description: Literature review. https://core.ac.uk/download/161432240.pdf (accessed on 12th July 2025).

26. Cole, S. A. (2020). Individual and collective identification in contemporary forensics. https://core.ac.uk/download/323082704.pdf (accessed on 12th July 2025).

27. Formosa, M. C. (2007). Atopic eczema. https://core.ac.uk/download/46602108.pdf (accessed on 12th July 2025).

28. Gauci, C., Pace, L., & Sammut, M. R. (2014). The attitudes, knowledge, and practices of Maltese family doctors in disease prevention and health promotion. https://core.ac.uk/download/46602512.pdf (accessed on 12th July 2025).

29. Jarrett, J. B., Moss, D., & Mounsey, A. (2017). Oral agent offers relief from generalized hyperhidrosis. https://core.ac.uk/download/98352896.pdf (accessed on 12th July 2025).

30. Jenevein, C. L. (2015). Texas physicians' awareness and utilization of genetic services. https://core.ac.uk/download/46720101.pdf (accessed on 12th July 2025).

31. Lieberman, M. R., Schwartz, Z., & Siegel, D. M. (2020). The evolving maintenance of certification process: Update on the financial status of the medical boards. https://core.ac.uk/download/287622748.pdf (accessed on 12th July 2025).

32. Lo Sicco, K., Novice, M., Novice, T., et al. (2022). The impact and implications of COVID-19 on using scalp cooling therapy for prevention of chemotherapy-induced alopecia. https://core.ac.uk/download/542715664.pdf (accessed on 12th July 2025).

33. Logan, S. (2019). Melanoma surveillance. https://core.ac.uk/download/215156030.pdf (accessed on 12th July 2025).

34. Mair, F. S., McMillan, S. S., Salehi, A., et al. (2017). Measuring the burden of treatment for chronic disease: Implications of a scoping review of the literature. https://core.ac.uk/download/96884695.pdf (accessed on 12th July 2025).

35. Nesbitt, T. S., & Young, H. M. (2017). Increasing the capacity of primary care through enabling technology. https://core.ac.uk/download/323070127.pdf (accessed on 12th July 2025).

36. Nicholson, S. (2025). Barriers to entering medical specialties. https://core.ac.uk/download/pdf/6716587.pdf (accessed on 12th July 2025).

37. Nødtvedt, A. (2007). Epidemiology of canine atopic dermatitis. https://core.ac.uk/download/11695161.pdf (accessed on 12th July 2025).

38. Patton, E. E. (2016). Nutritional factors associated with acne vulgaris. https://open.bu.edu/bitstream/2144/19444/1/Patton_bu_0017N_12304.pdf (accessed on 12th July 2025).

39. Ramirez, F., Heinrich, M., Leonti, M., et al. (2018). Medicinal flora of the Popoluca, Mexico: A botanical systematical perspective. https://core.ac.uk/download/159154488.pdf (accessed on 12th July 2025).

40. Sartorius, K. (2010). Hidradenitis suppurativa: Clinical studies with focus on evaluation. https://core.ac.uk/download/70338703.pdf (accessed on 12th July 2025).

41. Sullivan, K. M. (2017). Promotion of skin protection in children in Waterbury, VT. https://core.ac.uk/download/79664984.pdf (accessed on 12th July 2025).

PEDIATRIC CARE

9

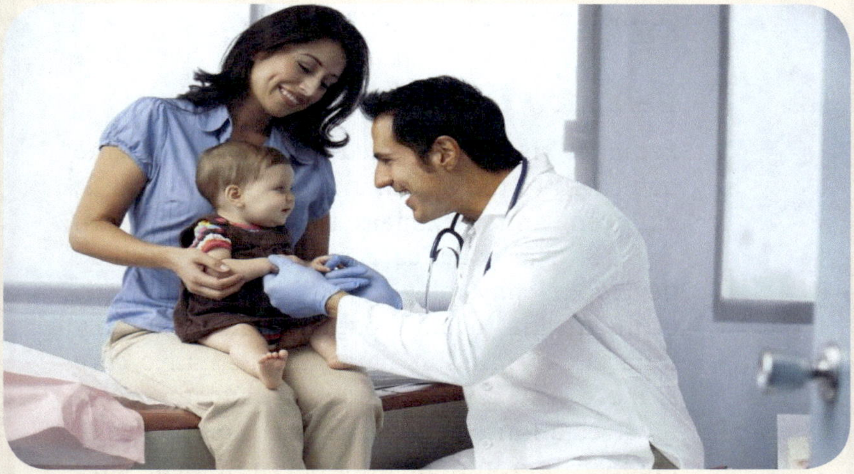

Introduction

In the medical sector, pediatric care is a key specialty that addresses the unique developmental, physical, and mental needs of children from infancy to young adulthood. The contribution of early intervention in pediatric institutions cannot be overstated, as many health issues identified in childhood have long-term effects on overall health and well-being throughout the life course. Pediatric practice encompasses many aspects, ranging from preventive health to the care of acute and chronic illnesses to mental health care. Because children are likely to have symptoms different from those of adults and might not be able to communicate their needs efficiently, pediatric professionals must have broad knowledge of child development principles. Hence, the need for individualized models of care and evidence-based interventions is a major priority for improving the quality of health outcomes among children. The complexity layer for pediatric care also fits within the domain of bereavement and mental health concerns, namely, the experience of loss among families that present with it. Bereaved

LEARNING OBJECTIVES

After studying this chapter, you will be able to:

1. Describe the historical development of pediatric care
2. Know the pediatric health issues
3. Understand the pediatric care settings
4. Understand the role of pediatric healthcare providers
5. Describe the family involvement in pediatric care
6. Understand the advances in pediatric care

parent interventions are particularly significant as they address the physical and emotional trauma of bereavement during those escalated periods of child development. Researchers have identified a range of interventions, from expressive arts therapy to holistic support systems incorporating health-care resources and peer networks, through systematic literature reviews. However, such interventions work to varying degrees, as research has documented, ranging from very weak to moderate in study strength.

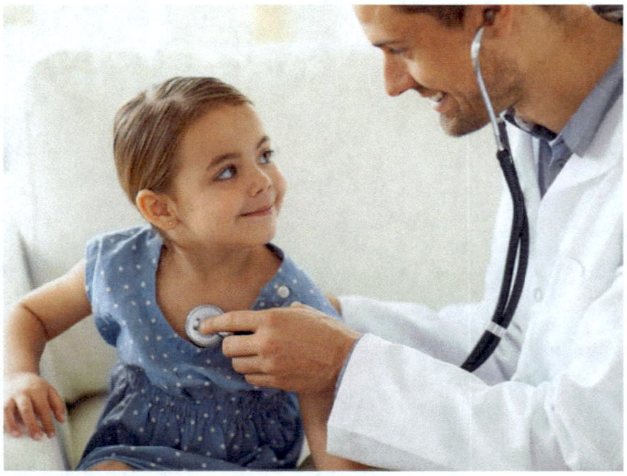

Figure 9.1. Pediatric care.

Source: https://centrichealthcare.org/wp-content/uploads/2021/08/546c7b_a368e4fa440e4ad29f7046cf1a2d0c32_mv2.jpg.

This variation indicates a crying need for stronger, more person-centered care strategies that clearly show theoretical justification and otherwise adequately address the multifaceted needs of bereaved parents, thereby supporting their psychological well-being after extreme loss (Boring et al., 2019). Pediatric mental health strategies to improve early intervention have emerged as essential components across all U.S. states. Colorado, Indiana, Massachusetts, and Rhode Island programs underscored joint initiatives to create robust mental health identification and intervention systems for children up to age 5. These initiatives demonstrate serious hindrances such as funding constraints and the need for effective cooperation among stakeholders. The results of these programs demonstrate the critical importance of cooperation among various sectors—schools, community groups, and health care—to create an enabling environment that fosters children's mental well-being. This integration not only encourages offering pediatric services but also highlights the importance of reform efforts to meet the diverse needs of children and families and foster even more holistic pediatric care (Lyman et al., 2010) (Figure 9.1).

Definition of Pediatric Care

Pediatrics is a specialized branch of medicine dedicated to the health and welfare of infants, children, and teenagers from birth through age 18. The practice recognizes the unique developing, physiological, and emotional needs of infant and juvenile patients and is notably different from adult medicine. Pediatric care is more than a series of clinical encounters; it involves an integrated approach incorporating medical, emotional, and psychological care tailored to the particular child and the family as a whole. Effective pediatric care requires healthcare providers to have an excellent understanding of children's diseases and disorders, as well as the environmental and social determinants associated with children's health. These considerations are central to creating an enabling environment that maximizes the physical and mental well-being of pediatric patients, with an emphasis on continuity of care across developmental stages. The model of effective pediatric care transcends traditional medical care and demands collaboration among sectors such as education and family support services. Pediatric care coordination in the recent literature is the efficient and organized integration of healthcare, school services, and community resources that together support the child's development. Implementing such a system is crucial in effective simplification of the complicated issues children face, particularly those with chronic conditions or developmental disabilities. This combined strategy, which bridges medical professionals with educational and family support systems, enables clinicians to create tailored interventions that enhance children's overall well-being. The importance of this collaborative process cannot be emphasized enough, as it facilitates early detection and treatment of health concerns, thus yielding better results for young patients and families (McAllister et al., 2009). A second level of complexity in the care of children is medication administration, since so many medicines are not formulated for children. Lack of available appropriate drugs for children creates serious problems for efficacious treatment, compliance, and general health outcomes in child populations. A Tanzanian survey illuminated pediatric prescribing and drug administration practices, including preferences for medicine sweetness and oral liquid preparation requirements among younger age groups. These results highlight the pivotal significance of pharmaceutical development that meets the unique needs and preferences of pediatric patients. It is necessary that healthcare systems respond to these findings, overcoming impediments to optimal administration and minimizing issues such as poor tolerability and risks of under- or over-dosing (Sachs et al., 2013). Therefore, the concept of pediatric care now encompasses not just the child's health but also the processes and structures that ensure effective and acceptable treatment.

Importance of Pediatric Care in Healthcare

Pediatric medicine plays a significant role in the general health system by virtue of its focus on the unique physical, emotional, and developmental needs of children. Compared to adults, youngsters undergo radical growth and development within their formative years that demand special medical attention to address prevention, diagnosis, care, and their respective phases of development. Acknowledgment by the healthcare system of these needs necessitates that comprehensive pediatric care be delivered that takes into account a child's overall health. As reiterated in contemporary models of health, including the Institute for Healthcare Improvement's Triple Aim, optimal pediatric care not only needs to improve patient experiences and outcomes but also to make healthcare more cost-effective and efficient. This strategic alignment is also essential to the strategy for addressing long-term child health pathways to the future adult population and for ensuring these children receive the best possible start in life towards a healthy life (Caron et al., 2019). Pediatric care can also deal with key social determinants of health disproportionately affecting young populations, particularly low-income and minority groups. Availability of quality care is often tied to socio-economic status, leading to health disparities that may be carried into adulthood. Trauma-informed care practices help pediatricians better meet the psychological needs of at-risk populations, ultimately improving health equity. A review of the implementation of trauma-informed behavioral health practices in pediatric primary care clinics points out that implementation is paramount to counter the many issues children and families face, especially when such families have limited resources. Apart from facilitating a quick response to traumatic stress by providers, implementation fosters a healthy, supportive healthcare environment, which is paramount to pediatric care in general (Aceves et al., 2021). Lastly, by emphasizing preventive care and early intervention, pediatric care is a central pillar in minimizing future healthcare costs and community health outcomes. If children receive appropriate preventive services, such as routine screenings and immunizations, the risk of developing severe illness later in life is significantly reduced. Through this vision-oriented method, the economic cost to the healthcare system that otherwise would be incurred in treating mature-stage disease is eliminated. Health systems that invest in pediatric care, in effect, guarantee the long-term viability of healthcare. Therefore, prioritizing pediatric care is not merely a moral imperative but also a sensible step in the interest of society as a whole, as it ensures healthier generations to come who can lead productive lives without the drag of prolonged health issues (Figure 9.2).

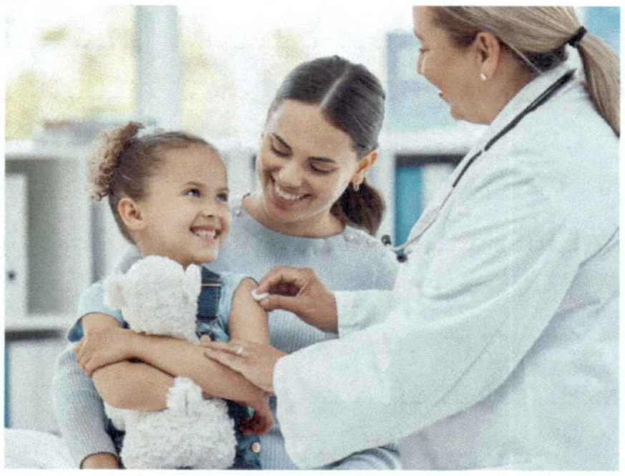

Figure 9.2. The vital importance of pediatric care.

Source: https://reddymedicalgroup.com/wp-content/uploads/2024/03/AdobeStock_606494893-1920w.webp.

9.1. Historical Development of Pediatric Care

Learning Outcome

1. Know the evolution of pediatric medicine
2. Understand the key figures in pediatric history
3. Describe the milestones in pediatric care practices

The historical development of pediatric care has evolved significantly over the centuries, reflecting changes in societal attitudes and advances in medical knowledge. In ancient times, children were often viewed merely as miniature adults, leading to inappropriate treatment and care. It was not until the late 19th century that pediatric medicine began to emerge as a distinct specialty. It was largely initiated by forerunners such as Dr. Abraham Jacobi, often termed the father of pediatrics in America. Jacob's initiatives towards the establishment of children's hospitals and his emphasis on the unique medical needs of children formed the foundation for pediatric treatment as it is known today. His contributions stressed the necessity of targeted interventions in the pediatric age group, resulting in the development of specialized child study and training in child health. Dramatic advances continued through the 20th century, with advancements in public health and Medicare. The establishment of the American Academy of Pediatrics in 1930 was pivotal as it unified the pediatricians to advance children's health and well-being. This period also saw the introduction of vaccines and antibiotics, which dramatically reduced child mortality from infectious diseases. Additionally, advances in pediatric research enabled a better understanding of pediatric diseases and the identification of psychosocial determinants affecting pediatric health. Preventive medicine and public health education were the main areas of concern, with pediatricians increasingly focused on achieving public health by promoting the wellness of children. These developments put greater emphasis on a balanced approach, treating not just the physical health of children but also their emotional and developmental needs. More recently, the field of pediatrics has expanded further to encompass cutting-edge technology and greater knowledge of chronic childhood diseases. The creation of platforms such as Tidepool, which aims to bring together diabetes device data with an open-source strategy, is the best example of how modern technology is being integrated into pediatrics. This device-agnostic method maximizes data availability and improves the interoperability of medical devices, thereby fostering innovation in chronic disease management, particularly for children with type 1 diabetes (Adi et al., 2015). Also, the call for preparedness in pediatric care during health emergencies, i.e., potential pandemics, is key to shedding light on adaptive approaches to healthcare. Reminders on vaccine dosages and management protocols also demonstrate advancements in pediatric care as practitioners strive to protect and improve children's health. As pediatric practice continues to evolve, it remains characterized by an activist philosophy, emphasizing synergy among diverse stakeholders to achieve integrated health outcomes for children (Figure 9.3).

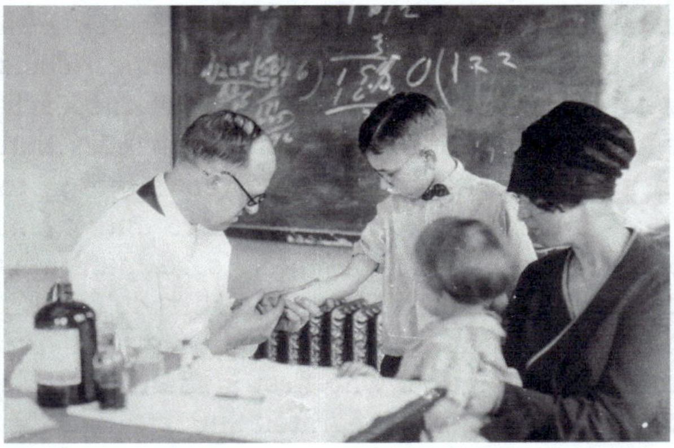

Figure 9.3. The history of pediatrics.

Source: https://globmed.co.uk/wp-content/uploads/2023/11/history_of_Paediatrics-2-scaled.jpg.

9.1.1. Evolution of Pediatric Medicine

The history of pediatrics has witnessed an enormous transformation from its early origins to the present. Historically, children were given the status of small adults and were administered the same drugs without considering their unique physiological and psychological requirements. With an increased understanding of child development, the position of pediatrics as a distinct branch came to the forefront. This shift made specialized techniques focused on children's developmental milestones, emotional growth, and preventive medicine a central part of pediatric practices. With advances in research and clinical practices, the profession has become increasingly evidence-based, leading to better health outcomes. The history of pediatric medicine is a witness to a long-term commitment to the study of the complexities of children's health and the all-around care needs of developing children, a prelude to more comprehensive and enhanced pediatric care in the medical systems of the contemporary world. Pediatric medicine in recent decades has been marked by a wave of technical advancements and collaboration in medical research. With the advent of sophisticated diagnostic tools, such as genetic testing and new imaging technology, medical professionals can diagnose a host of childhood diseases in time and with greater precision. These improvements have overhauled the treatment and management of child diseases, particularly the uncommon ones, which were previously challenging due to their elusive nature. The establishment of international programs and collaborative networks has also facilitated data sharing and the development of uniform protocols in pediatric research. Consequently, health practitioners can now engage in pediatric practice with improved methods that guarantee patient safety and ethical standards. Further innovations in technology reinforce the implementation of such innovations into pediatric practice to advance effective treatment and responsive healthcare provision. The discipline of pediatric oncology demonstrates most vividly the spectacular improvement in pediatric medicine, with emphasis on the impact of tailored treatment regimens and multidisciplinary care. Cancer in children, although less common than in adults, is a serious challenge to pediatric morbidity. Hence, the evolution of treatment modalities like chemotherapy, radiotherapy, and more modern targeted therapies represents a drift toward individualized treatment based on the particular needs of children. Furthermore, the psychosocial aspect of survivorship has gained greater acceptance, with emphasis on the necessity of psychological support and education for children undergoing cancer treatment. Concern for long-term side effects and quality of life in survivors has led current pediatric oncology to not only improve survival but also well-being following treatment. This focus on care of the whole person is a direct demonstration of the transformation of pediatric medicine as it shifts to meet the demands of an increasingly complex healthcare landscape, maintaining the priorities of children at the forefront of clinical practice (Goldblatt et al., 2019; Deb et al., 2025).

9.1.2. Key Figures in Pediatric History

The evolution of pediatric practice has largely been shaped by such pioneering practitioners whose efforts have advanced the treatment and knowledge of children's diseases. Dr. Benjamin Spock is well-known as one such iconoclast in the field. His publication of The Common Sense Book of Baby and Child Care in 1946 revolutionized parenting cultures and placed tremendous emphasis on a child-centered culture. Placing emotional attention ahead of physical attention, Spock's writings attracted an estimated 1 million professionals and parents, enabling them to design healthier homes. This shift in thinking not only cured short-term medical conditions but also opened a doorway to a more comprehensive child-development model in which the role of emotional health in children's medicine took center stage. Another historical pediatrician is Dr. Virginia Apgar, who is renowned for inventing the Apgar Score in the 1950s. The Apgar Score, used to evaluate the condition of newborn babies at birth, is an international standard today. Apgars contribution was particularly vital in the identification of newborn babies that urgently needed medical attention, leading to improved survival rates. Her commitment to infant and maternal health extended beyond this single innovation, as she also encouraged better training for pediatricians and the placement of neonatal intensive care centers. The ongoing use of the Apgar Score in hospitals and medical settings demonstrates how her work has endured, underscoring the importance of early medical intervention during critical periods of life. In the prevention of childhood obesity, recent research is a testament to the pioneering work of pediatricians of the past, who focused strongly on early intervention. The innovative work presented in today's trials clearly elucidates that obesity needs to be tackled from the prenatal period through the early childhood years, with a focus on the very important first 1000 days of life as a one-time chance for preventive intervention (Sarmiento et al., 2020). This focus has continuity with the previous work of prominent pediatricians who recognized the significance of the early environmental and nutritional influences that influence health outcomes. By continuing to focus on the role of prenatal care and infant well-being, modern pediatric care maintains continuity with earlier theory, further solidifying preventive practice and highlighting the legacy of the early figures who first made it possible to embrace a more integrated understanding of the child's health (Figure 9.4).

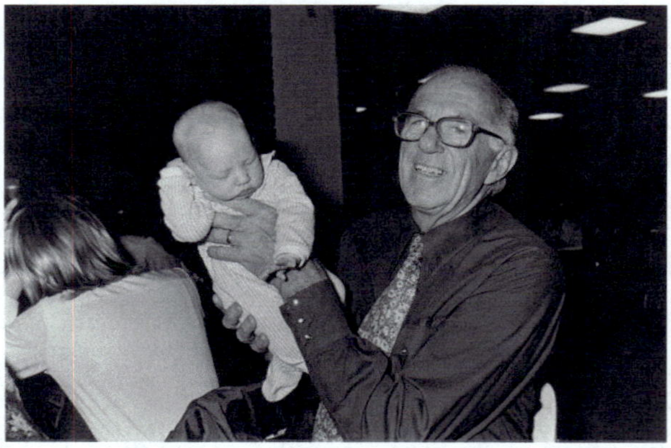

Figure 9.4. Dr. Spock holding baby, April 19, 1977.

Source: https://connecticuthistory.org/wp-content/uploads/2015/09/DrSpockBaby.jpg.

9.1.3. Milestones in Pediatric Care Practices

In pediatric practice, the emergence of developmental screening tools is a milestone that enhances early diagnosis and intervention.

Traditionally, developmental delay identification relied on subjective caregiver and primary care provider observations, which frequently resulted in delayed diagnosis. However, current advancements in developmental screening tools, as discussed in Drotar et al. (2008), have brought to the forefront the necessity of systematic and standardized approaches. This shift not only encourages more accurate identification of both general and specific developmental issues but also facilitates healthcare professionals in making informed decisions. Offering an interactive questionnaire with suggested tools enables a tailored screening process that is sensitive to variable individual needs. Therefore, the implementation of these tools is a key milestone in pediatric care, as children receive timely and appropriate interventions to maximize overall development. In addition, the creation of effective referral systems for developmental intervention is another key area of pediatric practices. Such systems help ensure that the process of linking children to required services is effective, thereby minimizing the delay between identification and intervention. As cited in Hagelow et al. (2010), efficient systems are characterized by the ability to organize complex care, maintain continuous support, and give feedback to the providers regarding patients' outcomes. This holistic method not only maximizes efficiency but also fosters effective interprofessional collaborations between families and healthcare providers. This collaboration is central in that it facilitates coordination of care by families via complex healthcare systems while providing children with comprehensive, age-specific care. Enhanced referral systems are a major milestone towards more responsive and coordinated pediatric practice. Beyond screening and referral success, the inclusion of evidence-based practices in pediatric care has significantly improved child health outcomes. Evidence-based practice guides practitioners to apply interventions supported by strong research, enhancing the efficacy and quality of care they provide to children. As an illustration, the transition from anecdotal practice to statistically based practice was evidence of the momentum toward transparency and accountability in pediatrics. By focusing on interventions proven effective through clinical trials, medical practitioners can establish an atmosphere that fosters optimal health and development in their pediatric patients. The ongoing interest in using evidence-based practice in the care of children also reflects a broader appreciation of the importance of ongoing improvement and innovation in meeting the diverse needs of children. These milestones constitute a critical nexus among science, pediatric health policy, and clinical practice in pursuit of the whole-child approach to pediatric care.

Test Your Knowledge

1. Who was Dr. Abraham Jacobi?
2. What is Benjamin Spock best known for?

9.2. Pediatric Health Issues

Learning Outcome

1. Know the common childhood illnesses
2. Describe the chronic conditions affecting children
3. Understand the mental health challenges in pediatrics

Addressing child health issues requires a multi-pronged approach encompassing not only physical health but also oral and mental health. Among the most glaring of these issues is that of dental caries in children, a problem that can lead to long-term health repercussions if not addressed. Children's oral health outcomes vary widely by geographic and socioeconomic factors, based on many studies, including recent findings in New Hampshire. New Hampshire is better than the nation's average in some areas, but the differences are substantial, particularly among low-income individuals. There are programs aimed at improving access to dental care, such as mobile dental clinics and school-based sealant programs, which are necessary to overcome barriers and deliver comprehensive oral health for children who are non-prioritized in usual healthcare settings (Jaffee et al., 2015). Another critical pediatric health issue area is the intersection of intellectual disabilities and oral health. People with intellectual disability are at increased risk of acquiring dental disease, not due to the pathology itself but due to the fact that most of these disorders impair their ability to provide proper self-care. These children tend to present with specific difficulties with seeking dental treatment, along with access barriers to the health system. Modern guidelines emphasize the need for personalized preventive interventions targeting this at-risk population, advocating that all caregivers, families, and health professionals work hand-in-hand to avert threats from poor oral hygiene and health. Through collaboration, they not only ensure individuals are educated but also encourage them to prioritize oral health in their agendas, ultimately fostering an enabling environment for effective health outcomes (Brugnoletti et al., 2015). Also, pediatric relevance extends to mental health and chronic disease, and it indicates a requirement for an integrated approach. Pediatric chronic disease patients, such as asthma or diabetes patients, are more likely to have anxiety and depression levels, which indicates the connection between mind and body. Proper pediatric care involves an understanding of these connections, promoting early intervention and whole-person management strategies. In addition, schools and communities can play a key role in prevention and intervention, providing vehicles for education and resource distribution. Through interdisciplinary collaboration among healthcare providers, educators, and families, pediatric care can be revolutionized to address the full spectrum of children's needs, ensuring that physical and mental health concerns are addressed and served effectively (Figure 9.5).

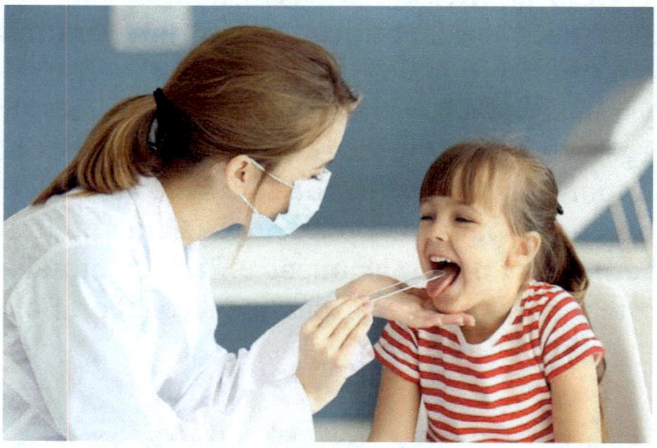

Figure 9.5. Common health issues in children.

Source: https://sa1s3optim.patientpop.com/assets/images/provider/photos/2330181.jpg.

9.2.1. Common Childhood Illnesses

Common childhood conditions often encompass a range of illnesses that vary in severity and duration, affecting the well-being of young individuals. Most common among them are upper respiratory infections (URIs), which are typically viral in etiology. The parents tend to misinterpret the symptoms, and therefore, there is a high rate of medical visits, along with the tendency to receive antibiotics despite the fact that such an infection is viral and cannot be treated with antibiotics. An improvement project in a particular study aimed to reduce inappropriate antibiotic prescribing in pediatric practice by increasing antibiotic avoidance from 66% to 82% through procedures supporting viral management and shared decision-making with guardians and parents (Lucas et al., 2017). The project highlights the importance of educating parents and healthcare providers in effectively managing common childhood illnesses. In addition to URIs, gastroenteritis is a prevalent childhood illness seen in pediatric practices. Inflammation of the stomach and intestines caused by viral gastroenteritis, most commonly norovirus or rotavirus, results in vomiting and diarrhea. This can lead to dehydration, particularly in younger children, and demands aggressive management and monitoring. Pediatric providers emphasize early treatment and the administration of oral rehydration solutions to compensate for fluid loss. Parent education is also necessary due to the fact that parents can be worried about their child's condition and create unnecessary visits to the emergency room. Therefore, these parental worries, together with educating parents regarding when additional medical treatment should be sought, can improve overall management and results for children who endure this common sickness. Another critical domain of consideration in pediatric care delivery is the emotional and psychological dimensions of chronic childhood illness, such as congenital heart disease (CHD). Researchers have shown that mothers with children with CHD report greater vigilance and stress compared to mothers whose children have no illness, with a clear impact on parenting actions (Carey et al., 2002). This kind of stress can have an impact on mother-child relationships and, consequently, the child's emotional and developmental milestones. Culturally sensitive and supportive interventions must be offered so that these families receive what they need to ensure their childis health. Furthermore, establishing a supportive environment can help normalize the incident for both the parent and the child, ensuring that their developmental needs are met while addressing the complexity of long-term care planning (Figure 9.6).

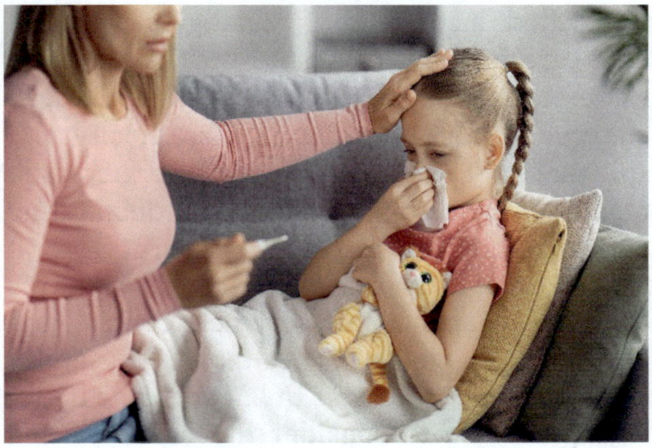

Figure 9.6. Common childhood illnesses.

Source: https://medanta.s3.ap-south-1.amazonaws.com/blogs/April2025/i4YU5YoW95UlKmETSt41HtsNfPk137-metac2h1dHRlcnN0b2NrXzIzMTI3NDQ3NDEuanBn-.jpg.

9.2.2. Chronic Conditions Affecting Children

Pediatric chronic illness is one of the big challenges of pediatric practice that not only impacts the health conditions of children but also their families and the healthcare system. Children with diseases like Type 1 diabetes, asthma, and sickle cell disease require ongoing care and very specialized care focusing on the developmental variations of children. The process of transfer from pediatric to adult care can be especially challenging for adolescents with chronic conditions, as indicated by a systematic review that reveals possible declines in glycemic control among those with Type

1 diabetes at this crucial transfer period. Effective management programs must address the challenges faced by pediatric patients, emphasizing age-specific learning, specialist education, and collaborative family engagement in care planning to achieve the best results (Bagnall et al., 2013). Sickle cell disease (SCD) is one of the chronic conditions that require continuous pediatric management and presents certain issues throughout childhood and adolescence. The complexity of SCD necessitates integrated management strategies that not only care for physical issues but also address the emotional and spiritual needs of children engaged. Evidence exists that religiosity and spirituality (S/R) are facilitators of increased quality of life among patients with debilitating chronic illnesses like SCD. Integrating S/R into interventions can offer patients multiple coping mechanisms, improve pain control, and encourage healthy use of healthcare. This multi-faceted view emphasizes the need for pediatric care providers to consider the whole-person character of managing chronic conditions and to modulate interventions appropriately (Clayton-Jones et al., 2016). Further, chronic conditions also have longer-range effects beyond clinical measures, with strong effects in everyday life on young patients and their families. Working with the emotional and psychological burden of chronic conditions calls for the involvement of a support network that includes medical staff but also educators, social workers, and community services. Families often struggle with complex healthcare systems and balance with their children's educational needs and healthcare. Effort coordination must exist that facilitates communication and coordination between various stakeholders in order to ascertain the provision of holistic physical, emotional, and developmental needs of children. Such a collaborative framework is critical in averting the long-term impact of chronic illness on the general well-being and quality of life for children (Figure 9.7).

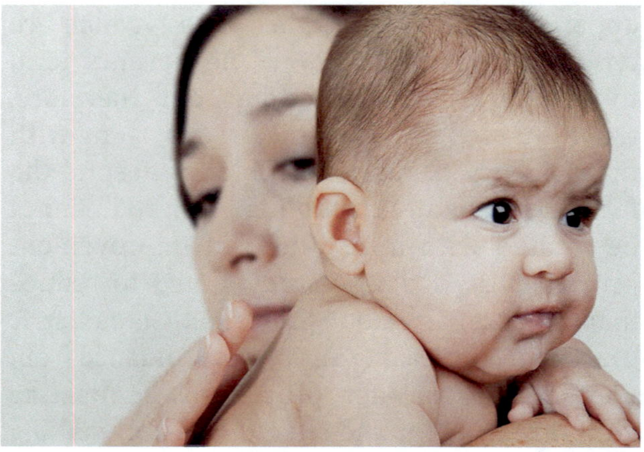

Figure 9.7. Combating chronic health conditions in children.

Source: https://cdn.cdnparenting.com/articles/2018/10/combating-chronic-health-conditions-in-children.jpg.

9.2.3. Mental Health Challenges in Pediatrics

Children's mental health disorders have become increasingly prominent in recent years, as the acceptance of psychological well-being as supplementary to bodily well-being in biomedical models has increased. Being early with detection and intervention is especially urgent because mental illnesses start to develop during childhood. Several efforts, some of which began in Colorado, Indiana, Massachusetts, and Rhode Island, sought to create systems for identifying and treating mental health issues in children up to age five. State programs reveal not just barriers, such as scarce funds and restrictions on training, but also the potential for change; cross-sector collaboration must become one of the keys to making interventions work. These cooperation strategies not only encourage community collaboration but also provide the foundation for sustaining pediatric mental health programs, thereby constituting a core element of comprehensive healthcare delivery to children (Lyman et al., 2010). Parental mental health significantly influences the emotional and developmental cycles of children and calls for a two-pronged approach towards both children and parents in pediatrics. Since maternal and paternal mental health problems, especially depression, can produce negative outcomes in children, these parental challenges must be addressed. New models for delivering services that address both generations can reduce these risks to healthy development. As examples, choices that combine parent mental health assistance with promoting positive developmental practices for children can improve overall outcomes. By reducing the influence of parental ill health, these approaches can help build a more stable backdrop for children and, over time, reduce behavior problems. Two-generation approaches like these value combined care within pediatric settings, so that the door can be opened to improved family life and child well-being (Fortuny et al., 2011). Moreover, mental health stigma within child populations generates significant barriers in front of treatment and support. Unawareness of many families regarding indicators and symptoms of mental health disorders among children leads to unnecessary delays in seeking help. Training interventions among healthcare providers and parents can greatly mitigate this stigma and create an environment where mental health is discussed without hesitation and allotted its rightful place. Training of healthcare professionals to recognize mental health problems is paramount; it transforms the pediatric healthcare environment to one where early intervention is promoted. Thus, children are exposed to interventions in time, an element that plays a critical role in determining their development trajectory. A better-supported, better-educated model of child care not only enhances current mental health problems but also lays the foundation for a healthier, more resilient future generation (Lyman et al., 2010) (Figure 9.8).

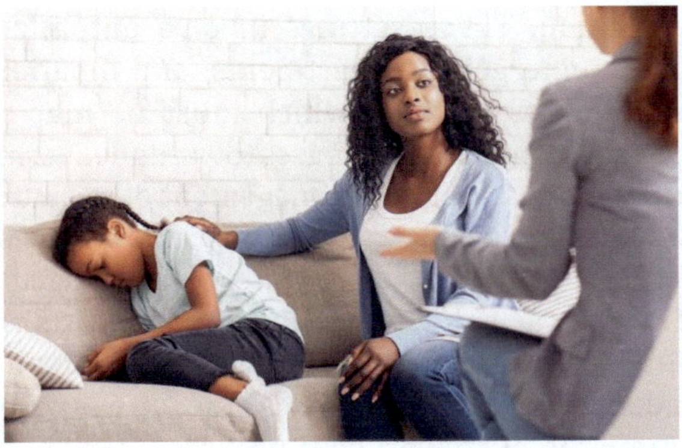

Figure 9.8. Prioritizing children's mental health.

Source: https://www.vachhanihospital.com/blog/wp-content/uploads/2024/01/Mental-Health-in-Pediatrics.jpg.

Test Your Knowledge

1. What are the 2 most common childhood illnesses?
2. What are the most common chronic conditions in children?

9.3. Pediatric Care Settings

Learning Outcome

1. Understand the role of primary care pediatricians
2. Describe the pediatric hospitals and specialty clinics
3. Learn about home health care for children

Pediatric healthcare settings are critical to the delivery of specialized care for children and adolescents, using a multidisciplinary model to address the unique issues of this population. These settings involve outpatient clinics, emergency departments, and inpatient departments, each of which must be met by specially formulated measures towards delivering the best treatment and management of pediatric patients. In the ED, for instance, the need for rapid assessment and timely intervention requires a robust antibiotic stewardship infrastructure, as a study showed that most ED leaders believe there is a need to set up ED-based antimicrobial stewardship programs (ASPs) to optimize care. These interventions have the potential to enhance the quality of pediatric care through improved decision-making and cautious antibiotic use, ultimately achieving better child health outcomes in emergency situations (Dayan et al., 2017). Pediatrics inpatient care also necessitates ongoing efforts to gain insights and assess patient and family satisfaction that can be instrumental in decision-making with regard to the quality of care provided. Hospitals are urged to use tools such as the Child Hospital Consumer Assessment of Healthcare Providers and Systems Survey, which enables performance measurement against national standards. But due to the importance of this information, many hospitals find it challenging to effectively use patient and family experience feedback to improve. Literature review findings point out that integrating best practices, such as having strong internal communication mechanisms for patient experience, is crucial to propel care quality and build a responsive healthcare culture (Hays et al., 2020). With lessons from these findings, pediatric care centers can cultivate a culture of improvement that directly benefits the families they serve. In pediatrics, the intersection of newer technologies played an important role in redefining healthcare delivery. Electronic health records (EHRs) are now essential tools in simplifying the documentation and communication of patients' health information between providers. The ability to create antibiograms and develop clinical care guidelines from data obtained from EHR systems demonstrates the value of technology in enhancing the quality of care in pediatric settings. Studies indicate a strong preference among pediatric ASP leaders and ED directors for EHR-integrated clinical decision support to implement ASPs, suggesting that these technologies not only streamline workflows but also promote adherence to best-practice guidelines. The technology is central to the development of pediatric care as it ensures that children receive timely, effective, and appropriate interventions throughout their healthcare journey (Dayan et al., 2017) (Figure 9.9).

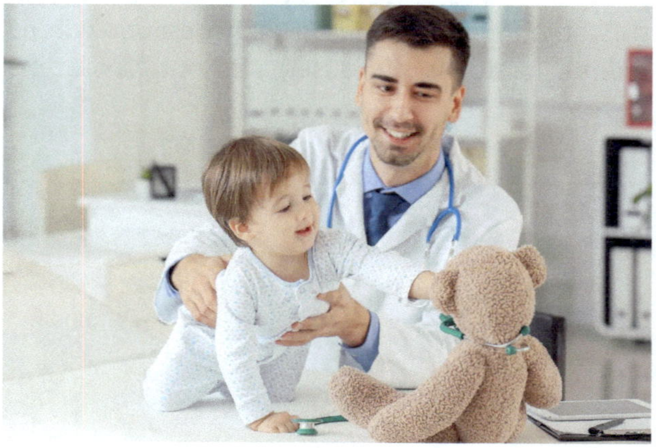

Figure 9.9. Pediatric care settings.

Source: https://sa1s3optim.patientpop.com/filters:format(webp)/assets/production/practices/f5fc7f2d8db672eba4a17daa93a50ed4134ebbd1/images/2623684.jpg.

9.3.1. Primary Care Pediatricians

The role of the primary care pediatrician is one that stands at the focal point of the broader canvas of pediatric care, specifically in the management of day-to-day illness, such as fever, so prevalent during childhood. The pediatricians are the first line of defense when parents bring in illnesses with fever. Their understanding of fever is not only how it acts at the clinical level, but also how it acts at the psychosocial level with families. Pediatricians do recognize the need to treat distress associated with fever, as per reports, but have difficulty translating clinical guidelines into practice.

These complications suggest the complex relationship between clinical information and everyday practice, particularly in primary care settings, where reassurance and education are key for parents caring for children's health (Miró-Bonet et al., 2025). Therefore, primary care pediatricians must place greater emphasis on parents' role and optimize their therapeutic strategy to more effectively treat fever in children. To the extent that they cure acute disease, primary care pediatricians have a fundamental responsibility for the long-term management of chronic respiratory conditions, such as asthma. The utility of office spirometry in the primary care office has emerged as an important topic of study in enhancing pediatric respiratory care. A study demonstrates that, after specialized training, pediatricians in primary care can perform spirometry in the office, with satisfactory results in a significant percentage of patients. This capacity for spirometry testing by primary care pediatricians not only increases the diagnostic precision but also promotes closer monitoring of asthma control in the comfort of a child's regular practice setting. Research has indicated that ongoing education and quality control are required to ensure the full potential of office spirometry, in support of specialist respiratory medicine and primary care collaboration. Multi-faceted care is facilitated by combined strategies, which is consistent with emerging children's needs. Moreover, primary care pediatricians' interaction with families extends beyond individual health conditions. Such rapport is essential in the development of preventive health habits and the encouragement of timely immunizations, which are significant drivers of public health outcomes.

Primary care pediatricians are teachers who provide families with evidence-based information regarding developmental milestones and health screening. By prioritizing preventive care, they can identify potential health issues before they become complex, further establishing themselves as promoters of overall health. In addition, through effective communication with families, pediatricians can intervene culturally and contextually to meet specific needs, ensuring care is both available and effective. As pediatric care continues to advance, the multifaceted role of primary care pediatricians remains essential in providing comprehensive health care that fully meets both short-term and long-term pediatric health needs, thereby enhancing the health of the entire population (Figure 9.10).

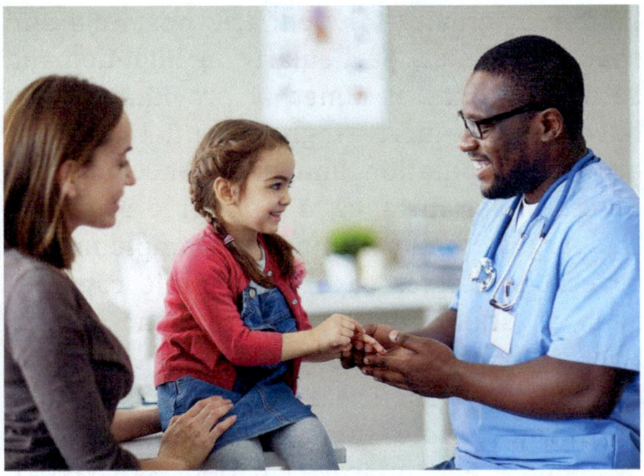

Figure 9.10. Primary care physician.

Source: https://kids1stpediatrics.net/wp-content/uploads/bfi_thumb/What-Is-a-Primary-Care-Physician-3a0aja3vnrecdxh1e0abcw.jpg.

9.3.2. Pediatric Hospitals and Specialty Clinics

Pediatric hospitals and specialty clinics are integral components of comprehensive pediatric care, specifically designed to address the unique medical needs of children. Unlike general hospitals, these facilities cater exclusively to the pediatric population, which allows for tailored treatment protocols and an environment that is developmentally appropriate for younger patients. The trained staff not only possess intensive knowledge about childhood illnesses and their presentations but are also capable of communicating effectively with children and their families. These abilities become useful in the management of complicated pediatric diseases, including chronic illnesses and birth defects. Children's hospitals have close interactions with multi-disciplinary teams, with continuity of care that not only includes medical treatment but also psycho-social support for families dealing with complex health experiences. This focus on total care is a response to the recognition that pediatric health is intricate, necessitating age-specific healthcare solutions with optimal outcomes for young patients. Care access is a matter of gravity for pediatric hospitals and specialty clinics, particularly in high-demand settings. Initiatives aimed at providing access have become increasingly essential with the growing population and prevalence of child illnesses. For instance, a task force at one of the largest pediatric hospitals implemented several strategies to expand clinic capacity, such as standardizing appointment lengths and utilizing a patient-oriented electronic scheduling system. These interventions resulted in a remarkable increase in appointment availability and improved patient satisfaction as captured on Press Ganey scores. Notably, the generation of over 53,000 extra appointments annually demonstrates the manner in which the streamlining of clinic schedules can benefit not only patient experiences but also increase hospital revenues. This two-pronged benefit identifies the significant impact operational efficiency can have on the provision of pediatric care and, by extension, the timely and effective delivery of medical services to children. The differing needs of child patients often require advanced care beyond the capabilities of general hospitals. Children's hospitals tend to treat complex medical cases, including those older than the traditional age cut-off, suggesting a broader range of care than is commonly assumed. For instance, teenagers with childhood-onset conditions continue to receive care in pediatric environments due to the sophisticated skills of professionals familiar with evolving care requirements. How challenging it is to transition from pediatric to adult care underscores the need for ongoing support and advocacy from the medical community. By bridging gaps in care, pediatric hospitals are able to maintain continuity available for adolescents with special health needs, as seen in the case of adult patients like a 26-year-old woman with CHARGE syndrome, who availed themselves of pediatric resources to access life-sustaining interventions. Pediatric hospitals and specialty clinics are, therefore, not only treatment centers but also integral components of an enabling system for lifelong health management (Figure 9.11).

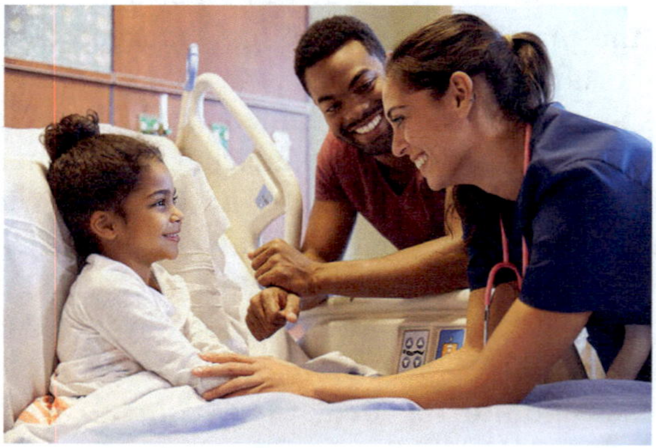

Figure 9.11. Pediatric specialties.

Source: https://www.uofmhealthsparrow.org/sites/default/files/styles/3_2_card_crop/public/2025-01/pediatric-neurosurgery-teaser-900x600.jpg?itok=iNiG-Cso.

9.3.3. Home Health Care for Children

The evolution of pediatrics has come to acknowledge the vital role of home health care for kids, particularly those with serious medical conditions or special health care needs. Home health care presents a choice to traditional hospital-based therapy, allowing kids to receive medical treatment in a familiar setting that facilitates comfort and emotional security. For those families providing care to individuals with chronic illnesses, such as asthma or diabetes, home health services enable ongoing surveillance and treatment that can lead to better health outcomes and reduced emergency room utilization.

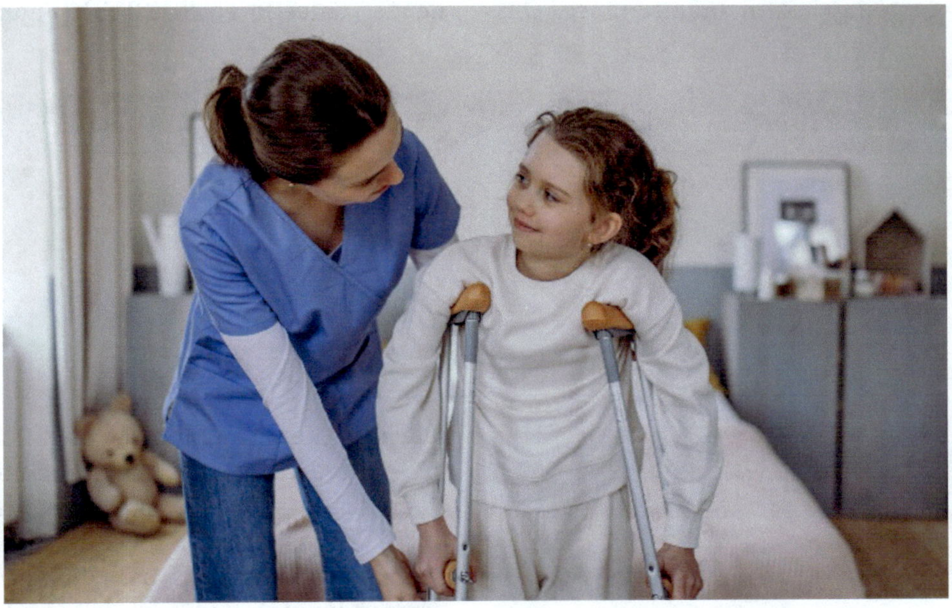

Figure 9.12. Home health care for children.

Source: https://kidscarehomehealth.com/wp-content/uploads/2023/06/KCHH-nurse-helping-girl.jpg.

Pediatric ambulatory care-sensitive conditions are under investigation to highlight the importance of accessible outpatient services, as more than 27% of these events began in acute care settings and often might have been managed within an immediate care system, highlighting the value of accessible home health models as a solution to divert care into more appropriate settings while minimizing unnecessary strain on emergency operations (Alpern et al., 2024). The growing need for care of increasingly complex children with special health care needs further illustrates the need for home health care. Improvements in medical technology have enabled the survival of many infants and children who had previously had life-threatening illnesses, producing an increasing population of children who need ongoing medical monitoring beyond routine developmental care. These children, at times classified as children with special health care needs (CSHCN), need highly intensive and coordinated care beyond what can be provided in standard pediatric clinics. Research has proven that home care is a good alternative for these children, allowing them to get specific interventions without additional stressors inherent in institutions. While families attempt to comprehend the complexities of these health requirements, home health care integration becomes a focal point for providing continuity of care and improving the overall quality of life for children and families (Caicedo et al., 2013). The quality of life for children and families has been shown to vary significantly by their care setting. Children observed in medical day care units tend to have better health-related quality of life (HRQL) scores than children in home health care, who are more likely to experience caregiving burden. Parents of children receiving home care often feel overwhelmed by the level of commitment required for ongoing health maintenance. On the other hand, the caregivers of children living in long-term care institutions experience less strain and therefore have more time to themselves and overall better well-being. These differences indicate the benefit of optimizing home health care utilization and suggest that with suitable support and services, families could enhance their quality of life yet remain capable of managing their children's health care needs (Caicedo et al., 2013) (Figure 9.12).

Test Your Knowledge

1. What is the role of primary care pediatricians?
2. What is the role of home health care for children?

9.4. Role of Pediatric Healthcare Providers

Learning Outcome

1. Describe the pediatricians and their responsibilities
2. Understand the role of nurses in pediatric care
3. Know the support staff and their contributions

Pediatric health professionals have a critical role in offering extended and specialist care to children, considering their unique needs at various stages of growth. The professionals, comprising nurses, allied health professionals, and pediatricians, can diagnose and manage a broad range of health issues affecting children, from acute illnesses to chronic conditions. For instance, timely diagnosis and intervention can significantly alter the trajectory of diseases such as asthma or obesity to achieve improved health outcomes later. The role of pediatric healthcare providers extends beyond medical therapy, as they typically serve as educators to parents, teaching them the nuances of children's health, preventive care, and developmental markers. Their leadership role in the healthcare system , with all aspects of physical, emotional, and social considerations being placed under the utmost importance on integrated approaches to the treatment of children, with all aspects of physical, emotional, and social considerations being brought into play. Interprofessional collaboration is another characteristic aspect of pediatric healthcare providers' roles, particularly in arranging transitions of care for adolescent patients with chronic diseases. As young people with the disease grow older, a switch from pediatric to adult care becomes increasingly urgent. This is especially reflected in the management of Type 1 diabetes, where evidence has highlighted the role of a properly planned transition if deteriorating outcomes, such as glycemic control, are to be prevented. Evidence from studies indicates that effective transitions incorporate youth-centered strategies, family involvement, and a consensus between pediatric and adult providers. Through the use of assigned transition programs and support systems, providers can, in some manner, buffer the difficulties patients face during this process. Such collaboration is instrumental, as it supports continuity of care and encourages self-management practices, laying the groundwork for successful long-term health management as these patients progress into adulthood and demonstrating the integral role of pediatric providers in doing so. Moreover, pediatric health professionals have a significant responsibility in addressing public health problems which target children in the contemporary world, such as the growing issue of childhood obesity.

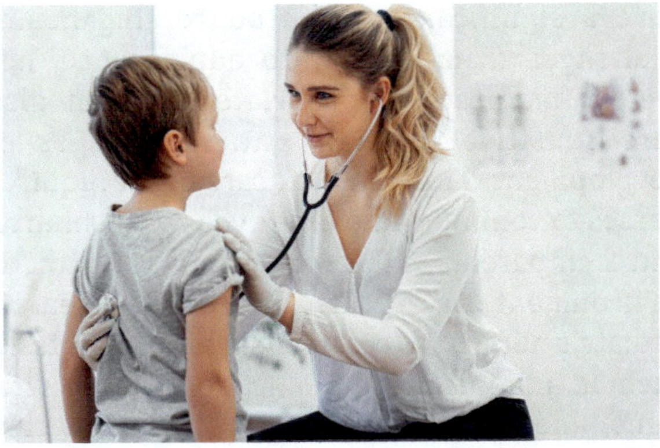

Figure 9.13. Role of pediatric healthcare providers.

Source: https://www.felixhospital.com/sites/default/files/2022-11/best-paediatrics-hospital-in-noida.jpg.

They should ensure they make contributions towards preventive health interventions because diseases that arise due to obesity can have lasting effects on a child's health. Pediatric health professionals are often involved in community activities, such as promoting physical activity and raising awareness in families regarding good nutrition and healthy lifestyle options. Strategies like those outlined in findings from organizations committed to childhood obesity highlight the collaborative roles of pediatric professionals within the healthcare system and community settings, indicating the impact of successful collaboration on health outcomes. These diverse roles illustrate the comprehensive nature of pediatric care, showing that medical practitioners not only heal illness but are also heavily engaged in public health programs, contributing to enabling children to receive preventive care to build a healthier world in the future (Murphy et al., 2008; Bagnall et al., 2013) (Figure 9.13).

9.4.1. Pediatricians and Their Responsibilities

Pediatricians' tasks extend beyond clinical assessment; they include a broader range of activities aimed at promoting children's health and well-being. Pediatricians have a crucial role in monitoring developmental milestones, conducting preventive visits, and offering vaccinations, all of which are vital in safeguarding children's development. In addition, they are primary care physicians who screen for and treat acute and chronic disorders. This generalist model integrates pediatricians into a child's healthcare team. Furthermore, they often work in collaboration with caregivers, parents, and multidisciplinary teams to provide children with individualized care that addresses their specific needs. Social determinants of health, such as socioeconomic status and resource availability, should be taken into account, as they greatly impact pediatric outcomes. Hence, their job requires continuous learning and staying abreast of the times to address new health problems in the pediatric age group. Lately, the role of mental health in childcare has come to be recognized more prominently. Pediatricians are now expected to screen for mental health conditions such as depression and anxiety that impact a child's well-being and development. This becomes all the more significant when considered in the context of adverse childhood experiences, where early identification has the ability to change a child's life trajectory. Advanced tools such as physiological measures of stress are the future, enabling pediatricians to better assess and address children's mental health needs. Incorporating the psychological dimensions of child health into their considerations has made the pediatrician's work a seamless blend of physical and mental care. This paradigm shift requires pediatricians to not only be taught to recognize symptoms but also to implement interventions that build resilience and mental health in children, taking a holistic approach to pediatric practice.

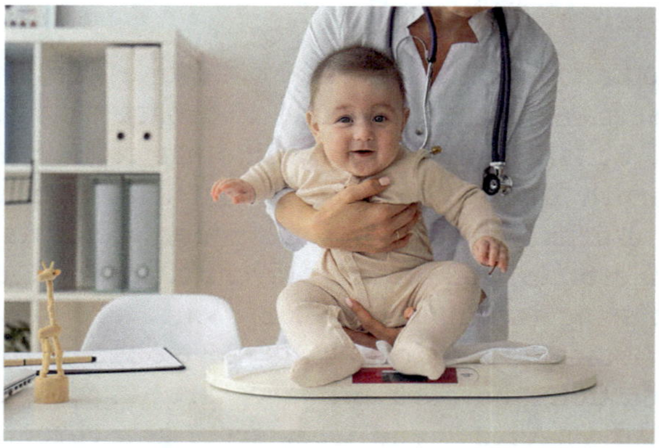

Figure 9.14. Duties and responsibilities of a pediatrician.

Source: https://drolfa.com/wp-content/uploads/2024/04/duties-and-responsibilities-of-a-pediatrician-1.jpg.

Furthermore, pediatricians play a vital role in addressing maternal mental health, most importantly postpartum depression, which can significantly affect mothers as well as children. Evidence indicates that maternal depression is likely to undermine parenting ability and thereby disrupt use of pediatric health care, thus making it important that pediatricians remain vigilant to this. Interventions aimed at enhancing pediatricians' knowledge and self-efficacy for identifying and responding to maternal mental illness have proved to be beneficial. For instance, education interventions are able to equip pediatricians with skills on how to properly identify symptoms and provide appropriate referrals, which have been shown to improve child and maternal health outcomes. As pediatricians advocate for holistic care that encompasses both child and maternal health, they help ensure healthier family lives and optimal child development in high-risk populations, as research on the topic elucidates (Agapidaki et al., 2013; Shonkoff et al., 2022) (Figure 9.14).

9.4.2. Nurses in Pediatric Care

Pediatric nursing work extends beyond the common clinical responsibilities to cover an integrated approach unique to the needs of children and families. Pediatric nurses have a significant role in addressing health challenges from infancy to adolescence, not merely medically appropriate care but also care sensitive to their patients' stages of development. This complex care often requires nurses to communicate effectively with children and their parents to foster a trusting, empathetic environment. As revealed by recent research, pediatric nurses are responsible for pivotal tasks such as administering medication, taking vital signs, and counseling families on health care management, while ensuring that the emotional and psychological needs of their patients are met. The multilateral contribution of nurses in pediatric settings is ultimately the factor that enhances the quality of care delivered to children and families. The emergence of pediatric nurse researchers (NRs) has been a revolution in the future of nursing in pediatric hospitals. Although relatively new, the role of NRs has been characterized by several significant tasks, including conducting research, shaping evidence-based practices, and supporting staff development in pediatric care. Evidence shows that the majority of NRs are based in children's hospitals for less than four years, a rapid shift in nursing research within this area. These researchers are particularly critical to addressing knowledge gaps in pediatric health outcomes and developing interventions tailored to children. Through the articulation of both shrievalties and the unique features of pediatric nursing studies, NRs' work forms a platform supporting the future development of nursing practice to meet the particular needs of pediatric patients and families, demonstrating the critical importance of research to improve child care (Balchunas et al., 2010).

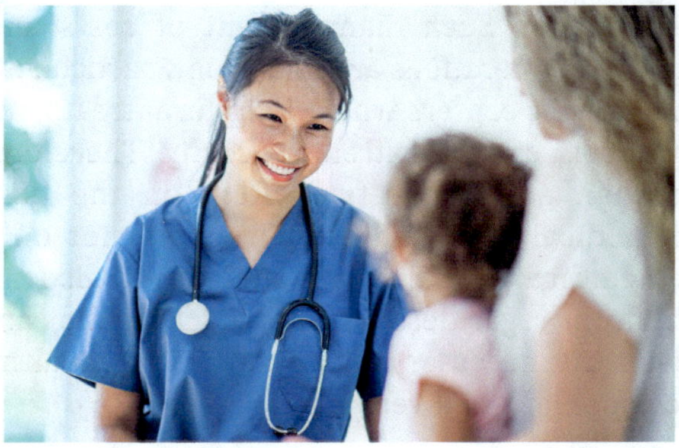

Figure 9.15. Role of nurses in pediatric care.

Source: https://lh5.googleusercontent.com/zXDFHGhlQH6X9ub2U_FcZQBr6b4F04-ykFYw4OV-KuV1k8-z9tnBEI5DTDZwclIlWpQ6l0qdFnRVu977KT53nqlNDR8qRAwVxjyO5YSc0BsL-ABe3yB4-IgPEJOvzItoddMWZS53=s0.

In pediatric palliative care, nurses make an invaluable contribution that is less likely to be referenced nationally in regard to roles and responsibilities. Such ambiguity can hinder the ability to provide holistic care within pediatric palliative teams, where there is some expectation for specialized nursing expertise to enhance overall patient and family experiences. A qualitative study of nurses employed in such teams shows that they perceive their work as essential to making children's and their families' lives simpler. However, nurses frequently express a sense of inadequacy because they cannot find time to address all required areas of care, indicating an incongruence between what they perceive as demanded of them and what is actually demanded. These issues call for more specific delineation of roles for pediatric palliative care teams, with an emphasis on the requirement for formal direction that permits whole-person, family-centered care (Eliseussen et al., 2024) (Figure 9.15).

9.4.3. Support Staff and Their Contributions

In pediatric health care, support staff are crucial in creating an entire person environment that fosters healing and development. Support staff comprises medical assistants, social workers, and administrative staff who all have essential roles to play in patient success. Their tasks extend beyond administration; they have an essential role in creating emotional connections with patients and families. This interpersonal aspect is particularly important in pediatrics, as a patient's psychological and emotional state can directly influence their healing process. Improved patient satisfaction through empathetic care and trust-building is achieved by support staff, allowing families to deal with challenging medical conditions more effectively. The coordination of care by the support staff is also teamwork, as it enables them to provide pediatric patients with holistic, individualized care.

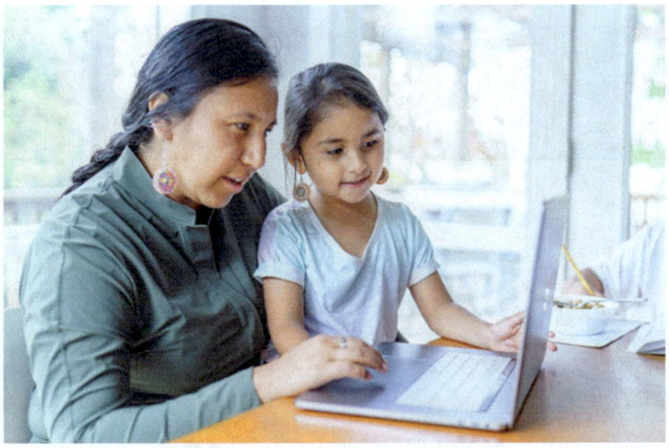

Figure 9.16. Support staff.

Source: https://professionals.adoptuskids.org/wp-content/uploads/2023/01/child-welfare-lived-experience-stock-675x441-1.jpg.

This is significant communication among various health practitioners, including doctors, nurses, and therapists, to coordinate care plans best suited for each child. Support staff , playing a central role as the link between families and medical staff, clarifying complex medical terminology in simple language, and acting in the best interests of the child. Such institutions like St. Jude Children's Research Hospital, which are renowned for their innovative approaches to treating cancer in children, set the precedent that having support staff included can lead to higher survival rates and healthier long-term outcomes for the patients, highlighting the critical function that must be filled by such jobs in the system of pediatric healthcare (Favuzza et al., 2018). Furthermore, support staff has a major financial and logistical impact on pediatrics, ensuring that services are available to children and families. Those programs that provide full-scope health coverage for children who fall outside public program eligibility indicate the immense control that support staff can exert over clinic operations and patient access (Farias et al., 2008). Through guaranteeing proper healthcare services for children, such professionals remove the barriers to treatment that would otherwise deter them. Such management of costs and control of operations are important, particularly in pediatric centers where long-term treatment protocols can be extremely costly. Therefore, through a collaborative effort on the part of medical staff and support staff, not only is healthcare quality enhanced, but also all children, regardless of their background, are given the necessary medical care for healthy development and recovery (Figure 9.16).

Test Your Knowledge

1. What is the role of the pediatrician?
2. What is the role of nurses in pediatric care?

9.5. Family Involvement in Pediatric Care

Learning Outcome

1. Understand the importance of family-centered care
2. Describe the communication between healthcare providers and families
3. Know the support resources for families

Involvement of the family in pediatric health care is a fundamental component that significantly influences patient outcomes and experiences. Family involvement not only improves the quality of health care but also enhances healing relationships between patients and health care professionals. Research has demonstrated that when families are involved in active medical decision-making, care plans more effectively prioritize patients' unique needs and desires. This collaboration can foster a sense of ownership and empowerment within families, which may lead to improved treatment adherence and greater satisfaction with care. Moreover, family-centered approaches have been associated with good health outcomes, as these intervention strategies allow the incorporation of family values and emotional support into the caregiving process, making the child's healthcare experience more holistic. Effective family engagement integration requires healthcare systems to implement systematic processes for collecting family experiences and feedback. One of the most effective tools for achieving this is the Child Hospital Consumer Assessment of Healthcare Providers and Systems Survey, which provides hospitals with a standardized measure of pediatric inpatient care through the family experience.

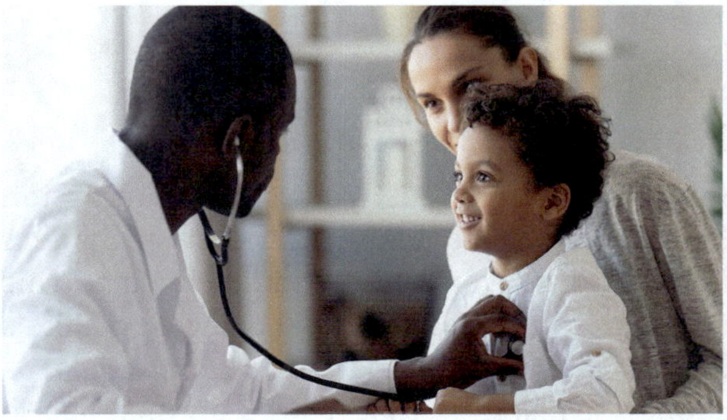

Figure 9.17. The role of the family in pediatric healthcare.

Source: https://www.waldenu.edu/media/5390/seo-2158-bs-african-american-pediatrician-353293868-1200x675.

Data gathered from experience surveys may enable hospitals to identify the strengths and weaknesses of their pediatric care. Converting such data into successful quality improvement projects remains a predicament for the majority of institutions. Hospitals should implement internal processes to track performance in patient and family experiences, thereby developing a culture of continuous learning and accommodation to maximize care delivery and outcomes in the pediatric setting (Hays et al., 2020). Furthermore, transforming pediatric practices into more family-centered medical homes can significantly increase access to care for children, particularly those with lower socioeconomic status. It is these non-profit agencies that have been instrumental in bringing this about, offering administrative services and funding for practices to develop integrated models of care. By facilitating pediatric practices' referrals to community support agencies and promoting interagency collaboration, these programs support more comprehensive models of health and social service support for families. The lessons learned from these projects reaffirm the importance of developing strong systems with family engagement and support as a high priority. Such programs are also important not only for augmenting immediate access to medical care but also in fostering long-term health outcomes, confirming families' central role in pediatric practice (Figure 9.17).

9.5.1. Importance of Family-Centered Care

Family-centered care (FCC) in pediatric practice is at the forefront of improving the well-being of treated children. Family-centered care recognizes that families play a key role in promoting their children's health and well-being; thus, it fosters cooperation among healthcare professionals, patients, and families. By placing the family as an essential member of the healthcare team at the forefront, FCC fosters open communication and shared decision-making, ultimately improving health outcomes. Those hospital environments that implement FCC principles indicate higher patient satisfaction and lower anxiety levels among families and patients, as families become more empowered to comprehend the complexities of healthcare and advocate for their child's needs. This partnership not only improves family well-being but also provides healthcare practitioners with all-important information about the patient's preferences and experience, making the care process far more enriching (Hays et al., 2020). There is a necessity to incorporate family-focused practices that become particularly clear in pediatric oncology. Being diagnosed with cancer is frightening for families, and there is a demand for specialist educational and emotional support programs that take into consideration their particular challenges. Systematic patient and family education is crucial since it is the foundation of informed decision-making and effective disease management. Education for pediatric oncology should ideally incorporate a multi-disciplinary approach that addresses three aspects: understanding the diagnosis and treatment options, psychosocial coping mechanisms, and hands-on interventions in care (Ahern et al., 2016). By creating an environment in which families feel they can complain and receive support, medical professionals foster family empowerment.

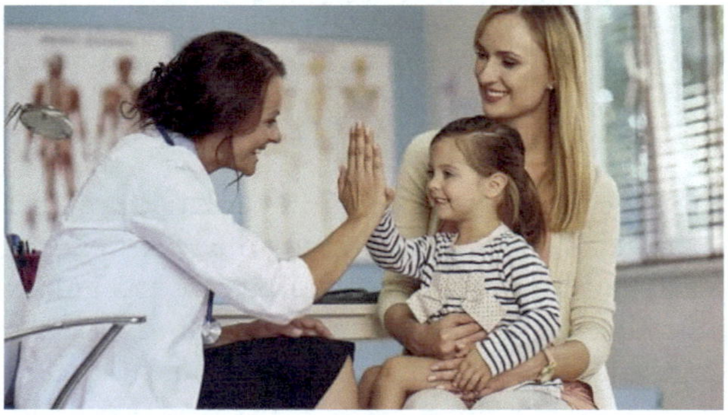

Figure 9.18. Importance of family-centered care.

Source: https://www.newportchildren.com/wp-content/uploads/PediatricianRelationshipNewport.jpg.

An educationally conducive environment like this improves the child's health outcomes and quality of life during the treatment period. Besides, effective family-centered care fosters ongoing mechanisms for feedback, enabling healthcare institutions to assess patient and family experience. This type of feedback is essential to identifying areas of improvement in care delivery and ensuring that families' voices become pivotal in shaping healthcare policies and practices. The application of the Child Hospital Consumer Assessment of Healthcare Providers and Systems Survey has been extremely promising for the realization of this aim, providing a systematic path to gather data on family experiences (Hays et al., 2020). But the persistent dilemma is how to tap into this information to stimulate positive quality improvement efforts. Seeking evidence-based practice, openness in the context of care delivery, and the integration of patient and family experience data into quality improvement programs will not merely transform pediatric care but also cement the essential role that families play in orchestrating their child's healthcare (Figure 9.18).

9.5.2. Communication Between Providers and Families

It is essential that good communication between families and healthcare providers is used to deliver quality pediatric care. This communication enables co-sharing of a child's health needs and the establishment of a cooperative setting that fosters optimal health outcomes. Open communication promotes trust and empowers families to become involved in their child's care. As providers impart information in a family-style manner, they not only convey medical details but also consider the emotional roles at play. This enhances caregiver satisfaction as families become more engaged in decision-making, ultimately aligning treatment plans with their individual values and preferences. Therefore, a provider's skill in communicating is not just a technical process; it is critical to delivering quality pediatric care founded on the child's overall needs and the family's issues. In treating chronic pediatric disease, continuity of care is more critical. Care disruptions, often the result of inordinate staff turnover, can severely dampen families' ability to engage with treatment regimens appropriately. Studies investigating this issue found that turnover stemming from compromised communication negatively impacts care plans and caregiver satisfaction, leading to medical errors and reducing treatment protocol compliance. Families that are having difficulty with inconsistent communication are more likely to face emotional issues with respect to coping with new care teams and the breakdown in trust that is essential for successful team collaboration in managing conditions like asthma or diabetes. Addressing these issues by utilizing improved measures of staff retention and a focus on continuous communication can enhance the overall quality of pediatric care with a more stable support network for their families. The COVID-19 pandemic revealed the need for robust lines of communication between families and healthcare workers, especially for children with special care needs. Changeable determinants such as shared decision-making and family-centered communication are instrumental in mitigating the risk of forgone care during the pandemic, as indicated by studies. These practices promote open lines of communication, allowing issues to be addressed and medical attention to be requested early. Responsive crisis care not only reassures families but also calls them in as active participants in decision-making regarding care, which is absolutely vital with children who have mental health needs. By adopting a collaborative model that engages parents and caregivers as active participants, providers can meet unpredictability head-on and reduce unwanted health outcomes. This dynamic reinforces that good communication is not only important in everyday practice but also in times of public health crises, hence becoming the cornerstone of quality pediatrics (Figure 9.19).

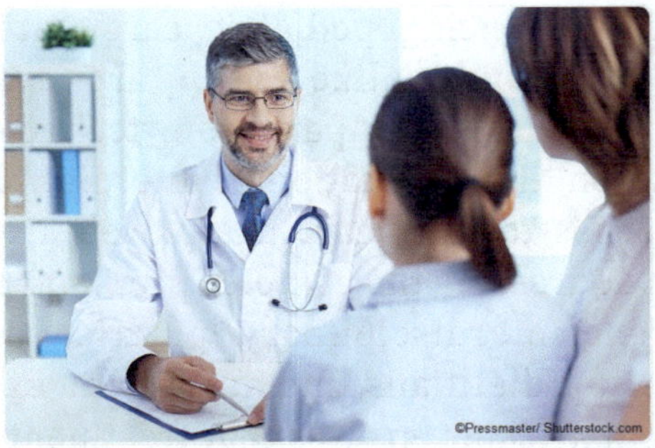

Figure 9.19. Communication between healthcare providers and families.

Source: https://www.news-medical.net/image-handler/picture/2017/6/Male_doctor%2C_patient_girl_and_mother_680x_-__Pressmaster.jpg.

9.5.3. Support Resources for Families

The intricate landscape of children's health demands solid support structures for families as they navigate health systems. Families are likely to experience a range of stressors in meeting their children's health care needs, thereby underscoring the imperative of ready access to supportive care. Family-centered care models are increasingly regarded as central to optimizing communication among healthcare teams, patients, and families. Such models are constructed through communication and collaboration to make sure that families are well-informed and actively involved in their child's treatment. According to Pansier et al. (2022), pediatric health providers can benefit from ongoing education on family and psychosocial care, which allows them to address not only medical needs but also the psychological and emotional well-being of children and families. These programs emphasize training and mentorship that place a robust emphasis on family dynamics in pediatric care settings. When offering solutions to mental disorders, which have taken off increasingly in pediatric patients, families need to be provided with adequate resources and information. Many families may struggle to detect mental health issues in their children, mostly due to their lack of proper awareness and access to suitable support services. As indicated by Singh et al. (2024), campaigns aimed at raising awareness of available mental health services significantly help address such issues. By establishing open channels through which parents can find mental health professionals and crisis intervention services, pediatric care providers can increase the likelihood of timely intervention. Parental educational programs are also necessary to equip parents with skills to control their children's mental health in the home setting, minimizing the stigma of seeking help and developing a facilitative environment that encourages candid discussions of mental health. In addition, the integration of these resources can significantly enhance the overall pediatric experience, offering families holistic support tailored to individual needs. The availability of mentorship programs and mutual understanding of mental health resources not only assists healthcare providers but also enables families to more effectively advocate for their children's diverse health needs. (Pansier et al., 2022) points out that psychosocial mentoring has been shown to enhance providers' confidence in delivering family-centered care, thereby improving clinical outcomes for children and families. Integrated with mental health resource lists and community outreach, these practices can yield higher educational attainment, emotional support, and a sense of community for families undergoing the process of pediatric care. Investing in family resource facilities, therefore, becomes a central solution to developing healthier conditions where children can grow.

Test Your Knowledge

1. What is the importance of family-centered care?
2. What is the purpose of communication between healthcare providers and families?

9.6. Advances in Pediatric Care

Learning Outcome

1. Know the technological innovations in treatment
2. Describe the research and development in pediatrics
3. Understand the role of preventive care and vaccination programs in pediatric care

The face of pediatric care is dynamically changing with revolutionary leaps toward maximizing therapeutic access and the level of interventions. Of these tech innovations, telehealth has revolutionized the delivery of care to pediatric patients. Teletherapy uses video conferencing technology to deliver therapy services to children, particularly those who may not have easy access to traditional interventions due to geographic or logistical constraints. This method is especially useful in children with developmental disorders, as early and stable therapeutic interventions are needed to ensure proper growth and development. Combining intervention program research on feeding and non-feeding problems in children, researchers highlight the importance of such developments in delivering necessary services to more customers, thereby enhancing pediatric care outcomes through individualized support systems (Luke et al., 2016). Apart from technological innovation, the application of interdisciplinary approaches to child care has played a crucial role in addressing the complex problems facing children. Interdisciplinary practice among therapists, dietitians, mental health experts, and pediatricians ensures that treatment plans are sensitive to children's complex problems. This teamwork model involves families in becoming active stakeholders in their child's care process, fostering communication among caregivers, and enhancing treatment plan adherence. Treatments, modalities, and care holism advancement not only develop clinical outcomes but also the psychosocial aspect of health, as it deals with the mental and emotional health of children. All these comprehensive approaches are a sustained step toward the profession evolving and improving the quality of child healthcare. As people become more aware of childhood health, early intervention and preventive care have taken center stage. The latest advances point towards addressing health issues before they become more serious conditions, thereby reducing hospitalization rates and improving quality of life among younger populations. Interventions based on nutrition, physical activity, and mental health are given greater importance, suggesting a proactive pediatric healthcare. Additionally, training programs for the identification of early signs of developmental disorders among parents and the general population provide greater access to care and timely interventions. By transitioning from a reactive healthcare model to proactive, preventive care, systems of pediatric care can position themselves to build healthier futures for kids, equipping them with the tools they need to thrive across all aspects of their development (Figure 9.20).

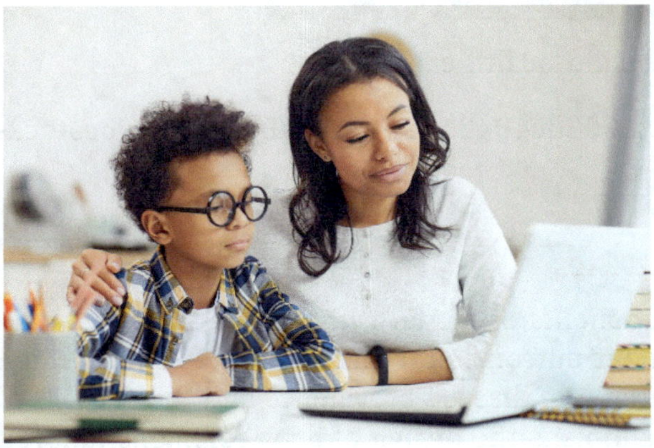

Figure 9.20. Pediatric teletherapy.

Source: https://qtxasset.com/quartz/qcloud5/media/image/fiercehealthcare/1631112267/GettyImages-1225545084.jpg/GettyImages-1225545084.jpg?VersionId=QGwhDoMnl5WqkA6yWuX5P8LxnNZD.0BX.

9.6.1. Technological Innovations in Treatment

Technological advances in treatment processes have revolutionized pediatric care, making medical treatments more effective and efficient for children. With the advent of precision medicine, medical professionals can now tailor treatment to children's unique genetic profiles as outpatients, leading to more effective and personalized care. For instance, genomic developments enabled the identification of individualized genetic markers associated with various pediatric diseases, thereby enabling targeted therapies to avoid harm while maximizing health gains. Not only does the personalized approach maximize the efficiency of treatment but also reinforce the importance of early interventions in the end, rewriting the traditional paradigms of pediatric health care. These advances are indicative of a shift from reactive to proactive medicine, with a focus on the potential to achieve long-term health through wise medical decisions and individualized strategies, as exemplified by the potential to cure disease and optimize health span in children (Terzic et al., 2019). In addition to precision medicine, technological advances have facilitated the easier integration of digital platforms into the treatment of children, significantly reducing patient monitoring and engagement. Telehealth has become extremely popular, allowing healthcare providers to reach patients in remote areas while providing timely consultations and interventions. This access can be particularly valuable for pediatric populations, where it can be challenging to attend regular clinic visits due to geographic or socioeconomic factors. Additionally, wearable technology and mobile health applications have enabled parents and caregivers to monitor their children's health metrics in real time, facilitating a team-based care approach. These technologies facilitate active involvement of families in the management of pediatric illnesses, thereby enhancing follow-through on treatment plans and ultimately better health outcomes. The integration of digital technologies thus not only enhances accessibility but also parental involvement in the patient care process. Along with these developments, however, come ethical issues that must be navigated cautiously, particularly the application of new therapies in pediatrics. As treatments involving genetic modification or neuromodulation attract attention, there are relevant issues regarding their suitability and possible impacts upon the autonomy and future decisions of a child. Healthcare professionals have to weigh the innovation of treatment technology against the ethical imperative to prioritize patient dignity and safety above all else, especially when considering an intervention that could alter the very nature of personal identity. The discourse of the moral implications of new pediatric interventions is multifaceted, with perspectives from healthcare providers, patients, and families. As noted, the harmony that currently exists between technology development and the ethics of pediatric interventions is critical to maintaining trust and integrity in the practice of medicine, such that technological growth is used to enhance healthcare without compromising ethics (Whitaker et al., 2018) (Figure 9.21).

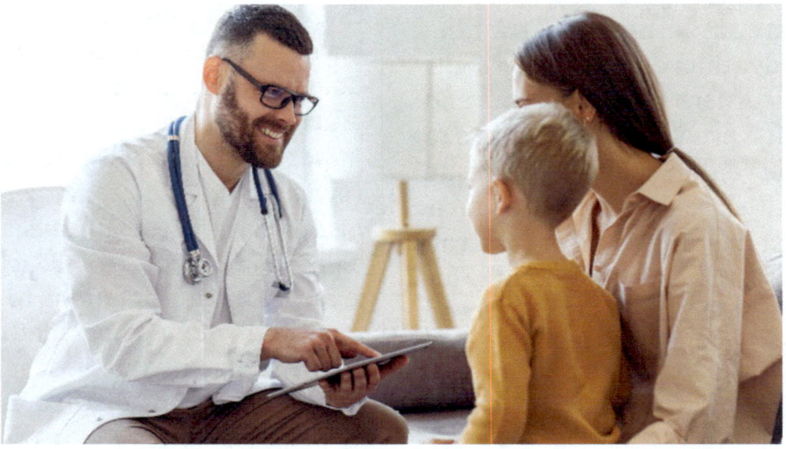

Figure 9.21. AI-driven medical research to improve child health care.

Source: https://assets.aboutamazon.com/86/83/2ab008dc4042affaae6155a80a3d/adobestock-doctor-ai-technology-child.png.

9.6.2. Research and Development in Pediatrics

Pediatric research and development are critical components of modern healthcare since not only do they drive medical science, but also improve patient outcomes for children. The sophisticated issues involved in pediatrics demand exclusive research into disease prevalence and the success of treatment in the pediatric population. An obvious example is the design of drug regimens tailored particularly for pediatric populations. For instance, a pharmacotherapeutic guide for treatment that defines the attributes of intravenous and oral drugs, including therapeutic classes, clinical indications, and potential adverse effects, is paramount for improving medication safety in children admitted to hospitals (da Cruz et al., 2024). Such guidelines enhance health practitioners' ability to provide informed, evidence-based treatment, significantly reducing the risk associated with pediatric pharmacotherapy. In addition, the value of research is not limited to pharmacological creation to address broader developmental aspects, such as early childhood literacy. Pediatric practice professionals are well-placed to enhance literacy as a vital aspect of child development. Studies have shown that shared reading practices promote positive infant-caregiver relationships, encouraging both attachment and cognitive growth (Klass et al., 2024). By integrating literacy promotion into well visits, healthcare providers can help create healthy home environments that foster social-emotional development and educational readiness. These efforts demonstrate how pediatric research not only addresses pressing medical issues but also enables greater developmental objectives that lead to healthier child life courses. In addition, collaboration among researchers, healthcare providers, and policymakers is the most important factor to adopt pediatric research and move it to practice. By focusing on the importance of policies that support access to good children's literature, for example, health practitioners can help address inequalities faced by children from less-resourced communities (Klass et al., 2024). The American Academy of Pediatrics (AAP) advocates for integrating literacy programs into pediatric education so that practitioners can more effectively address these developmental issues. With evolving research, it is required to bridge the gap between science and practice in the clinical field to deliver innovations that guarantee the all-around well-being of children. Through this interdisciplinary approach, the need for continuous research and development to transform pediatric care and enhance welfare becomes paramount.

9.6.3. Preventive Care and Vaccination Programs

Preventive checkups and immunization schedules are integral components of pediatric care that safeguard children's health against avoidable diseases. Vaccines are not just vital for the health of individual children but also for public health, as high levels of immunization lead to herd immunity. Herd immunity protects individuals who cannot be vaccinated, such as infants and children with certain medical conditions, by reducing the rate of vaccine-preventable illnesses within a population. Effective vaccination programs help reduce the incidence of diseases such as measles, mumps, and influenza, which can lead to severe complications or even death. Eradication of disease, as it would have to be without mass vaccination, would inevitably be followed by an increase in morbidity as well as in healthcare costs, making preventive vaccination efforts essential components of pediatric models of care. Despite scientific evidence of immunization's effectiveness, parental resistance remains a persistent issue despite high immunization coverage. Various studies indicate that parents are likely to decide based on conceptions of vaccine safety influenced by misinformation and anecdotal evidence.

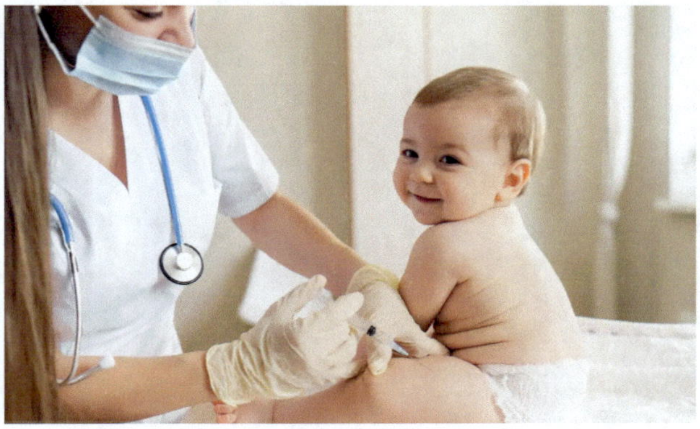

Figure 9.22. Newborn baby vaccination: protecting your child from deadly diseases.

Source: https://health-e.in/wp-content/uploads/2023/05/Newborn-Baby-Vaccination.webp.

For instance, in Juneau, Alaska, a study revealed that the sole significant factor in parental refusal of flu vaccination was their awareness of vaccine-related risks (Leder et al., 2015). This underscores the need for healthcare providers to adopt effective communication practices to dispel parental myths and fears about vaccines. By establishing a supportive atmosphere of trust and providing clear, evidence-based information, pediatricians can foster vaccination adherence, thereby improving community health and protecting vulnerable groups. Additionally, comprehensive preventive care programs extend beyond vaccines to cover regular health screening and education on healthy lifestyle choices. Childhood overweight, for instance, is a highly emergent condition that can be managed by preventive services through parents' education and early intervention. Multidisciplinary teamwork among healthcare providers, policymakers, and patients' advocates is required in the delivery of effective preventive programs (McCarthy et al., 2004). Preventive programs can have a profound impact on children's long-term health status by promoting frequent check-ups, dietary guidance, and physical exercise. By addressing all facets of health, from vaccines to nutrition, child care can make a significant difference in children's overall well-being, thereby contributing to a healthier future generation (Figure 9.22).

Test Your Knowledge

1. What is technological innovation in treatment?
2. What is the role of preventive care and vaccination programs in pediatric care?

SUMMARY

The synopsis of any comprehensive pediatrics review must capture the key principles that determine the special needs of this vulnerable group. Pediatric practice is not merely an offshoot of medical practice but a specialty in its own right that requires profound respect for the unique intricacies involved in the care of infants, children, and adolescents. Variables such as developmental stages, varying ability to understand medical information, and specific psychosocial dynamics necessitate that healthcare providers develop individualized strategies. In accordance with studies, particularly pediatric advanced care planning, incorporating family values and dynamics becomes the key to an effective treatment strategy. Experts must surpass the discomfort that besets the majority of people regarding end-of-life care, which poses challenges to enjoying well-crafted care models that respect patients' and families' preferences while maintaining thorough treatment. The role of new approaches in pediatric care cannot be overemphasized as well. Enhanced technology for liquid biopsies, i.e., cell-free DNA profiling, offers a glimpse of the potential of personalized medicine in the treatment of pediatric malignancies. These developments highlight an important step toward minimally invasive diagnostic techniques that could significantly enhance therapeutic decision-making. The promise of these developments lies not only in facilitating earlier disease detection and monitoring but also in improving prognostic assessment for pediatric patients. As pediatric oncology practice begins incorporating these approaches into standard care protocols, as noted in recent qualitative research, it is increasingly crucial that physicians remain up-to-date on their applications, benefits, and potential drawbacks; this vigilance will ultimately translate into improved clinical outcomes and better support for children facing severe health crises. In brief, the landscape of pediatric practice is evolving rapidly in the shadow of new technology and techniques, but still grappling with age-old ethical and functional concerns. The integration of pediatric advanced care planning, as highlighted by recent evidence, demands global effort from healthcare professionals in ensuring good communication and shared decision-making with families. As we navigate the gaps outlined in our analyses, collaboration among complex groups of clinicians, families, and policymakers will be required to fill them. Moreover, the knowledge that can be obtained from emerging technologies such as liquid biopsies is a promising future, presenting opportunities for personalized treatment protocols that could substantially enhance the lives of pediatric patients with devastating diseases. Thus, ongoing research and interdisciplinary discussion remain paramount in promoting the quality of care that children receive and in ensuring that their specific health needs are met with empathy and expertise.

The child health landscape is constantly evolving to meet the demands of advances in medical technology and a deeper understanding of the child's medical needs. Central to this evolution is an appreciation for the unique physiological and psychological needs of children as they fundamentally differ from those of an adult. Pediatric care encompasses an extensive range of services, from preventive health care to specialized treatments for complex conditions. This integral practice not only addresses short-term healthcare needs but also considers the future, keeping in mind the child's overall development. Excellent pediatric practice recognizes the importance of involving families and considering the affective and social aspects of pediatrics, fostering a setting in which holistic health can thrive. Practices in pediatrics are most significant, especially when severe conditions necessitate specialized interventions. For instance, patients admitted to pediatric intensive care units (PICUs) usually require a coordinated effort among various health care professionals to meet both medical and psychosocial needs. PICU admissions have broader implications than the short-term clinical result since families may suffer from severe emotional and functional challenges later on. Research also highlighted the point that while the majority of children recover from life-threatening illnesses, their families and they themselves are likely to experience a range of problems post-discharge. It is essential that the healthcare providers become aware of these concerns because they impact both the design of care protocols as well as the support systems available for families dealing with the consequences of a child's near-death illness (Coad et al., 2020). Moreover, a growing number of studies also focus on the importance of research in advancing pediatric practice. Studies such as those conducted by the Boston University Center for Global Health and Development aim to fill knowledge gaps regarding pediatric recovery trajectories, quality of life, and family relationships after critical care. Through the use of a mixed-methods design, researchers can gain a comprehensive picture of the variables that affect a child's recovery and the family's accommodation to changed circumstances. This focus not only improves clinical practice but also illuminates policy efforts to ensure higher standards of pediatric care. Last but not least, systematic research activities are necessary to inform strategies centered on the health and welfare of children throughout their lifetimes, so that the care of children renews its commitment to excellence and compassion (Fox et al., 2013).

KEY TERMS FROM THIS CHAPTER

- Antibiotic therapy
- Collaboration
- Diarrhea
- Pediatric care
- Pediatric oncology
- Pediatric research
- Screenings
- Asthma
- Diabetes
- Genetic testing
- Pediatric medicine
- Pediatric patients
- Pediatric services
- Vaccinations

CRITICAL THINKING QUESTIONS

1. **What is the most common cause of respiratory distress in newborns?**
   a. Pneumonia
   b. Meconium aspiration syndrome
   c. Respiratory distress syndrome (RDS)
   d. Transient tachypnea of the newborn (TTN)
2. **Which vaccine is typically given at birth?**
   a. Measles, mumps, and rubella (MMR)
   b. Bacillus Calmette-Guérin (BCG)
   c. Rotavirus vaccine
   d. Human papillomavirus (HPV) vaccine
3. **What is the recommended exclusive breastfeeding duration for infants?**
   a. 4 months
   b. 6 months
   c. 12 months
   d. 2 years
4. **What is the most common cause of diarrhea in children under 2 years?**
   a. Bacterial infection
   b. Viral gastroenteritis (Rotavirus)
   c. Parasitic infection
   d. Food allergy
5. **Which of the following is the most common congenital heart defect?**
   a. Tetralogy of Fallot
   b. Ventricular septal defect (VSD)
   c. Atrial septal defect (ASD)
   d. Coarctation of the aorta

Short Answer Questions

1. What age is pediatric for?
2. What is the importance of pediatric care in healthcare?
3. Who was considered the father of pediatrics?
4. What are the most common health issues for children?
5. What is the role of pediatric healthcare providers?

Answer to Critical Thinking Questions

1. (c); 2. (b); 3. (b); 4. (b); 5. (b).

REFERENCES

1. Sala-Hamrick, K. J., Isakson, B., Del Campo De Gonzalez, S., Cooper, A., Buchan, J., Aceves, J., Van Orton, E., Holtz, J., & Waggoner, D. M. (2021). Trauma-Informed Pediatric Primary Care: Facilitators and Challenges to the implementation process. *The Journal of Behavioral Health Services & Research*, *48*(3), 363–381. https://doi.org/10.1007/s11414-020-09741-1Adi, S., Arbiter, B., Blum, M., et al. (2015). A case study in open-source innovation: Developing the Tidepool platform for interoperability in type 1 diabetes management. https://core.ac.uk/download/323073561.pdf (accessed on 12th July 2025).
2. Agapidaki, E., Souliotis, K., Christogiorgos, S., Zervas, L., Leonardou, A., Kolaitis, G., Giannakopoulos, G., et al. (2013). A theory-based educational intervention to pediatricians in order to improve identification and referral of maternal depression: A quasi-experimental study. *Annals of General Psychiatry, 12*, 37. https://www.semanticscholar.org/paper/6e7c363fadd974c0a1d8d0e827d77327f11f31bf (accessed on 12th July 2025).
3. Ahern, J., Barakat, L. P., Bhatia, S., et al. (2016). Patient/family education for newly diagnosed pediatric oncology patients. https://core.ac.uk/download/213078812.pdf (accessed on 12th July 2025).
4. Alpern, E., Badaki-Makun, O., Bergmann, K., et al. (2024). Acute care utilization for ambulatory care-sensitive conditions among publicly insured children. https://core.ac.uk/download/649473321.pdf (accessed on 12th July 2025).
5. Astrahantseff, K., Chaali-Vlug, R., De Preter, K., et al. (2020). The pitfalls and promise of liquid biopsies for diagnosing and treating solid tumors in children: A review. https://core.ac.uk/download/286549310.pdf (accessed on 12th July 2025).
6. Bagnall, A., Day, R., & Kime, N. H. (2013). Systematic review of transition models for young people with long-term conditions: A report for NHS Diabetes. https://core.ac.uk/download/29018738.pdf (accessed on 12th July 2025).
7. Balchunas, M. K., Brock, L., Cavegn, B., et al. (2010). Nurse researchers in children's hospitals. https://core.ac.uk/download/213078811.pdf (accessed on 12th July 2025).
8. Borasio, G. D., Führer, M., Jox, R. J., et al. (2014). Pediatric advance care planning from the perspective of healthcare professionals: A qualitative interview study. https://core.ac.uk/download/77163303.pdf (accessed on 12th July 2025).
9. Boring, E., Dias, N., Haase, J. E., et al. (2019). A systematic literature review of the current state of knowledge related to interventions for bereaved parents. https://core.ac.uk/download/299809052.pdf (accessed on 12th July 2025).
10. Brugnoletti, O., Corridore, D., Cavallè, E., et al. (2015). Preventive strategies in oral health for special needs patients. https://core.ac.uk/download/54529526.pdf (accessed on 12th July 2025).
11. Caicedo, C. (2013). Children with special health care needs: Comparison of the effects of home care setting, prescribed pediatric extended care setting, and long-term care setting on child and family health outcomes and healthcare service use. https://core.ac.uk/download/46952373.pdf (accessed on 12th July 2025).
12. Carey, L. K., Fox, R. A., & Nicholson, B. C. (2002). Maternal factors related to parenting young children with congenital heart disease. https://core.ac.uk/download/213077045.pdf (accessed on 12th July 2025).

13. Caron, R. M. (2019). Co-producing healthcare in a volume vs. value-based healthcare system: Perspective of a parent of a patient and a health professions' educator. https://core.ac.uk/download/286641620.pdf (accessed on 12th July 2025).

14. Clayton-Jones, D. L., & Haglund, K. (2016). The role of spirituality and religiosity in persons living with sickle cell disease. https://core.ac.uk/download/213079099.pdf (accessed on 12th July 2025).

15. Coad, J., Colville, G., Curley, M. A. Q., et al. (2020). Study protocol for a multicenter longitudinal mixed methods study to explore the outcomes of children and families in the first year after pediatric intensive care: The OCEANIC study. https://core.ac.uk/download/323385694.pdf (accessed on 12th July 2025).

16. Das, D., Chakrabarty, T., & Halder, A. (2025). Effects of staff turnover on continuity of care in pediatric chronic disease management. *Journal of Neonatal Surgery*. https://www.semanticscholar.org/paper/27eed3011121608f4d9690093b696e2c40de82ee (accessed on 12th July 2025).

17. Dayan, P. S., Gerber, J. S., Hersh, A. L., et al. (2017). Current state of antimicrobial stewardship in children's hospital emergency departments. https://core.ac.uk/download/80495100.pdf (accessed on 12th July 2025).

18. Deb, T. R., & Jahan, A. (2025). A comprehensive study on various cancer occurred in pediatric units. https://core.ac.uk/download/656178867.pdf (accessed on 12th July 2025).

19. Drotar, D., Dworkin, P., & Stancin, T. (2008). Pediatric developmental screening: Understanding and selecting screening instruments. https://core.ac.uk/download/71353748.pdf (accessed on 12th July 2025).

20. Ehrenberger, K. A. (2023). Giving voice to cardiovocal syndrome: A 26-year-old woman with hypophonia and dysphagia. *Cureus, 15*. https://www.semanticscholar.org/paper/360d54f7ac1b675ddd386fbefc8297e57047d648 (accessed on 12th July 2025).

21. Eliseussen, J. N., & Grønli, M. (2024). Gjøre livene dere lettere: En kvalitativ studie om sykepleierens opplevelse av sitt ansvar og sin funksjon i et barnepalliativt team, og hvordan egen kompetanse nyttiggjøres i teamet. https://core.ac.uk/download/616581601.pdf (accessed on 12th July 2025).

22. Farias, A. J., Cousineau, M. R., & E-Nunu, T. (2008). Healthy Kids Program and the safety net: Perceptions of community clinic administrators. https://core.ac.uk/download/71351710.pdf (accessed on 12th July 2025).

23. Favuzza, A. (2018). Passion with purpose: A case study of St. Jude Children's Research Hospital. https://core.ac.uk/download/158246431.pdf (accessed on 12th July 2025).

24. Fortuny, K., & Golden, O. (2011). Improving the lives of young children: Meeting parents' health and mental health needs through Medicaid and CHIP so children can thrive. https://core.ac.uk/download/71357294.pdf (accessed on 12th July 2025).

25. Fox, M., & Rosen, S. (2013). Retention on antiretroviral therapy in low- and middle-income countries: Systematic review of papers and abstracts since 2008. https://open.bu.edu/bitstream/2144/23260/1/HDDP-16-retention-on-ART.pdf (accessed on 12th July 2025).

26. Goldblatt, J., Isasi, R., Jagut, M., et al. (2019). Model consent clauses for rare disease research. https://core.ac.uk/download/237010883.pdf (accessed on 12th July 2025).

27. Hagelow, G., & Silow-Carroll, S. (2010). Systems of care coordination for children: Lessons learned across state models. https://core.ac.uk/download/71355339.pdf (accessed on 12th July 2025).

28. Hays, R. D., Lerner, C., Palimaru, A., et al. (2020). A review of best practices for monitoring and improving inpatient pediatric patient experiences. https://core.ac.uk/download/287622168.pdf (accessed on 12th July 2025).

29. Jaffee, E. M., Speropolous, L., & Widmer, J. (2015). Oral health care access in New Hampshire. https://core.ac.uk/download/72048638.pdf (accessed on 12th July 2025).

30. Klass, P., Miller-Fitzwater, A., & High, P. C. (2024). Literacy promotion: An essential component of primary care pediatric practice: Policy statement. *Pediatrics.* https://www.semanticscholar.org/paper/5aaf56ecc42f36ce16aa335952e46fea6c66e7ec (accessed on 12th July 2025).

31. Leder, L. (2015). Vaccination hesitation: Investigation why parents decline pediatric influenza vaccines in Juneau, Alaska. https://core.ac.uk/download/162577318.pdf (accessed on 12th July 2025).

32. Lucas, S. H., Thompson, S., et al. (2017). Reducing antibiotic use in pediatric upper respiratory infection: A multifaceted parent-clinician approach. https://core.ac.uk/download/84064374.pdf (accessed on 12th July 2025).

33. Luke, T. A. (2016). The role of telehealth technology in the remediation of pediatric feeding disorders. https://core.ac.uk/download/211336814.pdf (accessed on 12th July 2025).

34. Lyman, D. R., Dougherty, R. H., & Holt, W. (2010). State case studies of infant and early childhood mental health systems: Strategies for change. https://core.ac.uk/download/71355034.pdf (accessed on 12th July 2025).

35. McAllister, J. W., Popp, J., & Antonelli, R. (2009). Making care coordination a critical component of the pediatric health system: A multidisciplinary framework. https://core.ac.uk/download/71352885.pdf (accessed on 12th July 2025).

36. McCarthy, D., & Leatherman, S. (2004). Quality of health care for children and adolescents: A chartbook. https://core.ac.uk/download/71354153.pdf (accessed on 12th July 2025).

37. Meduri, G. U., & Schwingshackl, A. (2016). Rationale for prolonged glucocorticoid use in pediatric ARDS: What the adults can teach us. https://core.ac.uk/download/323079960.pdf (accessed on 12th July 2025).

38. Miró-Bonet, R., Molina-Mula, J., & Vicens-Blanes, F. (2025). Discursive analysis of pediatrician's therapeutic approach towards childhood fever and its contextual differences: An ethnomethodological study. https://core.ac.uk/download/653728874.pdf (accessed on 12th July 2025).

39. Murphy, C. G., Alendy, C., Cooper, J., & Simpson, L. (2008). Childhood obesity: The role of health policy. https://core.ac.uk/download/71342400.pdf (accessed on 12th July 2025).

40. Pansier, B., & Zheng, A. (2022). Global child and family-centered care fellowship, education, and mentorship for pediatric healthcare professionals: A literature review. https://core.ac.uk/download/539123892.pdf (accessed on 12th July 2025).

41. Sachs, A. N., Nutt, C. T., Baguley, D., Notterman, D. C., Knoppert, D. M., Taylor, D. M., Ansah, E., et al. (2013). Children's medicines in Tanzania: A national survey of administration practices and preferences. https://core.ac.uk/download/11307828.pdf (accessed on 12th July 2025).

42. Salvi da Cruz, L. H. de Oliveira, Silva, A. C. S. S., Amarante, L. H., Ferreira, A. B. R., Góes, F., & de Rocha, B. C. O. (2024). Development of a pharmacotherapeutic assistance protocol in pediatrics: Contributions to nursing care. *Escola Anna Nery*. https://www.semanticscholar.org/paper/f9daba25763f64e64a9093e6729f17a9509364d0 (accessed on 12th July 2025).

43. Sarmiento, B. M. P., Díaz Rodríguez, M., Fernández Gutiérrez, M., et al. (2020). Effectiveness of a multifactorial intervention in the first 1000 days of life to prevent obesity and overweight in childhood: Study protocol. https://core.ac.uk/download/323288296.pdf (accessed on 12th July 2025).

44. Shonkoff, J., Boyce, W., Bush, N., Gunnar, M., Hensch, T., Levitt, P., Meaney, M., et al. (2022). Translating the biology of adversity and resilience into new measures for pediatric practice. *Pediatrics*. https://www.semanticscholar.org/paper/7dadef725df288b09b99a9ece81d91df91b58cf1 (accessed on 12th July 2025).

45. Singh, D. (2024). Mental health resources for pediatric patients. https://core.ac.uk/download/639243347.pdf (accessed on 12th July 2025).

46. Terzic, A., & Waldman, S. A. (2019). Health care evolves from reactive to proactive. https://core.ac.uk/download/213444739.pdf (accessed on 12th July 2025).

47. Volk, A., Davis, M. J., Abu-Ghname, A., Warfield, R. G., Ibrahim, R., Karon, G. N., & Hollier, L. (2020). Ambulatory access: Improving scheduling increases patient satisfaction and revenue. *Plastic and Reconstructive Surgery, 146*(5), 913–919. https://www.semanticscholar.org/paper/cc47dba14650d13c4c0951986b2de38c978a87d7 (accessed on 12th July 2025).

48. Whitaker, H. N. (2018). Attitudes on medical ethics of criminal neurointerventional treatment. https://core.ac.uk/download/213462108.pdf (accessed on 12th July 2025).

49. Wu, Q. L., & Brannon, G. (2023). Collaborative care and healthcare usage in families with pediatric patients during COVID-19: A secondary analysis of National Survey of Children's Health (NSCH) data. *Health Communication, 39*, 1053–1065. https://www.semanticscholar.org/paper/700510cac4d044bf42191e0b0f2b828bc1dbacae (accessed on 12th July 2025).

ADOLESCENT MEDICINE

10

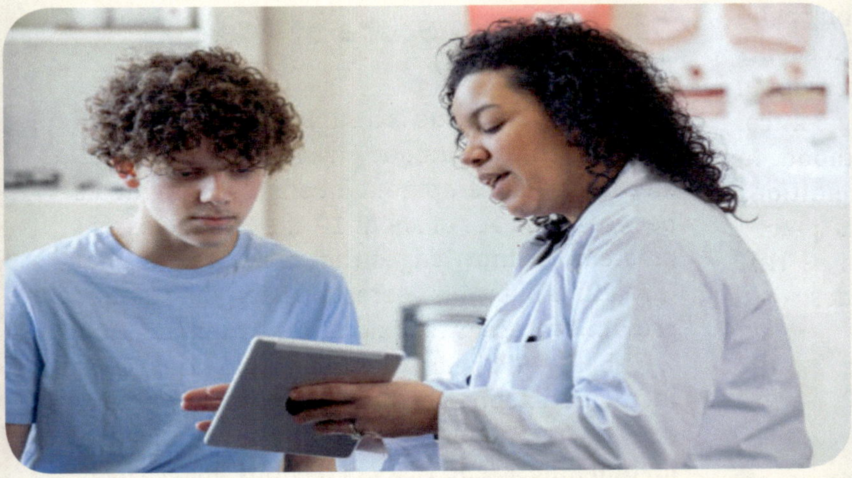

Introduction

The adolescent medicine specialty has an important role in addressing the unique healthcare needs of adolescents, a stage of life characterized by extensive physical, emotional, and social transformations. As the specialty evolved, it became apparent that adolescents faced health challenges specific to this age group, distinct from those of young children and adults. These consist of a wide array of issues ranging from mental disorders, drug use, sexual problems, and chronic illnesses. Given the transitional nature of adolescence, medical practitioners are compelled to use a developmental and integrative approach that addresses not only the biological aspects of care but also the psychosocial and behavioral aspects. Such a contextualized approach aims to provide comprehensive care, with interventions judiciously tailored to adolescents' developmental stages and associated problems. Also, the imperative for continuity in transition between child and adult health care cannot be overstated in the specialty of adolescent medicine. It has been documented that adolescents who have chronic illness typically

LEARNING OBJECTIVES

After studying this chapter, you will be able to:

1. Describe the physical development in adolescents
2. Know the mental health issues in adolescents
3. Describe the preventive health care for adolescents
4. Discuss the sexual and reproductive health
5. Know the impact of chronic illnesses on adolescents
6. Understand the role of technology in adolescent health

experience difficulty in such a transition, thereby leading to discontinuities in continuity of care that could have adverse impacts on health outcomes. Studies have pointed out that the lack of a proven model for transition may further affect the process of healthcare among adolescents with greater needs for health, such as palliative care recipients. (Adi et al., 2009) supports the variable quality of existing transition services and emphasizes the necessity of evidence-based guidelines to maximize best practices. By fostering cooperation among child and adult health care providers, adolescents can most readily benefit from an uninterrupted continuum of care, thereby maximizing control over disease conditions in early adulthood. In combating the dominance of disease conditions during adolescence, extensive focus is placed on the burden of some diseases, such as HIV, particularly in underserved communities.

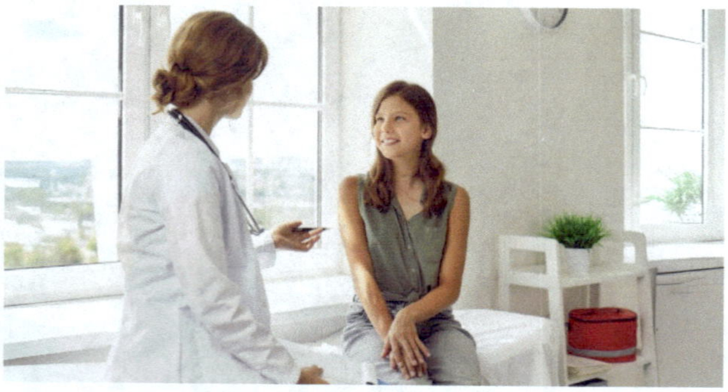

Figure 10.1. Adolescent medicine.

Source: https://baravkarclinic.com/wp-content/uploads/2025/04/Untitled-design-2025-04-18T171907.124.png.

Research conducted in Sub-Saharan Africa discovers that an impressive percentage of HIV-positive adolescents continue to experience difficulties with antiretroviral therapy adherence, resulting in adverse health outcomes. As acknowledged in Adejumo et al. (2019), a number of determinants influence adherence, including stigma, peer relationships, and caregiver support, indicating a complex interplay of social processes that must be considered in healthcare interventions. These problems illustrate the broader social context in which teens exist, and interventions that address not only the youth but also their community context are needed. By addressing these system-level problems and expanding educational opportunities and access to support, the field of adolescent medicine can establish settings that promote healthier outcomes for this group (Figure 10.1).

Definition and Scope of Adolescent Medicine

Adolescent medicine is a subspecialty dedicated to addressing the unique physical, psychological, and social development needs of individuals between the ages of about 10 and 21. Adolescent medicine acknowledges that teenagers are not tiny adults but rather persons undergoing unique growth processes that significantly impact their well-being and health. In this regard, adolescent medicine encompasses a wide range of items like the management of long-term disease, mental illness, and risky behaviors such as drug use and sex. As matters related to adolescents have lifelong implications, understanding the dynamics of this age group is crucial for providing effective medical care. Second, adolescent medicine confirms the importance of delivering care in a supportive environment that promotes communication, thereby developing a productive doctor-patient relationship critical to successful health outcomes. Adolescent medicine also extends beyond individualized self-care in addressing broader sociocultural and environmental determinants that shape young people's health. This specialty addresses systemic issues, including access to care, health disparities, and social determinants that influence the well-being of adolescents. For example, inadequate access to quality mental health care can hinder adolescents' ability to access timely care and support and, consequently, worsen their situations (Bagalman et al., 2013). In addition, the physical surroundings in which adolescents live and learn have profound impacts on their health outcomes. Contact with pollution and social violence are some of the environmental conditions that, as studies in green school violence argue, can significantly influence an adolescent's development and health (Barrett et al., 2016). Adolescent medicine thus prioritizes an integrated strategy, accepting that physical, emotional, and environmental health are interconnected. As the teenage population evolves, so too must the definition and scope of adolescent medicine to meet contemporary issues. Emerging technologies, such as telemedicine, have been increasingly integral to the provision of care, particularly for mental health care, which is normally difficult for teens to access. Additionally, the application of preventative services and health education is very important in addressing issues such as obesity, mental health, and drug abuse among adolescents. By focusing on integrated care in the sense of education on good life choices, teenage medicine aims to empower adolescents to take charge of their health. Moreover, continued research and policy development are required to promote quality adolescent care, as well as to address systemic issues, such as health care disparities. Ultimately, the practice of adolescent medicine is not only about improving individual health status but also about fostering a healthier next generation.

Importance of Specialized Care for Adolescents

The importance of specialized care for adolescents is underscored by the unique physiological, psychological, and social issues adolescents face during this stage of development. Adolescence is marked by rapid body change, including hormonal shifts that have severe impacts on mental health. Incidence of mood disorders such as depression is concerning; statistics show that close to 2 million adolescents experience major depressive episodes annually, with socioeconomic status increasing these disorders ((Hari et al., 2017)). This underscores the need for age-related interventions that account for the special needs of adolescents. By focusing on personalized care, healthcare providers can address both short-term health needs and long-term mental health effects, implementing more effective care that is responsive to the teen experience. In addition to areas related to mental health, specialized attention is indispensable for addressing the physical activity and lifestyle factors that affect overall well-being during adolescence. More sport specialization among children has also led to increased interest in its physical and psychological health consequences. Specialization early in life, where training begins as early as five or six years old, could generate far-reaching physical and emotional stress that could lead to burnout or injury (Hecimovich et al., 2004). As more adolescents engage in high-intensity training, there is a greater risk of neglecting other supportive factors such as symmetrical exercise and socialization. As such, special treatment must extend beyond intervention for physical injury to counseling for participation in safe sports and recreation. This holistic approach promotes not only physical well-being but also healthy stress- and anxiety-management skills, which are crucial during adolescence. In addition, specialized treatment is not limited to the clinical arena but also includes educational settings where teens are present for many hours. School-based mental health interventions are a vital channel for providing assistance, especially for low-income youth who are disproportionately impacted by mental health concerns ((Hari et al., 2017)). School-based programs can provide screenings and interventions and cultivate settings that support mental health. By integrating mental health training into school curricula, teachers can help young people become aware of signs of distress and foster help-seeking attitudes. These comprehensive measures empower young people to take responsibility for their own mental health and create supportive networks among both peers and teachers. A multi-dimensional approach combining clinical and school-based services fosters the mental and physical health needs of youths to create a resilient healthier generation (Figure 10.2).

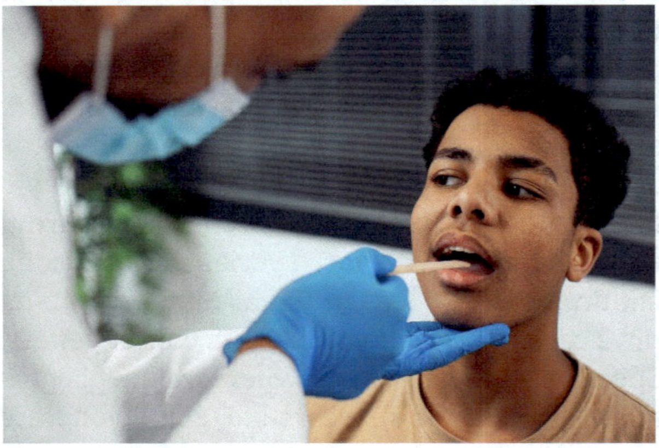

Figure 10.2. Adolescent care.

Source: https://rigbypediatrics.com/media/pdvc4or4/doctor-taking-care-afro-american-child-1.jpg.

Overview of the Developmental Stages in Adolescence

Adolescence is marked by intense developmental changes, both physical, cognitive, emotional, and social. Physically, the onset of puberty initiates a sequence of changes, including growth spurts, sexual maturation, and compositional changes. These are not uniform and significantly vary from person to person, influencing self-concept and interpersonal relationships. Cognitively, adolescents transition from concrete operational thought to more advanced, abstract thought, enabling them to visualize hypothetical scenarios, reflect on moral dilemmas, and comprehend the future consequences of their actions. This cognitive maturation is crucial because it provides the foundation for decision-making and for assessing risk, and thus is crucial to understand how these skills develop during adolescence. As teenagers strive to complete these tasks of development, the nature of their parent-child relationships may go a long way in influencing their emotional and behavioral growth, particularly for risk behavior associated with drug use (Ralston et al., 2012). Socially, the teenager is increasingly turning toward the external world to break free from parents, fostering development of peer relationships that either support or deter them. The effects of peer dynamics become very evident, as friendship is a source of identity exploration and social learning. At this stage, adolescents tend to struggle with acceptance and belonging, which in turn translates into behaviors that may involve experimentation with drugs or nonconformity in society. Such experimentation is influenced by both intrinsic developmental issues and external forces, including peer pressure. Proper studies, such as the present Adolescent Brain Cognitive Development (ABCD) Study, aim to identify protective and risk factors that influence such behaviors. This longitudinal study provides valuable data on how cognitive development and social milieus are connected, thereby informing effective intervention strategies for healthy adolescent development (Bartsch et al., 2018). The teenage growth phases bring with them the transition to young adulthood, where one consolidates identity, acquires autonomy, and forms defining life choices. The final stage is characterized by ongoing self-definition exploration, making lifestyle decisions, like learning and career pursuits. During the time adolescents solidify their experiences, they often experience serious psychological problems like depression and anxiety, which may be compounded by drug use. The interactive dynamics between developmental milestones and mental health outcomes underscore the importance of an integrated adolescent medicine model that incorporates physical and psychological health. Facilitating healthy environments—through family engagement, peer support groups, or access to mental health services—supports adolescents' navigation through this tumultuous life stage, facilitating healthier adult transitions.

10.1. Physical Development in Adolescents

Learning Outcome

1. Understand the growth spurts and changes in body composition
2. Describe the sexual maturation during puberty
3. Know the impact of nutrition and exercise on physical health

Physical growth in adolescence is a complex and multifaceted process that marks the transition from childhood to adulthood. This stage of formation, typically between 10 and 19 years old, is characterized by massive growth spurts, hormonal changes, and the development of secondary sexual features. This change not only encompasses height and weight gain but also the development of organs and systems to prepare the body for reproduction. It is essential for medical practitioners committed to providing comprehensive adolescent medicine to understand these changes. Physical and psychological growth during this phase may lead to a variety of outcomes in health, which demand certain educational interventions to raise awareness in adolescents regarding the changes they go through, as supported by research findings yielding great improvements in knowledge after targeted educational interventions (Jyoti et al., 2025). Besides, the physical alterations that adolescents experience are typically accompanied by changes in body image. Teenagers begin to wrestle with societal beauty standards and appearance, which affect their emotional well-being and self-esteem. These pressures can have the capability to trigger behaviors in an attempt to achieve an ideal body image, e.g., over-exercising or extreme dieting, which can put immense strain on health. It is critical that those who deal with teenagers are informed about these pressures and their probable consequences. For instance, there are teenagers who resort to changing their appearance regarding tattoos and piercings for reasons of identity or acceptance, demonstrating their ongoing inner turmoil (Ciampo et al., 2024). Broaching these issues sensitively but informatively is required to foster healthy habits and self-acceptance in teenagers. Taking into account physical development, appropriate education and communication are critical. The application of consistent programs may help adolescents better understand their bodies and the changes occurring in them.

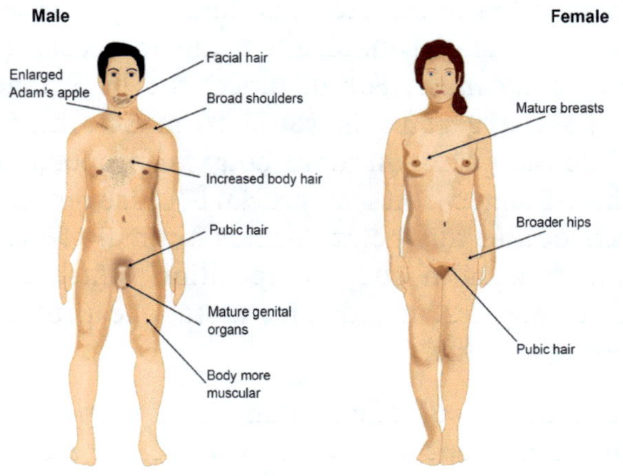

Figure 10.3. Puberty brings dramatic changes in the body, including the development of primary and secondary sex characteristics.

Source: https://cod.pressbooks.pub/app/uploads/sites/61/2021/01/image6.png.

As studies show, effective information sessions can significantly expand adolescents' knowledge of bodily changes, helping them navigate this unstable phase with greater ease and awareness. These programs not only offer young people information, but they also provide a safe environment in which young people are comfortable discussing their problems and experiences with a trusted adult or healthcare provider. This comprehensive approach to adolescent medicine prioritizes addressing physical growth challenges in the context of emotional and social care, ultimately supporting the development of healthier lifestyles and better mental health at this pivotal point in life (Jyoti et al., 2025). (Figure 10.3).

10.1.1. Growth Spurts and Changes in Body Composition

During adolescence, patients have sudden spurts of growth that essentially restructure body composition. Marked changes in height, weight, and body fat patterning accompany rapid physical development, with endocrine changes affecting most. The interplay between growth hormones and sex steroids initiates processes such as skeletal maturation and increases in lean body mass. For instance, the boys tend to have a greater increase in muscle mass, while the girls gain more body fat proportion. These biomechanics are crucial because optimal nutrition at this point enables optimal growth and changes in body composition, which can affect physical health and metabolic profiles throughout life.

Recognition of such changes is important for adolescent medicine providers because deviations from normal growth patterns can indicate underlying disease or malnutrition. Variability in body composition is also known to influence growth outcomes, particularly in adolescents with pre-pubertal short stature. Longitudinal analysis showed that children who reached normal height made substantially greater gains in body muscle mass index and total height than children who remained short-statured during this critical growth phase (Chun et al., 2025). This shows that not only the degree of improvement but even the body weight composition is a factor in achieving or maintaining maximum well-being in adolescence. The need to monitor alterations in body composition cannot be overstressed since it helps provide data on an adolescent's ongoing growth and potential health risks, including the potential of becoming obese and concomitant chronic diseases in the future. Body composition is also of significant concern in evaluating adolescents' health status, particularly obesity indicators. The World Health Organization has also proposed standards for assessing obesity, now recognized as essential in children, following the alarming rise observed across the globe in recent years (Park, 2024). Awareness of the causes and effects of growth spurts, and of their impact on body composition, enables health professionals to address the rising incidence of obesity and related health conditions effectively. A multidisciplinary approach that takes into consideration both physical growth and changes in body composition can provide a clear picture, and early interventions that affect long-term health consequences can be planned. Proper monitoring and encouragement of healthy growth in adolescence has to be a priority in adolescent medicine practice.

10.1.2. Sexual Maturation and Puberty

Puberty sexual development is a complex physiological process that transforms the individual from childhood to adulthood. It is at this stage that there are sharp hormonal changes that drive the development of secondary sexual characteristics, such as breast growth in girls and muscular development in boys. Additionally, the timing and pace of these developments could be controlled by various factors such as genetics, diet, and stressors. Adolescence typically starts in girls at the age of 9 to 14 years, and in boys at the age of 10 to 17 years, but occasionally there are variations leading to precocious or delayed puberty. For example, oligomenorrhea and abnormal uterine bleeding (AUB) may interfere with the usual course of sexual maturation among girls, particularly during high-stress conditions, for example, residence in areas of conflict, where environmental stresses may exacerbate such reproductive health problems (Dynnik et al., 2025). The role of environmental toxicants on sexual maturation has received more focus, particularly regarding chemicals like bisphenol

A (BPA). Studies have established a robust link between BPA exposure and precocious puberty, and this endocrine disruptor may hasten sexual maturation processes, mainly in females. The biological mechanisms by which BPA brings about these effects are still not fully understood, and the diversity of methods employed in research makes it difficult to draw conclusions of causality. However, the consequences are extensive for public health because exposure at these developmental windows is known to lead to premature puberty and long-term psychopathology (Pereira et al., 2025).

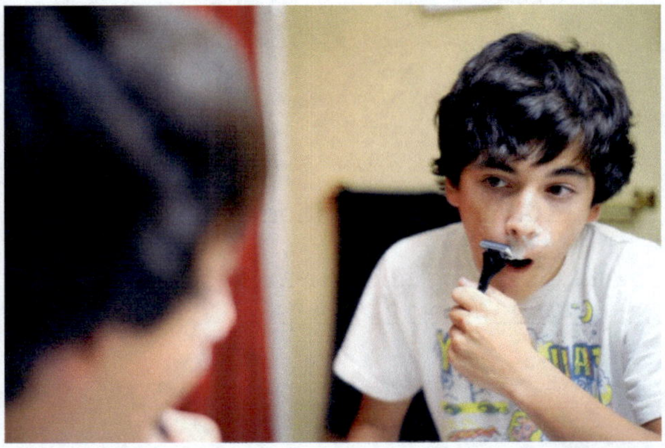

Figure 10.4. Males often start shaving during puberty.

Source: https://cod.pressbooks.pub/app/uploads/sites/61/2021/01/image7-1.jpeg.

These linkages must be understood to inform policy regulation designed to protect adolescents from harmful environmental exposures that have a profound effect on their physical and psychological well-being during this formative period of development (Pereira et al., 2025). When adolescents navigate the challenges of sexual maturation, their experiences are so much shaped by psychosocial as well as biological changes. Girls' menstruation and changes in boys' bodies can occur in parallel with heightened emotional sensitivity and social pressures that affect their self-concept and body image. Moreover, these physical changes may introduce new social processes, whereby adolescents become more conscious of their sexual selves and sexual relationships. Pressure on these negotiations may be added by external factors, for example, family disturbance or scholarly stress. Teenage medicine must then concentrate on integrated care that embraces both the medical and psychosocial dimensions of adolescence. Providing supportive settings can help empower healthier pubertal transitions, reducing risks of maladaptive adaptations to the widening emotional and physical landscape of adolescence (Dynnik et al., 2025) (Figure 10.4).

10.1.3. Impact of Nutrition and Exercise on Physical Health

The relationship between nutrition and physical health is particularly significant during adolescence, when there is such rapid growth and development. Proper eating habits formed at this foundational stage can lead to long-term benefits, including improved physical health and reduced risk of chronic diseases. Teenagers require adequate nutrition to allow for increasing metabolic demands, which will be supplemented by a balanced diet of fruits, vegetables, whole foods, and lean protein. For instance, evidence has shown that nutrition initiatives targeted at preadolescents can significantly improve health outcomes, as exemplified by a diabetes prevention camp that implemented a behavior-change intervention in a rural setting. These interventions demonstrate how deliberate nutrition education can yield positive behavior antecedents that lay the groundwork for long-term health benefits in youth (Mead et al., 2012). Physical fitness also complements the role of nutrition in promoting adolescent health, as it serves not only to keep the body physically fit but also to keep the mind. Sustained exercise enables weight management in adolescents, ensures healthy bones and muscles, and enhances heart health. Moreover, the environment is a significant exercise behavior. Available evidence on college students indicates that environmental predictors such as proximity to exercise facilities can influence physical activity frequency and weight control. Proximal female students to gym facilities had a greater exercise level, indicating the critical relationship between accessible environments and healthy lifestyle choices. These findings highlight how a supportive climate can maximize exercise behaviors and promote a general state of physical health during the developing phase of adolescence (Eisenberg et al., 2014). In the battle adolescents face with weight management and well-being, the relationship between diet and exercise becomes more evident. Effective interventions that target both dietary change and physical activity can maximize a general approach to adolescent health. Obesity prevention programs, such as those implemented in school or community settings, have been shown not only to alter short-term behaviors but also to affect healthy long-term habits. These programs underscore the importance of combined strategies that engage adolescents and their families and promote an integrated approach to healthier lifestyles. By tackling their issues through collaborative efforts in active living and nutrition education, health care professionals and educators can help empower young people to be more self-sufficient with the tools they need for a healthier future (Figure 10.5).

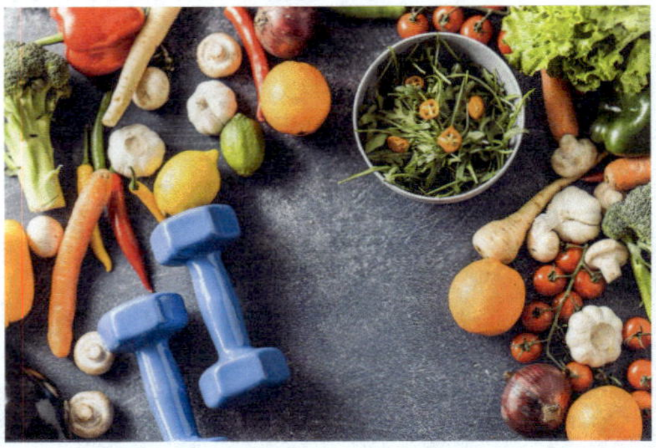

Figure 10.5. Role of nutrition in physical fitness.

Source: https://cms-api-in.myhealthcare.co/image/20220913125713.jpg.

Test Your Knowledge

1. What is the sexual maturation of puberty?
2. What is the impact of nutrition and exercise on physical health?

10.2. Mental Health Issues in Adolescents

Learning Outcome

1. Describe the common mental health disorders
2. Understand the role of social media and peer pressure
3. Know the strategies for promoting mental well-being

Teenage mental health gained more focus in the last decade, with increased pressures in the form of external stress adding to the natural issues within this age group. Academic pressure, social pressures through social media, and pressures from the family are major causes of increased instances of mental health conditions, including anxiety and depression. Evidence supports that, during the COVID-19 pandemic, adolescents all over the world suffered more mental health problems; for instance, one study revealed that high school students suffer from extreme mood shifts and tremendous levels of academic pressure compared to their middle school counterparts. These findings corroborate the requirement of instant awareness and specially formulated interventions on mental health that resonate with the particular pressures adolescents face in modern society. By establishing a culture that promotes openness and understanding around mental health, stakeholders can reduce stigma and promote healthier coping strategies among young people, thereby enhancing adolescent well-being (Gupta et al., 2024). Moreover, global reaction to adolescent mental health is shifting, and various countries are recognizing the benefits of systemic intervention and education. For instance, in 2019, the Philippines enacted its first mental health law, which reflects its aim to improve adolescent mental well-being through education. The legislative framework attaches great importance to incorporating mental health topics into school curricula, so that students learn relevant information to properly care for their own mental health. Similarly, Japan has also placed emphasis on educating mental health, incorporating it into their national curriculum to raise awareness about adolescent mental illnesses. All of these are necessary not only for equipping adolescents but also for cultivating a culture that appreciates the significance of mental health, thereby enabling young people to navigate their adolescence with strength and guidance (Ojio et al., 2024). In addition, coping strategies used by adolescents in the event of mental health challenges have a significant impact on their overall adjustment and well-being. A study of Indian adolescents during the pandemic revealed various coping mechanisms such as taking up new activities, spending time with family, and practicing meditation as stress management and anxiety devices. The diversification of the coping methods validates the idea that mental health is not only the lack of illness but also the development of emotional intelligence and resilience. Since schools and health facilities are working together to set up mental health programs, there is a need to incorporate these coping methods in the preventive approaches. By equipping adolescents with effective techniques to handle stressors, the likelihood of developing chronic mental health issues can be significantly reduced, fostering a generation that is more resilient in the face of adversities (Gupta et al., 2024) (Figure 10.6).

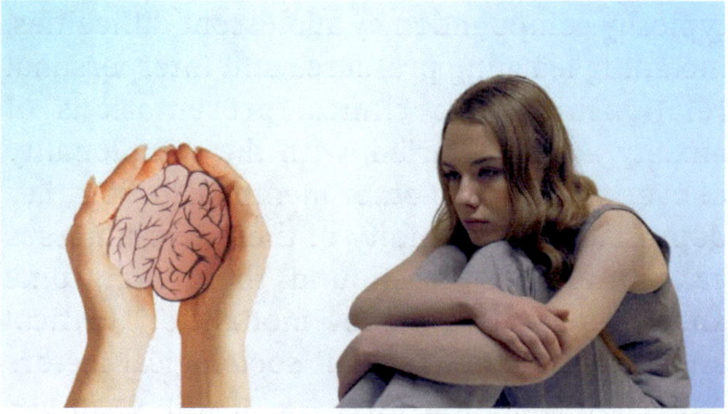

Figure 10.6. Mental health disorders in adolescents.

Source: https://nchstats.com/wp-content/uploads/2024/05/8-Statistics-on-Mental-Health-Disorders-in-Adolescents.jpg.

10.2.1. Common Mental Health Disorders (e.g., Anxiety, Depression)

Teenagers are especially susceptible to mental disorders, with the usual ones being anxiety and depression. It is important to understand how prevalent these disorders are so that effective intervention methods can be developed. Studies have shown depression to be the most diagnosed mental disorder in teenagers, occurring in around 32.12% of adolescent clinic patients, as seen in one study where data from 169 adolescent patients were observed in Lexington, KY. This population result underscores the fact that, across gender, ethnicity, or socioeconomic status, adolescents exhibit high rates of depressive symptoms. The recognition of this issue underscores the urgent need for accessible mental health treatment that is specifically tailored to adolescent populations to establish an environment for early intervention and continued support to avert long-term deleterious outcomes (Al-Alem et al., 2009). Anxiety disorders are also a specific concern for adolescent mental health, affecting about 13% of the population in various clinical environments.

Anxiety disorders exist in countless different forms, including generalized anxiety disorder, panic disorder, and social anxiety disorder, typically compounded by adolescent difficulties, including learning pressures and interpersonal relationships. The clinical presentations of anxiety are also varied, with the commonality of overlapping with other mental disorders, i.e., depression. Comorbidity of these two illnesses can sometimes compound their symptoms and influence treatment modalities. Critical knowledge of the inherent sociological factors and environmental stresses of, for example, living in urban versus rural settings is therefore essential to establishing effective treatment plans for anxious adolescents (Al-Alem et al., 2013).

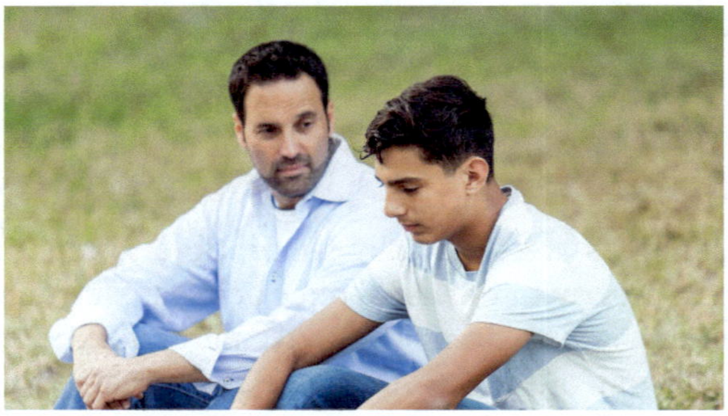

Figure 10.7. Anxiety disorders.

Source: https://raisingchildren.net.au/__data/assets/image/0025/48580/anxiety-disorders-teenagers.jpg.

The influence of mental disorders, such as depression and anxiety, and psychosocial factors complicates adolescent well-being. Factors such as exposure to violence, instability in families, and stress are likely to have a significant influence on mental disorder onset and development. Additionally, the clinical evidence depicts a concerning trend where the majority of adolescents fail to receive adequate mental health treatment. This gap in care calls for greater awareness and anticipatory efforts across school, community, and health systems to identify susceptible teenagers early on. Through interventions targeting causal factors and the delivery of specified interventions, it is possible to minimize the burden of these common mental disorders and improve psychological outcomes in vulnerable groups (Al-Alem et al., 2009) (Figure 10.7).

10.2.2. The Role of Social Media and Peer Pressure

The influence of social media on peer pressure has become increasingly prevalent in the discussion of teenage medicine. Social media sites such as Instagram, TikTok, and Snapchat, during their teenage years, shape their identities and interactions. Online time spent on these sites tends to foster social comparison, where teens measure themselves against filtered images of other people's lives. This tendency can exacerbate mental health disorders such as depression and anxiety, particularly since they are constantly seeking validation in the form of likes and comments. The unstable combination of social media exposure and peer pressure can heighten teenagers' sensitivity to perceived social acceptance and rejection, which in turn influences their self-esteem and emotional state, as highlighted in more recent public health discussions (Nelson et al., 2024). Moreover, social media normalization of harmful behaviors also has a material contribution to the use patterns of drugs among young people. Young people are exposed to idealized models of drug use by peers or celebrities, which can create a culture where this behavior is perceived as acceptable. Studies show that teens who extensively use social media are more likely to be drug abusers because these sites become breeding grounds for peer pressure and the fear of missing out (FOMO) (Kumar et al., 2024). This worrisome connection necessitates a comprehensive set of strategies that reach out to these influences, as they intersect with the teen medical problems of drug abuse and mental illness. By recognizing the significant role that social media plays in shaping adolescent behaviors and attitudes, healthcare providers are better positioned to offer prevention and intervention measures. With these influences in mind, it is more critical than ever that parents, educators, and policymakers encourage honest discussions about social media usage and potential consequences. Curricula centered on digital literacy and ethical online behavior can equip teenagers with the skills necessary to effectively resist peer pressure online. Encouraging sensitivity to the constructed nature of online personas might avoid the deleterious effects of social comparison and reduce academic susceptibility to peer pressure. Additionally, evidence-based practices can prioritize supportive environments as a focus for mental health and social media resilience (Kumar et al., 2024; Nelson et al., 2024). Ultimately, addressing the psychological components of social media and peer pressure not only improves adolescent health but also enhances overall community well-being (Figure 10.8).

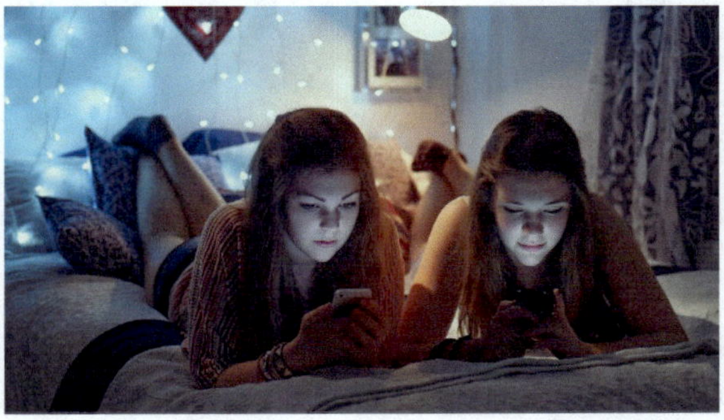

Figure 10.8. Social media affects your teen's mental health.

Source: https://ysm-res.cloudinary.com/image/upload/ar_16:9,c_fill,dpr_3.0,f_auto,g_faces:auto,q_auto:eco,w_500/v1/yms/prod/5ead84a9-6170-4d8a-ac3e-32cf417c24fe.

10.2.3. Strategies for Promoting Mental Well-Being

To properly promote mental well-being among adolescents, prevention efforts with specific plans that address their individual developmental needs have to be implemented. One broad strategy is educating adolescents on health literacy, which helps prepare them to make sound decisions about their mental health. Such programs can be integrated into school curricula, offering students the coping mechanisms that help them deal with the challenges of adolescence. By enhancing self-knowledge and resilience, these programs teach an appreciation of mental health issues, leading to an active approach in seeking help when necessary. Further, incorporating peer-led discussions regarding mental health issues can desensitize the talks that are normally stigmatized, making teens more receptive to sharing and providing them with the support networks required. Lastly, the application of educational techniques within the context of adolescent medicine is essential to fostering a prevention and awareness culture in mental health care. When used to their fullest potential, social media platforms can be extremely helpful in promoting mental wellness among adolescents. As social media is such a ubiquitous force in contemporary life, using it to raise awareness of mental illness can reach many people. Internet campaigns that disseminate messages and information related to mental health can help adolescents talk about emotional well-being. Further, constructing healthy online forums allows adolescents to bond with similar peers and talk about coping strategies and experiences, thereby fostering a sense of belonging. Through user-generated content, mental health organizations can construct community-based platforms that engage questions and reduce the stigma typically associated with mental illness. Encouraging the healthy consumption of these media is of utmost importance, as it can balance the negative impact, such as cyberbullying and anxiety, caused by unhealthy social media use (Kapoor et al., 2017). Research indicates that physical exercise through regular activity routines is also an important factor in enhancing the mental well-being of adolescents (Tom

Cás et al., 2016). Consistent physical activity promotes the release of endorphins, which may help reduce stress and anxiety. Schools and community centers can prioritize physical activity by offering diverse opportunities, such as sports, dance, and mindfulness activities like yoga, specifically designed for adolescents. By offering systematic environments for physical activity, communities can promote a more active lifestyle that results in improved mood and self-esteem. Also, working with mental health professionals to develop interdisciplinary wellness programs can be an excellent way to offer comprehensive support in meeting both the physical and psychological dimensions of health. Finally, incorporating physical activity as an integral part of adolescent medicine can significantly enhance mental well-being and help develop a more robust, self-assured generation (Figure 10.9).

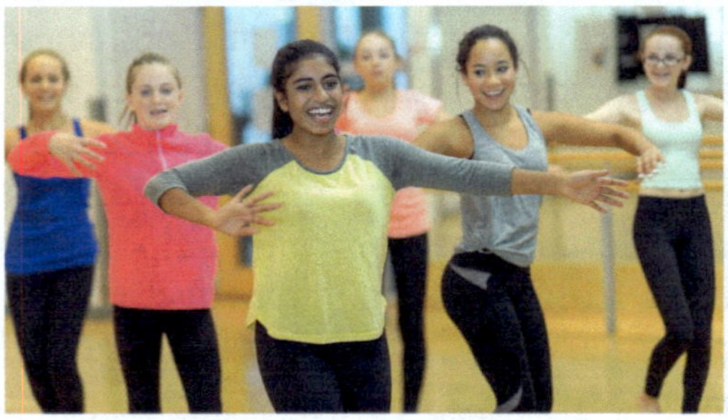

Figure 10.9. Strategies for Promoting Mental Well-Being

Source: https://images.moneycontrol.com/static-mcnews/2023/09/Easy-workout-routines-dance-workout-sessions.jpg?impolicy=website&width=770&height=431.

Test Your Knowledge

1. What are the 2 most common mental disorders?
2. Describe the strategies for promoting mental well-being.

10.3. Preventive Health Care for Adolescents

Learning Outcome

1. Understand the importance of regular health check-ups
2. Describe the vaccination schedules and recommendations
3. Screening for risky behaviors

Adolescent preventive health care is a significant consideration in addressing many health risk factors affecting youth. Since adolescents are experiencing a formative developmental period, they must endure a number of risks, including obesity, substance abuse, and psychological illness. Preventive care aims to mitigate these risks by initiating interventions and education early enough so that youth learn healthy behaviors. Research shows that factors such as insurance coverage significantly influence access to preventive care. In the absence of adequate insurance, teenagers are unlikely to undergo basic health screenings or counseling, which can lead to other medical issues. It is paramount that these systemic barriers be treated to ensure an equal health care environment for teenagers. Besides, promotion of preventive health care must encompass the social and cultural environments that influence health behaviors among adolescents. In sexual and reproductive health, preventive care is particularly critical, especially in the context of teenage pregnancy. The social context of teenage pregnancy is complex and mediated by socio-economic situations and sexual and relationship attitudes. Research has established that, while a myriad of interventions, such as programs, have been put in place, their impact on reducing teen repeat pregnancies is highly variable, ranging from significant reductions to no effects or even adverse effects. An integration of well-crafted sex education programs as well as youth development programs must be present to equip adolescents with the education and skills needed to make appropriate decisions. The results from intervention studies are consistent with the policy requirement to increase preventive health care in adolescent medicine, as emphasized by Rowlands et al. (2010). Ensuring that such interventions are evidence-informed can significantly improve health outcomes among adolescents. In addition, promoting mental health resources is a vital component of adolescent preventive health care. Because mental illness often emerges during this critical formative phase, it is critical to incorporate mental health testing and counseling as part of standard preventive care. Early detection and treatment of mental illness, such as depression and anxiety, can lead to more favorable prognoses as well as reduced long-term consequences. Schools and community organizations play a crucial role in providing resources and support, thereby creating an overall adolescent health model. The stigma of mental illness remains a problem, but it is essential in encouraging adolescents to seek help. While research shows the association of mental health with other risk areas like substance use and suicide ideation, integrated solutions become key in effectively meeting the overall health needs of adolescents (Figure 10.10).

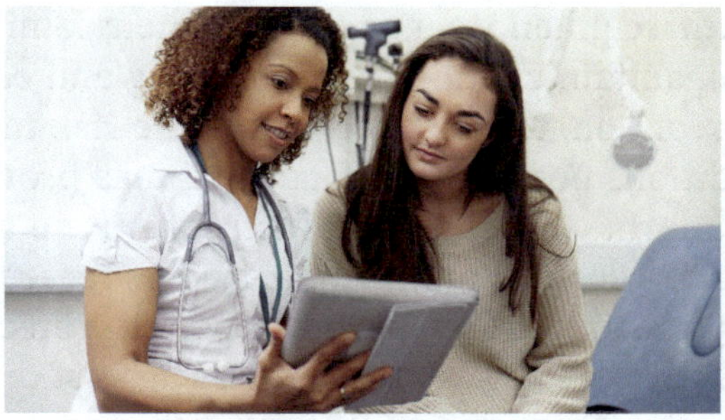

Figure 10.10. Preventive health care for adolescents.

Source: https://www.cdc.gov/healthy-youth-parent-resources/media/images/2024/11/shutterstock_284569505.jpg.

10.3.1. Importance of Regular Health Check-Ups

Regular check-ups are a critical component of adolescent medicine since they are a main prevention intervention. Over adolescence, the person undergoes remarkable physical, emotional, and social growth, making them extremely vulnerable to many health issues. Check-ups offer a structured opportunity for healthcare providers to assess adolescents' development and growth, during which they can detect potential health issues early on, such as obesity, diabetes, and mental illness. These visits enable health care providers to monitor vital signs, discuss food and exercise with adolescents, and treat any behavioral health issues that may arise during this time of transition. Emphasizing the importance of consistent health checks can lead adolescents to take an active role in their own care and develop habits conducive to long-term wellness. Secondly, regular health check-ups are important for detecting and controlling chronic conditions that could develop early in adolescence. Conditions such as asthma, attention-deficit hyperactivity disorder (ADHD), and developmental disorders can have a significant impact on the quality of life and schooling for adolescents as well. By incorporating regular check-ups into their health regimen, teenagers and their families can maintain continuous monitoring and early intervention, thereby decreasing the risk these conditions pose. Continuous visits also provide a platform where health practitioners are able to start a conversation with teenagers regarding risky practices such as drug use or unprotected sex in order to prevent and advise against them. This three-dimensional approach addresses not only physical health but also mental and emotional health, which is critical for these formative years.

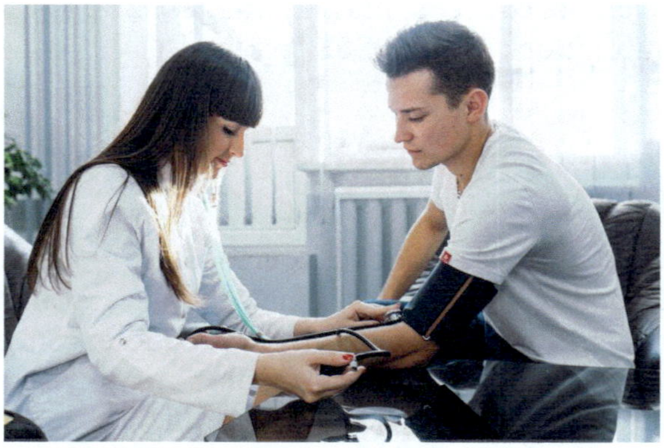

Figure 10.11. Regular health check-ups.

Source: https://max-website20-images.s3.ap-south-1.amazonaws.com/Regular_Health_Check_Ups_80ddc03670.jpg.

Routine health check-ups, aside from individual benefit, also contribute to public health outcomes by facilitating the overall detection of epidemiological trends among teen populations. Monitoring teen health status enables healthcare systems to identify emerging health issues and allocate appropriate resources to address them. As an example, periodic data collection at check-ups can detect trends in vaccine coverage, mental health concerns, and lifestyle habits across different groups. Public health interventions and policy actions are directed by the detection of these trends through check-ups in order to improve the health outcomes of adolescents. Moreover, these measurements can lead to interventions within schools and communities, yielding high benefits for health promotion activities and for the creation of healthy adolescent development-conducive environments. This greater understanding emphasizes the significant role that regular health check-ups can play not only in individual health but also in strengthening public health policy and systems (Figure 10.11).

10.3.2. Vaccination Schedules and Recommendations

Vaccination series are integral components of adolescents' health care, as they help reduce the risk of vaccine-preventable illness during a critical stage of development and growth. Recommendations from health authorities aim to provide adolescents with immunizations that protect against infection with human papillomavirus (HPV) and meningococcal disease. One investigation found incomplete immunization series among adolescents, with only 62.2% fully vaccinated against HPV and 44% against meningitis C in one geographic region (da Costa et al., 2024). These figures highlight the importance of adhering to vaccination schedules, as incomplete immunization not only exposes the individual to an increased risk of disease transmission but also compromises herd immunity and affects community health. Also, perceived hindrances to vaccination are largely responsible for the observed differences in follow-up to recommended timetables. Concerns regarding injections, social pressure, and administrative issues, such as distance to immunization services, account for low coverage levels in the majority of municipalities (da Costa et al., 2024). These are barriers to the necessity for targeted educational interventions and the utilization of more powerful communication approaches to educate parents and adolescents about vaccination advantages. By meeting the barriers directly, healthcare practitioners can develop a supportive environment that facilitates routine vaccination utilization. The promotion of vaccination not only advances individual health interests but also strengthens community immunity against public health issues. In adolescent medicine, the vaccine provider is key to optimizing vaccination rates. All healthcare providers who are involved in the care of adolescents, such as sports medicine physicians, are well-positioned to encourage vaccination as a normal part of health assessment. They are urged to assess vaccination status during sports and other activity-related preparticipation exams, thereby incorporating vaccination discussions into the care of adolescents. In such a manner, medical professionals can customize vaccination schedules in light of personal health profiles and some risks associated with sporting activity. Such a proactive approach not only maximizes compliance with recommended vaccination schedules but also improves overall health and performance among adolescents, enabling them to engage in full-fledged sports and social life.

10.3.3. Screening for Risky Behaviors (e.g., Substance Use)

Effective screening for high-risk behavior, including drug use, is an essential part of adolescent medicine. Early identification of high-risk behavior facilitates early intervention, which leads to better health outcomes in the long run. Adolescents are likely to engage in high-risk behavior due to the cumulative influence of development, social determinants, and the environment. Medical practitioners, therefore, have to utilize an integrative strategy in screening that considers the influences. Applying standardized assessment tools and questionnaires can potentially allow clinicians to gather essential information regarding the patterns of alcohol and drug use among adolescents. These wide-ranging assessments not only identify risk individuals but also yield essential information regarding underlying motivations for such alcohol and drug use. Proactivity is especially critical, as the effects of adolescent alcohol and drug use can continue into adulthood, exacerbating other health problems and yielding profound social repercussions. Besides, the veiled presentation of risky behaviors in adolescents calls for a tailored screening approach. For instance, symptomological differences across genders, particularly in disorders like ADHD, might influence the expression and observation of conduct. Under-referral and underdiagnosis of females have been indicated to be the results of gender bias in society, whereby they present with internalized symptoms masked by compensatory strategies (Young et al., 2020). This underscores the need to train health professionals to recognize such biases and screen more effectively across diverse adolescent populations.

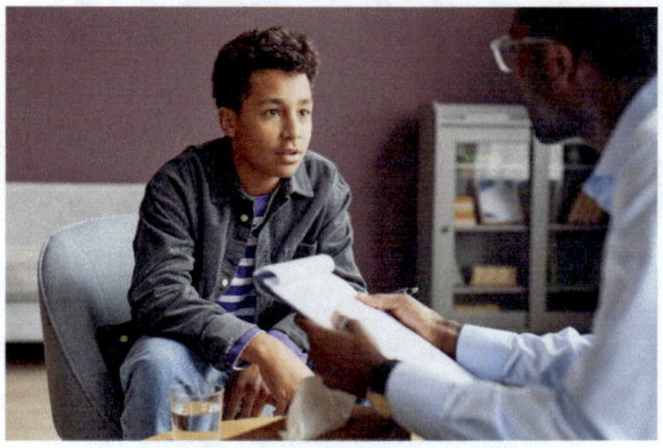

Figure 10.12. Screening for substance use.

Source: https://www.aap.org/globalassets/patient-care/substance-use--prevention/boy-talking-to-psychologist.jpg.

Eliminating such biases and awareness can contribute to ensuring that at-risk individuals get appropriate care, thereby facilitating improved long-term outcomes among youth. By establishing a non-biased, informed screening environment, practitioners can efficiently implement interventions and support systems to meet the specific needs of all youth. In addition to the acknowledgment of drug use, effective screening also entails evaluation of more general activity in lifestyle that may indicate increased risk, such as the degree to which gambling has become associated with addictive disorders. Emphasis on variables such as extended heavy use is likely to enable clinicians to assess the severity of the behavior and its potential health effects. This insight not only reduces stigma but also supports a public health response to stigma that emphasizes early intervention (Admin, 2020). By integrating this holistic practice into routine adolescent health screens, practitioners are able to build a stronger foundation for the identification of at-risk individuals. Ultimately, dangerous behavior can be addressed through regular and efficient screening, thereby enhancing health promotion processes in adolescent medicine and equipping youths with the tools for a healthier transition into adulthood (Figure 10.12).

Test Your Knowledge

1. What is the importance of regular health check-ups?
2. What vaccines are recommended for adolescents?

10.4. Sexual and Reproductive Health

Learning Outcome

1. Describe the education on safe sex practices
2. Understand the access to contraceptive methods among adolescents
3. Address issues of consent and healthy relationships

Reproductive and sexual health is central to adolescent medicine, as it is related to a range of problems facing young people during their adolescence. Adolescents have particular issues relating to sexual health, including access to information, education, and services that allow them to make informed decisions about their bodies. Such issues are most often compounded by stigma in society and the common lack of comprehensive sexual education in most communities. There is evidence that information delivery can have a significant impact on adolescents' perceptions and knowledge regarding sexual health. Interview-administered questionnaires, for instance, have been shown to induce embarrassment, resulting in underreporting of important mental health indicators like anxiety and depression, which are often associated with risky sexual behavior (Aziz et al., 2009). It is due to this reason that special interventions must be put in place to empower the teenagers by fostering a conducive environment that encourages open discussions on sexual and reproductive health. Sexual and reproductive health services must respond to the complex barriers adolescents encounter in their attempt to get such care. Access to healthcare remains a significant challenge, often hindered by economic constraints, insufficient health coverage, and poorly coordinated healthcare systems. For instance, studies examining healthcare services in urban environments reveal that adolescents are likely to face obstacles that limit their access to reproductive services, thereby affecting their health (Fox et al., 2003). Moreover, the disparities in the quality and accessibility of such services have been known to exacerbate health issues among disadvantaged groups, making it even more critical to include innovative programs that not only serve adolescents but also engage them. Through optimized delivery of healthcare services and overcoming system barriers, we are able to offer a model in which young people feel empowered to access the sexual health care that they require. In addition to accessibility, education plays a central role in optimizing sexual and reproductive health in young people. Sexual education initiatives address all elements of sexuality and empower youth with the knowledge necessary to direct their sexual life safely and responsibly. These curricula need to cover various subjects, including consent, contraception, sexually transmitted infections (STIs), and positive relationships. Provision of correct, appropriate, and age-appropriate information is necessary for preventing rates of unintended pregnancy and STIs among adolescents. Moreover, if such education is delivered in a non-judgmental, accepting environment, it fosters greater comfort and honesty, allowing genuine questions and discussions. The convergence of qualitative results suggests that adolescents want educational environments that respect their privacy and foster open dialogue, once more highlighting the role of educational models in affirming sexual and reproductive health outcomes (Aziz et al., 2009). An empowering education system will ultimately lead to more informed and healthier decision-making among adolescents, with beneficial impacts on their long-term health (Figure 10.13).

Figure 10.13. Sexual and reproductive health.

Source: https://www.svgrepo.com/show/326117/sexual-reproductive-health.svg.

10.4.1. Education on Safe Sex Practices

Safe sex behavior education is a significant component of adolescent medicine, given that it sensitizes adolescents and makes them responsible in their sexual life. Since adolescents are faced with complex social relationships, full sex education is required in order to minimize risks associated with unprotected sex. The incorporation of such programs can significantly affect adolescents' knowledge of sexually transmitted diseases (STIs) and contraceptive methods. Studies have indicated that teenagers with extensive sex education are most likely to be more knowledgeable about safe sex and have safer sexual behaviors in their lives. The presence of this connection serves to affirm the need for educational frameworks that not only emphasize abstinence but also informed consent, communication, and the use of protection in an attempt to establish a well-rounded awareness of sexual health among youth. Cultural transformations, particularly in dating practices, further complicate the adolescent sexual scene. The formation of dating cultures in most environments affects attitudes about sex among young individuals. For instance, from focus group interviews in Nepal, it was revealed that both urban and rural youth alike embraced dating more, which further fueled the high rates of premarital and extramarital sexual activity. Those who engaged in these forums noted that dating culture, as constructed by mass media, can offer an environment in which exploration and experimentation can take place. But this greater autonomy also necessitates the integration of discussions surrounding safer sex into the formal and informal educational frameworks. Talking about these shifts in culture through proper education is essential to instilling safe sexual habits in teenagers who have to navigate these new social spaces (Acharya et al., 2010). The debate about which kind of sex education is being taught in schools has deep implications for whether or not programs aimed at promoting safe sex practices are effective. Comprehensive-Based advocates for sex education feel adolescents must be taught about STIs and birth control, with the insistence that adolescents must be taught in order to prevent risky behaviors. Abstinence-only sessions only address abstinence as the sole safe sex practice. Stunning figures indicate a better percentage of teenagers experiencing negative outcomes from unprotected sex, as a measure of abstinence-only models' failures. Studies have shown that Comprehensive-Based participants are more educated on safe sex practices and are likely to use them safely to a certain degree, compared to needing more studies that yield statistically significant results. The ongoing debate around sex education eventually informs policies and practice decisions towards leading more healthy sexual outcomes among young people (Motherway et al., 2010).

10.4.2. Access to Contraceptive Methods

The issue of the accessibility of contraceptive methods to adolescents is one of the persisting problems in the practice of adolescent medicine. As the sexual health of adolescents continues to be a matter of mass public concern, recognizing the determinants of the availability of contraceptives is necessary. Adolescents present specific barriers based on the deficiencies of sexual education, the service shortages, and the reproductive health taboo culture. These barriers can actually obstruct young people's ability to make healthy decisions regarding contraception, which may result in negative health consequences. If effective forms of contraception are unavailable, youths will have to rely on risk-taking behaviors that can lead to unwanted pregnancies or the spread of STIs (Tripp et al., 2005). It is for this reason that these barriers must be addressed as a way of ensuring healthier sexual behavior among youths. Additionally, the variations in teen pregnancy and birth rates across various regions indicate the demand for available contraceptives. A comparative report of these rates in the United States, Canada, Australia, and New Zealand highlights the importance of good access to contraceptives in reducing these figures (Cheesbrough et al., 2002). For instance, in regions where there is widespread access to contraceptive services, adolescents tend to have lower rates of unwanted pregnancy and STIs.

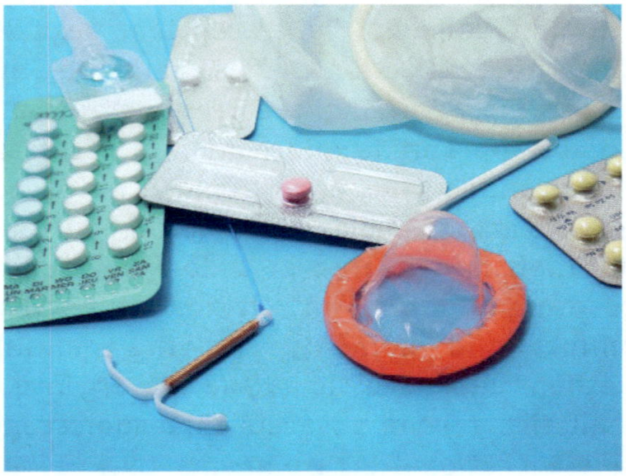

Figure 10.14. Access to contraceptive methods.

Source: https://knowledgesuccess.org/wp-content/uploads/2020/01/reproductive-health-supplies-coalition-m206W8HQJAQ-unsplash.jpg.

That means that available and also efficient contraceptive methods can empower youth so that they can exercise control over their reproductive health. Better access can be achieved through multi-faceted efforts, including policy reforms, improved financing of young people's health services, as well as education among the people. With a framework placed at access priority, youths are likely to engage in responsible sex and avoid the risks associated with risk behavior. In conclusion, expanding adolescent access to contraceptive methods is critical in the promotion of sexual health and well-being. Expanded access allows youth to have autonomy over their reproductive health, therefore reducing rates of unintended pregnancy and STIs. As stated earlier, the interconnectedness of sexual health and risk-taking activities increases the need for proactive education and resource investment. These stakeholders include policymakers, educators, and healthcare workers who must collaborate in breaking existing barriers to access to contraceptives. Through this cooperation, there can be a healthier next generation of adolescents that is educated and resourceful enough to care for their sexual health responsibly. As adolescents become more responsible for their health decisions, the potential for improved outcomes in the practice of adolescent medicine becomes more pronounced (Figure 10.14).

10.4.3. Addressing Issues of Consent and Healthy Relationships

In adolescent medicine, managing consent problems and healthy relationships is essential to adolescent development. Adolescents are at a point where they are trying to figure out who they are and what relationships are about, so it is important that they learn why consent matters. As they navigate romantic and friendship relationships, teenagers will have to know that consent is not merely a term but a continuous, reciprocal agreement that respects the agency of all individuals. Education about the topic makes them comprehend the complexities of relationships such that they can have wholesome interactions resulting in emotional and psychological well-being, which is a component of adolescent health defined in the scholarly work on adolescent health service status (Gootman et al., 2008). Besides, promoting a culture of wholesome relationships requires an integrated approach that includes both school programs and community outreach. Parents, schools, and healthcare providers can each play a vital role in helping teens navigate consent and relationship concerns. Strong programs would focus on open communication, empathy, and respect for boundaries as essential components of helping teens develop understanding and trust in others. Besides, with the health care system working to address the specific needs of adolescents, the inclusion of training providers in such efforts can enhance the quality of care they deliver. Such inclusion is in line with demands for enhanced primary care models addressing adolescent comprehensive health needs (Gootman et al., 2008). Ultimately, the implications of healthy relationships and informed consent bleed into broader social levels. Young people who are familiar with and apply these principles will be more likely to be positive contributors to healthier communities, reducing rates of relational violence and fostering respect for each other between individuals. New programs emphasizing consent education can also serve to dismantle harmful norms that deny healthy interactions, complementing research on healthcare systems in urban areas to assess the contribution of access to education and supportive services to adolescent development. By integrating consent and relationship health into adolescent medicine, the healthcare sector can be a force to be reckoned with in deciding the social and emotional destiny for many decades to come.

Test Your Knowledge

1. What is access to contraception?
2. How to address issues of consent and healthy relationships?

10.5. Chronic Illnesses and Adolescents

Learning Outcome

1. Describe the common chronic conditions affecting adolescents
2. Know the transition from pediatric to adult services
3. Understand the role of family support in managing chronic illnesses

Chronic illness is strongly impacting adolescents, weakening their physical health, mental stability, and interpersonal relationships. Research indicates that adolescents with chronic illness are at increased risk of engaging in unhealthy behaviors, including increased aggression and mental issues. For instance, the study on Thai adolescents during the COVID-19 pandemic identified that 38.3% of adolescents with chronic illness developed risk behavior that is associated with violence. In addition, they had reported high levels of emotional challenges over their healthy counterparts, suggesting that having a chronic disease can deepen vulnerabilities under such uncertain circumstances. This underscores the necessity of multidisciplinary healthcare strategies tailored to address the unique needs of this population, ultimately improving their well-being and addressing the psychosocial challenges they often endure during the adolescent phase of development (Thitamethee et al., 2024). In addition to the direct health effects, chronic illnesses also lead to immense psychological trauma in adolescents, necessitating innovative approaches to healthcare. Availability of mental health care is most important among this group, particularly those with chronic conditions. The current state shows that the majority of adolescents experience stigma, which makes it difficult for them to access support systems. Interventions focused on establishing supportive systems are therefore vital. One process that is becoming increasingly popular involves task-shifting, in which professionals other than mental health professionals, such as nurses, play a more participatory role in mental health treatment. The use of creative arts in such interventions has also proven highly effective. Interventions that involve art forms not only help alleviate mood changes but also promote a sense of belonging among adolescents who are afflicted with similar problems (Hoare et al., 2024). Moreover, the importance of peer support interventions cannot be overstated in addressing the multifaceted problems that accompany chronic diseases. Initiatives like Better Together demonstrated that creative space fosters valuable social interaction and emotional experience. Program participants offered feedback that revealed not only that creative engagement enriched their own outlook, but also that it exposed them to peers, building a support network. The implications of these findings are that interventions to include peer support, more specifically creative activity, would be useful channels for promoting mental health and resilience among young people with chronic conditions. Such new approaches need further exploration to develop holistic adolescent health care that continues to monitor the medical and psychosocial aspects of managing chronic illness (Hoare et al., 2024) (Figure 10.15).

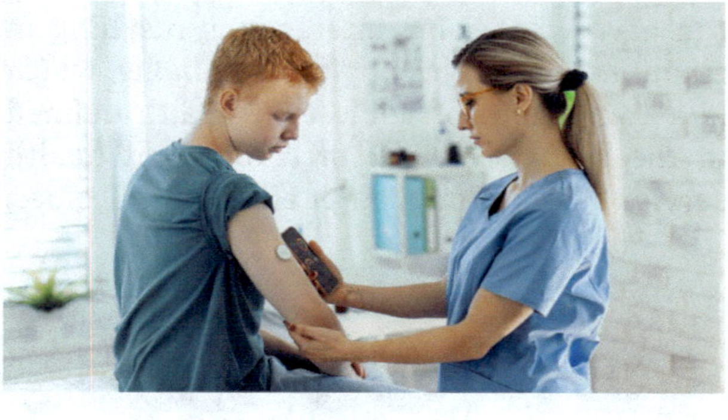

Figure 10.15. Adolescence and diabetes.

Source: https://healthenews.mcgill.ca/wp-content/uploads/2024/10/2024-10-11_Teen-and-diabetes-Adobe-stock_1080x566.jpg.

10.5.1. Common Chronic Conditions Affecting Adolescents (e.g., Asthma, Diabetes)

Adolescents get exposed to different chronic diseases, of which two are the most prevalent and include asthma and diabetes. Asthma, recurrent wheezing, shortness of breath, and chest tightness greatly affect the quality of life in adolescents. It typically occurs in adolescence, which might hinder physical activity and socializing, since these are key to developmental progress. The rising prevalence of asthma in teenagers has raised alarm among the medical community, especially as it requires constant upkeep and monitoring. Positive interventions include education about medication compliance and self-management strategies to decrease the severity of asthma attacks. The involvement of healthcare professionals is thus paramount in helping the teenagers understand their disease, the importance of following treatment protocols, and the identification of triggers that can precipitate attacks. On the other hand, type 1 and type 2 diabetes also present significant complications for adolescents. Both the diseases call for strict blood glucose level monitoring, diet control, and regular exercise. Type 1 diabetes tends to occur most frequently in childhood or early adolescence, while type 2 typically develops because of lifestyle reasons in adolescence, which coincides with obesity in this population. Recent evidence has demonstrated a strong association between diabetes and respiratory conditions such as COPD and asthma, with the influence of diabetes on respiratory health being multifaceted (Chen et al., 2024). In young people with diabetes, the likelihood of comorbidities underscores the importance of collaborative approaches to care that treat not only glucose management but also total health and well-being. Transition care for youth with ongoing conditions like diabetes and asthma poses particular challenges in the healthcare system. As they transition into young adulthood, they must transfer from pediatric to adult healthcare settings. The process is significant because abrupt changes can lead to negative health outcomes and increased morbidity. Programs to support this transition, such as those the COCCOS study focuses on, use the Experience-Based Co-Design approach to involve young people, their families, and healthcare professionals in designing enabling transition plans (Janssens et al., 2024). By incorporating such input from stakeholders, healthcare systems are better positioned to design comprehensive transition programs that address the specific needs of adolescents with chronic disease, ultimately leading to better health outcomes and disease management (Figure 10.16).

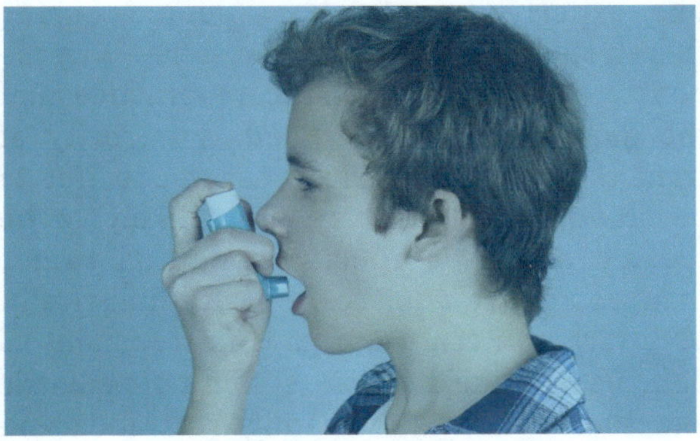

Figure 10.16. Adolescents with asthma.

Source: https://staymedical.com/wp-content/uploads/2025/05/clinical-trial-in-miami-for-adolescents-with-asthma.jpg.

10.5.2. Transitioning Care from Pediatric to Adult Services

Transition from pediatric to adult care is a critical process in adolescent medicine, particularly for chronically ill adolescents. Transition needs to be smooth to ensure continuity of positive health outcomes among these adolescents, so they do not experience a diminution in their health, which can be particularly apparent in the case of chronic illnesses like Type 1 diabetes. Evidence suggests that systematic transition practice, including the adolescent's developmental issues, self-care education, and family involvement, significantly enhances continuity of care. Neglect of cautious attention leaves young adults confused in adult health care systems, with deteriorating health and increased hospitalization. Given the complexity of managing dynamic health responsibilities, healthcare systems have a pressing need to develop standardized transition programs that address the unique needs of this population to streamline the transition process overall (Bagnall et al., 2013). Transition of care also raises concerns about continuity of care, particularly among adolescents with palliative care.

The experiences of young people during this transition can also be fairly diverse due to variation in healthcare practice and the quality of care provided. A majority of transition programs have been found not to be standardized and are more likely to be created around a specific condition rather than addressing adolescent health holistically. This variation can cause gaps in treatment as patients navigate disparate systems of pediatric and adult healthcare, creating frustration and a perception of abandonment. Interestingly, although some conditions, such as cystic fibrosis, have demonstrated successful models of care, for many other conditions, evidence is limited and further research is required to develop universally accepted guidelines for transition of care (Adi et al., 2009).

In addition, successful transitions are a product of collaboration among pediatric and adult providers, highlighting the role of multidisciplinary teams. Collaborative efforts with healthcare professionals from different specialties will ensure that transitions are developed to better match adolescents' needs, and that they receive proper guidance and support. A systematic review has shown that effective transition plans are more likely to include assigned transition coordinators and formal processes that facilitate communication between providers and patients. This interaction not only facilitates the understanding of the adult healthcare realm for young patients but also minimizes the likelihood of the emotional and psychological impact of this dramatic transition. According to these results, it is critical for health systems to invest in transition care strategies that are adaptable to diverse patient needs, ultimately resulting in better health status as patients transition from adolescence to adulthood (Adi et al., 2009; Bagnall et al., 2013) (Figure 10.17).

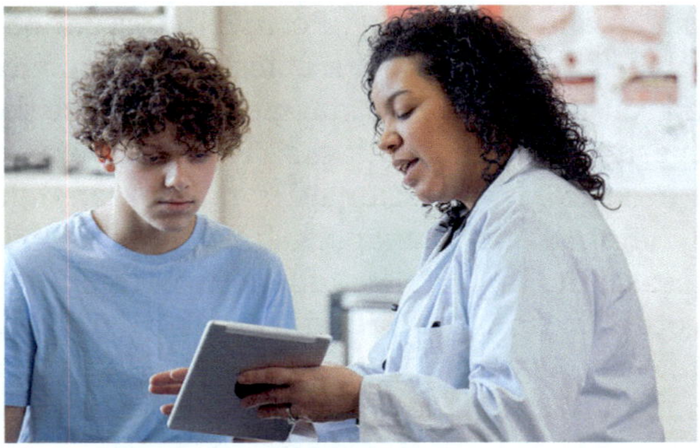

Figure 10.17. Transition from pediatric to adult care.

Source: https://ufhealth.org/assets/images/health-topics/_640x426_crop_center-center_line/4329770/pediatric-transition.jpg

10.5.3. The Role of Family Support in Managing Chronic Illnesses

In adolescent medicine, family support is a key factor in the successful management of chronic illness. While adolescents are grappling with the multifaceted physical and emotional challenges posed by chronic illness, their families are often the primary source of support and resources. Support can be provided in numerous ways, including emotional support, assistance with daily tasks, and support for proper health care. Family involvement not only helps buffer the stress of the illness but also fosters resilience in the adolescent, furthering their capacity to manage ongoing health problems. The resilience of the support system would most likely be attributable to the patient's capacity to adhere to treatment protocols and remain in mental health, thus highlighting the need for health care professionals to consider family life when formulating strategic care plans for the patient. Furthermore, the concept of family resilience is critical in chronic illness care for adolescents. Family resilience can aid in improved coping strategies, which are imperative in tackling challenges arising from chronic diseases. Systematic review has shown that predictors of family resilience, like social support and communication, help determine family resilience in caring for chronic illnesses (Suwanwong et al., 2025). These qualities not only allow families to manage day-to-day functioning but also establish harmony and direction. By working together, as families discuss and create concerted plans of management, they can optimize the adolescents' overall level of functioning and reduce the burden to caregivers. This collaborative approach can also foster a proactive environment, encouraging adolescents to take charge of their health and be more actively involved in their treatment. In the healthcare context, establishing a strong family support system is important to optimize treatment outcomes for children with chronic conditions. Physician providers must strive to involve family members in care plans in ways that empower them with the necessary knowledge and skills to provide supportive care. Educating the family on disease management and the importance of offering emotional support can empower them, and open communication with the healthcare providers enhances their capacity to handle crises as they arise. Importantly, appreciating the complexity of managing chronic illness can also call upon the healthcare providers to be sensitive to the psychological and social problems afflicting both the adolescent and the family. By finding solutions to such intricate issues, health systems can greatly enhance the delivery of a healing and resilient environment, ultimately leading to better chronic disease control in teens (Alsudairy et al., 2025) (Figure 10.18).

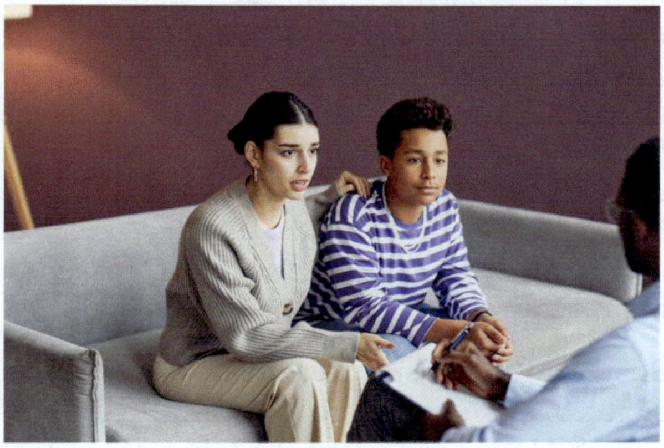

Figure 18. Role of family support in managing chronic illnesses.

Source: https://willowcreekbh.com/wp-content/uploads/2024/06/iStock-1463773199.jpg.

Test Your Knowledge

1. What are the common chronic conditions affecting adolescents?
2. What is the role of family support in managing chronic illnesses?

10.6. The Role of Technology in Adolescent Health

Learning Outcome

1. Describe telemedicine and its benefits for adolescent patients
2. Know the health apps and their impact on health management
3. Understand the risks associated with technology use

The link between technology and adolescent health has been a key area of study in adolescent medicine. With the increasing digital innovations, their effects on the health and well-being of young people are becoming increasingly deep. Technology has a dual function as an agent promoting health and as a potential risk. On the positive side, telemedicine and mobile health applications provide unprecedented access to health resources for teens, enabling them to receive guidance, track conditions, and engage in preventive care (Gootman et al., 2008).

On the negative side, technology penetration enables adolescents to become victims of cyberbullying and unhealthy habits related to excessive screen use. Thus, a harmony between using technology for health benefits and safeguarding against its detrimental effects is necessary to achieve a healthier generation of young people. Moreover, the inclination of young people towards gambling and gaming behavior illustrates the subtle way technology impacts their health. Recent studies have shown that there is a bifurcation in attitudes towards gaming and gambling across age groups, with evidence of a knowledge gap in regards to risks and benefits of both phenomena. For instance, one study in the case of Portuguese adolescents revealed that they perceive game-playing as an addiction, while young adults consider it positively, as a means to enhance interpersonal skills (Alexandre et al., 2014).

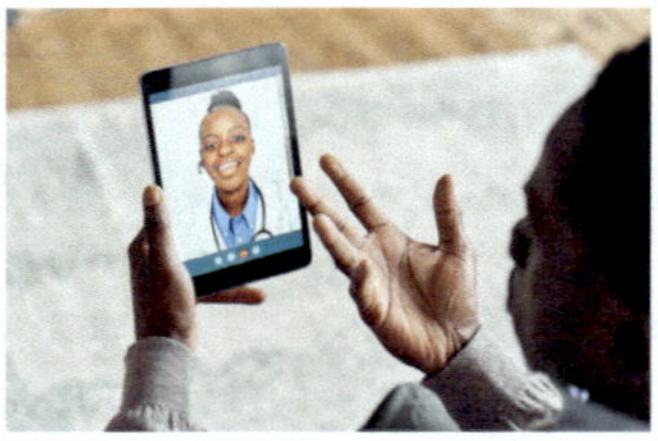

Figure 10.19. The role of technology in adolescent health.

Source: https://www.nepad.org/sites/default/files/styles/521_800/public/2023-08/800X50~1_1.PNG?itok=KNuvHXTm.

Such a contrast underscores the need for targeted interventions to address the problems adolescents encounter in the virtual environment.

By recognizing these differences, medical professionals can more effectively tailor their approaches to teach adolescents about the safe use of technology and healthy lifestyle choices that correspond to their level of development. In general, technology's role in adolescent health is a complex mix of promises and limitations that warrants significant scrutiny in adolescent medicine.

As health care systems strive to improve services for this population, technological uptake must be complemented by an appreciation of the drawbacks of digital participation. Goals for adolescent health improvement include technological adoption, as well as the implementation of whole-of-policy interventions that promote positive behavior. By fostering an environment that includes education, community, and stable primary care, one can leverage technology's potential while mitigating its adverse effects to achieve healthier adolescents overall (Gootman et al., 2008) (Figure 10.17).

10.6.1. Telemedicine and Its Benefits for Adolescent Patients

In the field of adolescent medicine, telemedicine is now a revolutionary way of accessing health care services for teenage patients. Teenagers are likely to encounter unique health conditions, including mental illness and chronic diseases, so telemedicine provides an uncomplicated way to receive specialized care without the barriers of traditional in-office visits. Through technology, health practitioners can provide consultations, make diagnoses, and follow up on treatment from a distance, thereby improving patient adherence and engagement. Notably, research has proven that telemedicine has the capacity to significantly improve health outcomes such as treatment adherence and quality of life, particularly among adolescents with chronic illnesses such as asthma. Besides, the COVID-19 pandemic has accelerated the integration of telehealth services, necessitating innovative solutions for health delivery and thereby incorporating telemedicine as a crucial aspect of modern adolescent medicine (Garriga-Baraut et al., 2025). Promoting active patient engagement in healthy environments is a core element of adolescent health. Telemedicine allows stronger relationships between adolescents and their healthcare practitioners, making it easier to establish strong support systems. As youth patients are more likely to be assisted by peers and other adults who are not their parents, telemedicine can bridge the divide between medical practitioners and these critical support systems.

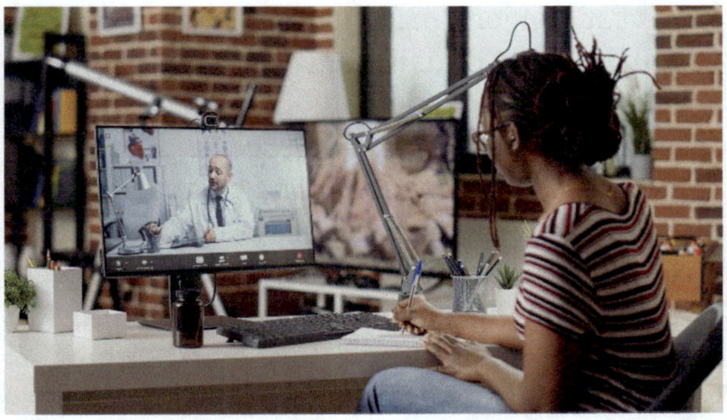

Figure 10.20. Adolescent telehealth services.

Source: https://enhancehealthgroup.com/wp-content/uploads/2024/03/sick-patient-talking-doctor-telehealth-videocall-conference-using-computer-with-webcam-medical-consultation-online-videoconference-remote-telemedicine-virtual-meeting-scaled.jpg.

Using virtual communication platforms, clinicians can assess and expand a patient's support network, ultimately resulting in healthier outcomes. Moreover, engaging teens in their care through telemedicine can make it easier for them to manage their health conditions more effectively. This is extremely significant for developing autonomy, a very essential component of adolescent development, and can lead to increased self-efficacy in managing their health (Karcher et al., 2025). Despite the clear advantages, introducing telemedicine for use with teen patients is not without challenges. Problem areas such as technological barriers, variation of digital literacy, and restricted access to necessary devices can preclude equal access to healthcare. In addition, the requirement of standardized protocols and evidence-based guidelines tailored to the adolescent population ranks high. Telemedicine has shown promise in some areas, but further study is required to better understand its overall potential, particularly regarding cost-effectiveness and long-term care. Resolving these issues is critical to optimizing telemedicine's utility in adolescent medicine, to ensure that such a novel strategy not only enhances the accessibility of care but also provides equitable, quality care to all adolescents, especially those in disadvantaged zones (Garriga-Baraut et al., 2025) (Figure 10.20).

10.6.2. Health Apps and Their Impact on Health Management

The advent of health applications has introduced an all-encompassing revolution in the practices of managing health, particularly among younger people who are increasingly technology savvy. Cellular applications offer state-of-the-art solutions that enhance access to health information, facilitate communication among patients and healthcare professionals, and improve adherence to health regimens. With the increasing popularity of smartphones among younger people, these applications have the potential to provide tailored health information, monitor fitness parameters, and even offer psychological support. Evidence indicates that treatment can be improved by the utilization of telecommunications technology, such as smartphones, to increase access to mental health services and reduce treatment barriers, particularly for adolescents who may be stigmatized about help-seeking (Susick et al., 2011). Thereafter, the inclusion of health applications in young people's medicine not only renders adolescents active participants in their own health but also generates an active culture of health management. Health applications in primary care complement the clinician's role by facilitating an integrated model of young people's health. These applications can be used to enable communication between providers of health and adolescents to speed up check-ins and streamline chronic condition care among the adolescent population. With technology, health applications can help adolescents adhere to treatment regimens, thereby improving overall health outcomes. Furthermore, such technological advances facilitate clinicians to monitor adolescent patients' progress via data collected through apps, which can lead to more personalized care strategies (Nesbitt et al., 2017). However, a rigorous evaluation of these technologies is required because disparities in smartphone and health app access can limit equitable access to health for adolescents from different socioeconomic backgrounds. Although there are benefits to health apps for teen medicine, there are still challenges to their effective use. Most adolescents may be unfamiliar with the various functions of health apps, thus requiring initial training and subsequent support for optimal use. In addition, privacy concerns about data and the credibility of health-related information may discourage teen users from adopting these technologies. Pilot trials of smartphone use have been encouraging but often identify the need for larger studies to establish efficacy and user acceptability (Susick et al., 2011). Resolving these concerns is vital to maximizing the full potential of health apps in managing adolescent health care and promoting a better model of care, ultimately achieving better health outcomes for this critical population (Figure 10.21).

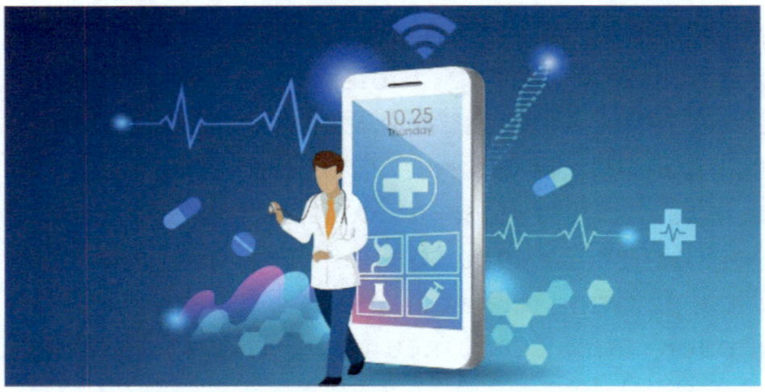

Figure 10.21. The impact of health apps on the healthcare industry.

Source: https://authorselvi.com/wp-content/uploads/2023/07/mobile-health-app.jpg.

10.6.3. Risks Associated with Technology Use (e.g., Cyberbullying)

The integration of technology into daily life among adolescents has ushered in both potential and great dangers, particularly to mental health. Leading the list of dangers from technology use is cyberbullying, which has increased with the spread of social media. Adolescents sometimes vulnerable to peer pressure and comparison will likely undergo a great deal of emotional distress through persecution online. Psychological effects of cyberbullying are devastating, resulting in depression, anxiety, and low self-esteem for victims. According to evidence in the literature, excessive use of platforms like Instagram serves to enhance this effect, creating an image of a double-edged sword where technology engages people in terms of social connections on one hand while exposing them to adverse interactions on the other (Balamurugan et al., 2025). In adolescent medicine, it is essential to understand the complex relationship between technology use and its impact on mental health. From the current literature, it is evident that social media can promote healthy networks and unhealthy lifestyles among vulnerable groups (Balamurali, 2025). For instance, LGBTQ teens and individuals who are already experiencing mental health problems are at a higher risk because the experience of being cyberbullied is more likely to intensify feelings of loneliness and anxiety. In addition, the impact of technology on teen mental health extends beyond direct harassment; it also includes issues such as addiction to digital screens and the negative impacts on sleep habits and academic performance. Knowing these complex risks enables healthcare providers to tackle adolescent welfare with an all-encompassing strategy. To efficiently counter the risks involved in technology usage and ensure healthier experiences for adolescents, a balanced approach is necessary. This involves establishing digital literacy curricula aimed at teaching youth about safe online behavior and the need to recognize abusive behaviors such as cyberbullying. Holistic measures must also include fostering open communication among parents, teachers, and adolescents about the potential negative effects of technology. Being open to responsible use and education on technology, adolescents can learn to deal more effectively with the world of technology. Moreover, advancing culturally responsive interventions and ethical practices in e-health services will consolidate support systems responsive to the needs of this community, generally promoting resilience and well-being in the fast-digitalizing world (Balamurali, 2025) (Figure 10.22).

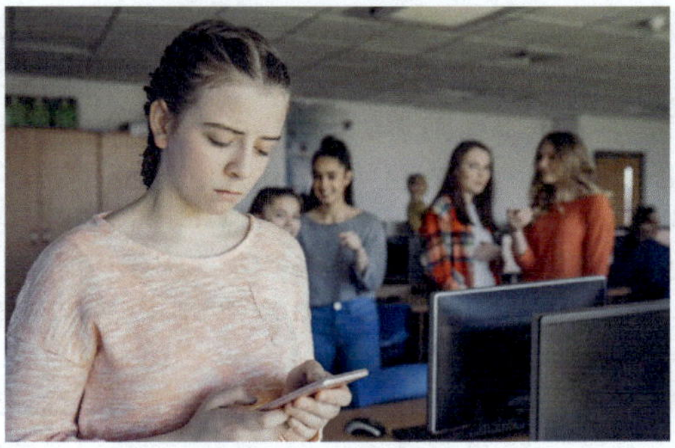

Figure 10.22. Cyberbullying.

Source: https://canyoncreekbh.com/wp-content/uploads/2024/06/cyberbullying-1200x800.jpg.

Test Your Knowledge

1. What is the role of telemedicine in adolescent healthcare?
2. What risks are related to technology use?

SUMMARY

In summary, research in adolescent medicine reveals a complex environment that requires constant scholarly attention and innovative solutions. As young people navigate the complexities of their growth stage, their health behaviors and interactions with the healthcare system are greatly influenced by shifting social patterns and technology. The emergence of online health information, and indeed particularly through social media, is a double-edged sword. While it offers adolescents a site to draw on peer life and share personal stories, it also introduces problems regarding the credibility and reliability of the information accessed, given users' ability to recognize authentic sources (Bloor et al., 2013). It calls for ongoing research to develop resources that guide adolescents through the often confounding online world of health information. Also, the involvement of adolescents in health decision-making is critical to instill a sense of empowerment and ownership of their health condition. The transition from passivity to active participation in physical exercise within a school environment is a specific example that illustrates the priceless role that structured environments play in instilling healthier behaviors in young people (Brooks et al., 2006). Teenagers not only gain from formal programs but also flourish when encouraged to be part of creating such projects. With healthcare professionals and educators working on developing solutions that appeal to this age group, it is necessary to know about their individual experiences and points of view. Engaging them in health policy discussions, curriculum development, and wellness programs will help create more responsive and efficient solutions. Finally, inclusion of adolescent medicine in global health educational efforts assumes a holistic interpretation of well-being that transcends the physical. Diet, mental health, and reproductive health are all top-end tenets of paradigms on adolescent health. By advocating for full-scale efforts, stakeholders can address the numerous challenges that adolescents face today. This demands unified action by healthcare providers, schools, and families to create enabling environments conducive to healthy growth and development. In the long term, as adolescent health terrain evolves further, responsive and evidence-informed actions will play a key role in meeting new challenges and developing resilient, health-oriented adolescents.

Adolescent medicine encompasses a broad array of health issues specific to teenagers and tailored to meet their physiological, psychological, and social needs. Among the salient issues highlighted, the prevalence of mental illness conditions such as depression and anxiety has been a dominant concern and most often triggered by external forces and social media pressures. It is critical to recognize these psychiatric disorders, which can impact the general well-being, education level, and later health outcomes of teenagers. A multidisciplinary approach, in coordination with healthcare providers, teachers, and families, is critical to fostering effective coping strategies and enhancing resilience among teenagers. Early identification and treatment of these concerns can lead to more effective interventions and better outcomes. Another key aspect of adolescent medicine is the increasing number of chronic conditions, such as obesity, diabetes, and asthma, due to lifestyle habits and environmental factors. The presentation emphasized that adolescents lack the necessary awareness and skills for making the right health-related decisions. Therefore, nutrition, physical fitness, and chronic condition self-management health education programs are of vital significance. As much as teenagers need to be encouraged to engage in preventive health practices, such as annual screenings and immunizations, it is equally important to address the rising prevalence of these chronic diseases. By providing young adults with information and resources, healthcare providers can significantly impact teenagers' health status over their entire lifespan and promote a culture of wellness and prevention. Besides, the integration of oral health under the umbrella of adolescent health is a very commonly overlooked but vital component. This is so in the case of systemic diseases that can present in their oral manifestations. A case in point is adolescent gingival conditions as a possible harbinger of more serious conditions like acute lymphoblastic leukemia, and therefore requiring early detection and control. As recent research has shown, collaborative care between dental practitioners and medical professionals is key to successfully managing these cases. Greater awareness among pediatricians and dentists of the oral signs of systemic diseases ensures that adolescents receive thorough care, thereby enhancing their long-term health and well-being, as seen in the results of (Yang et al., 2025). The discussion outlines the importance of collaboration among healthcare practitioners to address the complex health challenges prevalent during adolescence.

KEY TERMS FROM THIS CHAPTER

- Abstract thinking
- Adolescent medicine
- Antiretroviral therapy
- Anxiety
- Chronic illnesses
- Depression
- Medical care
- Mental health
- Obesity
- Palliative care
- Peer pressure
- Sexual health
- Sexual maturation
- Social violence

CRITICAL THINKING QUESTIONS

1. **What is the most common cause of death in adolescents globally?**
   a. Infectious diseases
   b. Road traffic injuries
   c. Suicide
   d. Cardiovascular diseases
2. **What is the primary characteristic of puberty in males?**
   a. Development of facial hair
   b. Enlargement of the testes
   c. Deepening of the voice
   d. Increased muscle mass
3. **Which of the following is the most commonly diagnosed mental health disorder in adolescents?**
   a. Bipolar disorder
   b. Schizophrenia
   c. Anxiety disorders
   d. Substance use disorders
4. **Which vaccine is recommended for adolescents to prevent certain types of cancer?**
   a. HPV vaccine
   b. Hepatitis A vaccine
   c. Varicella vaccine
   d. MMR vaccine
5. **What is the most common nutritional deficiency in adolescents worldwide?**
   a. Vitamin D deficiency
   b. Calcium deficiency
   c. Iron deficiency
   d. Protein deficiency

Short Answer Questions

1. What is adolescent medicine?
2. Why is specialized care important for adolescents?
3. Explain the physical development in adolescents.
4. What are the mental health issues in adolescents?
5. What is the role of technology in adolescent health?

Answer to Critical Thinking Questions

1. (b); 2. (b); 3. (c); 4. (a); 5. (c).

REFERENCES

1. Regmi, P. R., Van Teijlingen, E. R., Simkhada, P., & Acharya, D. R. (2010). Dating and sex among emerging adults in Nepal. *Journal of Adolescent Research*, *26*(6), 675–700. https://doi.org/10.1177/0743558410384735Adejumo, A., Ankrah, M., Bernays, S., et al. (2019). Factors impacting antiretroviral therapy adherence among human immunodeficiency virus-positive adolescents in Sub-Saharan Africa: A systematic review. https://core.ac.uk/download/287581306.pdf (accessed on 12th July 2025).

2. Adi, Y., Carter, Y., Doug, M., et al. (2009). Transition to adult services for children and young people with palliative care needs: A systematic review. https://core.ac.uk/download/44454.pdf (accessed on 12th July 2025).

3. Al-Alem, L., Omar, H. A., & Salous, A. (2009). Trends in mental health of an adolescent medicine clinic patient population. https://core.ac.uk/download/232583688.pdf (accessed on 12th July 2025).

4. Al-Alem, L., Omar, H. A., & Salous, A. (2013). United States: Mental health issues in an adolescent medicine clinic patient population. https://core.ac.uk/download/232583689.pdf (accessed on 12th July 2025).

5. Alexandre, J., Calado, F., & Griffiths, M. D. (2014). Mom, Dad it's only a game! Perceived gambling and gaming behaviors among adolescents and young adults: An exploratory study. https://core.ac.uk/download/30650469.pdf (accessed on 12th July 2025).

6. Alsudairy, N., Alhijji, N., Aljafar, B., Alanazi, A., Alshaikh, S., Alsultan, D., Hijab, Z., et al. (2025). A comprehensive review of the impact of medications in family medicine on the health of pregnant women and children: Risks and benefits. *International Journal of Medicine in Developing Countries*. https://www.semanticscholar.org/paper/df7de2829db606765c6927b5f3ea725092cd8ee3 (accessed on 12th July 2025).

7. Appleton Gootman, J., Sim, L. J., & Lawrence, R. S. (2008). Adolescent health services: Missing opportunities. https://core.ac.uk/download/71349202.pdf (accessed on 12th July 2025).

8. Aziz, C., Cheung, M., Cowan, F. M., Fu, H., Hermens, H., et al. (2009). Difference in prevalence of common mental disorder as measured using four questionnaire delivery methods among young people in rural Zimbabwe.

9. Bagalman, E., & Heisler, E. J. (2013). The mental health workforce: A primer. https://core.ac.uk/download/18615793.pdf (accessed on 12th July 2025).

10. Bagnall, A., Day, R., & Kime, N. H. (2013). Systematic review of transition models for young people with long-term conditions: A report for NHS Diabetes. https://core.ac.uk/download/29018738.pdf (accessed on 12th July 2025).

11. Balamurali, R. (2025). The role of social media in shaping adolescent mental well-being: A comprehensive review on its pros and cons. *Adolescent Psychiatry*. https://www.semanticscholar.org/paper/e6d0e7ae6c94e37d566ec506fb27c2bb04bd656f (accessed on 12th July 2025).

12. Balamurugan, G., & Vijayarani, M. (2025). Filtering reality: Navigating Instagram's influence on adolescent mental health. *Journal of Education and Health Promotion, 14*, 913–919. https://www.semanticscholar.org/paper/9bbb5173e827e55d163fd1ccf78417a64a17d087 (accessed on 12th July 2025).

13. Barrett, K., Lynch, M., & Stretesky, P. (2016). Green criminology and the reconceptualization of school violence: Comparing green school violence and traditional forms of school violence for school children. https://core.ac.uk/download/41072521.pdf (accessed on 12th July 2025).

14. Bartsch, H., Conway, K. P., Feldstein Ewing, S. W., et al. (2018). Adolescent brain cognitive development (ABCD) study: Overview of substance use assessment methods. https://core.ac.uk/download/323065853.pdf (accessed on 12th July 2025).

15. Bloor, M., Borzekowski, D. L. G., Boyd, D., Buckingham, D., Charmaz, K., Conrad, P., Denzin, N., et al. (2013). What young people want from health-related online resources: A focus group study. https://core.ac.uk/download/16460260.pdf (accessed on 12th July 2025).

16. Brooks, F., & Magnusson, J. (2006). Taking part counts: Adolescents' experiences of the transition from inactivity to active participation in school-based physical education. https://core.ac.uk/download/1638107.pdf (accessed on 12th July 2025).

17. Cheesbrough, S., Ingham, R., & Massey, D. (2002). Reducing the rate of teenage conceptions: A review of the evidence (US, Canada, Australia & NZ).

18. Chen, J., Zhang, X., & Sun, G. (2024). Causal relationship between type 2 diabetes and common respiratory system diseases: A two-sample Mendelian randomization analysis. *Frontiers in Medicine, 11*. https://www.semanticscholar.org/paper/b0c6a6978b90ca33d0c28e944905d0381b8596c8 (accessed on 12th July 2025).

19. Chun, D., Kim, S. J., Suh, J., & Kim, J. (2025). Body composition changes and catch-up growth in pre-pubertal children with short stature: A longitudinal retrospective cross-sectional cohort study. *Journal of Clinical Research in Pediatric Endocrinology*. https://www.semanticscholar.org/paper/2ee9cf8449b2b91762a8af4cfc490f2d7b504ef2 (accessed on 12th July 2025).

20. Ciampo, L., & Ciampo, I. (2024). The changing body: Importance of adequate adolescent development. *Journal of Advances in Medicine and Medical Research*. https://www.semanticscholar.org/paper/fc1c121646687fb42c969106172ca84bc8cc38e4 (accessed on 12th July 2025).

21. Dynnik, V. D., Dynnik, O., Verhoshanova, O. G., Druzhynina, A., Havenko, H., & Novokhatska, S. (2025). The impact of the war in Ukraine on the physical and sexual development of girls with menstrual disorders. *Child's Health*. https://www.semanticscholar.org/paper/40d72ef55b61f15bc1383b630dfa3ab2b396a974 (accessed on 12th July 2025).

22. Eisenberg, D., Kapinos, K. A., & Yakusheva, O. (2014). Obesogenic environmental influences on young adults: Evidence from randomized dormitory assignment. https://core.ac.uk/download/213088472.pdf (accessed on 12th July 2025).

23. Fox, H. B., Shejavali, K. I., & McManus, M. A. (2003). Is the health care system working for adolescents? Perspectives from providers in Boston, Denver, Houston, and San Francisco. https://core.ac.uk/download/71352449.pdf (accessed on 12th July 2025).

24. Garriga-Baraut, T., Méndez-Brea, P., Alvarez-García, O., Cabrera-Freitag, P., Fernández-Cortés, S., Sanchís-Merino, M. E., & Tomás-Pérez, M. (2025). A telemedicine care protocol for pediatric and adolescent patients with asthma after the COVID-19 pandemic. *Exploration of Asthma & Allergy*. https://www.semanticscholar.org/paper/c11a525aff6bedd5ddc8e3e35cc9c8e40daed7bf (accessed on 12th July 2025).

25. Gupta, M., Sarangi, R., Sharma, S., & Patnaik, L. (2024). Mental health issues and lifestyle changes associated with the COVID-19 pandemic in adolescents: A cross-sectional study in selected schools of Eastern India. *Journal of Education and Health Promotion, 13*. https://www.semanticscholar.org/paper/48b0f4e148b5489587e66b8cba6c9ec8cc63ff12 (accessed on 12th July 2025).

26. Hari, G. (2017). Depression in low-income adolescents: Guidelines for school-based depression intervention programs. https://core.ac.uk/download/130354083.pdf (accessed on 12th July 2025).

27. Hecimovich, M. (2004). Sport specialization in youth: A literature review. https://core.ac.uk/download/11234954.pdf (accessed on 12th July 2025).

28. Hoare, J., Sher, R., & Cullen, K. R. (2024). Using creativity and the arts to promote mental health in youth living with HIV in South Africa. *Southern African Journal of HIV Medicine, 25*. https://www.semanticscholar.org/paper/d7ed99a7979ba07d96efc151437011932a5bc379 (accessed on 12th July 2025).

29. Janssens, N., Van Wilder, L., Van Hecke, A., Van Hoorenbeeck, K., Vanden Wyngaert, K., De Smedt, D., & Goossens, E. (2024). COCCOS study: Developing a transition program for adolescents with chronic conditions using experience-based co-design. A study protocol. *PLOS ONE, 19*. https://www.semanticscholar.org/paper/275b7e07f70a571c651cc44ed6cc4f940d0e32f3 (accessed on 12th July 2025).

30. Jeong, J., Franchett, E., Ramos de Oliveira, C. V., Rehmani, K., & Yousafzai, A. K. (2021). Parenting interventions to promote early child development in the first three years of life: A global systematic review and meta-analysis. *PLOS Medicine, 18*, e1003602–e1003602. https://doi.org/10.1371/journal.pmed.1003602 (accessed on 12th July 2025).

31. Jyoti, K., Mahajan, S., Singh, D., & Gupta, A. (2025). Awareness of physical changes occurring in adolescent period: An interventional study among girls 13–17 years of age in rural field practice area, Government Medical College, Amritsar. *International Journal of Community Medicine and Public Health*. https://www.semanticscholar.org/paper/504ad12caf4ef9a7b24092dd68cc04c027c8cf34 (accessed on 12th July 2025).

32. Kapoor, K. N., Tamilmani, K., Rana, N. P., Patil, P. P., Dwivedi, Y. K., & Nerur, S. (2017). Advances in social media research: Past, present, and future. *Information Systems Frontiers, 20*, 531–558. https://doi.org/10.1007/s10796-017-9810-y (accessed on 12th July 2025).

33. Karcher, M. J., & Zaff, J. F. (2025). Connecting in a disconnected world: Tools for health professionals to assess and expand adolescent patients' connectedness and webs of support. *American Journal of Lifestyle Medicine*. https://www.semanticscholar.org/paper/ec2612c4f76dad3ae36c0dec46eb1b01056d0139 (accessed on 12th July 2025).

34. Kumar, R., Kumar, V., Latif, A., & Shah, S. A. (2024). Social media addiction: Psychological impacts on future generations. *Qlantic Journal of Social Sciences*. https://www.semanticscholar.org/paper/2744e0eb8baa23d15073272ca1fa6b30c07cbd9f (accessed on 12th July 2025).

35. Mead, A. S., Nagy, M. C., & Nagy, S. (2012). Utilizing community resources to reduce the presence of type 2 diabetes in rural youth. https://digitalscholarship.unlv.edu/cgi/viewcontent.cgi?article=1060&context=jhdrp (accessed on 12th July 2025).

36. Motherway, C. (2010). Sex education: The effectiveness of comprehensive-based compared to the effectiveness of abstinence-only. https://core.ac.uk/download/56322974.pdf (accessed on 12th July 2025).

37. Nelson, K., Adindu, A., Otaniyen, P., Onochie, O. E., Oyedemi, D., Akubuiro, C. O., et al. (2024). The influence of social media on adolescent mental health and substance abuse patterns. *World Journal of Advanced Research and Reviews*. https://www.semanticscholar.org/paper/394dd6fbed31695685c6fd44ff1c7656515dd49d (accessed on 12th July 2025).

38. Nesbitt, T. S., & Young, H. M. (2017). Increasing the capacity of primary care through enabling technology. https://core.ac.uk/download/323070127.pdf (accessed on 12th July 2025).

39. Ojio, Y., Shiozawa, T., Gregorio, E., Leynes, M. C., Hernandez, P. M. R., Estrada, C. A., Fuyama, T., et al. (2024). An international interdisciplinary approach to developing video educational materials promoting mental health literacy among adolescents in the Philippines. *Early Intervention in Psychiatry, 18*, 1047–1054. https://www.semanticscholar.org/paper/56f36d0a9ff4e2cfc2f5fd22833c05c86e3bb150 (accessed on 12th July 2025).

40. Park, J. G. (2024). Brief commentary based on article "A case report on changes in body composition in an adolescent obese patient treated with complex Korean medicine treatment with modified fasting, and space spinal conduction exercise and manipulation." *Journal of Alternative, Complementary & Integrative Medicine*. https://www.semanticscholar.org/paper/f3eefa089963add71e535daeb514d3911ec0afed (accessed on 12th July 2025).

41. Pereira, N. F. L., Kavalek, D. S., Zanardo, L. G., Guerra, T. C., & Lima, M. R. (2025). Ne health: Bisphenol A and early puberty, a systematic literature review. *Revita de Gestapo Social e Ambiental*. https://www.semanticscholar.org/paper/52bc8c2781fd21654e32a8f9189991c69d09d5a6 (accessed on 12th July 2025).

42. Ralston, E. S., Spoth, R., & Trudeau, L. S. (2012). Effects of parent-child affective quality during high school years on subsequent substance use. https://core.ac.uk/download/46603610.pdf (accessed on 12th July 2025).

43. Rowlands, S. (2010). Social predictors of repeat adolescent pregnancy and focused strategies. https://core.ac.uk/download/1352762.pdf (accessed on 12th July 2025).

44. Roy, D., Ghosh, R., Dubey, S., Jana Dubey, M., Benito-León, J., & Ray, B. K. (2020). Neurological and neuropsychiatric impacts of COVID-19 pandemic. *Canadian Journal of Neurological Sciences / Journal Canadien des Sciences Necrologies, 48*, 9–24. https://doi.org/10.1017/cjn.2020.173 (accessed on 12th July 2025).

45. ScienceOpen Admin. (2020). *Journal of Behavioral Addictions*. https://doi.org/10.14293/s2199-1006.1.sor-socsci.clnpyry.v1 (accessed on 12th July 2025).

46. Susick, M. (2011). Application of smartphone technology in the management and treatment of mental illnesses. https://core.ac.uk/download/12206606.pdf (accessed on 12th July 2025).

47. Suwanwong, C., & Raksat, D. (2025). Navigate chronic illness: Antecedents and consequences of family resilience—a systematic review and meta-analysis. *The Family Journal*. https://www.semanticscholar.org/paper/240a4015fb67b3699a951643bf19e31bc37a787a (accessed on 12th July 2025).

48. Thitamethee, P., Likhitweerawong, N., Louthrenoo, O., & Boonchooduang, N. (2024). Chronic conditions and resilience: Adolescent health behaviors in the midst of the COVID-19 pandemic in Thailand. *Global Pediatric Health, 11*. https://www.semanticscholar.org/paper/8e1b8f08c69917665cecf1a4bc4ecd9f535e2504 (accessed on 12th July 2025).

49. Tomás, C., Oliveira, E., Ferreira Sousa, D. C., Chupel, M. U., Furtado, G. E., Rocha, C., & Teixeira, A. (2016). Proceedings of the 3rd IPLeiria's International Health Congress. *BMC Health Services Research, 16*. https://doi.org/10.1186/s12913-016-1423-5 (accessed on 12th July 2025).

50. Tripp, J., & Viner, R. (2005). ABC of adolescence: Sexual health, contraception, and teenage pregnancy. https://core.ac.uk/download/1670599.pdf (accessed on 12th July 2025).

51. Vaghef-Koodehi, A., & Lapizco-Encinas, B. (2025). Dielectrophoresis in carcinoma diagnosis: Recent developments and applications. *Electrophoresis*. https://www.semanticscholar.org/paper/b224772b0ee524895c9a69aa0a07e2672201281d (accessed on 12th July 2025).

52. Venhorst, A., Gärtner, B., Hollander, K., & Meyer, T. (2022). Vaccinations in athletes. *Deutsche Zeitschrift für Sportmedizin/German Journal of Sports Medicine*. https://www.semanticscholar.org/paper/2c042cf48377a8926541c5ec534d910f535e1541 (accessed on 12th July 2025).

53. Verissimo da Costa, C., Sáfadi, M. A. P., de Moraes, J. C., Gondim, J. B., Bezerra, A. M. F., Azevedo, D. D. M., Bezerra, K. K. S., et al. (2024). Vaccination situation of adolescents and factors associated with the incomplete vaccination scheme in the eight-health region of Paraíba, Brazil. *CONTRIBUCIONES A LAS CIENCIAS SOCIALES*. https://www.semanticscholar.org/paper/5f2a70048c5df4482ee86e3aae2b7e029cb20ef0 (accessed on 12th July 2025).

54. Yang, G., Tu, Y., Hu, W., & Feng, X. (2025). 10-year follow-up of adolescent leukemia diagnosed through gingiva: A case report. *Clinical Advances in Periodontics*. https://www.semanticscholar.org/paper/04f33f104f9d525e3aa1f0fd6917e1c01ca97c5e (accessed on 12th July 2025).

55. Young, S., Adamo, N., Ásgeirsdóttir, B. B., Branney, P., Beckett, M., Colley, W., Cubbin, S., et al. (2020). Females with ADHD: An expert consensus statement taking a lifespan approach providing guidance for the identification and treatment of attention-deficit/hyperactivity disorder in girls and women. *BMC Psychiatry, 20*. https://doi.org/10.1186/s12888-020-02707-9 (accessed on 12th July 2025).

WOMEN'S HEALTH

11

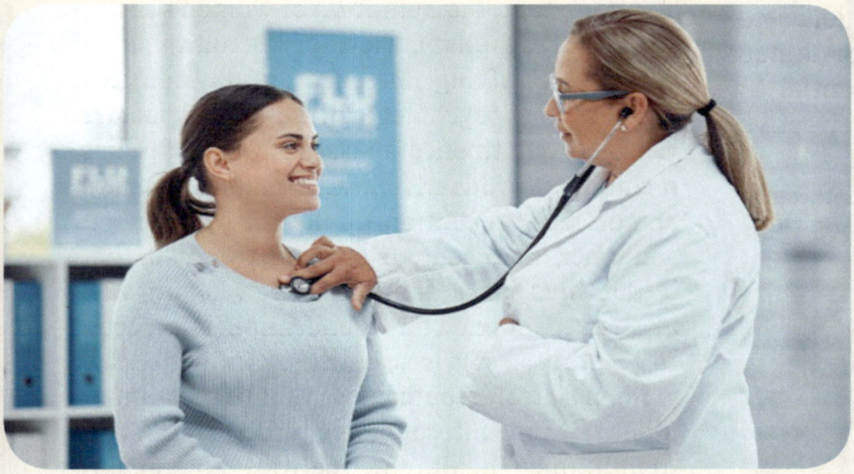

LEARNING OBJECTIVES

After studying this chapter, you will be able to:

1. Describe the reproductive health
2. Understand the mental health of women
3. Know the chronic diseases
4. Understand the nutrition and lifestyle
5. Understand the access to healthcare
6. Describe the health disparities

Introduction

The discussion on women's health has drawn increasingly more attention from scholars, policy-makers, and healthcare professionals over recent years. The multifaceted notion of women's health is significant, as it encompasses a broad spectrum of issues that extend beyond reproductive health. Gendered social norms, economic inequalities, and healthcare service access are just a few of the most pertinent determinants of women's health outcomes. Inclusion of these variables into one concept allows for consideration of both the physical and psychological aspects of health and thereby a more successful integrated investigation of the particular health concerns that are experienced by women. This integrated framework not only underscores the importance of meeting specific health needs but also identifies the system barriers that hinder women's access to quality care and services, necessitating special policies and interventions to improve overall health outcomes for women (Kanyinga et al., 2007). As we continue into the complexities of women's health, it can be seen that cultural, social, and economic determinants have a significant impact on health habits and access to treatment. Women in the majority of societies are disproportionately impacted by socioeconomic limitations that reduce their ability to address health as a priority. For example, the persistence of gender discrimination within the workforce continues economic disparities that further marginalize women, thereby impacting their health outcomes. Similarly, community stigma for some of the illnesses, like mental illness and reproductive health, most likely leads to underreporting, incorrect diagnosis, or undue treatment. Because of this, it is essential to identify these factors to enable effective policy and program planning that will address women's own needs, foster fair access to care, and promote a setting that will improve their health (Turgoose et al., 2019).

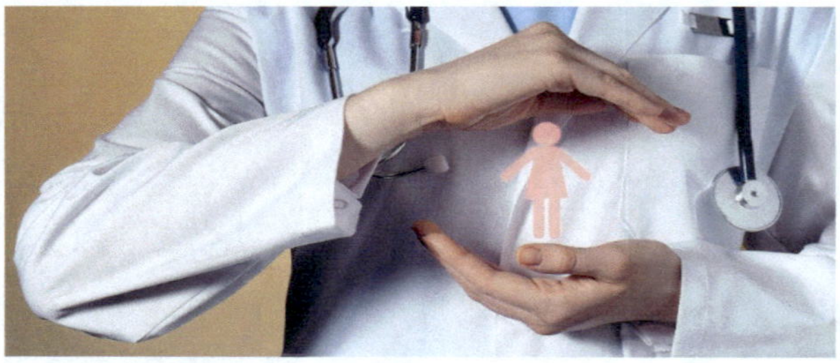

Figure 11.1. Women's health.

Source: https://www.care2curephysiotherapyclinic.com/wp-content/uploads/2023/06/11.jpg.

In addition, gender-sensitive interventions have proven successful across various health settings. Given the specific health risks and needs posed by women, clinicians can design programs that not only address symptoms but also incorporate preventive care and educational components. For instance, interventions aimed at women's mental health, maternal health, and chronic disease management have had a significant impact on alleviating health disparities, which are based predominantly on intersectional factors like race, socioeconomic position, and place. Such targeted interventions also empower women by improving their health literacy and enabling them to make informed decisions about their health. Lastly, by focusing on women's health holistically, society can strive to achieve health equity, where women are treated with care and support so they can live healthy and productive lives (Kanyinga et al., 2007) (Figure 11.1).

Definition of Women's Health

To understand the definition of women's health is to take a holistic view of its multifaceted nature, identifying not only the physiological but also the psychological and social factors. Women's health encompasses a range of issues, including reproductive health, maternal health, and disease prevention, applicable to women in a manner that is unique to them. On top of that, it identifies social determinants of health, such as socioeconomic status, education, and access to healthcare services, as major influencers of women's health outcomes. It is important to identify these interdependent factors in order to minimize health inequalities and ensure women's health receives the significance it should within the overall healthcare framework. By focusing on individual and population health, women's health has to expand its definition to encompass all stages of life, as health is a continuous process and is subject to multiple contextual factors. Moreover, the dynamic nature of women's health stresses the importance of evidence-based recommendations to help health professionals deliver integrated care. While the prenatal care guidelines are important tools for practitioners, a critical review of these protocols reveals imbalances in the delivery of key educational components. For instance, the guidelines reviewed between 2005 and 2009 highlighted significant deficits in addressing women's distinctive health needs, highlighting the importance of an individualized system for prenatal care (Forristal et al., 2009). Such systemic alertness not only compromises the effectiveness of health delivery but also highlights the need for a paradigm shift in favor of women as active subjects of their own health experience. Integrating education, care, and informed decision-making into practice is important to define women's health in a holistic, responsive framework attuned to their diverse experiences. Also, activism and women's health intersect to highlight the importance of accessible healthcare practices. Activism on the internet, for example, such as the movements that emerged from the Disability March, has demonstrated how marginalized voices can serve as a unifying force for advocacy of accessibility and inclusion in the context of health issues (Bora et al., 2018). Disabled activists, for example, navigate the contradictions of their identities, which shape their approaches to health-related concerns and advocacy for policy changes. This calls for healthcare systems to be attuned to the various facets of women's health, where social identity, like disability, becomes significant in determining health outcomes. This attunement not only raises awareness of women's health issues but also fosters a more inclusive environment that amplifies the voices and demands of all women, thereby enriching the broader discourse on women's health (Figure 11.2).

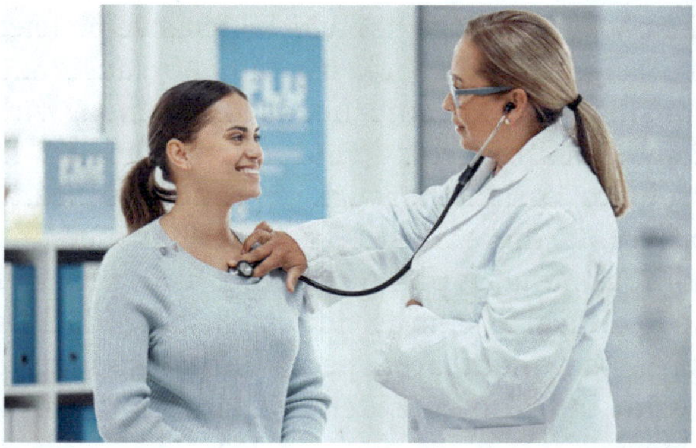

Figure 11.2. Redefining the focus of women's health.

Source: https://emi.parkview.com/media/Image/Dashboard_835_womens_heart_health_3_23.jpg.

Importance of Women's Health in Society

The significance of women's health in society transcends simple individual well-being; it is a cornerstone of public health and social equity. Women's health is intricately linked to maternal and child health outcomes, workforce participation, and community stability. When women are healthy, they can participate fully in society, contribute to economic development, and support the next generation through better parenting. Moreover, poor health among women can lead to profound societal repercussions, including increased healthcare costs, reduced productivity, and greater dependency on social services. As such, prioritizing women's health is not merely a personal issue but a societal imperative that fosters sustainable development and social cohesion. Understanding the complexities surrounding women's health is essential, particularly for marginalized groups. For instance, women with disabilities face unique challenges that often go unaddressed in broader health discussions. Research indicates that over one in ten women of reproductive age identifies as having a disability, yet they often encounter stigma, inadequate health care, and societal misconceptions about their reproductive capabilities (Clark et al., 2019). Addressing these disparities is crucial for fostering inclusivity and ensuring that all women have equal access to health resources. By emphasizing the necessity for tailored healthcare solutions and accessible information, society can empower women with disabilities to assert their reproductive rights and achieve positive health outcomes. Organizations such as the International Council on Women's Health Issues (ICOWHI) play a vital role in advocating for women's health globally. ICOWHI focuses on participation, empowerment, and research to improve the health of women and girls, recognizing the interconnectedness of gender issues and health outcomes (Meleis et al., 2011). Their efforts to facilitate education and promote community engagement underscore the importance of collaborative approaches to tackling women's health challenges. By engaging a multidisciplinary network of health providers and advocates, they aim to address the unique needs of women, fostering an environment where equitable access to health is not just an ideal but a reality. This comprehensive framework not only enhances healthcare delivery but also contributes to improved societal health, thereby illustrating the integral role that women's health plays in overall community well-being (Figure 11.3).

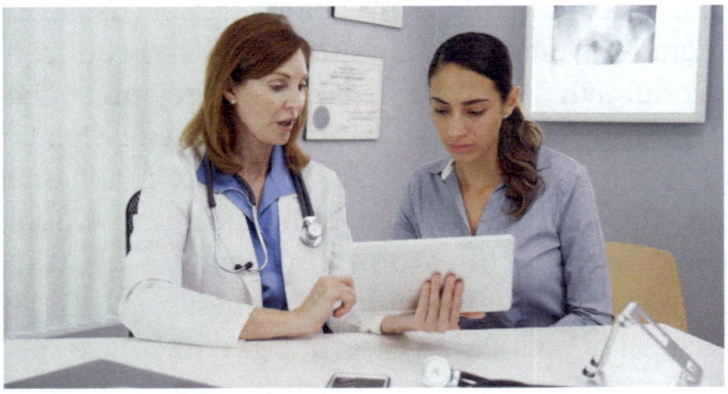

Figure 11.3. Importance of women's health.

Source: https://hunterhealth.org/wp-content/uploads/2023/05/AdobeStock_222222657-scaled.jpeg.

11.1. Reproductive Health

Learning Outcome

1. Know the menstrual health and disorders
2. Understand the access to a diverse range of contraceptive options
3. Describe the pregnancy and maternal health

Reproductive health is a multifaceted subject that encompasses a wide range of issues, including prenatal care, complications of pregnancy, and women's rights to decide about their reproductive lives. Among the most significant issues of reproductive health is access to quality healthcare services, which includes education regarding risks of pregnancy and the consumption of drugs. Research indicates that state legislation regarding drinking alcohol while pregnant more closely mirrors an anti-abortion agenda than public health concerns. This divergence could lead to the failure to provide adequate services for women, endangering their lives and those of the unborn (Roberts et al., 2019). Therefore, women can be stigmatized and coerced away from appropriate care or help, hence validating the need for policies that address women's health comprehensively and not politically. Fostering the complexity of the reproductive health debate is that of women with disabilities, who find it extremely challenging to access reproductive healthcare. Since over 10% of the reproductive-aged women have some disability, their dreams towards motherhood are as much as those of their non-disabled counterparts. But women with disabilities are often subjected to unique stigma and discrimination that could impede them from accessing health care services. The blogs authored by the women offer the required stories about adaptation to reproductive health issues, shedding light on their experiences of pregnancy and motherhood (Clark et al., 2019). The disparity among the services provided in healthcare, along with the social prejudice, is the background against which inclusive policies are required that look beyond the cause and consider the specific needs of women with disabilities regarding reproductive health. In order to design thorough reproductive health programs, there must be a more informed and compassionate policy-making and practice of healthcare. This is not only about dealing with the medical aspects of reproductive health but also considering the socio-cultural determinants of women's choices and access to care. Empowering women through education, awareness, and support networks can reduce the stigma and obstacles to their empowerment, particularly among vulnerable populations such as those with disabilities. By integrating findings from personal data and existing studies, stakeholders can create effective interventions that enhance reproductive health outcomes for all women. Ultimately, the solution is an integrated approach that acknowledges women's problems and aspirations to support women's health and respect and protect reproductive rights (Figure 11.4).

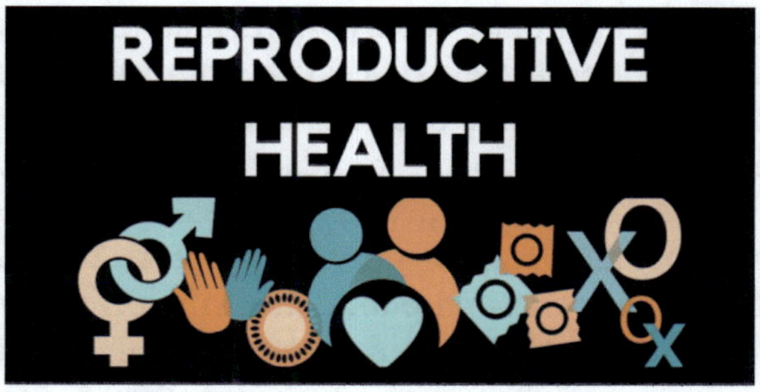

Figure 11.4. Reproductive health.

Source: https://s3.ap-south-1.amazonaws.com/24x7-cors/cover/a92db570-10ee-11ee-a6ae-759a325aa8dd_1235x330.png.

11.1.1. Menstrual Health and Disorders

Menstrual health is a component of women's global health that affects the quality of life and everyday functioning of women considerably. Menstrual disorders like premenstrual syndrome (PMS) affect a large group of women, and holistic health education and management are required. PMS consists of a variety of affective and somatic symptoms that appear in cycles, with consequences on mood, behavior, and bodily well-being before menstruation. Research has shown that nearly 63% of female university students report that they have had PMS, and 42.5% of them report severe PMS symptoms. Symptomatic presentations such as irritability and bloating of the abdomen suggest that PMS can seriously disrupt usual activities and emotional stability, and therefore, there is a strong rationale for awareness and intervention approaches in educational settings (Akiki et al., 2018). The effects of PMS extend beyond intrinsic discomfort, influencing learning performance and social relationships. PMS affects learners by reducing concentration, increasing absenteeism, and reducing engagement in learning activities, leading to poorer grades and fewer learning opportunities. A research study on female health science students revealed the prevalence to be 60.8% for PMS that impacts significant things in life, such as physical well-being and psychological states (Kustriyanti et al., 2020). This is an evident correlation between menstrual disorder and overall health quality, suggesting that it is important to intervene in menstrual health for the empowerment of women and success in education. Schoolsmust therefore recognize the significance of menstrual health in creating favorable learning environments for women students.

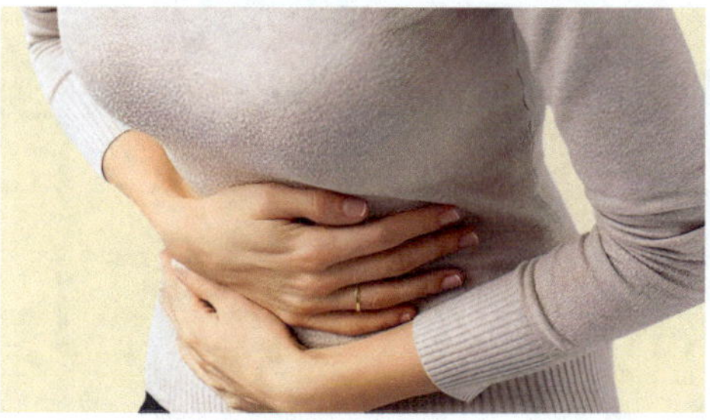

Figure 11.5. Menstrual disorders.

Source: https://drkaminiraohospitals.com/images/services/menstrual-disorder-treatments.jpg.

Awareness of the complicated nature of menstrual disorders can enhance management and treatment interventions. Obesity, consumption of caffeine, and drug use have also been suggested as contributors to the severity of PMS symptoms. Such findings put more focus on lifestyle interventions, including diet and stress reduction, to alleviate the sufferings of PMS. By raising awareness of the impact of these lifestyle factors, healthcare providers can implement preventive interventions to improve menstrual health. This holistic strategy not only assists in managing menstrual disorders but also contributes to improved physical and mental well-being in women, underscoring the crucial intersection of menstrual health within the broader context of women's health (Figure 11.5).

11.1.2. Contraception Options and Access

Availability of a broad range of contraceptive methods is at the core of women's health and empowerment. Safe and effective contraception allows women to make informed decisions regarding family planning, thereby increasing their quality of life and economic security . Various methods, including barrier methods, hormonal contraception, and long-acting reversible contraceptives (LARCs), allow women to have a sense of freedom to choose what best fits them in terms of lifestyle, health needs, and personal preference. Even with access to these means, there are still hindrances, particularly in low-income populations where access to reproductive health services might be limited. Healthcare providers have a very important role in providing access to and educating women about these means. Access to contraceptives through public health is pivotal in attaining better health, greater autonomy, and a lower incidence of unwanted pregnancies. Evidence indicates that educational interventions have a positive impact on the use of contraceptive methods, especially among adolescents.

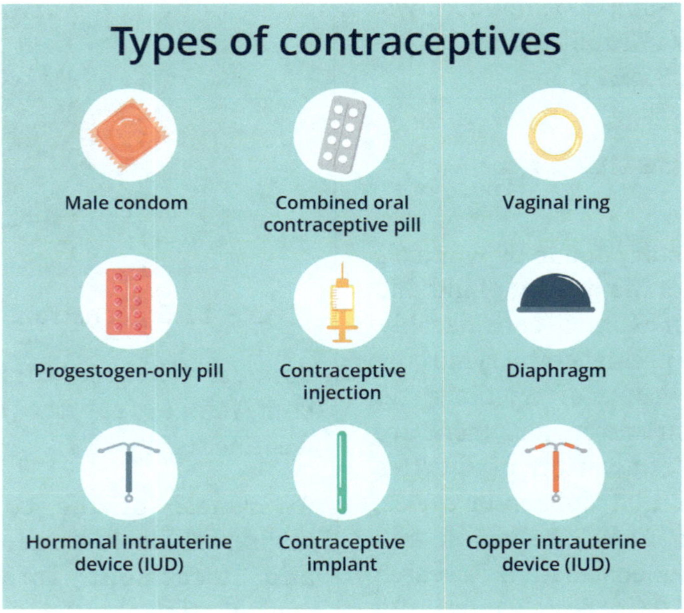

Figure 11.6. Types of contraceptives.

Source: https://media.healthdirect.org.au/images/inline/original/hd_types-of-contraceptives-67342c.png.

Research pointed out that adolescents presenting for care usually show a high interest in acquiring information on preventing pregnancy, yet many feel that there is a deficiency of effective educational tools in health facilities. For instance, the dissemination of an educational video to a group of emergency department patients increased the enthusiasm for LARCs in teenage girls significantly, and this suggests that some kinds of education can increase awareness and utilization of effective contraceptive techniques. Such practice not only teaches young women about alternatives such as intrauterine devices (IUDs) and implants but also plugs significant loopholes in the health care system that habitually shortchange vulnerable groups. Home-based transmission of focused information can bridge information gaps and improve adoption rates of contraception among younger age groups. The role of well-trained health workers in delivering such educational interventions cannot be overemphasized. In rural Uganda, tubal ligation performed by well-trained clinical officers was shown to be associated with high patient satisfaction and low complication rates. This result underscores the potential of task-sharing to enhance access. If women are able to obtain safe, effective family planning care close to home, not only do they gain more options, but they also trust the health system. Enabling an ethnically diverse group to provide such services can help reduce barriers that women face in receiving contraception, fostering a culture where educated reproductive health decisions are the norm rather than the exception, which in turn can result in improved overall health outcomes for women all over the world (Figure 11.6).

11.1.3. Pregnancy and Maternal Health

The complexities of pregnancy and maternal health necessitate a multifaceted process of understanding the variety of factors that affect mothers' and children's outcomes. There is evidence to indicate that maternal mental health is at the hub of the perinatal period, and significant correlations between psychiatric illness and maternal as well as fetal health. For instance, studies show that females being admitted to specialist mother and baby units are those with the most severe mental illness, such as non-affective psychosis, affective psychosis, and non-psychotic depressive episodes, which are linked with higher risks of adverse developmental outcomes among children. Specifically, almost a third of children whose mothers have had psychiatric admissions during pregnancy are known to be at potential risk of adversity, underscoring the critical need for targeted interventions and support mechanisms during this vulnerable point in life (Cantwell et al., 2017). Furthermore, public policy on maternal health also plays an important part in determining pregnancy outcomes and the overall health of mothers and children. More recent studies of the regulation of alcohol consumption during pregnancy have made it clear that most state policies actually have their roots in an anti-abortion perspective and not in concern for the public good.

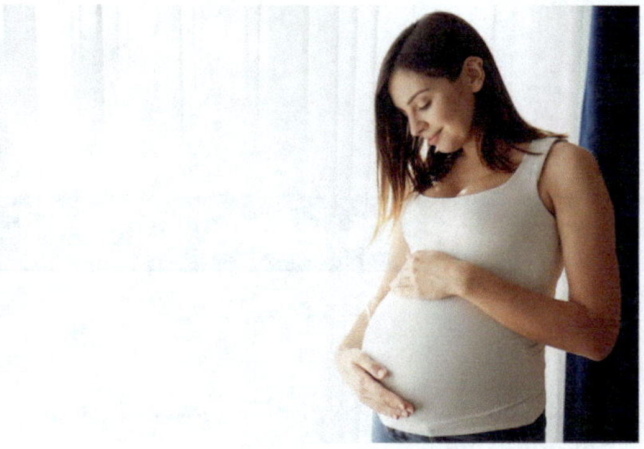

Figure 11.7. Maternal health during pregnancy.

Source: https://www.metropolisindia.com/upgrade/blog/upload/2023/05/Maternal-Health-During-Pregnancy.jpeg.

The alarming pattern here is that the emphasis on the mother's behavior has the potential to subvert the larger picture of pregnancy health. For example, the refusal to acknowledge abortion as a solution for severely alcohol-dependent mothers risks exacerbating health hazards for both mothers and children. In addition, the concern regarding alcohol abstinence counseling during pregnancy has the perverse effect of inhibiting constructive public health discussions toward reducing harm caused by substances (Roberts et al., 2019). Addressing the interconnected problems of maternal health and pregnancy, an integrated strategy must thus be employed to include mental health care and policy reform that prioritizes evidence-informed best practices. Aligning mental health care with prenatal care would allow healthcare workers to help pregnant women better manage their mental health, potentially enhancing developmental success for children. Moreover, encouraging public policies that focus on education and harm reduction regarding drug use during pregnancy can offer healthier environments for mothers and infants. With policymaking and societal attitudes ongoing, it is imperative that maternal health policy addresses women's comprehensive needs, thereby improving families' and generations' overall health landscape (Figure 11.7).

Test Your Knowledge

1. What are the common menstrual disorders?
2. What are the options for contraception?

11.2. Mental Health

Learning Outcome

1. Know the prevalence of mental health issues among women
2. Understand the impact of societal pressures on women's mental health
3. Describe the resources and support systems available

Women's mental well-being is a key area to consider, particularly within the perinatal period, that is, the time from pregnancy until shortly after delivery. Herein, women become susceptible to mental illnesses such as depression and anxiety. Research has indicated that these conditions have serious, long-lasting impacts not only on mothers but also on infants and families. The suffering that occurs during this period is not a personal issue; rather, it poses serious public health concerns. As more is learned by society about these issues, interventions have been established to enhance the psychological well-being of pregnant women, which suggests that mental health interventions play an imperative role in ensuring healthy outcomes for women and their babies (Jomeen et al., 2016). The development and implementation of group interventions to address perinatal mental health have emerged as a successful means. Interventions of this sort have been known to emphasize psychological frameworks such as cognitive behavioral therapy and mindfulness, which are tailored to meet the demands of pregnant women. Qualitative research has shown that the majority of the participants find these group settings helpful since they provide reassurance and, in turn, make them feel a sense of normalcy in their lives. However, although some studies report encouraging quantitative outcomes, the evidence remains insufficient to support these interventions universally. This highlights the necessity for ongoing research to refine these interventions so that they are responsive to the diverse needs of women who are striving to navigate mental health problems at such a developing phase of their lives (Jomeen et al., 2016). The broader consequences of women's mental health extend to many aspects of society and affect gender equality and economic engagement. Organizations dedicated to advancing women's rights have recognized the inherent connection between mental health and women's well-being and empowerment. They are striving to create systemic shifts that benefit mental health outcomes by stopping issues such as discrimination on the basis of gender and non-recognition of women's value contributions. Investment in women's mental health benefits not just the individual but also enhances , community resilience, and social cohesion. Therefore, the response must be multi-faceted, harmonizing mental health care with broader support for women's rights and voices, thereby ensuring a holistic approach to women's health (Figure 11.8).

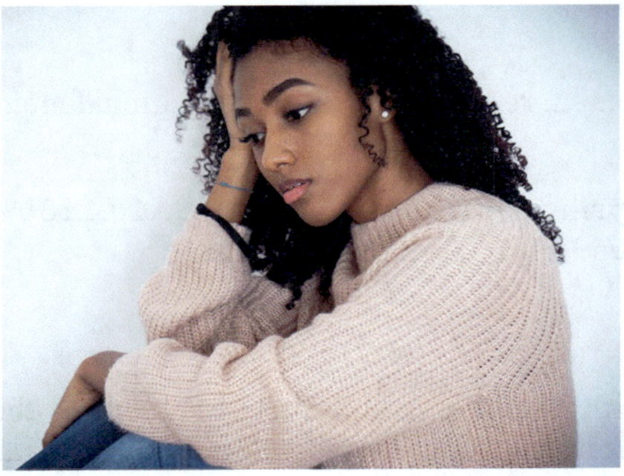

Figure 11.8. Women's mental health.

Source: https://www.kernodle.com/wp-content/uploads/2020/08/Kernodle-OBGYN_Womens-Mental-Health.jpeg.

11.2.1. Prevalence of Mental Health Issues Among Women

The prevalence of mental illnesses among women is an issue of utmost concern in the area of women's health, necessitating a comprehensive account of the particular causes that are responsible for the imbalance. Studies indicate that there is a higher likelihood of mental illnesses affecting women compared to men, particularly with regard to anxiety, depression, and post-traumatic stress disorder (PTSD). For instance, the postpartum period is particularly challenging, with the majority of women reporting PTSD symptoms concerning giving birth, which has a negative effect on their relationship with their infants. This association indicates the intricate interplay between maternal health and mental health, imposing the importance of early intervention and treatment to safeguard both the mothers and the children (Anđelinović et al., 2020). Furthermore, mental health and culture cross paths to have a considerable impact on prevalence rates. Women of African descent, particularly those residing in the United States and territories, experience victimization at frightening levels of intimate partner abuse that contributes to mental illness. Multisite analysis concluded that, among these women, lifetime IPA prevalence is stunningly high, with rates of 45% reported in some areas. The mental health impacts of violence of this nature are so significant that there are increased rates of depression and anxiety reported among survivors. An appreciation of these demographics' unique challenges can help guide targeted interventions, not just enhancing mental health, but also attempting to reduce rates of intimate partner violence (Bertand et al., 2014). Women's mental health is multidimensional, transcending personal experience and becoming intertwined with deeper societal issues and systemic inequalities. Access to mental health care remains a limitation for the majority of women, particularly marginalized women who may face additional stigma or economic restriction. Such disparate access often results in untreated mental illness, perpetuating cycles of suffering and disrupting overall well-being. Furthermore, socio-economic context significantly affects mental health outcomes, with lower socio-economic status women usually experiencing further stressors that accumulate psychological distress. This intricate interplay of mental health problems highlights the necessity of multisectoral, community-based interventions that focus on prevention as well as treatment and an awareness of the specific needs of women in varied social and cultural contexts (Figure 11.9).

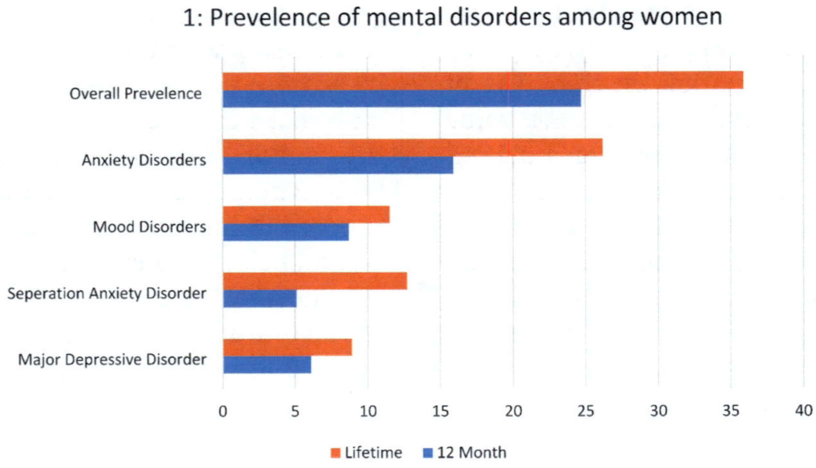

Figure 11.9. Prevalence of mental disorders among women: results from the Saudi national mental health survey.

Source: https://media.springernature.com/full/springer-static/image/art%3A10.1186%2Fs12889-024-20069-9/MediaObjects/12889_2024_20069_Fig1_HTML.png?as=webp.

11.2.2. Impact of Societal Pressures on Women's Mental Health

The effect of social pressures on women's mental health is profound and intricate, affecting their sense of self and emotional state. With social definitions of body image and femininity in a constant state of flux, women are most often exposed to unrealistic expectations that can lead to mental illness in the form of eating disorders. Research indicates that the cultural constructions of gender play a key role in the etiology of such disorders, which tend not to be treated in treatment centers. From talking with women and observing their lives, one realizes how their self-worth and identity are shaped by social expectations. These have explained some of the pressures which necessitate bringing in feminist methodologies into treatment interventions, and this is evidenced by the criticisms by women of the traditional biomedical model of treatment. Therefore, an examination of these pressures in society in detail is crucial in explaining their connection to women's mental health and the effectiveness of treatment modalities used today (Bartky et al., 2016). In addition to this, society's expectations dictate not only women's body image issues but also uphold the ideals of motherhood and family roles. Women with diseases such as female genital fistula illustrate the extreme effects of these pressures. For others, a desire to fit society's idea of childbearing significantly impacts their mental health. Research has established that support from the partner, financial status, and social stigma associated with infertility further increase feelings of isolation and distress among such women. Personal experiences lead them to navigate complex emotional realms governed by social expectations, influencing their well-being following treatment. It is an acknowledgment of the mental effects of these social norms that can guide medical practitioners in creating improved counseling methods responsive to women's unique experiences and mental health trajectories (Barageine et al., 2025). This dance between societal forces and mental health reflects the far-reaching significance of integrating balanced methods that prioritize women's overall well-being. By combining the social context and feminist theory in mental health treatments, professionals are better positioned to help women combat external pressures. Both the alleviation of mental distress and the permitting of a healthier and empowering discourse on women's identity must take into account societal demands. As researchers and practitioners continue to dig deeper into these overlapping arenas, it is apparent that a well-informed approach must be inclusive of the larger societal forces that structure women's lives. It is a recognition of the significant role such pressures play that can lead to new approaches to facilitating women's mental well-being in the context of a more complicated social environment, requiring treatment modalities that will more effectively communicate with women's lived experience and reality (Bartky et al., 2016) (Figure 11.10).

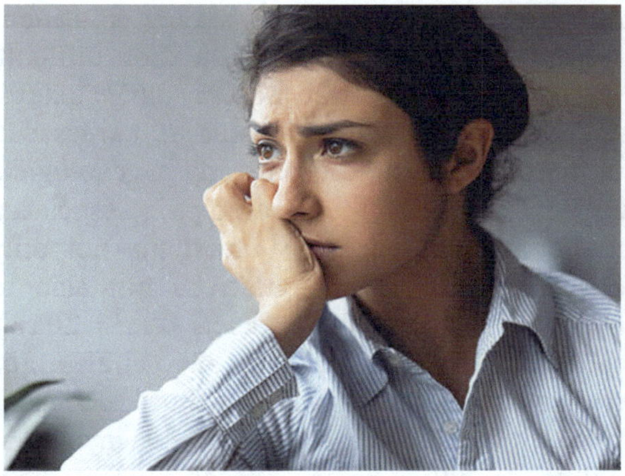

Figure 11.10. Societal pressures on women.

Source: https://shaadi.org/wp-content/uploads/2021/08/Societal-Pressures-on-Women.jpg.

11.2.3. Resources and Support Systems Available

Availability of good-quality health facilities and support systems continues to be central to the overall health of women. These include educational services, healthcare facilities, as well as advocacy groups. Some of the lead organizations devoted to women's health include the International Council on Women's Health Issues (ICOWHI). This is a multidisciplinary professional and advocacy network committed to enhancing the quality of life and health for girls and women worldwide. Through facilitated participation and the empowerment of women through education and advocacy, ICOWHI embodies the kind of support system needed to address the varied health issues faced by women, from reproductive health to chronic disease management (Meleis et al., 2011). Through such joint efforts, the stigma associated with women's health can be minimized, creating a culture that recognizes and values their distinct health requirements. The accessibility of full-range prenatal care (PNC) facilities is crucial in the process of supporting pregnant women. Adequate prenatal services are intended to provide women with the necessary evaluations and informative guidance throughout pregnancy. A comparison of multiple sets of PNC guidelines underscores the inconsistency and gaps in education prevalent in these guidelines. Even though the primary focus usually falls on medical evaluation and laboratory tests, educational material relevant to prenatal care often remains insufficient (Forristal et al., 2009). This surveillance underscores the need to prioritize women's individual learning needs in prenatal care, and practitioners are advised to maintain a commitment to individualized care. By talking through each woman's educational needs and conducting clinical exams, health workers can foster an integrated approach to improving long-term health outcomes. Support networks, such as community health programs and peer counseling programs, are also critical to improving women's health. These systems provide a space for women to speak with one another, sharing information and resources most relevant to their health problems. Community organizations have a tendency to offer access to mental health care, nutritional guidance, and preventive medicine, thereby filling gaps in traditional healthcare systems. Empowering women through peer-based programs not only fosters an encouraging environment but also promotes active health management. By integrating community support with existing health care, the general effectiveness of the resources available to women can be maximized, so they can receive comprehensive care that is tailored to their unique experiences and situations, an essential component often hyped by agencies like ICOWHI (Meleis et al., 2011).

Test Your Knowledge

1. What is the prevalence of mental health disorders in women?
2. What is the impact of societal pressures on women's mental health?

11.3. Chronic Diseases

Learning Outcome

1. Know the common chronic diseases affecting women
2. Describe the risk factors specific to women
3. Know the prevention and management strategies in women's health

Chronic disease is a pervasive problem for women's health that significantly impacts their quality of life and overall well-being. Diabetes, hypertension, cardiovascular disease, and autoimmune disease especially and disproportionately occur in women, adding complications to their health trajectory. Moreover, the pathogenesis of these illnesses is multifactorial, with complex interactions among genetic, endocrine, and lifestyle factorsand differs so , and it differs widely between women. This intersectionality calls for specialized healthcare plans to treat chronic diseases appropriately among varied populations. For instance, socioeconomic, ethnic, and educational disparities in health can exacerbate the spread of such diseases, highlighting rightly the need for in-depth research and intervention strategies specifically targeting women's health (Afaf I Meleis et al., 2011). It is also important to understand the psychological nature of chronic diseases for women's health, since mental health most likely becomes associated with chronic physical disease. Women with chronic illness are more susceptible to developing depression and anxiety, which further makes treatment of the disease and taking medication difficult. The stigma of mental health and societal expectations of women's roles as carers can deter women from accessing any psychological support. Moreover, the chronic pain associated with conditions such as vulvodynia not only contributes to physical distress but also to emotional distress (Georgescu et al., 2016). Fixing these interdependent challenges requires a holistic strategy that addresses physical and mental health in ways that healthcare policy encompasses mental well-being as an integral component of chronic disease management. Public health initiatives designed to improve women's health must be prevention and education-focused on chronic diseases. Education-based programs with lifestyle components, i.e., diet and exercise, can potentially decrease the risk of chronic disease onset. Additionally, greater awareness of chronic disease symptoms and signs is essential for ensuring early diagnosis and treatment, thereby reducing the long-term burden and its associated health costs. Empowerment of women through community mobilization can assist in building a culture of preventive health care, promoting early intervention and regular use of health services. Organizations such as the International Council on Women's Health Issues (ICOWHI) play a pivotal role in raising awareness and conducting studies to strengthen healthcare systems for women globally (Meleis et al., 2011). Therefore, managing chronic diseases based on a gender-sensitive approach could be a more effective public health intervention towards enhancing the general welfare of women(Figure 11.11).

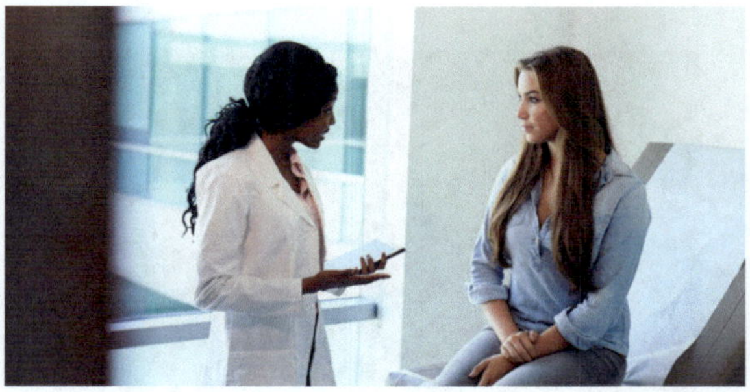

Figure 11.11. Chronic disease.

Source: https://doh.sd.gov/media/lird0jsz/doh-library_assets50.jpg?width=768&height=394&v=1d99e4033cae210.

11.3.1. Common Chronic Diseases Affecting Women

Chronic diseases profoundly impact women's health, posing challenges to diagnosis and treatment that are in many ways unique. Some of the most prevalent conditions to affect women include autoimmune diseases such as rheumatoid arthritis and lupus, which affect them disproportionately compared to men. These diseases can also present with any number of disabling symptomologies such as joint inflammation, fatigue, and organ failure. The pathophysiology of autoimmune disorders has a tendency to complicate the treatment regimens, requiring a multidisciplinary treatment system that incorporates both traditional medical therapies and non-traditional methods. Appropriate care for such chronic conditions typically involves pharmacologic management, lifestyle modifications, and psychiatric interventions to enhance patients' quality of life. Another chronic illness that significantly affects women's health is vulvodynia, which is a chronic pain disorder affecting the vulvar region. This condition is underdiagnosed and poses enormous challenges to early diagnosis. The etiology of vulvodynia is multifactorial, encompassing hormonal, infectious, inflammatory, and psychological factors, but no single cause has been identified (Georgescu et al., 2016). The immense effect of vulvodynia on the emotional and physical health of these women emphasizes the need for research and an evidence-based approach to treatment. As healthcare workers work on developing improved management programs, the integrated and patient-focused strategy used in responding to the unique needs of each patient, as well as improving health outcomes, is essential. Chronic illness extends beyond individual illness issues to encompass broader implications for the community, particularly where women's specific health issues globally are considered. These organizations, for example, the International Council on Women's Health Issues (ICOWHI), lead the crusade for improved health care and greater awareness of women's chronic illnesses. They launch campaigns that aim to educate women, conduct research, and campaign with the objective of improving the quality of life for women across the globe (Meleis et al., 2011). By promoting greater awareness of chronic diseases among women, these agencies are at the forefront of reducing health disparities and promoting equal access to healthcare resources. The resolution of the multidimensional profile of women's chronic diseases thus requires a multi-stakeholder response from healthcare providers, researchers, and policymakers dedicated to enhancing women's health (Figure 11.12).

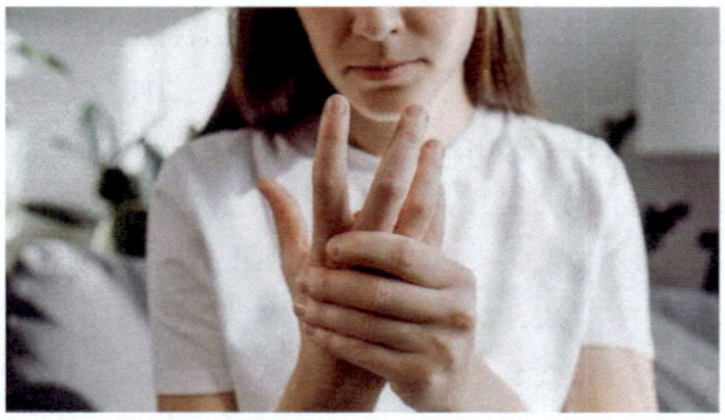

Figure 11.12. Autoimmune diseases in women.

Source: https://images.news18.com/ibnlive/uploads/2025/05/Image-2025-05-02bd145ee9c7c1caa9f5c71e86b72dee-16x9.png?impolicy=website&width=640&height=360.

11.3.2. Risk Factors Specific to Women

Pinpointing those risk factors distinct for women is central to the successful resolution of their health inequalities. Among the major issues is disability that significantly impacts reproductive health. More than 1 in 10 women of reproductive age report experiencing a disability of any type, which may complicate pregnancy and motherhood experiences. These women are likely to be subjected to stigma and stereotypes that will restrict their access to necessary healthcare services, thus leading to poor reproductive healthcare (Clark et al., 2019). As such, certain healthcare interventions therefore need to consider the particular needs of disabled women, both the physical challenges they are likely to face as well as the social factors that affect their health status. By acknowledging these complexities, clinicians can better respond to them and develop interventions that ensure equal access to reproductive health services. A further area of concern is the occurrence of mental illness in the perinatal period, which disproportionately affects women. Evidence indicates that women with pregnancy-related psychiatric illness, such as non-affective and affective psychosis, are not only more likely to be admitted to specialist maternal and baby units but are also at additional risk from their psychiatric history (Cantwell et al., 2017). The implications of these admissions extend beyond short-term maternal well-being, as almost a third of children whose mothers had such admissions are known to be at risk of adversity. This speaks volumes for the necessity of holistic health systems that take into account both maternal mental health and child development. Implementing massive support systems for pregnancy and after will help minimize long-term effects on children and mothers, reflecting a deeper sensitivity to the health of women. Socioeconomic status also plays a crucial role in determining the risk to women's health.

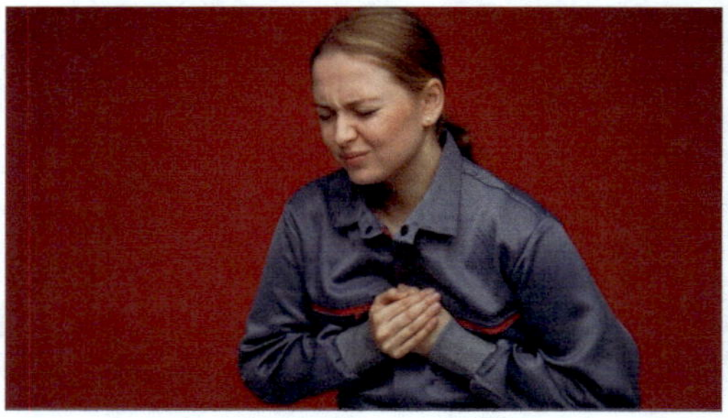

Figure 11.13. Risk factors for heart disease in women.

Source: https://www.hindustantimes.com/ht-img/img/2024/06/13/550x309/MixCollage-13-Jun-2024-08-38-PM-1910_1718290784140_1718290804647.jpg.

For instance, studies have shown that women in poor neighborhoods are most likely to experience serious psychiatric issues, further complicating their maternal health pathways (Cantwell et al., 2017). These socioeconomic inequalities typically deny quality healthcare services, resulting in profound disparities in health outcomes. Understanding the intersectionality among socioeconomic status, mental health, and women's reproductive health is important to developing improved policy and interventions. As we proceed with the discussion of women's health, it is important that these complex considerations and comprehensive solutions be developed, facilitating equity and access for all women, regardless of their conditions (Figure 11.13).

11.3.3. Prevention and Management Strategies

Effective management and prevention strategies in women's health are increasingly well accepted as pivotal to improved health outcomes. Interventions encompass a range of health promotion and prevention activities that disproportionately affect women. A successful approach is encouraging screening for illnesses such as cervical cancer, for which human papillomavirus (HPV) is more sensitive than older methods like cytology. Prioritizing the removal of obstacles to screening engagement, particularly for underserved groups, is a significant means of constructing health equity. Such programs as those that incentivize women to be screened regularly for HPV, for instance, stand to greatly extend coverage and, as an indirect effect, reduce morbidity from cervical cancer, and complement other broader public health goals such as promoting accessibility and prevention in women's health care. The second key aspect of effective management practices is the use of holistic and sustainable methods to women's healthcare. Organic farming practices, as defined in a critical analysis, highlight ecological health as integral in wellness, particularly in maternal and child wellness. Sustainable agriculture not only offers improved nutrition but also supports the achievement of global health equity targets by addressing environmental consequences related to agrochemical products. This is in line with women's health policies that focus on creating healthier communities through environmental conservation and ensuring equal access to safe food. Putting these principles into practice requires a coalition of health practitioners, policymakers, and communities to develop frameworks that advance ecological sustainability and women's health. Also, new methods such as vaginal self-collection devices for HPV testing are being explored as promising means of enhancing uptake of cervical cancer screening. These devices provide women, particularly those in resource-limited communities, with more privacy and autonomy and may lead to enhanced screening uptake. Notwithstanding that, there are challenges in how to handle results for high-risk HPV-positive women with clear guidelines on triage and follow-up. Education regarding the implications of a positive HPV result is important in strengthening women's health decisions and increasing health literacy. Management measures such as these emphasize the necessity for health systems to respond effectively to the nuances of women's health issues, increasing both prevention levels and post-diagnostic care, as addressed in recent studies (Castanon et al., 2013) (Figure 11.14).

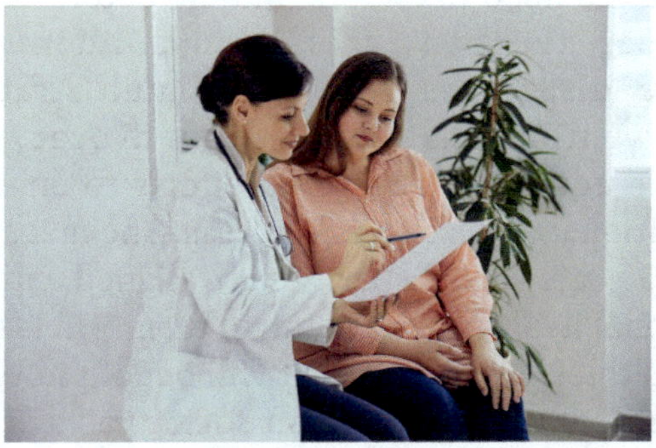

Figure 11.14. Prevention and management strategies in womens health.

Source: https://wp04-media.cdn.ihealthspot.com/wp-content/uploads/sites/433/2023/12/iStock-1492726899-1.jpg.

Test Your Knowledge

1. What are the common chronic diseases affecting women?
2. What are risk factors for women?

11.4. Nutrition and Lifestyle

Learning Outcome

1. Understand the importance of nutrition in women's health
2. Describe the exercise and physical activity recommendations
3. Know the impact of lifestyle choices on overall health

The intricate interaction between diet and lifestyle is the key to determining women's health outcomes. Food consumption, physical activity, and lifestyle habits are frequently potent determinants of conditions such as obesity, diabetes, and cardiovascular disease. It is made evident through studies that the majority of women face health inequality because of socio-economic status, education, and whether they have access to healthy foods. These disparities are further fueled by cultural beliefs that shape dietary behavior; therefore, there is a need to understand the determinants of poor nutrition across groups. Addressing these disparities requires a multistrategic intervention that combines advocacy for health equity with targeted efforts to enhance nutritional education and access. The measures to eradicate such disparities are aligned with the national health agenda and, in turn, will lead to a healthier population that will benefit not only individual women but also society as a whole (Borysova et al., 2012). Perinatal nutrition is an important component of women's health that impacts both maternal and child health. Diet during pregnancy and postpartum in women can impact fetal development, growth, and later health. Immigrant women in particular will be navigating complex cultural ground when it comes to dietary habits that will complicate their nutrition at these stages. They carry culturally-inscribed attitudes toward correct eating habits, yet are new to environments that run counter to such habits. A comprehensive ethnographic study identified overarching themes encompassing health beliefs, food consumption during the antenatal and postnatal periods, and the socio-economic determinants influencing these women's choices. An understanding of such variables is crucial in the formulation of culturally responsive nutritional advice that not only respects native traditions but also promotes the greatest health gains to mothers and children (Davey et al., 2016). The convergence of lifestyle and nutrition is further illustrated through the operation of socio-environmental variables on women's health.

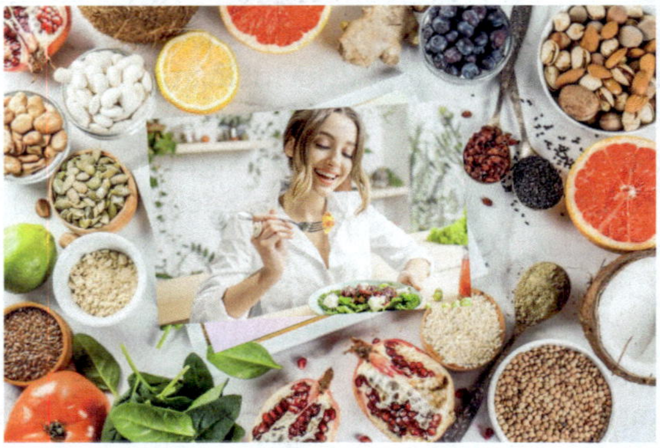

Figure 11.15. Women's health and nutritional needs.

Source: https://consumer-voice.org/wp-content/uploads/2023/03/Womens-Health-and-Nutritional-Needs.png.

Patterns of lifestyle, for instance, the degree of physical activity and styles of stress management, are generally set by job demands, family life, and social relationships. Physically active women have a lower likelihood of contracting chronic illness, demonstrating the profound interconnection between lifestyle and health status. In addition, mental well-being and stress can have an adverse effect on eating patterns, leading to unhealthy food habits that perpetuate ill health. To enhance these interconnected aspects of women's well-being, integrative health interventions must tackle nutrition, lifestyle factors, and socio-cultural processes on an integrated level. By fostering healthy settings and promoting healthier lifestyles, communities can empower women to make informed choices favorable to their health and well-being (Borysova et al., 2012) (Figure 11.15).

11.4.1. Importance of Nutrition in Women's Health

Nutrition is a critical factor in women's well-being, playing a central role in the understanding of many physiological and psychological aspects of health. Proper nutritional intake is essential during distinct phases of life, such as adolescence, pregnancy, and menopause, as these stages are characterized by individual dietary requirements. For instance, pregnant women require more of some nutrients like folic acid, iron, and calcium to provide for fetal development and safety against prematurity and other complications. Not only does a balanced diet meet these increased nutritional requirements, but it also promotes overall well-being by reducing the risk of chronic diseases such as obesity, diabetes, and cardiovascular disease. Despite the identified benefits, the majority of women remain under-informed about their nutritional requirements, highlighting the need for comprehensive education and specialized dietary counseling that addresses women's distinct health needs across the life course (Forristal et al., 2009). Furthermore, nutrition has a direct bearing on women's mental health and can potentially play a role in mood disorder prevention. Evidence highlights that a diet rich in fruits, vegetables, whole grains, and healthy fats can enhance cognitive functioning and overall mental well-being. Nutrient deficiencies, particularly of vitamins and minerals such as B vitamins, omega-3 fatty acids, and magnesium, have been linked with increased anxiety and depressive symptoms. Therefore, adopting a healthy diet is essential not only for overall well-being but also for women's mental strength. Further, interventions targeting the psychosocial determinants of food choice, such as socioeconomic position and stress, can empower women to make improved choices. Programs aimed at improving access to wholesome foods, particularly among low-income populations, are needed to provide equal health outcomes for all women (Bermúdez-Millán et al., 2017). Generally, the role of nutrition in women's health extends beyond physical health to include emotional and mental health. This combined strategy is needed to address issues such as maternal health and the long-term effects on women and their families. For example, proper nutrition before and during pregnancy significantly influences women's and infants' health, as well as the course of children's lifelong health. Emphasizing nutrition education and dismantling system-level obstacles to access will enable us to establish an environment in which women can achieve optimal health. Empowering interventions that target women through nutrition not only enhance health benefits but may also reduce the incidence of conditions such as preterm birth, thereby contributing to healthier communities (Forristal et al., 2009; Bermúdez-Millán et al., 2017) (Figure 11.16).

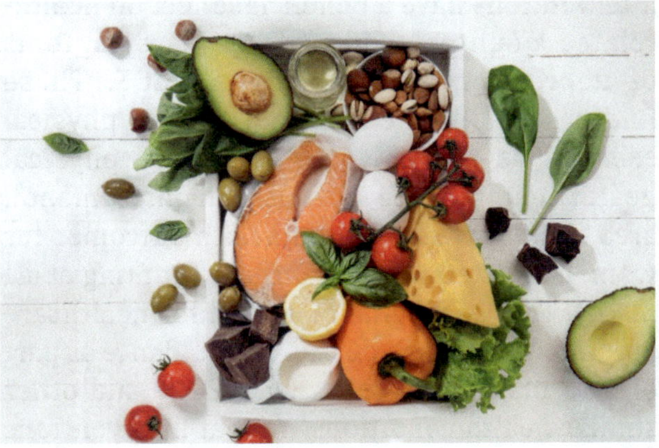

Figure 11.16. The importance of nutrition in women's health.

Source: https://gynobmedgroup.com/wp-content/uploads/2024/05/ketogenic-low-carbs-diet-food-selection-white-wall.jpg.

11.4.2. Exercise and Physical Activity Recommendations

Exercise and physical activity are important components in promoting women's health, contributing to physical and mental well-being. Current recommendations indicate that women should have at least 150 minutes of moderate-intensity aerobic exercise each week, in addition to muscle-strengthening activities on 2 or more days. These recommendations are imperative in the prevention of lifestyle conditions such as obesity, cardiovascular disease, and cancer. Further, exercise has also been shown to have benefits in reducing anxiety and depressive disorders, a disease that disproportionately afflicts women. Integrative thinking about mothers' health further emphasizes the importance of physical activity because exercise can spur healing in the postpartum months and overall quality of life for new mothers, as documented in various interdisciplinary studies on maternal health (Fox-Harding et al., 2024). In addition, women with specific health conditions, such as polycystic ovary syndrome (PCOS), are likely to gain benefits from tailored programs of exercise. It is evident that physical activity interventions have a beneficial effect on health-related quality of life as well as symptoms of depression and anxiety in PCOS. These findings emphasize the dual role of physical exercise as not only a strategy for physical health maintenance but also an instrumental area for improving mental health outcomes for women afflicted with the disease (Banting et al., 2014). This is a signal of a need for healthcare practitioners to include exercise guidance as part of care plans for women with PCOS and other similar health conditions, so that interventions are evidence-based and individualized for this group of people. Culturally specific exercise programming is another critical element of women's health and physical activity counseling. These interventions must address the diverse backgrounds, preferences, and barriers of women across ethnic, racial, and socioeconomic groups. Community-based interventions that incorporate culturally acceptable practices can be effective in enhancing participation rates and promoting a favorable climate for exercise. For example, neighborhood sport-based group fitness classes honoring heritage or dance can not only promote physical health but also enhance social connection. By ensuring exercise prescriptions are flexible and inclusive, we can more effectively address the complexity of women's health and support better health outcomes within the diverse extent of women's lives (Fox-Harding et al., 2024) (Figure 11.17).

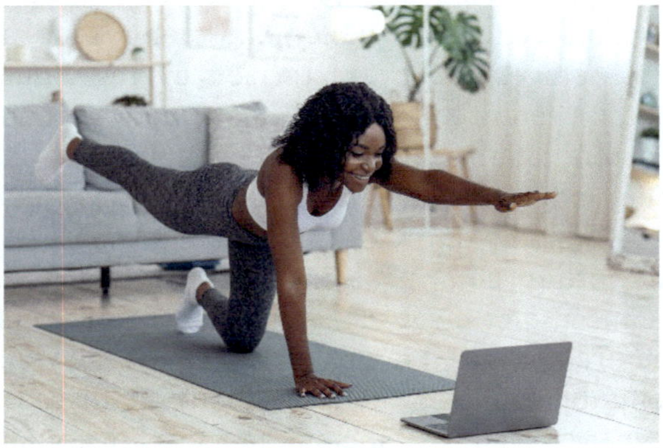

Figure 11.17. Physical activity and women's health.

Source: https://www.factsaboutfertility.org/wp-content/uploads/2021/05/AdobeStock_370378983-scaled.jpeg.

11.4.3. Impact of Lifestyle Choices on Overall Health

This connection between risk behaviors and general health is a major area of research in women's health. Diet, physical exercise, and risk behaviors such as heavy drinking and smoking significantly determine women's overall well-being across their life cycle. Women also experience a number of health issues that compound these problems, such as hormonal changes during menstruation, pregnancy, and menopause. Susceptibility to disease resulting from diet is promoted by socio-economic status and cultural attitudes towards body image. The ill effects of lifestyle can manifest in various forms, including physiological conditions as well as mental illnesses. The perception of these interdependencies can lead women to adopt healthier lifestyles that directly benefit quality of life, thereby highlighting the crucial need for public health campaigns focusing on lifestyle modification and preventive education techniques specifically aimed at women (Borysova et al., 2012). Diet and physical exercise are not the sole areas of concern, though, as mental health also plays a most critical role in delineating overall health outcomes for women. Stress, anxiety, and depression can be consequences of lifestyle patterns, for example, work-life conflicts and caregiving tensions. The high rate of these diseases among women is often compounded by lifestyle disorders like insomnia, unhealthy eating, and lack of exercise, creating a vicious circle of illness. Addressing these stressors not only improves mental health but can also positively affect physical health outcomes. Greater awareness of interconnected mental and physical well-being prompts women to embrace holistic approaches towards wellness. Since it is in society that pressures can be maximized and harmful tendencies refined, specific interventions aimed at building resilience and coping skills might successfully prepare women to actively manage their health (Davey et al., 2016). Perinatal food culture also illustrates the impact of lifestyle on women's health. Immigrant women, for instance, may bring culturally entrenched nutritional concepts of adjusting to new conditions under which traditional practices are compromised. Adapting can lead to more adverse nutritional consumption as previous eating patterns become impractical because of the accessibility or affordability of foods to which they are accustomed. Understanding how these cultural food habits relate to health outcomes will help improve maternal and child health. There is evidence that using culturally competent health and nutritional care can lead to healthier eating habits among migrant women and, therefore, enhance their overall well-being during this critical stage in their lives. This puts emphasis on managing women's health through effective interventions that are attuned to cultural diversity, as it pushes for health equity (Borysova et al., 2012) (Figure 11.18).

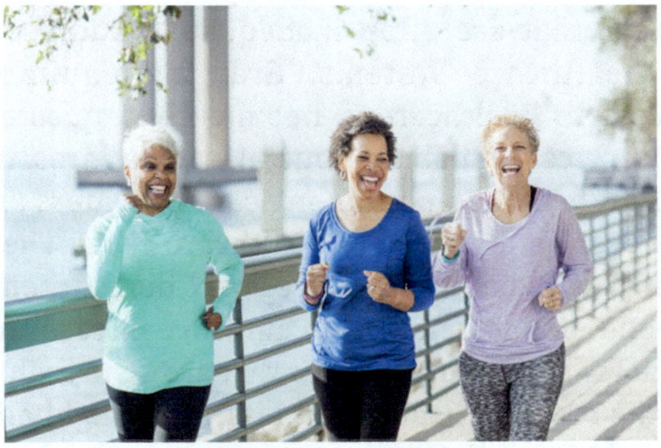

Figure 11.18. The power of simple lifestyle changes.

Source: https://www.ideafit.com/wp-content/uploads/files/Lifestyle%20Changes-1024x683.jpg.

Test Your Knowledge

1. What is the importance of nutrition in women's health?
2. What is the impact of lifestyle choices on overall health?

11.5. Access to Healthcare

Learning Outcome

1. Know the barriers to healthcare for women
2. Understands the importance of health insurance coverage
3. Describe the role of community health programs

Access to healthcare is a fundamental component of women's health, as it significantly influences well-being and health outcomes. Inequalities in access exacerbate existing health inequalities, particularly among marginal populations. Socio-economic status, immigration status, and residence could present barriers for women in accessing vital health care. Women equally face unique challenges, like reproductive health needs, that are often inadequately addressed in healthcare systems. Granting equitable access to healthcare is not merely a question of service availability but also of addressing cultural competency among care providers and the economic impact of healthcare costs. These complex dynamics of issues will demand end-to-end policy reforms to improve access and address systemic injustices that are so prevalent in the realm of healthcare. Literature highlights that intersections of immigration, race, and gender play a significant role in affecting the degree to which women are able to access healthcare services. For instance, qualitative studies that probed women refugee claimants' experiences in Canada revealed pronounced immigration status barriers, health coverage barriers, and also discrimination within the healthcare system (Gateri et al., 2019). These barriers not only compromise access to reproductive health services like prenatal and postnatal care but also indicate broader issues in the delivery of healthcare to vulnerable groups. The findings point to historical and socio-political causes and thus require intervention that specifically addresses the particular context of these women. Thus, a consideration of equal access also needs to include the underlying social and structural inequities that perpetuate these barriers. Furthermore, there is an essential knowledge gap in communication research between healthcare providers and women that is essential to improving access to care (Cooper et al., 2022). As many women have complex health conditions like endometriosis and menopause, the connection between communication and healthcare accessibility is established. Women often complain of being misunderstood or not listened to during physician encounters, resulting in delays in diagnosis and treatment. Addressing these communication deficiencies is essential to enhancing the patient experience and giving women rightful and timely care. Building frameworks that prioritize effective communication can empower women, enhance health literacy, and support healthier outcomes, thus emphasizing the importance of bottom-up reforms in healthcare policy and practice (Figure 11.19).

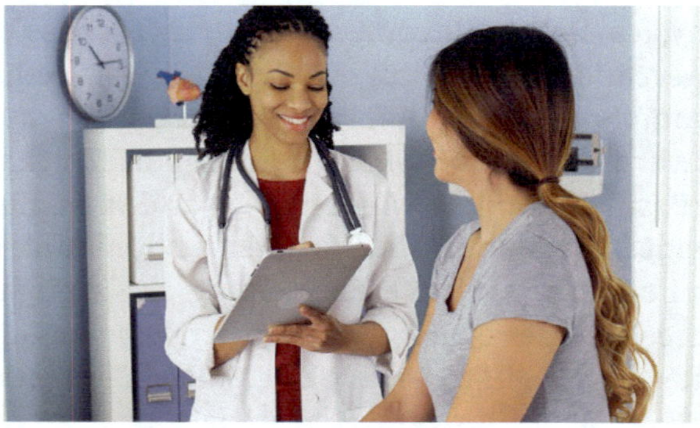

Figure 11.19. Healthcare access in rural communities.

Source: https://www.ruralhealthinfo.org/assets/2632-9902/healthcare-access-tw.jpg.

11.5.1. Barriers to Healthcare for Women

Access to healthcare remains a central concern for women, particularly when they are from marginalized communities. Various system and structural barriers stand in the way of accessing and seeking proper medical care. For instance, societal stigma makes it difficult for women to navigate interactions with healthcare providers, leading to discomfort or avoidance of care. It is difficult for most women to articulate their healthcare needs, especially in situations involving reproductive health. The insufficiency of belief in training health professionals to address the needs of different populations, such as sexual and gender minorities, also contributes to these problems. Studies indicate that only a few obstetric anesthesia fellowship programs include mandatory education to address the needs of these vulnerable populations, suggesting a gap between training and practice (George et al., 2020). Education shortages of this kind can foreclose upon women's access to adequate care and necessitate the reformulation of curricula to better equip providers to serve varied female populations. Budget constraints also significantly affect women's access to health care services. The majority of women, particularly those with limited incomes, are not adequately insured by health insurance, which restricts their access to effective and timely medical treatment. Women refugee claimants, for example, encounter complicated barriers that are not just a function of their immigration status but also a lack of awareness about available healthcare services. Such circumstances thus highlight their unavailability to receive adequate prenatal or postnatal care, jeopardizing their health and that of their children (Gateri et al., 2019). The convergence of socioeconomic status with healthcare access points to the multifaceted obstacles faced by the majority of women accessing public systems. The imperative need, therefore, is to address economic disparities to ensure equitable access to healthcare, which further underscores the necessity of an intervention policy that addresses gender, income, and health intersectionality. Cultural and linguistic barriers also pose concrete obstacles to women's access to care. Many multicultural women can experience challenges in gaining access to the healthcare system, as they will either lack knowledge or have culturally different beliefs that are incompatible with prevailing medical practice. These barriers are subsequently compounded by a healthcare system that lacks culturally competent professionals. These deficiencies will inevitably lead to miscommunication, misunderstandings, and a general sense of alienation in the health care environment. Women may feel marginalized or discriminated against, thus inhibiting them further from receiving care. To overcome such obstacles, the healthcare system must invest in employee training to effectively handle and resolve cultural sensitivities. By establishing a culture that is receptive and inclusive of diverse value systems, the health sector can significantly improve women's overall health outcomes, ensuring all women have access to the care they need (Figure 11.20).

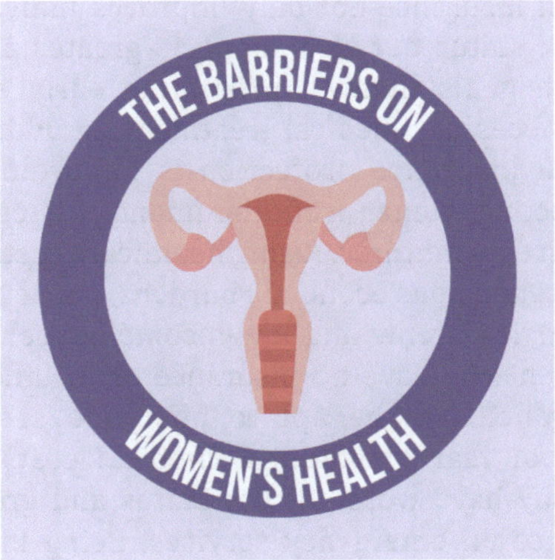

Figure 11.20. Significant barriers to women's health.

Source: https://static1.squarespace.com/static/5855cbd2ff7c50433c31de7b/585d3698414fb5e3548578ff/628e85a71197227675b9b1c8/1654105253522/the+barriers+on+women%27s+health.png?format=1500w.

11.5.2. Importance of Health Insurance Coverage

Availability of affordable health insurance coverage is necessary in a bid to offer women's health for various groups. Women, in particular, will have certain health needs, for instance, reproductive health issues, chronic illness, and mental illness that require continued and extensive treatment. Without adequate health insurance coverage, most women would go without preventive care, such as screenings and vaccinations, that could help reduce these risks. Research indicates that covered women are more likely to use basic services such as prenatal care and regular checkups than those without coverage. These services are particularly important for minority women who, according to (Jones et al., 2015), experience high health disparities, which can be exacerbated by not being covered. Therefore, providing health insurance not only improves individual health status but also supports greater public health goals through promoting early entry into necessary medical treatment. In addition, health insurance protection is important for protecting women from the financial effects of health expenditures. Rising healthcare costs can place enormous economic burdens, particularly on single parents and low-income households. Women who have no insurance or insufficient insurance will be apt to postpone seeking care for fear of potential medical costs and thereby have worse health status and greater reliance on emergency services. Being in this vulnerable position only underscores the necessity of comprehensive health insurance coverage that includes reproductive health services, preventive care, and chronic disease management. Illustrations in Jones et al. (2015) reveal that minority women, who are less likely to access quality care, have poorer health outcomes when accessing the healthcare system without the cover of insurance, pointing out the importance of health coverage in safeguarding women's health. Health insurance coverage may also significantly affect women's reproductive choices and family well-being. In families where members live with chronic illness, access to necessary treatments and preventive care through insurance is critical. Among couples who plan to have children, awareness of health management decisions becomes critical, particularly among those whose partners are living with HIV serodiscordance. Studies have shown that when physicians successfully remove barriers to safer conception methods, including PrEP, improved health and well-being for both partners can be ensured. These dynamics emphasize the importance of comprehensive health insurance coverage that not only permits individual access to care but also family health choices. It is thus important that adequate insurance coverage be prioritized as part of public health initiatives aimed at improving women's health outcomes in diverse communities (Figure 11.21).

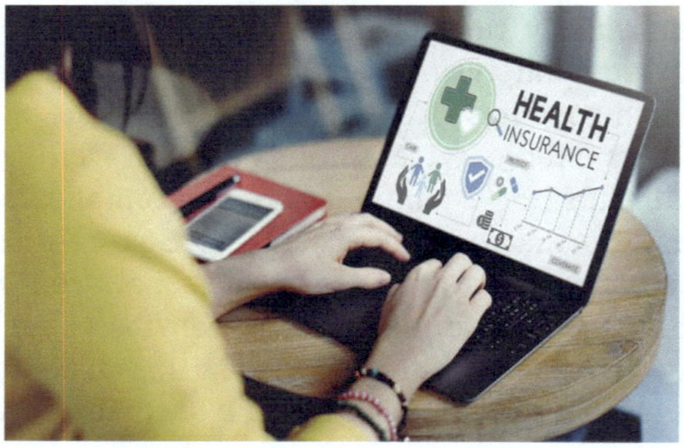

Figure 11.21. Health insurance for women.

Source: https://cdn.turtlemint.com/wp-content/uploads/health-insurance-policy.jpg.

11.5.3. Role of Community Health Programs

Community health programs are essential to enhancing women's health by addressing specific health needs and barriers faced by women in different communities. By focusing on preventive care, such programs facilitate access to important health services, including screening for cervical and breast cancers, reproductive health services, and mental health services. Further, they tailor their interventions to fit the specific cultural, socioeconomic, and environmental contexts of their populations of concern. Such interventions usually involve educational activities that raise people's awareness of their health issues, enabling women to make informed decisions about their health. The International Council on Women's Health Issues' article stresses the need for participation, advocacy, and research to effectively promote women's and girls' health globally, reinforcing the fact that community health programs are central to achieving balanced health outcomes. Community health programs also establish valuable resources and support systems that empower women. By integrating health education into economic and social initiatives, these programs not only encourage healthy practices but also enhance women's self-determination and autonomy. Programs, for instance, can engage in training in skills and educational workshops, equipping women with the tools that are not solely health-oriented, strengthening resilience in other aspects of life. As noted from observations of adolescent girls' outlooks, education is a powerful driver of better health, social, and economic performance, thereby helping arrest the cycle of poverty and ill health. The removal of barriers to education and health access is necessary, given that these elements are inextricably linked and underscore the need for integrated interventions within community health systems. Finally, community health programs have impacts that extend beyond individual-level health benefits, effecting broad social change. By mobilizing community resources and engaging communities in health promotion efforts, these programs foster collective action to better health practices, ultimately leading to greater community well-being. This model of collective action fosters cooperation among healthcare providers, educators, and community groups, generating sustainable results that are appropriate to culture and community. The synergy created in these partnerships not only enhances women's health but also promotes awareness of women's rights and healthcare needs. Initiatives carried out by agencies such as the International Council on Women's Health Issues demonstrate the potential of community health programs to advocate for systemic interventions that provide gender equity and enhance the quality of life for women and girls around the world.

Test Your Knowledge

1. What is the importance of health insurance coverage?
2. What is the role of community health programs?

11.6. Health Disparities

Learning Outcome

1. Describe the socioeconomic factors affecting women's health
2. Understand the racial and ethnic disparities in health outcomes
3. Know the strategies to address health inequities

Health disparities are among the key barriers to achieving optimal health outcomes among women, particularly those in low-income communities. The gap in access to health facilities, quality of treatment, and health outcomes typically results from socioeconomic status, race, and geographic location. For instance, research has indicated that facilities that deal with high proportions of vulnerable women experience longer follow-up times for abnormal mammograms, which can delay diagnosis and treatment of breast cancer. Interestingly, those facilities that were categorized under long follow-up had a high proportion of women diagnosed with advanced cancer. This reflects the interaction between health equity and institutional resources and demonstrates that women within disadvantaged groups are exposed to compounded issues in accessing appropriate and timely health care services, thereby impacting their overall health trajectory (Kaplan et al., 2019). Another major characteristic of women's health disparities is the high prevalence rates of lower initiation of breastfeeding among African American women. The application of traditional one-to-one prenatal care has been shown to fail to adequately support such women and, as a result, to extend the health disparities present. A new approach referred to as Centering Pregnancy has been discovered to increase initiation of breastfeeding, to increase the chances of success among African American participants by a potential 71%. This population-focused model not only provides prenatal care but also fosters community and support among mothers, illustrating how targeted interventions can successfully bridge healthcare disparities. This evidence also highlights the necessity of culturally tailored healthcare interventions that are sensitive to the particular needs of different populations to ensure better health outcomes and reduced disparities (Garnier-Villarreal et al., 2018). Addressing health disparities in women's health requires a strategy that involves policy changes, community involvement, and increased investment in healthcare resources. Ensuring equal access to preventive care, such as mammograms and prenatal care, is paramount to achieving health equity. Healthcare facilities that serve vulnerable groups need to be prioritized by policymakers as a focus of funding, and training needs to equip healthcare providers to deliver culturally competent care. In addition, there may be community-initiated programs to raise awareness and educate about access services so that women can approach care proactively. Lastly, these problems being solved at the system level lead to improved health outcomes, reduced disease diagnosis rates at late stages, and a more equitable healthcare setting for all women, regardless of their background or circumstances (Garnier-Villarreal et al., 2018; Kaplan et al., 2019) (Figure 11.22).

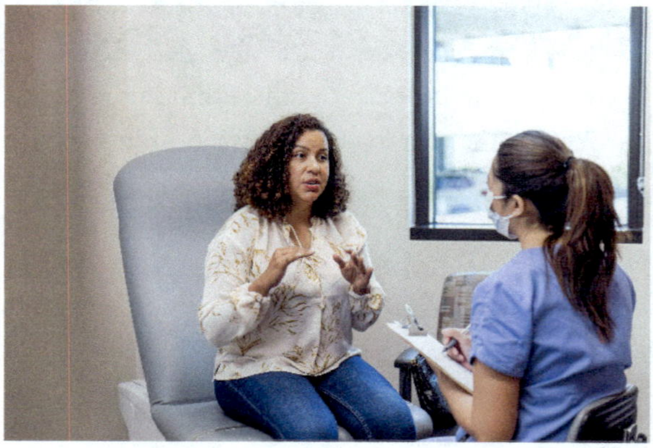

Figure 11.22. Health disparities.

Source: https://wellnessatnih.ors.od.nih.gov/news/PublishingImages/GettyImages-1421938936-min.jpg.

11.6.1. Socioeconomic Factors Affecting Women's Health

Socioeconomic factors play significant roles in determining women's health outcomes and have strong implications on their access to healthcare, nutritional status, and overall well-being. Persons in lower socioeconomic levels often find themselves having obstacles that prevent them from accessing necessary medical services, potentially leading to unresolved conditions and adverse health outcomes. Limited education is also associated with a deficiency in health resource and preventive care knowledge, which has a tendency to lead to a high incidence of chronic diseases in disadvantaged women. Besides, budgetary constraints can lead to delays in receiving medical care, aggravating existing health issues. The consideration of socioeconomic status in women's health discourse highlights the requirement for systemic change working to address such imbalances so that all women, regardless of their economic standing, have equitable access to quality care and education. The socioeconomic determinants of women's health also involve the impact of intimate partner violence (IPV), which disproportionately occurs among women in economically disadvantaged environments. Evidence has shown that economic insecurity stress increases the risk of IPV, hence contributing to negative health outcomes, such as mental illness and physical injury. Women involved in abusive relationships, in most instances, are in such situations due to a lack of economic resources or shelter after leaving. This complex intersection of economic susceptibility and IPV underscores the necessity of comprehensive policies that not only address women's health in a straightforward sense but also address the socioeconomic determinants increasing the risk of violence. As has been noted by studies, social determinants of health have a significant influence on the status of pregnant women, further underscoring the necessity of the intervention ((Quintanilla et al., 2016)). The state-level policy also influences the disparities in women's health outcomes, with the most significance in policies that address substance use and reproductive health issues. Politics-driven restrictions avoid public health mandates and have a detrimental effect on women's health outcomes when they are pregnant. For instance, policies highly influenced by anti-abortion prejudice can discourage pregnant women from obtaining critical counseling on alcohol consumption, thereby leading to public health outcomes, including fetal alcohol spectrum disorders (Roberts et al., 2019). If healthcare policies fail to benefit the interests of women's health through evidence-based practice, they perpetuate habits of ill health and socioeconomic disadvantage. Therefore, the promotion of overall health policies grounded in scientific evidence rather than politicized agendas is crucial to improving women's health status across all spheres of life.

11.6.2. Racial and Ethnic Disparities in Health Outcomes

Racial and ethnic variations in health outcomes present a massive challenge in the arena of women's health, particularly within marginalized groups like American Indian and Alaska Native (AI/AN) women. These variations are also exacerbated by multiple socio-economic determinants, access to healthcare, and cultural notions influencing health-seeking behavior. For instance, a study revealed that obstetricians-gynecologists (Ob-Gyns) had knowledge of health disparities among non-pregnant AI/AN women but not in pregnant AI/AN patients. This is a cause of the cycle of poor care, and therefore, amplification of training among healthcare providers is necessary to enhance services for these groups (Jones et al., 2015). Finally, addressing these disparities must be done at two levels: increasing provider education and establishing trust between AI/AN communities and the healthcare system to improve health throughout their reproductive lives. The impact of racial and ethnic disparities permeates beyond maternal health to affect the broader landscape of women's health issues, including chronic disease and mental illness. Evidence shows that certain populations have uneven rates of disease incidence of conditions such as diabetes and cardiovascular disease, which can have catastrophic effects on a woman's overall health. Perhaps most prominently, these kinds of disparities are often spurred by a wide range of social determinants of health, including education, income, and community setting. Furthermore, the complexity of such issues underscores the necessity of intersectional approaches to analyzing women's health disparities, since no single factor predicts health outcomes. By considering these health disparities holistically, it is possible to identify effective interventions and policy changes that can reduce the burden of disease among minority women and provide equal health opportunities (Borysova et al., 2012). Racial and ethnic health disparities among women must be approached with interventions that also address past traumas and systemic disparities that have led to mistrust of healthcare systems. For instance, AI/AN communities most often present medical institution mistrust due to a tradition of marginalization, as well as mistreatment. Furthermore, this tradition is known to lead to hesitation in accessing care, which may ultimately influence women's health outcomes at key times such as pregnancy and postpartum. Therefore, it is crucial that healthcare providers not only be aware of these disparities but also go out of their way to establish rapport with underrepresented groups. Interventions to raise cultural competency and community engagement can potentially foster cooperation and trust, leading to improved healthcare outcomes for marginalized women. In setting policies that facilitate such enabling systems, we can work towards eradicating inequalities and making quality healthcare accessible to all women, as they are entitled to (Figure 11.23).

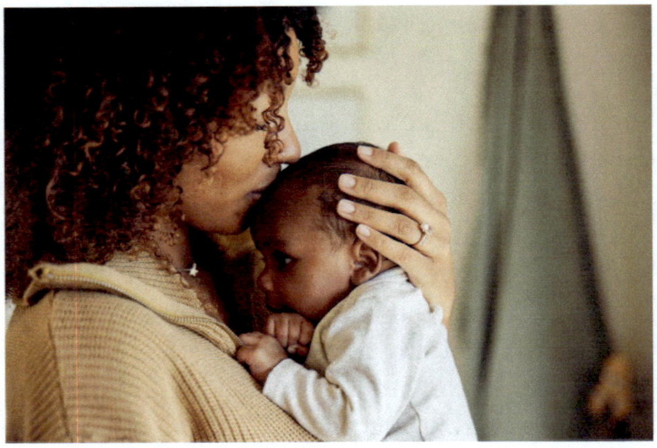

Figure 11.23. Racial and ethnic disparities in maternal and infant health.

Source: https://upriseri.com/wp-content/uploads/2023/01/Mom-and-Baby-scaled.jpg.

11.6.3. Strategies to Address Health Inequities

Health inequities, particularly in women's health, must be addressed through an intersectoral response that includes educational interventions, community engagement, and policy reform. Education plays an important role in empowering women with the information they need to access the healthcare system effectively. Heightening awareness through campaigns about available healthcare services and preventive interventions has a tangible effect on women's health outcomes. For instance, the inclusion of culturally relevant information in educational materials enhances comprehension across diverse populations and makes the materials more inclusive. Moreover, the use of community health workers can help link mechanisms between healthcare practitioners and vulnerable groups to fortify trust as well as facilitate open communication. These efforts aim to empower women so they can voice their health needs, thereby addressing widespread disparities in access to and outcomes of health across different populations (Bendera et al., 2025). In addition to education, community engagement is also a primary method of averting health inequities in women's health. Local organization and group involvement in multistakeholder health programs ensures interventions that consider the unique concerns of a given population. For example, partnerships with grassroots women's advocacy organizations enable the identification of health concerns disproportionately affecting vulnerable populations, leading to specialized outreach. By providing safe spaces for discussion, these initiatives also encourage women to speak up and report their experiences and health concerns. Grassroots involvement increases the likelihood that interventions will be appropriate to the culture and more likely to reduce health inequity. Lastly, community-based interventions are instrumental in addressing gaps in health care and raising awareness regarding women's health issues through an integrated approach (Forristal et al., 2009). Policy reform also plays an active role in achieving health equity for women. Policy action with enhanced access to total healthcare service, such as reproductive health and mental health care, is key to dismantling systemic barriers that constrain women's health. Governmental programs that finance community health programs and develop facilitating regulatory environments can empower the utilization of equitable healthcare policy. In addition, advocacy for policies that address the socioeconomic determinants of health, such as housing, education, and work, will contribute to better global health outcomes for women. To that end, health equity is not merely a call to focus on the delivery of care but also on the consideration of overall policies that lead to disparities. Thus, a multi-factorial process that includes education, community participation, and policy intervention is critical in addressing health inequities among women (Forristal et al., 2009).

Test Your Knowledge

1. What is the role of socioeconomic factors in determining women's health outcomes?
2. What are racial and ethnic disparities in health outcomes?

SUMMARY

As this journey of women's health draws to a close, it is evident that tackling the numerous issues affecting women calls for an integrative approach that is sensitive to physical, mental, and social spaces. Women's health issues are likely to cross over with societal issues around wealth, education, and healthcare access, and therefore necessitate the formulation of extensive health policies that are focused on equity and inclusiveness. Additionally, understanding specific groups' experiences, such as those of wāhine Māori, is significant for acknowledging the particular barriers and opportunities in the health system. By critically analyzing these aspects, stakeholders can build environments that promote women's health outcomes across different contexts. Such an in-depth understanding forms the foundation for further research and policy development to enhance women's well-being and health. With regard to women's health, it is essential that education and support systems in the community are made central. Based on the research, women who hold the view that education is a door to empowerment are likely to serve as reference points for future generations. Especially, wāhine Māori demonstrate the dynamics by earning academic degrees and finding jobs that set a precedent for their children. Their existence, founded on a dense cultural background, illuminates how multigenerational engagement, for instance, the caregiving roles of grandfathers and other males, is beneficial to children's well-being and resilience. Connecting and capitalizing on such family and societal relationships has the potential to improve health interventions and create a collective energy toward improving women's overall health. Finally, systemic change to women's health will entail coordination among several sectors, including health care, education, and social services. Research on marginalized communities indicates an immediate necessity for culturally relevant programs that address specific obstacles women, particularly solo parents like the wāhine Māori, face. By applying the recommendations and findings of such studies, policymakers can enhance support networks and resources for women. Additionally, these endeavors must be active, continually evolving to meet emerging challenges and societal changes. In doing so, women's diverse health needs and experiences will be dealt with comprehensively, making the population even healthier in the years to come.

The dynamic tension between gender identity and health outcomes is of prime concern in women's health discourse. By recognizing that health problems cannot be delineated from the socially constructed nature of gender, researchers are increasingly demanding approaches that transcend the biomedical model. As explained in descriptions of eating disorders, the biopsychosocial model is frequently employed, but the social and cultural aspects are not adequately addressed. By examining the lives of those with anorexia and bulimia, it is apparent that their understanding of these conditions is heavily shaped by social gender roles and expectations. Examining feminist critiques can enrich treatment frameworks by calling for integration of these factors into therapeutic practice. This integration of social identity and health underscores the need to consider broader cultural factors when formulating intervention and support systems for women with these problems (Bartky et al., 2016). Another significant sphere of women's health is the use of holistic nutrition strategies, such as organic farming, in health paradigms. Evidence indicates that organic agriculture not only enhances productivity in the developing world but also supports sustainable health programs that are of benefit to people and communities. Ecology, Health, Care, and Fairness, as IFOAM's principles, demonstrate commitment to fair food systems that enhance health outcomes alongside addressing environmental sustainability concerns. Agro-chemical product impacts have a propensity to expand health inequalities, particularly for vulnerable groups. Therefore, organic agriculture offers a relevant solution to these challenges through supporting health-promoting practices, enabling women, particularly in the Global South. Organic agriculture aims to examine the relationships among sustainable agriculture practices and women's health through holistic policy measures that embrace future generations and biodiversity (Vaarst et al., 2010). Moreover, engaging women in conversation regarding their health conditions helps to foster a more thorough examination of the systemic nature of their conditions. Examining such issues through a feminist lens enables a more dynamic discussion of the sociocultural determinants shaping health scenarios. Empowering women to express themselves can reveal discrepancies in prevailing treatment regimes, particularly in mental health, which is inherently susceptible to social expectations and social pressures. By highlighting gender as a key theme, health practitioners can make interventions more relatable to women's lived experiences and ultimately disrupt biomedical paradigms that usually dominate clinical environments. This interaction may also introduce a range of alternative views on good practice grounded in feminist theories aimed at making health systems more inclusive and responsive. Such a redefinition of women's health is not only important for facilitating personal well-being but also for promoting broader societal change (Bartky et al., 2016).

KEY TERMS FROM THIS CHAPTER

Abdominal bloating
Cardiovascular disease
Gender discrimination
Hypertension
Menstrual health
Pregnancy
Reproductive health
Angry outbursts
Chronic disease
Hormonal contraception
Maternal care
Mental health
Premenstrual syndrome
Reproductive rights

CRITICAL THINKING QUESTIONS

1. **What is the most common cause of maternal mortality worldwide?**
   a. Eclampsia
   b. Postpartum hemorrhage
   c. Pulmonary embolism
   d. Sepsis
2. **At what age is cervical cancer screening with Pap smears recommended to begin?**
   a. 18 years
   b. 21 years
   c. 25 years
   d. 30 years
3. **Which of the following is a risk factor for developing osteoporosis in women?**
   a. Early menopause
   b. Obesity
   c. Sedentary lifestyle
   d. Both a and c
4. **What is the most common type of breast cancer?**
   a. Lobular carcinoma *in situ* (LCIS)
   b. Ductal carcinoma *in situ* (DCIS)
   c. Invasive lobular carcinoma
   d. Invasive ductal carcinoma
5. **Which contraceptive method provides the longest duration of action?**
   a. Oral contraceptive pills
   b. Copper intrauterine device (IUD)
   c. Injectable progestins
   d. Contraceptive patch

Short Answer Questions

1. What is the meaning of women's health?
2. What is the importance of women's health?
3. What is the reproductive health?
4. Write the names of three chronic diseases.
5. What is the meaning of access to healthcare?

Answer to Critical Thinking Questions

1. (b); 2. (b); 3. (d); 4. (d); 5. (b).

REFERENCES

1. Christy, C., Zeina, A., Safaa, D., & Shafika, A. (2018). Factors Associated with Premenstrual Syndrome and its Different Symptom Domains among University Students in Lebanon. *International Journal of Women S Health and Wellness*, *4*(1). https://doi.org/10.23937/2474-1353/1510068Anđelinović, M., Ayers, S., Matijaš, M., et al. (2020). The role of posttraumatic stress and depression symptoms in mother-infant bonding. https://core.ac.uk/download/288395676.pdf (accessed on 12th July 2025).
2. Bachrach, L., Patel, S., Tebb, K., et al. (2020). Adolescents' acceptance of long-acting reversible contraception after an educational intervention in the emergency department: A randomized controlled trial. https://core.ac.uk/download/305124071.pdf (accessed on 12th July 2025).
3. Banting, L., Conte, F., Stepto, N., et al. (2014). Mental health and physical activity in women with polycystic ovary syndrome: A brief review. https://core.ac.uk/download/33476327.pdf (accessed on 12th July 2025).
4. Barageine, J., El Ayadi, A., Getahun, M., et al. (2025). Understanding women's pregnancy intentions, decision-making, and factors influencing reproductive choices after genital fistula repair in Uganda: A qualitative study. https://core.ac.uk/download/650677658.pdf (accessed on 12th July 2025).
5. Bartky, S. L., Baumgardner, J., Bordo, S., Boskind-White, M., Boughtwood, D., Burns, M., et al. (2016). 'Blindness to the obvious'? Treatment experiences and feminist approaches to eating disorders. https://core.ac.uk/download/41993831.pdf (accessed on 12th July 2025).
6. Bazzi, A. R., Biancarelli, D. L., Drainoni, M. L., et al. (2018). Implementing a pre-exposure prophylaxis intervention for safer conception among HIV Sero discordant couples: Recommendations for health care providers. https://digitalscholarship.unlv.edu/cgi/viewcontent.cgi?article=1714&context=jhdrp (accessed on 12th July 2025).
7. Bendera, S., Gordon, R., Kadzamira, E., et al. (2025). Promoting girls' education in Africa – The design and implementation of policy interventions. https://core.ac.uk/download/pdf/6443151.pdf (accessed on 12th July 2025).
8. Bermúdez-Millán, A., Prost, A., Singh, A., Singh, A., Al-Riyami, A. A., Picklesimer, A. H., Donovan, B., et al. (2017). Conceptualizing pathways linking women's empowerment and prematurity in developing countries. *Annals of General Psychiatry, 12*, 37. https://www.semanticscholar.org/paper/6e7c363fadd974c0a1d8d0e827d77327f11f31bf (accessed on 12th July 2025).
9. Bertand, D., Bolyard, R., Callwood, G. B., et al. (2014). Intimate partner violence among African American and African Caribbean women: Prevalence, risk factors, and the influence of cultural attitudes. https://core.ac.uk/download/323064368.pdf (accessed on 12th July 2025).
10. Bora, D., Brady, E., Li, H., Salvi, et al. (2018). Slacktivists or activists? Identity work in the virtual disability march. https://core.ac.uk/download/187423879.pdf (accessed on 12th July 2025).
11. Borysova, M. E., Mitchell, O., Sultan, D. H., et al. (2012). Racial and ethnic health disparities in incarcerated populations. https://digitalscholarship.unlv.edu/cgi/viewcontent.cgi?article=1141&context=jhdrp (accessed on 12th July 2025).
12. Cantwell, R., Langan-Martin, J., Martin, D., et al. (2017). Admission to psychiatric hospital for mental illnesses 2 years prechildbirth and postchildbirth in Scotland: A health informatics

approach to assessing mother and child outcomes. https://core.ac.uk/download/84915858.pdf (accessed on 12th July 2025).

13. Castanon, A., Lorincz, A., Sasieni, P., et al. (2013). New strategies for human papillomavirus-based cervical screening. https://core.ac.uk/download/30696532.pdf (accessed on 12th July 2025).
14. Chowdhury, C., Gordon-Maclean, C., Dusitsin, H. Q., et al. (2013). Safety and acceptability of tubal ligation procedures performed by trained clinical officers in rural Uganda. https://core.ac.uk/download/19163248.pdf (accessed on 12th July 2025).
15. Clark, L., Dearden, S. E., Guo, J. W., et al. (2019). What women with disabilities write in personal blogs about pregnancy and early motherhood: Qualitative analysis of blogs. https://core.ac.uk/download/323075970.pdf (accessed on 12th July 2025).
16. Cooper, A., Csontos, J., Edwards, A., et al. (2022). A rapid evidence map of women's health. https://core.ac.uk/download/544094405.pdf (accessed on 13th July 2025).
17. Davey, C., Higginbottom, G. M. A., Osswald, B., et al. (2016). Understanding South Asian immigrant women's food choices in the perinatal period. https://core.ac.uk/download/42510445.pdf (accessed on 13th July 2025).
18. Forristal, A., American Academy of Pediatrics and the American College of Obstetricians and Gynecologists, Armstrong, T. M., Declercq, E. R., Joyce Roberts, Kirkham, C., et al. (2009). A critical appraisal of guidelines for antenatal care: Components of care and priorities in prenatal education. https://core.ac.uk/download/213087165.pdf (accessed on 12th July 2025).
19. Fox-Harding, C. (2024). Maternal health considerations: Highlighting and advancing opportunities for improved maternal health. https://core.ac.uk/download/621356924.pdf (accessed on 13th July 2025).
20. Garnier-Villarreal, M., Hanson, L., & Robinson, K. M. (2018). Effectiveness of Centering Pregnancy on breast-feeding initiation among African Americans: A systematic review and meta-analysis. https://core.ac.uk/download/213086165.pdf (accessed on 13th July 2025).
21. Gateri, H. W. (2019). Exploring barriers refugees and refugee claimants experienced accessing reproductive health care services in Toronto. https://core.ac.uk/download/188194501.pdf (accessed on 13th July 2025).
22. George, R. B., & MacCormick, H. (2020). Sexual and gender minorities educational content within obstetric anesthesia fellowship programs: A survey. https://core.ac.uk/download/287623797.pdf (accessed on 13th July 2025).
23. Georgescu, S. R., Mitran, C. I., Mitran, M. I., et al. (2016). Vulvodynia: An under-recognized disease. https://core.ac.uk/download/144552984.pdf (accessed on 13th July 2025).
24. Goldstein-Siegel, E., Cardinal, L., & Greene, M. E. (2010). Girls speak: A new voice in global development. https://core.ac.uk/download/71358264.pdf (accessed on 13th July 2025).
25. Jomeen, J., Jones, C., & Wadephul, F. (2016). The impact of antenatal psychological group interventions on psychological well-being: A systematic review of the qualitative and quantitative evidence. https://core.ac.uk/download/151161190.pdf (accessed on 13th July 2025).
26. Jones, K. M., Lannon, S. M., Raglan, G. B., et al. (2015). Obstetrician-gynecologists' knowledge of health disparities and barriers among American Indian/Alaska Native women in Washington

State. https://digitalscholarship.unlv.edu/cgi/viewcontent.cgi?article=1352&context=jhdrp (accessed on 13th July 2025).

27. Kanyinga, K., & Mitullah, W. (2007). The non-profit sector in Kenya: What we know and what we don't know. https://core.ac.uk/download/75779663.pdf (accessed on 13th July 2025).

28. Kaplan, C., Karliner, L. S., Kerlikowske, K., et al. (2019). Mammography facilities serving vulnerable women have longer follow-up times. https://core.ac.uk/download/323079508.pdf (accessed on 13th July 2025).

29. Kustriyanti, D., & Rahayu, H. (2020). Prevalence of premenstrual syndrome and quality of life among health science college students. https://core.ac.uk/download/480550077.pdf (accessed on 13th July 2025).

30. Matipou, R. (2017). The highs and lows of sole parenting experienced by wāhine Māori: A thesis presented in partial fulfilment of the requirements for the Master of Philosophy (Health) at Massey University, Palmerston North, New Zealand. https://core.ac.uk/download/148645804.pdf (accessed on 13th July 2025).

31. Meleis, A. I., Teitelman, A., Beaglehole, R., Breman, J. G., Sampselle, C., et al. (2011). The health of women and girls determines the health and well-being of our modern world: A White Paper from the International Council on Women's Health Issues. https://core.ac.uk/download/10908168.pdf (accessed on 12th July 2025).

32. Quintanilla, B. P., McDonald, S., Pollock, W., et al. (2016). Social determinants and maternal exposure to intimate partner violence of obstetric patients with severe maternal morbidity in the intensive care unit: A systematic review protocol. https://core.ac.uk/download/305121417.pdf (accessed on 12th July 2025).

33. Roberts, S. C. M. (2019). The presence and consequences of abortion aversion in scientific research related to alcohol use during pregnancy. https://core.ac.uk/download/323073633.pdf (accessed on 13th July 2025).

34. Turgoose, D. (2019). Change that lasts is a chance for change. https://core.ac.uk/download/287585408.pdf (accessed on 13th July 2025).

35. Vaarst, M. (2010). Organic farming as a development strategy: Who are interested and who are not? https://core.ac.uk/download/10929428.pdf (accessed on 13th July 2025).

36. Victorian Women's Trust. (2011). Annual report 2009/2010. https://core.ac.uk/download/75785046.pdf (accessed on 13th July 2025).

OBSTETRICS IN FAMILY MEDICINE

12

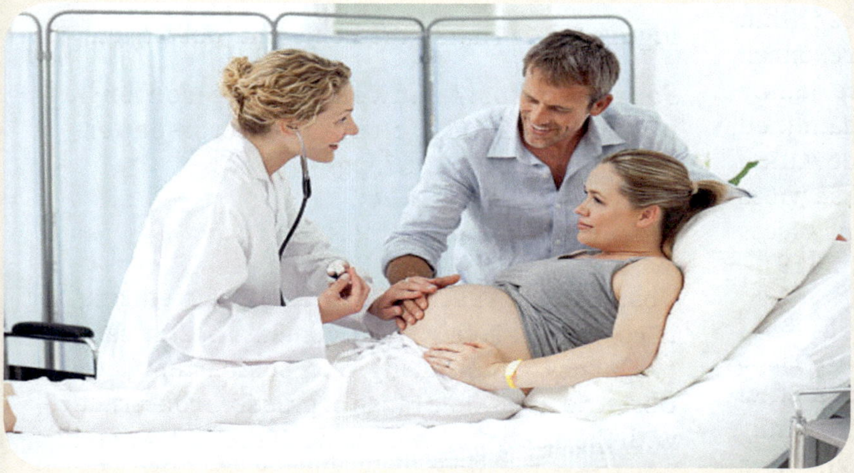

LEARNING OBJECTIVES

After studying this chapter, you will be able to:

1. Understand the scope of practice for family physicians in obstetrics
2. Know the benefits of integrating obstetrics into family medicine
3. Describe the challenges faced by family physicians in obstetrics
4. Know the current trends in obstetrics within family medicine

Introduction

The integration of obstetrics into family medicine is an integrated model of care that emphasizes continuity and whole-person care throughout a patient's life. Family medicine physicians are best positioned to provide the sophisticated services that women require throughout their reproductive lifespan, from preconception counseling to prenatal care and postpartum follow-up. The family medicine practice today requires professionals not only to care for obstetric patients but also to establish relationships beyond the delivery room. Family doctors, for instance, are able to provide a conducive environment for teaching women on important issues like maternal diet, mental health, and family planning, which has a conducive environment for both child and mother health outcomes. This varied involvement not only enhances patient satisfaction but also offers contributions to improved overall measurements of health in the community, showcasing the integral nature of family medicine in obstetric care. Furthermore, challenges exist in family medicine obstetrics, particularly regarding educational preparedness and the specific needs of obstetric care. Family medicine residents may have limited access to obstetric training compared to their peers in obstetrics and gynecology, and therefore they may differ in competency and confidence when caring for pregnant women and during delivery. This training gap needs to be closed when family physicians are intent on delivering full-spectrum care, including obstetric care. Furthermore, the arrival of newer models, such as Direct Primary Care, only complicates obstetric practice within family medicine. Highlighted in research into DPC practices, increasingly more family physicians are focusing on more streamlined modes of care, possibly leading to a deviation in the means of delivery of obstetrical services in the end, with implications for patient access and quality of outcomes (Ablah et al., 2019).

Moreover, the importance of recognizing and controlling environmental health risks during pregnancy has become a fundamental component of obstetric care provided by family physicians. To be specific, lead exposure is a critical environmental concern whose effects on both maternal and fetal well-being can be detrimental.

One research study on Vermont lead screening practices found that very few maternity care providers are appropriately screening pregnant patients for lead exposure, indicating a need for improved educational materials and standardized procedures (Berkman et al., 2017). The inclusion of appropriate screening methods and environmental risk education in family medicine practice enables doctors to adequately prepare their patients for such problems. This active role not only enhances the education of the providers and patients but also promotes a more educated approach to pregnancy management, ultimately resulting in improved maternal and neonatal health outcomes (Figure 12.1).

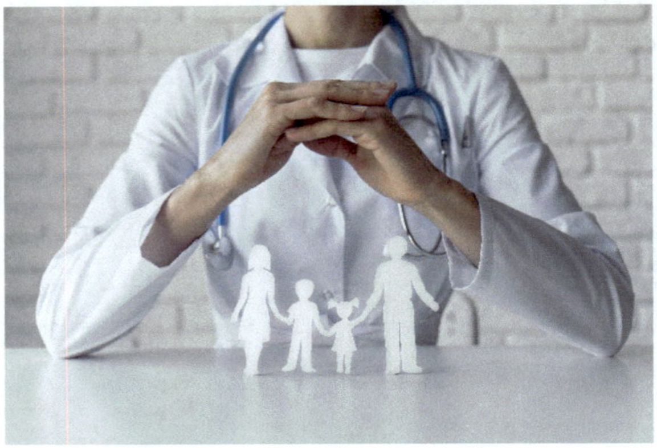

Figure 12.1. Family medicine and obstetrics.

Source: https://mdwell.com/wp-content/uploads/2023/12/close-up-doctor-paper-family-min-2048x1367.jpg.

Definition of Obstetrics

Obstetrics, a specialized branch of medicine, is concerned solely with women's health care, pregnancy, childbearing, and postpartum care. Obstetrics is a whole range of practices concerned with the safety and well-being of the mother and fetus throughout the process of reproduction. Obstetrics has traditionally been part of family medicine, as it addresses not only the physiology of reproductive health but also psychological and social outcomes entailed. In both capacities, thus, obstetric care is frequently provided by family medicine doctors, who serve as primary sources and link patients with needed services. Family medicine practitioners must have knowledge of obstetrics to offer comprehensive care that includes preventive care and health education tailored to women undergoing the transformative processes of pregnancy and childbirth. In examining obstetrics, the greater social forces on maternal health should be examined. Complications such as pregnancy and DV are major risk factors that have a harmful influence on fetal and maternal outcomes. Systematic review of literature in Nigeria raised concern regarding high prevalence rates of DV among pregnant women, which ranged between 2.3% and 44.6% during pregnancy (Alo et al., 2017). Such identification broadens the vision of obstetric care beyond clinical management to include social determinants and psychosocial interventions. In family practice, this means developing strategies not only to monitor obstetric health but also to mitigate the effects of social determinants, making patients more resilient against abusive environments. Thus, the inclusion of these aspects can lead to improved maternal health outcomes and more resilient family relationships. Furthermore, the obstetrics practice is constantly in interaction with cultural environments and medical norms. For instance, in Nepal, healthcare providers are required to navigate varying cultural ideas of when to give birth, possibly contrary to standard medical practice. Negotiation of these opposing perspectives plays a crucial role in achieving successful pregnancy outcomes despite working within patients' beliefs (Brunson et al., 2018). Therefore, obstetrics must adapt to disparate settings and practices while retaining an evidence base. Family medicine practitioners, particularly in obstetric care, are tasked with this delicate balance—practicing evidence-based care and remaining sensitive to the patient's unique cultural environment. This type of practice not only enhances the quality of care but also fosters patient trust and compliance, ultimately improving maternal and infant health outcomes (Figure 12.2).

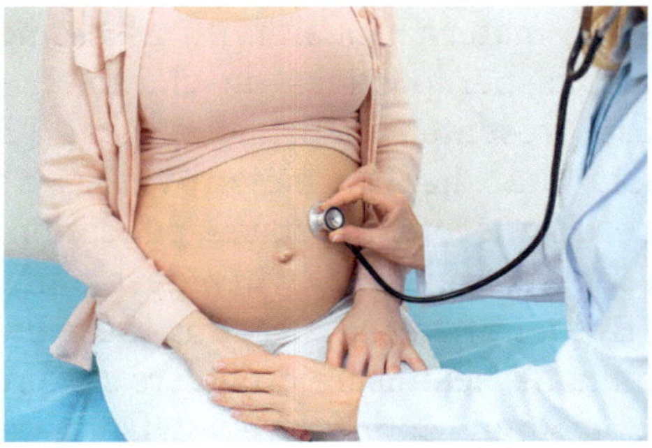

Figure 12.2. Obstetrics.

Source: https://southlakeobgyn.net/wp-content/uploads/2021/12/What_Is_Obstetrics_637740344424475023.png.

Role of Family Medicine in Obstetrics

Family practice plays a significant role in obstetrics by bridging the gap between specialist maternal care and primary care. Family physicians, as the first-contact caregivers, are best placed to provide complete prenatal care, enabling early identification and management of potential complications. This ongoing relationship supports customized care that addresses not only the physical needs of mother and fetus but also social and psychological dimensions of health. By continuing through pregnancy, family medicine doctors are trained to enable women to make autonomous decisions about their own health and that of their new baby. Such an integrative approach is particularly pertinent to addressing health inequities in ways that enable family doctors to provide culturally relevant care that considers several socioeconomic determinants of maternal well-being. The importance of understanding local dynamics further gains prominence when analyzing the roles of traditional birth attendants (TBAs) within society. Despite limited funding for training TBAs, TBAs are key figures in maternal and newborn health care, particularly where access to skilled birth attendants is limited. Literature review indicates that TBAs are integral figures in the process of giving birth in developing countries, with a thin line between traditional practices and biomedical ones (Adamson et al., 2010). Here, family medicine practitioners can liaise with TBAs to ensure their work integrates with clinical care, benefiting the overall patient experience. Such collaboration not only gives traditional knowledge its due respect but also transmutes the gap between biomedical interventions and culturally derived practices in order to achieve effective maternal health outcomes. Furthermore, the cost-effectiveness of safe motherhood interventions necessitates that family physicians advocate for and deliver extended obstetric care in their practices. It has been estimated that a significant percentage of maternal deaths can be prevented using cost-effective antenatal and community-based interventions (Jowett M). Preventive medicine is at the core of family medicine and can drastically reduce maternal mortality rates through routine screening, educational outreach, and community health programs. By prioritizing family doctors' access to general obstetric care, uninterrupted and quality maternal care can be made accessible to all women, including those in need of advanced intervention. Such proactive involvement ensures not just improved healthcare but also adherence to the very essence of family medicine, which is to comprehensively maximize wellness from birth to old age, including the perinatal stage (Figure 12 .3).

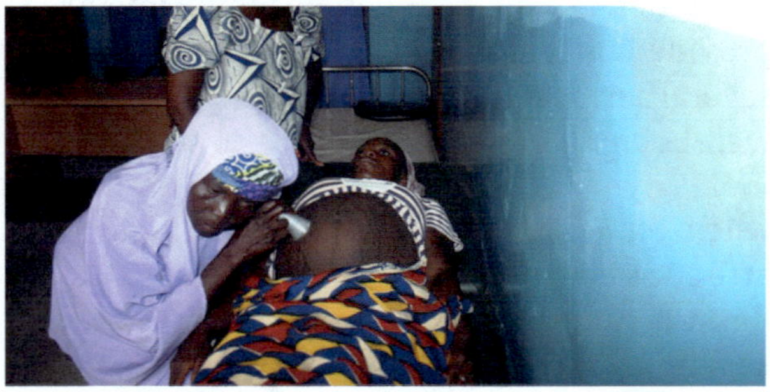

Figure 12.3. Traditional birth attendants.

Source: https://www.theelephant.info/wp-content/uploads/2020/02/tba-1.jpg.

Importance of Integrated Care in Maternal Health

The concept of integrated care plays a critical role in enhancing maternal health, particularly in obstetrics in family medicine. Integrated care is an overarching system that combines several healthcare services to provide high-level, patient-centered care throughout pregnancy, childbirth, and postpartum. The model facilitates seamless coordination among midwives, obstetricians, and other physicians, which is important for meeting the various needs of pregnant women. As confirmed by recent studies, multidisciplinary team collaboration not only improves the health status of mothers and newborns but also facilitates the detection and management of early pregnancy-associated complications. Through gap bridging among service providers, integrated care offers a platform for maternal health to thrive, ultimately leading to healthier families and communities. Also, integrated care emphasizes the need for cultural competency in maternity care, the recognition that women from different cultures may have varying expectations and experiences that go with childbearing. This aspect is important to note when examining the process of childbirth among different communities. For instance, the role of midwifery has deep roots in cultures and remains highly applicable in contemporary maternity care in America. Understanding the evolutionary context of delivery, as outlined in Dunham et al. (2016), enables health care providers to respect and incorporate existing customary practices when delivering modern obstetric care. Integrated care, by instilling sensitivity to cultural nuances, can potentially ensure that maternal health care is adequately modified to cater to the unique preferences of individual women, thereby instilling confidence and overall satisfaction with health care. Finally, coordination of care extends beyond the immediate perinatal time frame because interoperative care models consider the social determinants of health that affect maternal health. An assessment of the various perspectives on childbirth, such as those presented in Brunson et al. (2018), suggests that healthcare providers should consider socioeconomic status, education level, and resource availability when developing care plans. By identifying and treating these broader determinants, healthcare providers can produce an increasingly supportive environment for pregnant and giving women. What results is an improved inclusive practice that not just improves the clinical result but also optimizes the psychological health of the mothers. Integrated care thus contributes meaningfully to the facilitation of healthy pregnancies, the reduction of maternal health inequalities, and the accomplishment of the overall goal of enhancing family medicine.

12.1. Scope of Practice for Family Physicians in Obstetrics

Learning Outcome

1. Describe the prenatal care services
2. Understand the labor and delivery management
3. Describe the postpartum care and support

The scope of practice in obstetrics among family physicians creates an exciting intersection of primary care and specialist maternal care. Family physicians are best positioned to offer holistic care to women throughout their childbearing years, encompassing prenatal, intrapartum, and postpartum care. This combined approach allows family doctors to address not only the pregnant woman's physical medical needs but also her psychosocial needs in care to promote better health outcomes. However, the extent of obstetric services provided by family physicians can vary substantially based on training, institutional capacity, and individual comfort levels. As the landscape of health care delivery continues to change, it is desirable to understand the role of the family physician in obstetrics so that practice can be adapted to shifting patient and community needs. A thorough examination of the family physician's educational background and training is adequate to establish heterogeneous experience with obstetric care. The majority of family medicine residency programs offer training in obstetrics, but the nature and extent of the training vary significantly. A study examining direct primary care practices finds that only 3% of family physicians reported obstetric services among their services, suggesting a potential service gap (Ablah et al., 2019). This low involvement may be due to varying residency curricula and the rising likelihood that obstetrics will be specialty-specific. Family physicians who include obstetric care in their practice can not only enhance continuity of care but also develop worthwhile patient-physician relationships that lead to improved patient satisfaction and outcomes. Additionally, family medicine practice in obstetrics also intersects with cultural and ethical concerns that influence reproductive health choices. Family physicians are typically the first to address family planning, pregnancy plans, and responsible childbearing. Employing methods such as natural family planning may enable patients to become better-informed decision-makers regarding reproductive health (Fehring et al., 2017). Being able to discuss and implement fertility awareness creates an integrated model that allows physicians to tailor care to specific patient values and needs. Finally, the obstetric scope of practice for family physicians emphasizes integrative care, placing the unique needs of patients first and adapting to a changing paradigm in healthcare delivery (Figure 12.4).

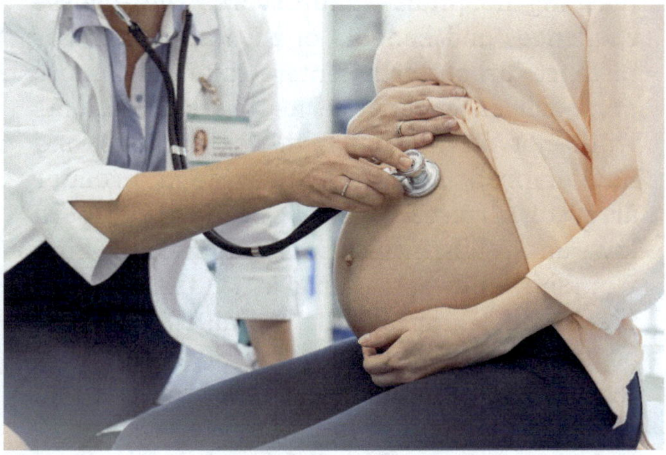

Figure 12.4. Obstetrician-gynecologist.

Source: https://www.verywellhealth.com/thmb/T7Kcq-UQfN4PjS25L8IGGPKliBI=/1500x0/filters:no_upscale():max_bytes(150000):strip_icc()/doctor-using-stethoscope-on-pregnant-patients-stomach-595348651-59932a7968e1a2001113f56d.jpg.

12.1.1. Prenatal Care Services

Prenatal care is a crucial component of obstetric services in family medicine, as it emphasizes early and continuous care throughout pregnancy. Prenatal services monitor the well-being of the mother and fetus and intervene when complications may arise during pregnancy. Good prenatal care involves routine check-ups, ultrasounds, and blood work for preeclampsia and gestational diabetes, which are useful for identifying risks that can affect maternal and fetal health. Education on nutrition, exercise, and childbirth is also frequently provided, equipping pregnant mothers with the knowledge to make healthy decisions regarding themselves and their unborn children. Emphasizing thorough prenatal care sets the stage for successful pregnancy outcomes and ensures a healthy setting for family development. The availability and delivery mode of prenatal care services can also differ significantly depending on the healthcare model adopted. Comparative research across models—e.g., those at city birth centers, safety-net clinics, and not-for-profit teaching hospitals—underscores the diverse challenges and benefits of each approach. For instance, urban birth centers can offer a more personalized experience for low-risk patients while not driving out high-risk patients, and not-for-profit hospitals provide a broader array of services to meet the needs of both low- and high-risk patients. Importantly, both women's and providers' attitudes towards these models improve the overall effectiveness of prenatal care. Investigation of these varied experiences can shed light on the strengths and weaknesses inherent in different care settings, facilitating more thoughtful policy decisions aimed at optimizing maternal health outcomes (Cook et al., 2009). Moreover, prenatal care services increasingly emphasize the necessity of culturally attentive care that addresses the unique needs of diverse groups. It is critical to consider cultural, socioeconomic, and linguistic variables in effective communication between healthcare providers and pregnant women. Adapting prenatal programs to incorporate these aspects could maximize patient satisfaction and adherence to medical recommendations, leading to better maternal-fetal health outcomes. Programs that allow flexible scheduling, language support, and education in more than one language are models that excel. As more family practitioners learn about the disparities, fighting them with evidence-based interventions will do much to enhance the quality of prenatal care available to all women, regardless of their background. Such commitment to inclusive care is part of success in the sense of having equity in maternal healthcare (Nichols et al., 1950) (Figure 12.5).

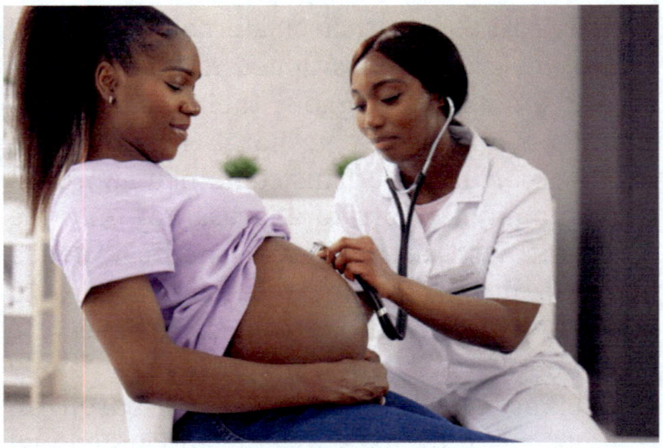

Figure 12.5. Prenatal care services.

Source: https://carestlhealth.org/wp-content/uploads/2021/06/PrenatalCare1_CareSTLHealth-1024x683.png.

12.1.2. Labor and Delivery Management

Effective labor and delivery management is an important domain of obstetrics, having a direct bearing on infant and maternal health outcomes. As family medicine doctors are taking an increased role in maternity services, learning about labor management dynamics becomes a necessity. Effective management involves the observation and assessment of the progress of labor, management of potential complications, and psychosocial care for pregnant women. Studies show that the intervention of trained birth attendants can reduce maternal mortality significantly, indicating the necessity for experts' intervention at the time of giving birth. Additionally, the application of patient-centered approaches enhances the quality of childbearing, allowing women to voice their preferences while ensuring safety and efficiency. The labor care continuum not only highlights the medical aspects but also addresses the emotional aspects of women, and, in doing so, formulates an elaborate view of childbirth within family medicine. One key aspect of labor management is addressing the dynamic interplay between biomedical interventions and customary practices, such as those of Traditional Birth Attendants (TBAs). In most developing countries, the traditional birth attendant has been a key provider of birthing care. During this shift towards promoting skilled birth attendance, it becomes necessary to evaluate the effectiveness of TBA training courses and their impact on maternal and child health outcomes. Education of TBAs, along with community mobilization, can help integrate an approach in which indigenous practices are seen as important, and this is done alongside up-to-date medical data. Such an integrated approach becomes particularly critical in areas where indigenous beliefs influence childbirth behavior, as it promotes teamwork among healthcare providers, patients, and families, thereby enhancing the uptake of safe birthing practices (Adamson et al., 2010). With evolving patterns of childbirth, awareness of the evolutionary and historical contexts of labor and delivery management is also equally important. The history of midwifery, dating back to ancient traditions, continues to influence modern concepts of childbirth. In the multilevel healthcare systems of the contemporary era, it is increasingly realized that human childbirth is complemented by skilled intervention, as outlined in recent literature on integrating midwifery into obstetric care. This emphasis allows healthcare professionals to be mindful of the anatomical and behavioral changes that occur at birth while promoting innovative practices that respect cultural guidelines. Harmony between biomedical intervention and traditional intervention can lead to effective labor management, yielding more positive outcomes. Emphasis on culturally congruent practices that respect both the evolutionary past and modern medical knowledge is crucial for providing comprehensive maternity care in family medicine (Dunham et al., 2016) (Figure 12.6).

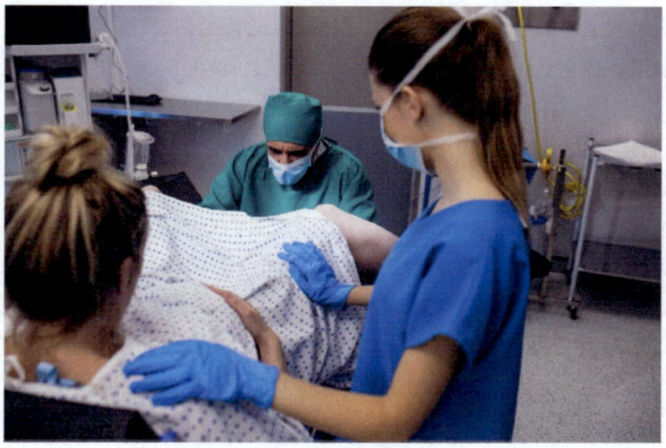

Figure 12.6. Labor and delivery.

Source: https://mdwell.com/wp-content/uploads/2023/12/gynecologist-performing-ultrasound-consultation-2-min-2048x1365.jpg.

12.1.3. Postpartum Care and Support

The postpartum period, typically characterized by significant physical and emotional disturbances, demands integrated care and counseling for new mothers. Postpartum care, in family medicine, extends beyond the immediate physical recovery from birth to encompass psychological well-being. Evidence indicates that postpartum depression (PPD) affects a significant percentage of women, with prevalence rates highlighting the importance of early identification and intervention. Styles of attachment have also been linked to the level of severity in postpartum depression, thereby emphasizing the importance of psychosocial factors in the treatment plan. The realization that females with a Fearful-Avoidant attachment style can be more vulnerable to PPD emphasizes the need for focused intervention strategies to enhance maternal-infant attachment as well as address associated emotional disturbances (Aceti et al., 2015). To promote postpartum care effectively, screening protocols for mental health conditions have undergone a dramatic change. Guidelines of the American College of Obstetricians and Gynecologists and the United States Preventive Services Task Force currently recommend universal postpartum depression screening, illustrating a dramatic change in clinical practice (Brown et al., 2017). This proactive approach aims at the early identification of vulnerable women during the postpartum period and hence enables early interventions and curbs the long-term effects of untreated depression for mothers as well as babies. In particular, tools like the Edinburgh Postnatal Depression Scale are pivotal to such screening efforts as they provide a systematic means for assessing maternal mental health. It is imperative that postpartum care be delivered effectively by well-informed, well-trained health providers who have the capacity to implement these guidelines. Providing all forms of care at this vulnerable phase of a woman's life is also paramount. Moreover, implementing these practices in family medicine necessitates collaboration between health providers, mental health professionals, and social support systems. Families are integral to the postpartum recovery process, and family members' or partners' education can lead to increased comprehension and empathy towards women's struggles. Crafting educational materials that highlight the importance of postpartum mental health, such as brochures and community education sessions, can empower women and their families in accessing help and recognizing the signs of postpartum depression. As evident in quality improvement projects of healthcare systems like the Alaska VA Healthcare System, awareness and proper screening can go a long way to support care systems for new mothers and therefore maternal and infant health (Brown et al., 2017) (Figure 12.7).

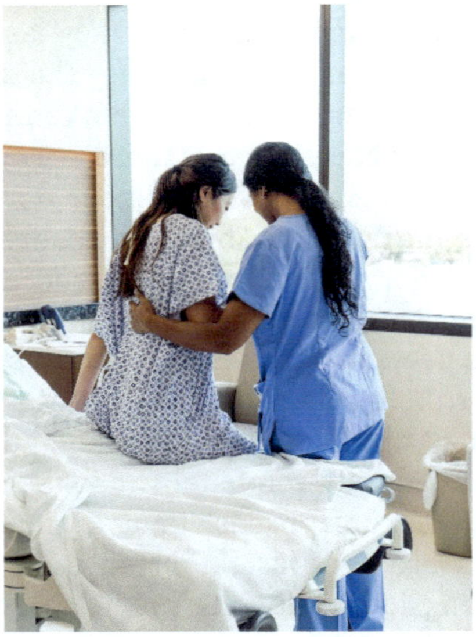

Figure 12.7. Postpartum care and support.

Source: https://akm-img-a-in.tosshub.com/indiatoday/images/story/202408/new-moms-are-turning-to-postpartum-care-centres--a-trend-india-is-embracing-235054981-3x4.jpg?VersionId=Esz_5axpCmSqA97rw3QXARY.ePiT._EG.

Test Your Knowledge

1. What are prenatal care services?
2. Explain the labor and delivery management.

12.2. Benefits of Integrating Obstetrics into Family Medicine

Learning Outcome

1. Understand the continuity of care for patients
2. Describe the holistic approach to maternal and child health
3. Know the improved health outcomes for families

The integration of obstetrics within family practice offers a comprehensive model of care, allowing family physicians to provide overall care throughout the patient's life cycle. Continuity facilitates better understanding of personalized health stories since family physicians are best placed to address the physiological, psychological, and social components of maternal health. By ensuring care for women during pregnancy and thereafter, such providers are in a position to identify and avert potential health risks that accompany childbirth, thus deepening the maternal-fetal bond. Moreover, this model enhances a more family-oriented care approach, with effective communication and collaboration among family members. It allows patients to be engaged with their healthcare decisions actively, evoking a sense of ownership that is particularly important at life-changing times like giving birth, supporting the theory that giving birth can be enhanced by knowledge and prolonged support, evident in the evolutionary importance of understanding attendance while giving birth (Dunham et al., 2016). Having obstetrics integrated in family medicine is especially useful for rural and resource-deprived areas, where specialist obstetric care may not be readily available. Family physicians with obstetric training can address this deficiency, ensuring pregnant women receive appropriate and timely antenatal care, which is essential for optimal maternal and fetal outcomes. Therefore, this integration can potentially reduce maternal and infant morbidity and mortality rates in low-resource communities. The family physicians can also address other health concerns, such as chronic diseases, mental illness, and social determinants of health, thus adding a wholesome dimension to the unique problems of pregnant women. This three-part model of care embodies the ethos of community health, namely that healthcare is not merely reactive but proactive and culturally sensitive to meet diverse patient needs.

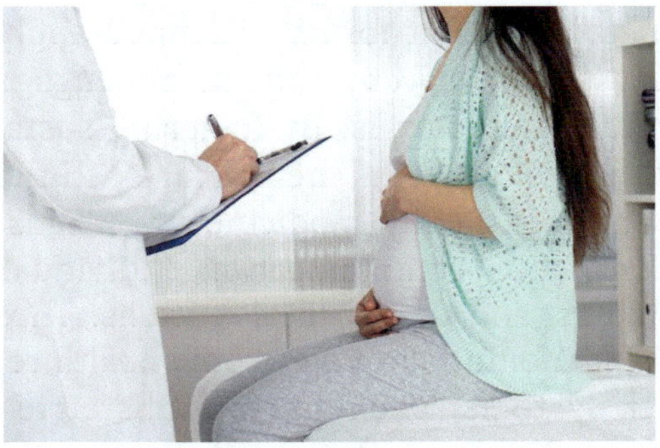

Figure 12.8. Benefits of integrating obstetrics into family medicine

Source: https://sa1s3optim.patientpop.com/assets/images/provider/photos/2286173.jpg

Additionally, the inclusion of obstetrics within the scope of family medicine is in keeping with the natural family planning (NFP) ethics that respect the body's natural rhythms. Fertility education can enhance the patient-doctor relationship and facilitate discussions of responsible parenthood in ways that respect the dignity of the individual (Fehring et al., 2017). NFP education can be done by family doctors so that couples are instructed on how to determine fertile and infertile periods. Education of this kind empowers couples with the information they need to make informed decisions about family planning, promoting open communication and respect within relationships. In addition to its ethical and spiritual benefits, NFP can also be medically advantageous, as tracking menstrual cycles can indicate potential medical issues. Thus, this synergy between obstetrics and family medicine not only promotes healthier pregnancies but also encourages a culture of life that honors the reproductive process and bonds families further (Figure 12.8).

12.2.1. Continuity of Care for Patients

Continuity of care is a vital component of best obstetric practice in family medicine, and it addresses the maintenance of the health of the mother and child throughout the prenatal and postnatal stages. It forms a planned approach to health care whereby patients are engaged in their care trajectories. By fostering sustained continuity between healthcare clinicians and patients, family medicine physicians can facilitate open communication, individualized care plans, and timely interventions. Through the implementation of electronic health record (EHR) systems, such as the Obstetric and Neonatal Ontology (OntONeo), this continuity becomes less difficult through interoperable data that is necessary for tracking maternal and neonatal health outcomes longitudinally. This integrated systematic data collection not only supports optimal clinical decision-making but also promotes health literacy among expectant families, thereby improving perinatal outcomes and patient satisfaction (Almeida et al., 2016). Maternity care delivery models, such as those in city birth centers, safety-net clinics, and teaching hospitals, reflect different strategies for obstetric continuity of care. Every environment is exposed to unique populations and faces similar challenges that impact the level of care being provided. Safety net clinics will see lower-resourced populations and must contend with fiscal constraints while still trying to maintain a cohesive care plan. Teaching hospitals, conversely, may have more robust resources and skilled care but can struggle with regard to their higher staff and patient volume. It is essential to note these differences, as continuity of care can vary enormously depending on the setting in which it is offered. Attitudes of both healthcare professionals and women towards these alternative models of care give excellent insight into what aspects of continuity are most valued, further informing best practice in obstetric care (Cook et al., 2009). Furthermore, optimal continuity of care in obstetrics demands a multidisciplinary approach. Family physicians, obstetricians, midwives, and support staff must communicate with each other to make certain that all aspects of a patient's care are thoroughly discussed. There is a special need for these groups to communicate during periods of precarious transition, i.e., from prenatal to labor and delivery, and subsequently to the postpartum period. Efficient communication and sharing of patient information between providers allow a holistic understanding of each patient's history and medical concerns. The deployment of universal protocols and uniform guidelines is also a critical factor contributing to this continuity. In the long run, a harmonized approach not only reduces the risk of medical errors but also reinforces patients' trust in the system, underscoring the pivotal role of continuity as an obstetric determinant of favorable outcomes (Figure 12.9).

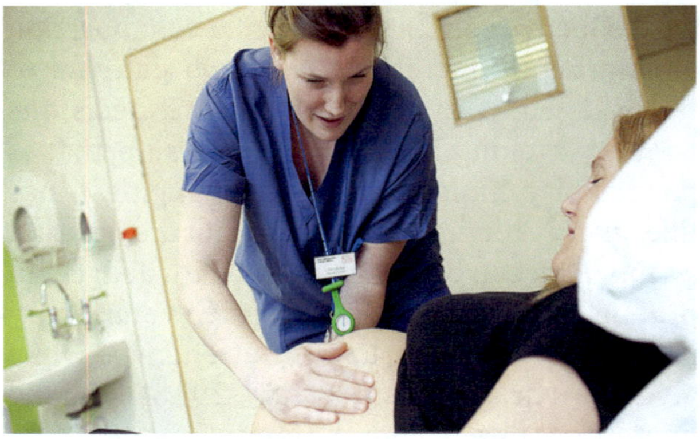

Figure 12.9. Midwife continuity of care model linked to positive experiences during pregnancy.

Source: https://www.kcl.ac.uk/ImportedImages/Schools/Nursing/00-new-cms-templates/780x450px/midwifery-taster-day-780x450.x1d4f6f46.jpg?crop=780,440,0,5.

12.2.2. Holistic Approach to Maternal and Child Health

A holistic approach to child and maternal health recognizes that the physical, emotional, and social health of women and children are interdependent. The vision extends beyond the immediate medical needs of pregnancy and birth to encompass such determinants as mental health, culture, and support systems within the community. The inclusion of traditional birth attendants (TBAs) in maternal and child health reflects this comprehensive model, especially in the developing world, where skilled medical facilities might not be readily available. Although criticized for their inability to lower the rates of maternal mortality, TBAs have a crucial function of caring for women at every stage of their reproductive cycle, offering culturally appropriate care that is consistent with community norms. Thus, a sensitive balance must be achieved between traditional practices and evidence-based medical care such that TBAs are adequately trained, and there is active involvement of the community in order to enhance the outcome of child and maternal health (Adamson et al., 2010). Perinatal mental health is an integral part of comprehensive maternal care, and it also has a great impact on maternal as well as child outcomes. There is evidence indicating that perinatal mental disorders may disrupt maternal-infant attachment and lead to adverse developmental outcomes among children. Detection and response to these mental health conditions are important in a system of comprehensive maternal health. The evidence does, however, indicate that inadequate training in the performance of mental health interviews can undermine the effectiveness of healthcare providers in responding appropriately to mothers. For instance, student midwives do not feel confident enough to recognize and manage perinatal mental health issues, which reflects a deficiency in education with emphasis on physical, rather than psychological, well-being. Incorporating a robust curriculum with training in perinatal mental health can empower the midwife and enhance their ability to provide fully holistic care (Jarrett et al., 2017). Community participation is key to the success of an integrated maternal and child health strategy. Such participation by national organizations, healthcare workers, and families generates an enabling context in which women are encouraged to use prenatal and postnatal care. In particular, culturally sensitive health education can decrease risky traditional practices while promoting desirable ones. Community health programs based on mothers' own feedback can identify the specific needs and interests across different populations and therefore optimize the overall impact of maternal healthcare programs. A focus on cooperation among healthcare professionals, families, and community members can lead to innovative solutions that improve access to care, raise mental health awareness, and promote health practices for both mothers and children. This comprehensive system of care is required to advance healthy outcomes and enable all children and all mothers to thrive (Figure 12.10).

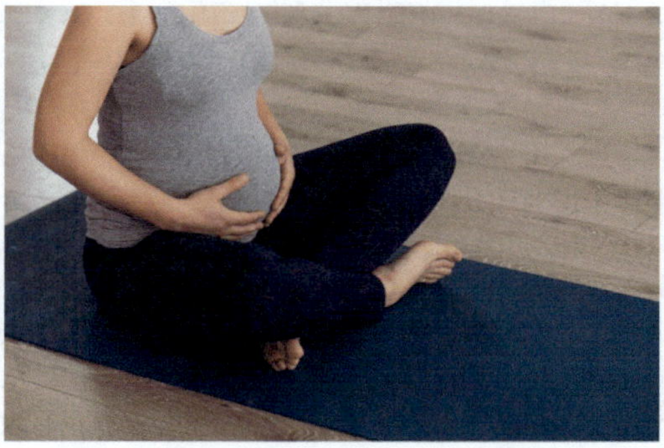

Figure 12.10. A holistic approach to maternal-child health.

Source: https://gomohealth.com/wp-content/uploads/2024/11/A-Holistic-Approach-to-Maternal-Child-Health-From-a-Wellness-Expert.png.

12.2.3. Improved Health Outcomes for Families

The intersection of obstetrics and family medicine is relevant to improving health outcomes for families. One of the main features is attention to shared care models that prioritize the use of informed attendants for delivery. The care ensures not only mothers' physiological and behavioral needs but also a safe birthing experience. The presence of highly trained practitioners can reduce birth complications, leading to less morbidity and mortality among mothers and newborns. In such a scenario, both medical proficiency and culturally competent care can be of significant help to families. For instance, integrating midwifery into contemporary obstetric practice can help bridge the gap between medical intervention and traditional practice, providing integrated care that aligns with evolutionary principles applicable to childbirth (Dunham et al., 2016). In addition, shared decision-making (SDM) becomes an imperative strategy to enhance health outcomes, particularly for complicated care scenarios such as previable births. Such situations are laden with ethical and individual values in decision-making regarding life support for infants born at the margin of viability. By applying decision support tools (DSTs) that empower families with information and personalized narratives, care providers can improve the quality of decision-making. Feedback from both patients and providers has indicated a need for materials that couple fact-based knowledge with families' actual experience, which helps build connection and trust. Ultimately, this SDM model facilitates not only enhanced decision-making outcomes but also stronger family bonds through shared connections regarding the care experience (Bauer et al., 2019). Merging successful obstetric practices with family medicine can yield long-term health gains for families, especially as they navigate the complications associated with childbirth. The merging of user-centered design for DSTs into the clinic environment is one such example, as it takes into account the desires and needs of patients and providers alike. By facilitating open articulation of options and understanding of potential consequences, these techniques will help bridge the gap between family values and clinician advice. These new ways are at the core of achieving common goals of health and well-being in family systems, ultimately creating healthier family relationships. With increasing research and development in family medicine, evidence-based practice according to the unique needs of families will be vital to enhancing health outcomes and delivering comprehensive, compassionate care (Bauer et al., 2019) (Figure 12.11).

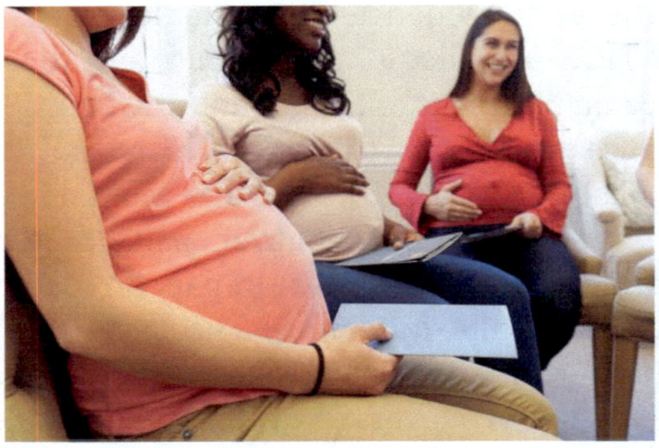

Figure 12.11. Improving health for women by better supporting them through pregnancy and beyond.

Source: https://www.commonwealthfund.org/sites/default/files/styles/hero_image_desktop/public/Immigrant%20pregnant%20women.jpg?itok=INZ43s2Y.

Test Your Knowledge

1. What is continuity of care for a patient?
2. What is the holistic approach to maternal and child health?

12.3. Challenges Faced by Family Physicians in Obstetrics

Learning Outcome

1. Know the limited training opportunities
2. Balance the family medicine and obstetric responsibilities
3. Navigate the healthcare policies and regulations

Family physicians who choose to include obstetrics in their practices face challenges that can directly affect their ability to provide holistic care. Among the major challenges is balancing the demands of obstetrics with other areas within their family medicine scope. This dual responsibility requires family doctors to be skilled not only in prenatal care but also in a broad spectrum of medical issues affecting diverse patient populations. This emphasis on obstetrics can therefore normally detract from their ability to fully engage in routine family practice, and thereby lead to professional burnout and job dissatisfaction. The weight of these duties has the potential to generate a tension that will discourage new practitioners from coming into obstetrics altogether, again exacerbating the issue of access to care for pregnant women in many communities. The second significant barrier is the evolving healthcare policy environment and the consequent effect on obstetric practice within family medicine. Regulatory developments can impose additional bureaucratic requirements on family physicians that divert valuable time and money from seeing patients. The insurance reimbursement arrangements for obstetric care can be complex and unpredictable, leaving family physicians unablezxc to sustain economically viable practices. Policy changes and healthcare reform initiatives can create uncertainty, leading physicians to be hesitant in providing care to obstetric patients. In such a situation, family physicians may be at a loss to balance maintaining obstetric care, particularly in underserved areas where such care would be invaluable. Such dilemmas further illustrate the intricacies of the layers in the practice of family physicians who do obstetrics, where extraneous considerations will largely shape their participation in this essential aspect of practice. Finally, the physical and emotional demands of obstetric care present an ongoing challenge to family physicians. The uncertainty of labor and delivery can lead to undue stress, requiring physicians to be available at a moment's notice, eliminating their work-life balance. Beyond the logistical challenges, family physicians also typically bear the emotional burden of complications during pregnancy and childbirth. Dealing with adverse outcomes can have a profound effect on their mental health and professional confidence. Support structures, such as mentorship programs and organized support networks, are crucial in addressing these emotional challenges but are not always readily available. There is a need to build an educated and resilient workforce in family medicine, as sustained support and training can mitigate some adverse impacts on physicians in obstetrics, thereby enhancing general job satisfaction and retention in the field (Figure 12.12).

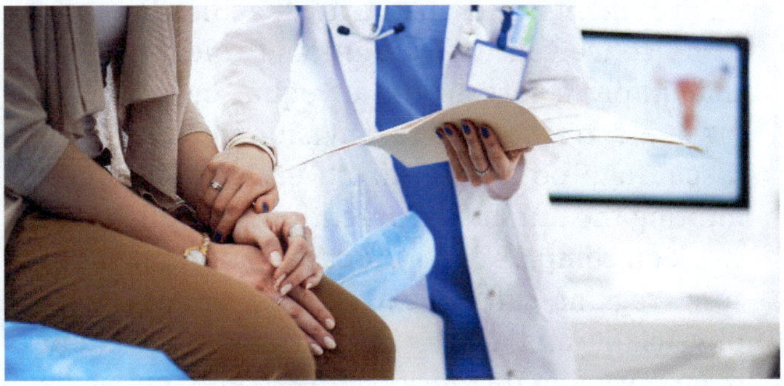

Figure 12.12. Challenges faced by family physicians.

Source: https://www.mobileodt.com/wp-content/uploads/2020/03/shutterstock_757171732-scaled.jpg.

12.3.1. Limited Training Opportunities

The obstetric environment in family medicine is largely shaped by limited training opportunities, which can hinder professional development among future providers. The majority of medical students would be eager to pursue extended obstetric training, but availability is often limited. Importantly, special training programs often prioritize metropolitan or established medical facilities at the expense of rural and underserved areas, leaving them with limited educational resources. This inequality not only affects the population of physicians but also affects patient access to quality maternal care, creating a cycle that perpetuates disparities in healthcare services from one region to another. As identified in the literature, the shifting demographics of the medical workforce, including the increased numbers of female physicians seeking specialized practice, highlight the need to expand training opportunities so they can more adequately reflect the needs of the served populations (Higgins-Opitz et al., 2017). Other cultural norms and organizational biases may also play a part in discouraging trainees who wish to pursue obstetrics. Some specialties are envisioned as gendered professions in most environments, and obstetrics specifically tends to be conceived with traditional roles in mind that imply a foreclosing of equal opportunity for male trainees. The envisioned roles may discourage both sexes from entering, thereby limiting the number of practitioners available to work on complex obstetric cases. Additionally, in some regions, cultural expectations about female physicians and travel restrictions deter them from pursuing further training to enhance their practice and career prospects. Such disparity calls for profound reform that enhances access to obstetric training for family medicine to ensure it is an amenable setting in which all physicians can acquire skills without being constrained by past gender assumptions (Higgins-Opitz et al., 2017). Studies of the outcomes of existing training programs have demonstrated that methods such as family-centered rounds (FCR) can provide frameworks to enable knowledge acquisition in medical students, including those learning obstetrics. Reports from institutions adopting reforms to FCR indicate a potential positive correlation between new teaching styles and student performance on critical exams, although more research is required to confirm these findings in the obstetrics arena. This means that reconsidering the educational practices and integrating them into training curricula can reverse some of the current constraints. In the end, by diversifying the training paradigms and making them inclusive, the practice of family medicine can equip practitioners with the skill set for providing full obstetric care in a way that patients are guaranteed to receive quality care, irrespective of their geographical or cultural location.

12.3.2. Balancing Family Medicine and Obstetric Responsibilities

Blending obstetric responsibility with family practice presents unique challenges for providers in a multifaceted discipline. Family practice addresses all aspects of care, and physicians must remain up to date on a myriad of topics. This diversity is generally at odds with the increasing demands of obstetric care, which can be quite physically and emotionally demanding. The declining population of graduates coming forth for family medicine, noted by (Cronau et al., 2004), is a sign that reflects more worry about the sustainability of undertaking both family medicine and obstetric obligations. Physicians must adopt strategic actions in carrying out these duties in a manner that does not compromise the quality of services being delivered to expectant women and their overall patients. By specializing their skill sets through specialized training and attending support educational programs, family medicine physicians can better fulfill their dual roles and improve patient outcomes. Gender and cultural challenges also contribute to the obstacles to balancing obstetrics and family medicine roles. While more women are entering the medical field, particularly in family medicine and obstetrics, the profession's classic gender roles are becoming more dynamic. Research has found a "gendered" understanding of specialties, with obstetrics widely regarded as a female-dominated area, as reported in (Higgins-Opitz et al., 2017). These cultural patterns may possibly influence how upcoming family practitioners approach specialty and role adaptation. Female physicians may also face unique challenges, e.g., workplace expectations regarding work-life balance.

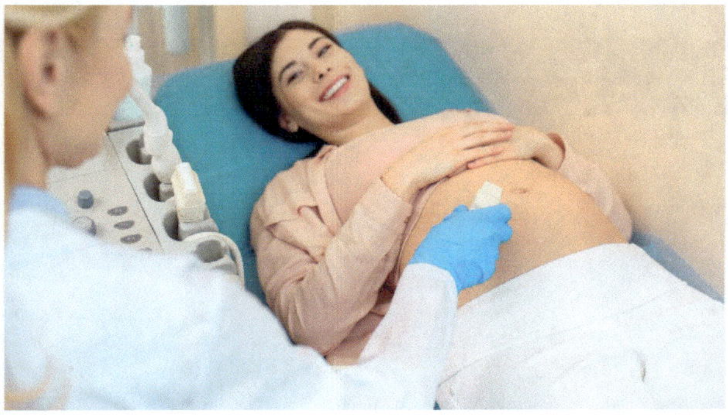

Figure 12.13. Obstetric responsibilities.

Source: https://cdn.careeronestop.org/OccVids/OccupationVideos/29-1218.00.jpg.

The ability to navigate these factors is crucial to fostering a professional environment that supports diversity and inclusion, which ultimately shapes the retention and success of physicians specializing in family medicine and obstetrics. The efforts to build supportive networks and teaching structures are critical in fostering a balanced focus on family medicine and obstetric practice. The conduct of mentorship programs and externships, as highlighted by Cronau et al. (2004), can support prospective family medicine doctors in gaining appreciative exposure to obstetric practice during training. The programs not only foster interest in the specialty but also enable doctors to provide competent, sensitive responses when managing obstetric cases. Lastly, providing specialized assistance that accounts for the unique challenges of fulfilling these responsibilities will enhance overall satisfaction and proficiency in family medicine and obstetrics. With ongoing changes in health needs, such programs are necessary to create a diversified medical pool well-positioned to deliver comprehensive care to diverse patient populations (Figure 12.13).

12.3.3. Navigating Healthcare Policies and Regulations

With the evolving context of obstetrics in family medicine, maneuverability of healthcare policy and regulation remains an ongoing priority for healthcare providers. With persistent discrepancies in maternal health outcomes, particularly among diverse populations, there is a need to monitor the frameworks that guide care provision. The effective application of those policies needs to be prioritized because they determine funding, resource allocation, and standard-setting in care. For example, efforts to expand the accessibility of maternal health services have been found to notably decrease maternal mortality rates, as demonstrated by India's recent progress, which serves to exemplify the potential influence of organized healthcare policies on health outcomes. However, despite the seen improvement, maternal morbidity remains a problem, indicative of strict adherence to regulations and particular interventions to deal with these ongoing complications (Naeve et al., 2017). Doctors also have to engage with policy models to actively improve maternal health care. This collaboration demands an interdisciplinary understanding of the rules that guide obstetric practices, such as patient safety, quality care, and treatment protocols. For example, innovative approaches to maternal management, such as the use of misoprostol for the prevention of postpartum hemorrhage, emphasize the need for careful policy interventions for better dissemination.

Institutional support from organizations such as the John D. and Catherine T. MacArthur Foundation illustrates how strategic funding can mobilize efforts to enhance effective interventions. Through investment in health interventions and research-based research in the community, stakeholders not only enhance the quality of care but also contribute to an overarching improvement in maternal health standards, which encourages enhanced health outcomes on a population-wide basis (Otive-Igbuzor et al., 2014). Lastly, the intertwined dynamics of healthcare policies and regulations, and how they impact obstetric services, must remain under close examination and reform. As family medicine physicians navigate through this difficult terrain, they should be attuned to dynamic changes in maternal health policies at home and abroad. Ongoing advocacy and evidence-guided debate by healthcare providers, policymakers, and communities are needed to ensure that obstetric interventions remain compatible with contemporary needs and evidence-based care. Furthermore, as new evidence and treatment options emerge, continued policy revisions will be needed to enable proper implementation and thereby enhance the environment for maximum maternal health outcomes and reduced health disparities across disparate populations (Naeve et al., 2017; Otive-Igbuzor et al., 2014).

Test Your Knowledge

1. What is a specialized training program?
2. What does the MacArthur Foundation support?

12.4. Current Trends in Obstetrics within Family Medicine

Learning Outcome

1. Understand the rise of telemedicine in prenatal care
2. Emphasize the patient-centered care
3. Know the innovations in obstetric practices

The obstetric world of family medicine is undergoing transformation, with major drivers including models of innovative care delivery, such as Direct Primary Care (DPC). DPC practices are unique in their emphasis on patient-centered care, allowing family physicians to practice whole-person care without the constraints of traditional insurance billing. A recent study found that 88% of practices reported reduced membership charges since 2005, and a considerable decline in insurance claims from 75% to 11% (Ablah et al., 2019). These reforms reflect a growing pattern among family medicine practitioners to pursue an overall model of preventive medicine and long-term patient interaction, one that is especially beneficial for addressing maternal and neonatal health outcomes within the core obstetric competence. With the focus on preconception care gaining momentum in family medicine, many practitioners are adding educational modules to promote improved maternal health through lifestyle interventions. Recent research portrays that being overweight or obese in mothers is strongly correlated with poor outcomes during pregnancy and post-pregnancy (Holleran et al., 2017). This understanding led to the development of directed educational materials for health care professionals to empower them to have suitable conversations with childbearing women. By placing emphasis on preconceptional nutrition, family medicine physicians can take a frontline role in guaranteeing healthy outcomes and preventing complications throughout pregnancy and thereby addressing the growing rates of obesity and its subsequent consequences in obstetric populations. Additionally, technology integration in obstetric care has become a top trend in family medicine. Use of electronic medical records (EMR), telemedicine platforms, and patient portals gives family physicians unprecedented ability to enhance care continuity and patient activation. Increased access to digital resources enables greater control over prenatal care, providing families with timely information and advice. This trend not only optimizes the doctor-patient relationship but also facilitates active family involvement in their own care, particularly at the vulnerable phases of pregnancy and delivery. As such, technological advances are fast becoming ubiquitous, they are bound to revolutionize the future of obstetrics in family medicine so that care is always responsive, effective, and patient-centered (Figure 12.14).

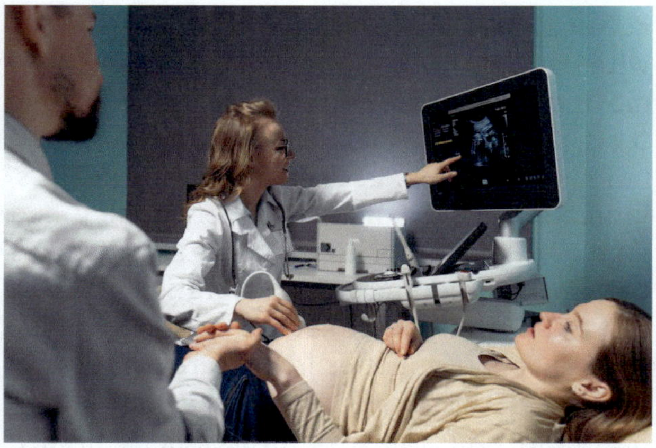

Figure 12.14. Current trends in obstetrics.

Source: https://ummeedurologyandgynecology.com/wp-content/uploads/2024/04/gynecologist-performing-ultrasound-consultation_23-2149353025.jpg.

12.4.1. Rise of Telemedicine in Prenatal Care

The integration of telemedicine in prenatal care has been a turning point in the mode of delivery of obstetric services, making it more convenient and efficient for pregnant women. Telemedicine uses technology to bridge the gap between patients and healthcare providers, particularly for underserved populations. It is an essential enhancement, especially for women who lack access to specialist care due to geographical or socio-economic barriers. With online consultations, healthcare providers can better track the well-being of expectant patients, enabling timely interventions and reducing the need for in-person visits. Telemedicine also helps patients educate themselves about prenatal care, keeping them actively involved in their path to wellness and improving outcomes for both mothers and newborns. The growing application of telemedicine in prenatal care also helps address high-stakes complications that could arise during pregnancy. For example, cases of placenta accreta spectrum require complex management plans, best managed by interdisciplinary teams. It may be difficult to implement this in resource-poor settings. And yet, telemedicine provides a framework for communication between patients and expert medical teams, so that women can receive the care they need wherever they are. As noted, the addition of professional interdisciplinary teams is associated with improved clinical outcomes, and telemedicine facilitates this by enabling remote consultation and management. Consequently, the use of telemedicine can significantly enhance the care of high-risk pregnancies with better outcomes for both mothers and children. The future of prenatal telemedicine looks promising, with studies still working to optimize its application across various settings. Initial evidence indicates that telemedicine not only expands access but also enhances patient satisfaction, as women prefer the convenience and reduced travel burden of virtual encounters. Moreover, as telemedicine platforms evolve and incorporate more advanced technologies, such as artificial intelligence and remote monitoring equipment, the potential for more individualized and effective prenatal care continues to expand. Subsequent lines of investigation will likely be aimed at the long-term consequences of telemedicine on neonatal and maternal outcomes, particularly in multicultural socioeconomic settings. Emphasis on the requirement that telemedicine practices be appropriate to the specific needs of disparate populations will be key to furthering prenatal care within the broader context of obstetrics within family medicine (Figure 12.15).

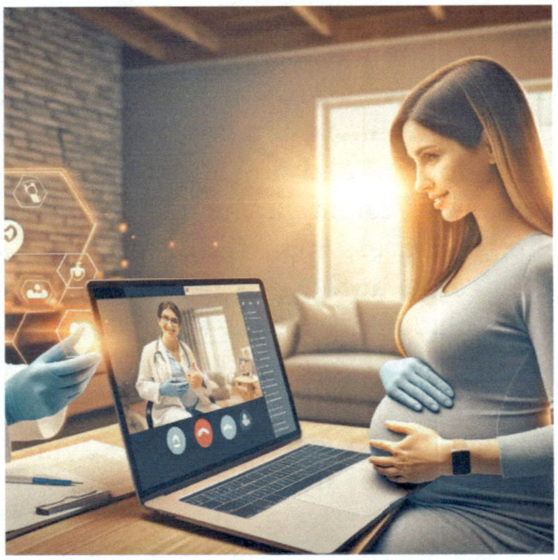

Figure 12.15. Rise of telemedicine in prenatal care.

Source: https://importikaah.com/cdn/shop/articles/DALL_E_2024-01-30_12.34.05_-_A_revised_and_accurate_depiction_of_Embracing_Telehealth_for_Prenatal_Care__A_New_Era_of_Maternal_Health_focusing_on_a_pregnant_woman_using_telehea.png?v=1706598303.

12.4.2. Emphasis on Patient-Centered Care

Patient-centered care is the most vital factor in improving the quality of care delivery in contemporary obstetrics and family medicine. The approach centers on patients' values, wishes, and choices, therefore, turns them into active participants in their care. In obstetrics, this is even more essential because women and families must make extremely engaged decisions regarding pregnancy and giving birth. Wherever healthcare providers facilitate shared decision-making (SDM), particularly in intimate issues such as previable delivery, they help patients express their preferences and values in the most effective way. Not only does this create trusting relationships among providers and patients, but also enhances the quality of care experience, which is most essential in the obstetric setting where emotion and uncertainty prevail. The use of user-centered design values in developing decision support tools (DSTs) can also improve patient-centered care in obstetrics. Involving patients and their families in the design ensures that practitioners develop tools better suited to their needs. Findings show that prototypes like tablet apps and family testimonial videos can effectively deliver unbiased information and comprehensible alternatives for delivery and care (Bauer et al., 2019). This initiative is part of the broader vision of health interventions becoming more patient-centered and aligned with patients' lived world and aspirations. The move towards more interactive and didactic tools not only enables easier communication but also facilitates decision-making processes, ultimately making mutual understanding and improved maternal and neonatal outcomes possible. Furthermore, the integration of cross-cultural training into medical curricula is key to developing patient-centered care practices in obstetrics. Educational systems that equip future healthcare professionals with such skills through which they can effectively communicate with diverse cultural backgrounds make provision of more egalitarian care (Weissman et al., 2007). By raising awareness about the necessity of making healthcare plans sensitive to unique cultural environments, obstetric professionals can create a more inclusive environment, promoting the diverse needs of the patients. Such a cultural competency promise not only strengthens the patient-provider bond but also improves health outcomes by ensuring that care systems are culturally responsive to diverse perspectives. Ultimately, a patient-oriented, culturally respectful model of holistic care is essential to achieving better health equity in family medicine obstetrics (Figure 12.16).

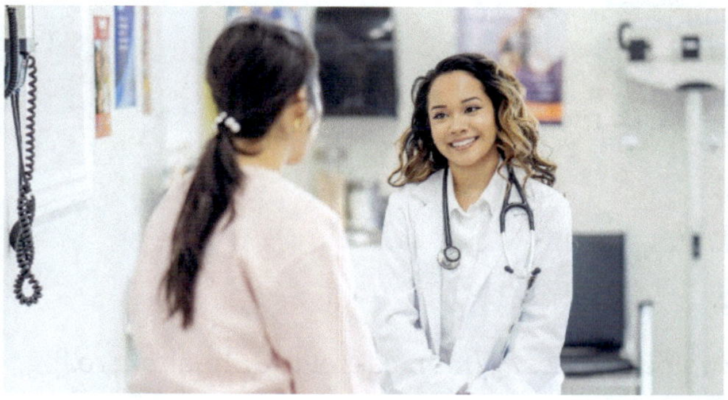

Figure 12.16. Patient-centered care.

Source: https://media.licdn.com/dms/image/v2/D4E12AQH7M1VWpyZ2tg/article-cover_image-shrink_720_1280/article-cover_image-shrink_720_1280/0/1722984056983?e=2147483647&v=beta&t=zMqd58nx9SH15vY6p_SHqjXEcta_yVgpNEgBUabeLeU.

12.4.3. Innovations in Obstetric Practices

Obstetric practice has been revolutionized by technological advances that bring modern medicine into harmony with the distinct physiological requirements of childbirth. Historically, midwifery has been central to providing care to women during the birthing process, with individual attention that directly addresses hormonal and physiological functions. As highlighted by more recent evaluations, the overlap between economic modernization and midwifery has reshaped the landscape of maternity care, precipitating a clash between the ancient traditions and the biomedical technologies. This conflict, unless properly managed, is bound to generate disparities in care which undermine the qualitative character of childbirth. Therefore, combining modern interventions with midwifery principles may create a space that meets both emotional and biological needs, ultimately improving maternal outcomes (Dunham et al., 2016). Family medicine clinicians can then apply such innovations to support childbirth as a quintessentially human encounter while still accommodating the complexity of patients' backgrounds. Modern technology has provided obstetric clinics with equipment that considers both fetal and maternal safety throughout pregnancy and childbirth. Innovations such as telemedicine have emerged as crucial tools, particularly for rural communities and underserved populations, enabling health practitioners to remotely monitor pregnancies and expedite interventions when needed. These innovations have been helpful in reducing complications since healthcare teams can make informed decisions on the basis of real-time data. Moreover, case studies from more than one healthcare organization demonstrate that cooperative learning and best-practice sharing will lead to top-notch improvements in patient safety across the board. For instance, combining information sharing and new procedure protocols has been said to enhance the obstetric team's clinical expertise directly at the expense of health outcomes (Blumenthal et al., 2006). By integrating these innovations into everyday practice, family medicine not only addresses the immediate healthcare needs but also has a reproducible model of integrated maternal care. The intersection of obstetric innovations and family medicine also presents a driving force for cultural competence in maternity practice. Understanding patients' diverse backgrounds is central to developing tailored approaches that respect individual desires and social norms. Culturally congruent innovations in obstetric care can lead to improved patient satisfaction and compliance with care. Doula programs or culturally responsive models of care, for instance, respect birthing traditions and care preferences of various ethnic groups, thereby improving the overall care experience. This not only fosters trust among healthcare providers and families but also reaffirms the importance of context in maternal health. By implementing these innovations in family medicine, clinicians can ensure that obstetric care is not only technically sound but also profoundly empathetic and responsive to the needs of the communities they serve (Dunham et al., 2016) (Figure 12.17).

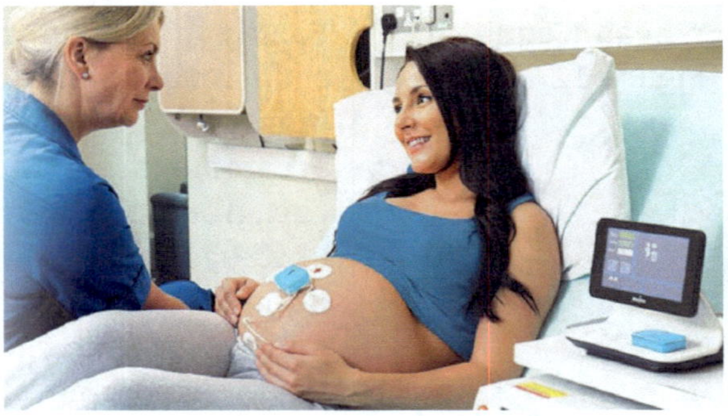

Figure 12.17. Wireless electronic fetal monitoring.

Source: https://emag.medicalexpo.com/wp-content/uploads/sites/9/monica-novii-GEHealthcare.jpg.

Test Your Knowledge

1. What is the rise of telemedicine?
2. What is patient-centered care?

SUMMARY

Briefly, the integration of obstetrics into family medicine provides a continuum of maternal and child care, with a focus on continuity of care throughout pregnancy. Such a model is compatible with closer provider-patient relationships, leading to better maternal and child health outcomes. By paying attention not only to the physiological but also to the psychological demands of pregnancy, family medicine providers are ready to identify and treat such problems as perinatal depression. Studies indicate that the severity of depression is linked to attachment styles, particularly among mothers, and highlight the need to include such psychological factors in early interventions in the framework of quality care (Aceti et al., 2015). Such a multi-dimensional strategy becomes imperative to ensure that pregnant women are not only provided with medical care but also emotional and psychological care during this sensitive phase of life. Furthermore, the problems that confront diverse groups, including minority communities, within the healthcare system also need to be addressed. Muslim women in America, for instance, highlight some specific cultural and religious barriers that might prevent access to appropriate obstetric care. Valuing special problems based on culture-informed perceptions of healthcare, family medicine can better adapt to create a more comprehensive practice. This change is required to create a setting in which all women are enabled to seek care and express their health needs. Obstetric cultural competence guarantees that clinical professionals are able to meet the specific needs of their patients, thereby achieving enhanced health outcomes and guaranteeing maternal care access equity (Seeger et al., 2015). Ultimately, integrative practices and cultural awareness will have to be the central focus for the future of obstetrics in family medicine. The professionals will have to ensure both strong care and cultural competence as the course of the profession continues to shift due to changing patient care. Such a foresight will improve patient satisfaction, but above all, create trust in the healthcare system, key to successful interventions for health. Furthermore, with evidence increasingly focusing on the interconnectedness of body and mind throughout pregnancy, psychological assessment and intervention as part of routine obstetric practice becomes increasingly important. This model of combined care promotes the underlying principle of family medicine: treating the whole person to achieve optimal outcomes for both mothers and babies in a rapidly diversifying population.

The inclusion of obstetrics in family medicine is essential to providing comprehensive care for women throughout their childbearing lifespan. Family medicine practitioners are uniquely positioned to meet the full range of needs of their patients, including prenatal care, labor and delivery, and postpartum care. This ecumenical approach enhances continuity of care, and this is most essential for the woman who experiences a complicated pregnancy or other issues. For instance, frequent contact between a patient and his or her family physician provides a background of trust and communication, enabling the more effective management of conditions such as gestational diabetes or hypertension. Preventive obstetric care in family medicine not only focuses on routine screening and preventive measures but also addresses mental health issues, which might be significantly impacted during pregnancy and in the postpartum period. Learning strategies among family medicine doctors in obstetrics can be greatly enhanced with innovative teaching methods that are effective in acquisition and retention. Traditional lectures are not effective in engaging learners, particularly in such a practical and dynamic specialty like obstetric emergencies. Consequently, institutions have devised interactive learning materials, such as board games, to facilitate near-peer learning. Evidence indicates that these interactive methods yield higher satisfaction and perceived educational gain than conventional lecture presentations, with respondents rating their experience positively (Chen et al., 2019). The inclusion of game-based learning enables family medicine residency programs to create an interactive learning environment that facilitates discussion and skill application, thus enhancing residents' preparedness to handle clinical scenarios encountered in practice. Pregnancy-associated domestic violence (DV) is a significant public health problem that needs to be recognized in family practice. Evidence shows a troubling prevalence of DV among pregnant women, so screening and intervention programs by family doctors are recommended (Alo et al., 2017). The nuances of such a sensitive subject require that healthcare professionals be well-equipped with the tools to evaluate risk factors, provide support, and refer patients to trained resources. Effective communication and a thorough understanding of the prevalence and mechanisms of abuse can enable physicians to effectively advocate for their patients. Integrated holistic care through family medicine puts practitioners in a unique position to influence not only maternal and fetal health outcomes but also the social determinants of health that impact women's health throughout pregnancy and their lifetime.

KEY TERMS FROM THIS CHAPTER

- Biomedical practices
- Community health
- Domestic violence
- Fetal health
- Gynecology
- Holistic approach
- Labor management
- Labor trajectory
- Maternal nutrition]
- Obstetric care
- Postpartum care
- Postpartum depression
- Prenatal care
- Psychosocial support

CRITICAL THINKING QUESTIONS

1. **Which of the following is the earliest biochemical marker of pregnancy?**
   a. Progesterone
   b. Estradiol
   c. Human chorionic gonadotropin (hCG)
   d. Alpha-fetoprotein (AFP)
2. **At what gestational age is a fetal heartbeat usually detectable by transvaginal ultrasound?**
   a. 4 weeks
   b. 6 weeks
   c. 8 weeks
   d. 10 weeks
3. **Which of the following is a sign of preeclampsia?**
   a. Elevated fasting blood sugar
   b. Proteinuria and hypertension
   c. Elevated amniotic fluid index
   d. Increased fetal movements
4. **Which of the following conditions is an absolute contraindication to vaginal delivery?**
   a. Breech presentation
   b. Prior cesarean delivery
   c. Placenta previa
   d. Gestational diabetes
5. **What is the first-line management for gestational diabetes?**
   a. Insulin therapy
   b. Dietary modification and exercise
   c. Metformin
   d. Immediate delivery

Short Answer Questions

1. What is obstetrics in family medicine?
2. Define the obstetrics.
3. What is the role of family medicine in obstetrics?
4. What is the importance of integrated care in maternal health?
5. What are innovations in obstetric practices?

Answer to Critical Thinking Questions

1. (c); 2. (b); 3. (b); 4. (c); 5. (b).

REFERENCES

1. Ablah, E., Dong, F., Rowe, K., et al. (2019). Direct primary care in 2015: A survey with selected comparisons to 2005 survey data. https://core.ac.uk/download/210549115.pdf (accessed on 13th July 2025).
2. Meuti, V., Aceti, F., Giacchetti, N., Carluccio, G. M., Zaccagni, M., Marini, I., Giancola, O., Ciolli, P., & Biondi, M. (2015). Perinatal depression and patterns of attachment: a critical risk factor? *Depression Research and Treatment, 2015*, 1–9. https://doi.org/10.1155/2015/105012Adamson, P., Armstrong, P., Bajpai, S., et al. (2010). Birthing practices of traditional birth attendants in South Asia in the context of training programmers. https://core.ac.uk/download/10898961.pdf (accessed on 13th July 2025).
3. Almeida, M., Elkin, P., Farinelli, F., et al. (2016). OntONeo: The obstetric and neonatal ontology. https://core.ac.uk/download/131214730.pdf (accessed on 13th July 2025).
4. Alo, A. O., Ameh, N., Ameh, N., Ameh, N., Ansari, U., Arisi, R. O., Centre for Reviews and Dissemination, et al. (2017). The prevalence of domestic violence among pregnant women in Nigeria: A systematic review. https://core.ac.uk/download/153536469.pdf (accessed on 13th July 2025).
5. Bauer, N., Edmonds, B. T., Hoffman, S. M., et al. (2019). Creation of a decision support tool for expectant parents facing threatened periviable delivery: Application of a user-centered design approach. https://core.ac.uk/download/227054358.pdf (accessed on 13th July 2025).
6. Berkman, A. M., Bradstreet, M., Davis, W., et al. (2017). Prenatal lead exposure risk assessment by Vermont maternity care providers. https://core.ac.uk/download/215154184.pdf (accessed on 13th July 2025).
7. Blumenthal, D., & McCarthy, D. (2006). Committed to safety: Ten case studies on reducing harm to patients. https://core.ac.uk/download/71350251.pdf (accessed on 13th July 2025).
8. Brown, E. L. (2017). Postpartum depression screening of women veterans in Alaska quality improvement project. https://core.ac.uk/download/286607496.pdf (accessed on 13th July 2025).
9. Brunson, J., & Tamrakar, S. R. (2018). Exploring biomedical, temporal, and embodied perspectives on the timing of birth in central Nepal. https://core.ac.uk/download/212890686.pdf (accessed on 13th July 2025).
10. Chen, E. H., & Silverio, L. M. (2019). L&D in the ED: A game-based approach to learning high-risk obstetric emergencies. https://core.ac.uk/download/323074437.pdf (accessed on 13th July 2025).
11. Cook, A., & Palmer, L. (2009). Providing maternity care to the underserved: A comparative case study of three maternity care models serving women in Washington, D.C. https://core.ac.uk/download/71348405.pdf (accessed on 13th July 2025).
12. Cronau, H., & Haines, D. J. (2004). Medical student summer externship program: Increasing the number matching in family practice. https://core.ac.uk/download/pdf/85923.pdf (accessed on 13th July 2025).
13. Dunham, B. (2016). Home birth midwifery in the United States: Evolutionary origins and modern challenges. https://open.bu.edu/bitstream/2144/29008/1/Dunham%20HN%20Midwifery%20for%20BU%20Open%20Access.pdf (accessed on 13th July 2025).

14. Fehring, R. (2017). Fertility care services. https://core.ac.uk/download/213072882.pdf (accessed on 13th July 2025).
15. Heh, V., Kimbrough, T. N., Ryan, M. S., et al. (2016). Family-centered rounds and medical student performance on the NBME pediatrics subject (shelf) examination: A retrospective cohort study. https://core.ac.uk/download/79821854.pdf (accessed on 13th July 2025).
16. Higgins-Opitz, S. B., & McLean, M. (2017). Male and female Emirati medical clerks' perceptions of the impact of gender and mobility on their professional careers. https://core.ac.uk/download/196605352.pdf (accessed on 13th July 2025).
17. Holleran, A. R. (2017). The impacts of preconception nutrition on pregnancy: An educational module promoting preconception care. https://core.ac.uk/download/84397645.pdf (accessed on 13th July 2025).
18. Jarrett, P., Jomeen, J., & Martin, C. R. (2017). The development and initial validation of the Perinatal Mental Health Awareness scale in student midwives. https://core.ac.uk/download/151162285.pdf (accessed on 13th July 2025).
19. Jowett, M. (2025). Cost-effective safe motherhood interventions in low-income countries: A review. https://core.ac.uk/download/pdf/6406578.pdf (accessed on 13th July 2025).
20. Naeve, K., Ved, R., & O'Neil, S. (2017). An examination of the maternal health quality of care landscape in India. https://core.ac.uk/download/89473010.pdf (accessed on 13th July 2025).
21. Nichols, M. R. (1950). Carney hospital's maternity service plan: A study of one hundred and eleven patients admitted to the Carney hospital's prenatal clinic during the months of May, June, July, 1949. https://open.bu.edu/bitstream/2144/4845/1/Nichols_Margaret_1950_web.pdf (accessed on 13th July 2025).
22. Nieto Calvache, Á. J. (2024). Placenta accreta spectrum in low- and middle-income countries: Usefulness of telemedicine. https://core.ac.uk/download/631133582.pdf (accessed on 13th July 2025).
23. Otive-Igbuzor, E., Wells, E., Azasi, E., Coeytaux, F., Potts, J., Danmusa, S., Tibebu, S., et al. (2014). Scaling up access to misoprostol at the community level to improve maternal health outcomes in Ethiopia, Ghana, and Nigeria. https://core.ac.uk/download/80511060.pdf (accessed on 13th July 2025).
24. Seeger, D. M. (2015). Muslim women and United States healthcare: Challenges to access and navigation. https://core.ac.uk/download/148922727.pdf (accessed on 13th July 2025).
25. Sherman, B., Landers, G. M., & Zhou, M. (2007). An assessment of health care safety net services in seven metropolitan Atlanta counties. https://core.ac.uk/download/71344364.pdf (accessed on 13th July 2025).
26. Weissman, J. S., Betancourt, J. R., & Kim, M. K. (2007). Resident physicians' preparedness to provide cross-cultural care: Implications for clinical care and medical education policy. https://core.ac.uk/download/71354412.pdf (accessed on 13th July 2025).

INDEX

D

E

F

G

H

I

L

M

S

T

U

V

W